A Thesaurus of Medical Word Roots

Horace Gerald Danner, Ph.D.

Forward by John Stephen Naulty, M.D.

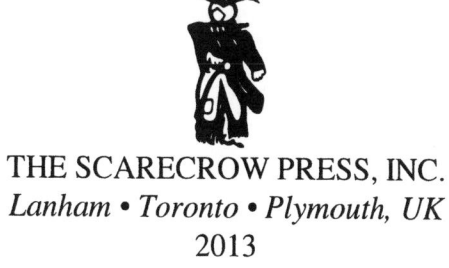

THE SCARECROW PRESS, INC.
Lanham • Toronto • Plymouth, UK
2013

Published by Scarecrow Press, Inc.
A wholly owned subsidary of The Rowman & Littlefield Publishing Group, Inc.
4501 Forbes Boulevard, Suite 200, Lanham, Maryland 20706
www.rowman.com

10 Thornbury Road, Plymouth PL6 7PP, United Kingdom

British Library Cataloguing in Publication Information Available

Library of Congress Cataloging-in-Publication Data

Library of Congress Cataloging-in-Publication Data Available

ISBN Cloth: 978-0-8108-9154-8(cloth : alk. paper)

Printed in the United States of America

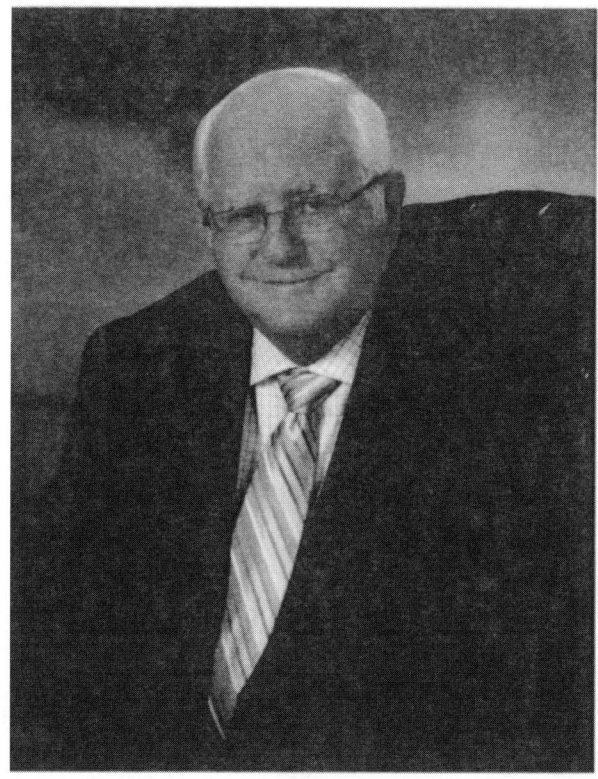

HORACE G. DANNER RECEIVED A B.A. IN SOCIAL SCIENCES FROM THE UNIVERSITY OF THE PHILIPPINES, QUEZON CITY, IN 1955, WHILE STATIONED IN THE PHILIPPINES WITH THE U. S. AIR FORCE. PRIOR TO JOINING THE MILITARY AT THE OUTBREAK OF THE KOREAN CONFLICT, HE STUDIED AT TROY STATE UNIVERSITY, TROY, ALABAMA.

BEFORE RECEIVING THE PH.D. IN EDUCATIONAL PSYCHOLOGY FROM AMERICAN UNIVERSITY, WASHINGTON, D.C., IN 1973, HE DID POSTGRADUATE WORK AT UNIVERSITY OF VIRGINIA, AND AT GEORGE WASHINGTON UNIVERSITY, WASHINGTON, D.C.

HE HAS TAUGHT IN THE PUBLIC SCHOOL SYSTEM OF FAIRFAX COUNTY, VIRGINIA, IN THE FIELDS OF MUSIC AND ENGLISH. HE HAS ALSO TAUGHT LITERATURE AND WRITING FOR NORTHERN VIRGINIA COMMUNITY COLLEGE, AT ITS ALEXANDRIA, ANNANDALE, LOUDOUN, AND MANASSAS CAMPUSES. IN ADDITION, HE TAUGHT TECHNICAL WRITING AT MONTGOMERY COLLEGE, ROCKVILLE, MARYLAND.

A RETIRED AIR FORCE CHIEF MASTER SERGEANT, HE WAS A WRITER AND EDITOR WITH THE AIR FORCE INTELLIGENCE SERVICE. AFTER RETIRING FROM THE MILITARY, HE TAUGHT TECHNICAL AND BUSINESS WRITING AT UNIVERSITY OF MARYLAND UNIVERSITY COLLEGE, COLLEGE PARK. HE HAS ALSO TAUGHT WRITING AT NATIONAL DEFENSE UNIVERSITY, FORT MCNAIR, WASHINGTON D.C.

HE IS THE AUTHOR OF THE AWARD-WINNING ACADEMIC VOCABULARY BOOK *Discover It! A Better Vocabulary, a Better Way*. THE AWARD WAS PRESENTED BY THE ASSOCIATION OF EDUCATIONAL PUBLISHERS, IN 2005. HE IS ALSO THE AUTHOR OF *The English Tree of Roots: and Words from around the World*. IN ADDITION, HE HAS WRITTEN *Horace's Quick List of Latin and Greek Prefixes and Combining Forms*. A REVISED AND UPDATED VERSION OF *Discover It!* IS SUBTITLED *The Ultimate Vocabulary Builder*.

HE LIVES IN OCCOQUAN, VIRGINIA.

FROM THE FOREWORD BY JOHN STEPHEN NAULTY, MD, INTERNATIONALLY ACCLAIMED PROFESSOR OF ANESTHESIOLOGY

As a pleasant surprise, I found it to be extremely enjoyable to read this stimulating work in a sort of "drunkard's walk," bouncing from root to root as whimsy took me. Using the thesaurus provided a constant surprise—a feeling of "I didn't know what *that* word really meant!" For example, *amygdale*, meaning "tonsil," originally meant "almond," because of the tonsil's shape being similar to that of an almond; and *pancreas*, literally "all flesh."

Dr. Naulty recommends this thesaurus to all health-care professionals as well as others who are interested in the vocabulary of medicine.

To my grandchildren, Nathan,
Alissa, Margaret, Donna,
Susan, and Madeline

A Thesaurus of Medical Word Roots

Acknowledgments

The author is thankful to so many professionals that it would be difficult to list them all. Without any intention of slighting anyone, the author is most deeply indebted to the writer of the foreword, the technical adviser, and final formatter.

The writer of the foreword, John Stephen Naulty, MD, the medical director of Woodbridge Medical Pain Management Solutions, Woodbridge, Virginia, is an internationally known professor of anesthesiology and the author of over 100 books and scientific papers. He has taught at the Naval Medical Research Institute and the Uniformed Services University, both in Bethesda, Maryland; Harvard Medical School; George Washington University, Washington, DC; The Pennsylvania Hospital, Philadelphia; and Yale University.

In the course of years that I've worked on this project, I have been assisted by Ron Evry, Computer Technician, Arlington County Public Schools, Arlington, Virginia. Ron is also a gym mate, friend, and neighbor. In addition, one of my former students at University of Maryland, Chris Cruz, has helped me on numerous occasions. With a graphics artist background, Chris is now a registered cardiovascular invasive heart specialist at Virginia Hospital Center, Arlington, Virginia.

A very special thanks go to two health care professionals, namely M. Scott White, DC, Woodbridge Chiropractic Clinic, Woodbridge, Virginia; and John S. Naulty, MD, listed above. Working together, they relieved me of almost unbearable neck and back pain. Without their professional care, I am not sure I could have finished this work, certainly not in comfort.

Amanda Hollins, President and Chief Financial Officer, Constellation Software Engineering, a business partner and friend of one of my former students at University of Maryland, has been most beneficial in helping with the formatting. Most of the work she did by email, but on two occasions, she drove sixty miles from her home on the Chesapeake Bay in Maryland to come to Occoquan, Virginia, to solve some tricky formatting problems. She is both a delight to know and to work with.

I am extremely grateful to Andreas K. Bolos, an LDS missionary, who was visiting. He straightened out a table, and in doing so, noticed that not all the pages were consistent in width. Of course, he didn't rest until he had made certain that all pages were uniform. I am also grateful to Elder Ryan Bramwell for his expertise in formatting.

Finally, I am appreciative to Ron Evry for his help in uploading the book to CreateSpace.

Foreword

I vividly recall my first day of medical school. The first thing the dean said when greeting us was the usual terrorizing speech: "Look to the left, look to the right; one of you will not be here at the end of the year." (As you can tell by this, I attended medical school before the "be nice to students, we're all in this together" movement of modern medical education existed.)

The dean then proceeded to babble for an hour or so in what seemed to me incomprehensible Greco-Roman gibberish, describing the future course of our medical education over the next four years. Barely one word in three was one with which I was familiar, and I did that well only because I had listened to 21 years of Catholic Latin by that time, and could puzzle out, somewhat slowly and haltingly, some of his words. I remember asking, "Why is he talking like that?" It appeared he was speaking a strange language that had a few familiar words used in unusual ways as well as many unfamiliar ones.

My classmates were equally bewildered, except for one lucky chap who had gone to St. John's College in Annapolis, Maryland, where the students were required to have a "classical" education. He helped translate for us in a hoarse whisper, explaining that the dean was speaking a strange conglomeration of English, Greek, and Latin. At the end of that day, I was convinced that doctors talked like that just to bewilder and impress patients with their arcane knowledge. How wrong I was!

My classmates and I then spent the next four years learning that new language. I spent a great deal of time with a medical dictionary, repeatedly looking up related, similar, but still unfamiliar words. As we learned it, we found that this language was beautiful, carefully constructed, precise, and wonderfully expressive. It was a language understood all over the world, across generations, even centuries, of medical literature, and has proven itself able over the subsequent 40 years since medical school to absorb and express entirely new concepts with no difficulty whatever.

During this learning process, I gained, by painful repetition, a rough idea of how medical words were constructed. But, lacking the insight this volume provides, I did not really understand how medical terminology is created. In my own field, anesthesia, entirely new drugs, procedures, diseases, complications, and conditions have appeared on an almost monthly basis, and they have been incorporated into our vocabulary with extreme clarity and with absolutely no difficulty. How this difficult task has been accomplished is the subject of this work.

Dr. Danner has constructed a thesaurus of medical roots that is an incredible achievement. It presents, in a clear and concise way, the roots of medical words and how they are used to construct the words we all use and understand on a daily basis. Using it will allow the student of medicine to use and understand our painfully acquired language in an extremely precise and clear manner. Knowledge of the roots of medical terms and their combinations allows one to immediately understand any medical terminology without resorting to a dictionary lookup, or in today's usage, "googling" the word.

As a pleasant surprise, I found it to be extremely enjoyable to read this stimulating work in a sort of "drunkard's walk," bouncing from root to root as whimsy took me. Using the thesaurus provided a constant surprise—a feeling of "I didn't know what *that* word really meant!" For example, *amygdale*, meaning "tonsil," originally meant "almond," because of the tonsil's shape being similar to that of an almond; and *pancreas*, literally "all flesh."

In my own field, pain medicine, I have to read many other doctors' referral notes, in which I find a great deal of imprecise descriptions of painful and perceptual states. Much of this confusion relates to the simple root *esthes*, meaning per Dr. Danner, "feeling, perception." From this root, as I found on page 238, one can prefix the root with *an-*, a negative, and get *anesthesia*, absence of feeling. One can then enter the world of my colleagues' imprecision with its combination with other prefixes, for example, *dis-*, a negative, gives us *disesthesia*, a feeling of discomfort. Adding the prefix *hyper-*, above, gives us *hyperesthesia*, heightened sensation, and *hypo-*, below, gives us *hypoesthesia*, decreased sensation. Amputees may have *pseudoesthesia*, a false sensation in an absent limb. The thesaurus lists many other examples.

I frequently read notes that confuse these states of sensation, which could be quickly resolved by understanding the way these root words were combined and the precise terms constructed.

Familiarity with these roots and their combinations gives the practitioner a powerful tool to precisely describe disease states in a clear and unequivocal way. I would like to send just this section to my referral doctors, but I fear my zeal for precision would be resented. Perhaps they will purchase and use this volume. I know I will.

John Stephen Naulty, MD
Medical Director
Woodbridge Medical Pain Management Solutions
Woodbridge, Virginia

Preface

There was a single reason for compiling this thesaurus: to provide a comprehensive list of medical word roots, or elements, as well as examples of words from those roots. I considered placing every medical word into each family of roots that composed the word, e.g., *epiplomphalocele* would have been placed under *epiploon*, omentum; *omphalos*, navel; and *kele*, hernia. It soon became evident that this would be an impossible undertaking in a one-volume thesaurus.

Consequently, the thesaurus was made comprehensive in the diversity of roots, rather than the number of families into which individual words were placed. Whereas many medical words comprise a number of roots, e.g., *hydromyelomeningocele*, I chose generally to list words with not more than three roots. If users desire to know the meaning of a root in a particular word not listed, they should look up that particular root in the "Element" column. To conserve space, the most common prefixes are not listed as a separate family; instead, they are included with the roots to which they are attached. Prefixes and initial combining forms, together with examples, are listed in a separate section, Appendix B.

Words and roots used in a general vocabulary were included only when they had specific medical applications. For example, *mobilize* was listed because in the medical lexicon, it means "to make mobile or capable of movement." For those wishing to consult a thesaurus of word roots in general, *A Thesaurus of Word Roots of the English Language* is recommended, which is now being revised.

The following explanation should assist users in obtaining the maximum benefit from the thesaurus.

The main body of the thesaurus is divided into four columns. In the first column, "ELEMENT," the roots are listed alphabetically; where the root has different forms, the most common form is listed first, followed by the others in alphabetical order. When two elements, usually a prefix and root, e.g., pericard-, produced a number of words, that combination is often listed as a separate entry. Consequently, *pericard-* is listed under SIMPLE ROOT; *endopericarditis* is listed as a PREFIXED ROOT; and *pericardectomy* is listed under LEADING ROOT COMPOUND.

The second column, "FROM," gives the original language from which the root is derived, mainly Greek but also Latin, together with the original word and meaning.

The third column, "MEANING," contains the generally accepted medical meaning of the root.

The last column, "EXAMPLES," is divided into several categories, which follow a paradigm. The first two categories listed are SIMPLE ROOT (the root itself together with non-medical suffixes) and PREFIXED ROOT (where the root is preceded by a prefix, e.g., *synergy*, where *syn-* is the prefix and *erg* is the root). Prefixed roots are listed in alphabetical order of the prefixes themselves, e.g., *peroral* precedes *perioral*, and *asepsis* precedes *antisepsis*.

A root is variously defined in the following dictionaries: *Webster's New World Dictionary* indicates it as the fundamental element of a word or form, exclusive of all affixes (prefixes and suffixes) and inflectional phonetic changes, e.g., *-ed* of *waited*; *-er* of *healthier*. *American Heritage Dictionary* indicates a root as a word or word element from which other words are formed.

Some authorities regard prefixes as those elements that come invariably at the beginning of the word, for example, in *autobiography*, auto- means *self*; Greek homo-, *same* (Latin homo- means *man*); hetero-, *different*. In this book, however, prefixes are considered as those elements that change the meaning of a root and are properly prepositions and adverbs in Greek and Latin. For simplicity, common numerical prefixes are included along with the grammatical prefixes.

The next category in the paradigm is LEADING ROOT COMPOUND, where the root under consideration comes at the beginning of a word comprised of at least two roots, e.g., if the root under consideration is *episio-*, vulva, *episioelytrorrhaphy* is listed as Leading Root Compound, with *episio* leading the compound, followed by *elytro*, vagina; and finally by *rhaphe*, suture; thus, *episioelytrorrhaphy* means "the suturing of the vulva and the vagina."

The next category is TRAILING ROOT COMPOUND, where the root under consideration comes after another root, thus most likely at the end of the word. However, for the sake of simplicity, this category includes any word where the root under consideration follows another root. For example, on page 302, in the *myos*, muscle, family, there is listed *fibromyalgia*, where *my* trails *fibro*, even though *algos*, pain, is the ultimate element.

In each category, the element not under consideration is listed in parentheses along with its meaning. For example, under the family *ped*, child, *pediatric* is listed as Leading Root Compound; consequently, *iatr* trails or follows *ped*. Therefore, after the entry *pediatric, pediatrics, pediatrician, iatrein,* to heal, is listed after the entry. Only in cases where the root's meaning is obvious is the meaning not given. Different forms of the same word within a list are indicated by {curly brackets}. Not all dictionaries agree on derivative words; some dictionaries indicate those words placed within curly brackets as entries themselves.

In cases where another root or roots have the same or a similar meaning, they are listed under CROSS REFERENCE. For example, Greek *thes* is cross-referenced to *pon, stas, stet*. In many cases where None is indicated, there are in fact other roots that do approximate the root's meaning. However, because of pagination constraints, it was necessary to omit them. Consequently, I focused on roots pertaining mainly to the body. There are also ROOT NOTES in cases where the meaning of the root is different from the original meaning or where there are interesting aspects to the root's background. For example, *aniso* is considered a root itself; however, *aniso* combines the prefix *an-* not + *isos* same. Consequently, the meaning of *aniso* is "not the same," and can be found in *anisogamete, anisomeric, anisotropic*.

In many cases, I gave explanatory notes or a short definition of the word. These definitions and notes are given for one of several reasons: to differentiate a particular word from a similar word; to give backgrounds of interesting words; or to break up the simple listing of words. These definitions and explanatory notes should not be construed as comprehensive, but simply as notes of differentiation or as pointers to understanding.

It should be stressed that this thesaurus is designed for a user to refer to when an unknown medical word of mainly Greek or Latin origin is encountered. By seeing other words in the same family, users can better associate, and therefore, better remember the meaning of the root. Psychologists have shown that when one associates an unfamiliar word with a familiar one, the learning is more readily absorbed, and thus remembered.

In the case of words comprised of two or more elements, users are encouraged to formulate their own definitions. To solidify the learning process, users should see if their definitions appear to fit the context of these particular words as the words are used in their textbooks or in their professional reading or practice. Users may also wish to consult a medical dictionary to see how closely their own definitions match those of the dictionary. See List of Works Consulted for a list of some of the medical references consulted.

Users are encouraged to write additional words in the blank space to the left of the word categories. The blank space can also be used for recording one's own definitions or for notes on particular words.

The thesaurus concludes with three indispensable features: the English to Roots Index (Appendix A), the List of Prefixes (Appendix B), and the List of Suffixes and Common Endings (Appendix C).

Although this thesaurus has been checked by computer for typographical errors, it is possible that errors may have still gone unnoticed. It is requested that any such errors be brought to my attention so that they can be corrected in any ensuing editions. Please send any comments and suggested additions, corrections, or suggestions to me at PO Box 614, Occoquan, VA 22125. My home telephone number is 703-491-5283, and my email is imprints5283@comcast.net.

Table of Contents

A

Element	From	Meaning	Examples
a-, an-	Greek prefix	negative, privative	See Appendix B for examples of words with this prefix. Others are listed with the roots to which it is attached. CROSS REFERENCE: ab-, in-[2]
ab-, abs-	Latin prefix	away, negative	See Appendix B for examples of words with this prefix. Others are listed with the roots to which it is attached. CROSS REFERENCE: a-, in-[2]
abdom	Latin *abdomen*	belly, abdomen	SIMPLE ROOT: abdomen (that portion of the body which lies between the thorax and the pelvis) {abdominal} abdominous (having a large abdomen) PREFIXED ROOT: endoabdominal (*endon* within) extra-abdominal (*extra* outside) intra-abdominal (*intra* within) subabdominal (*sub* below) transabdominal (*trans* across) LEADING ROOT COMPOUND: *abdomin*: abdominalgia (*algos* pain) *abdomino*: abdominocentesis (*kentein* to puncture) abdominocyesis (*kyesis* pregnancy) abdominocystic (*kystis* bladder) abdominogenital (*genere* to produce) abdominohysterectomy (*hystera* uterus + *ektome* excision) abdominohysterotomy (*hystera* uterus + *tomy* incision) abdominopelvic (pelvis) abdominoperineal (perineum) abdominoplasty (*plassein* to form) abdominoposterior (*posterior* back) abdominoscopy (*skopein* to examine) abdominoscrotal (*scrotum* bag: testicle pouch) abdominothoracic (*thorax* chest) abdominouterotomy (*uterus* womb + *tomy* incision) abdominovaginal (vagina) abdominovesical (also called *vesicoabdominal*) (*vesica* bladder) TRAILING ROOT COMPOUND: dorsabdominal (*dorsum* back) iliolumbocostoabdominal (ilium + *lumbus* loin + *costa* rib, side) inguinoabdominal (*inguen* groin) lateroabdominal (*lateris* side) lumboabdominal (*lumbus* loin) nephroabdominal (*nephros* kidney) rectoabdominal (rectum) thoracoabdominal (thorax) tuboabdominal (pertaining to the oviduct and the abdomen) uteroabdominal (uterus) vaginoabdominal (vagina) vesicoabdominal (also called *abdominovesical*) (*vesica* bladder) CROSS REFERENCE: cel[1], lapar, stoma, ventr

Element	From	Meaning	Examples
ac-	Latin prefix	to, toward	See ad- under Appendix B for examples of words with this prefix. Others are placed with the roots to which it is attached. CROSS REFERENCE: ad-
acanth	Greek *akantha* thorn, prickle	thorny, spiny	SIMPLE ROOT: acantha (the spine; the spinous process of a vertebra) acanthaceous (bearing prickles or spines) acanthion (tip of anterior nasal spine) acanthor (a larva with an anterior circlet of hooks and spines) PREFIXED ROOT: *acanth*: hexacanth (also called *oncosphere*) (*hexa* six) *acanthoma*: paracanthoma (*para* abnormal + *oma* tumor) *acanthosis* thorny condition: hyperacanthosis (or, acanthosis; hypertrophy of the prickle layer of the skin) (*hyper* above) paracanthosis (*para* abnormal) pseudoacanthosis (resembling acanthosis) (*pseudes* false) LEADING ROOT COMPOUND: *acanth*: acanthesthesia (a sensation as of a pinprick) (*esthesia* feeling) acanthoid (thorny; spiny; of a spinous nature) (*eidos* form) acanthoma (benign tumor of the skin) (*oma* tumor) acanthosis {acanthotic} (*osis* condition) *acantho*: acanthocephalan (a phylum of thorny-headed worms) (*kephale* head) acanthocytosis (*kytos* cell + *osis* condition) acanthokeratodermia (hypertrophy of the skin's corneous layer; also called *hyperkeratosis*) (*keras* horn + *dermia* skin condition) acantholysis {acantholytic} (*lyein* to loosen) acanthopelvis (a pelvis with the crest of the pubes very sharp) acanthopodia (toothlike pseudopodia in some ameba) (*podos* foot) TRAILING ROOT COMPOUND: *acanthoma* prickly tumor: adenoacanthoma (*adenos* gland) hidroacanthoma (*hidros* sweat) keratoacanthoma (*keratos* horn—horny tissue) melanoacanthoma (*melanos* dark) syringoacanthoma (*syringos* pipe, tube) *acanthosis*: zoacanthosis (a cutaneous eruption due to introduction into the human skin of hair, bristles, stingers, etc. of lower animals) (*zoon* animal + *osis* condition) CROSS REFERENCE: None
acin	Latin *acinus* grape	smallest division of a gland	SIMPLE ROOT: acinar (pertaining to or affecting an acinus or acini) acinose (made up of acini; acinar), acinous acinus (a small saclike dilatation, particularly one found in various glands; pl., acini) {acinic} PREFIXED ROOT: interacinar (or, interacinous) (*inter* between) intraacinous (*intra* within) panacinar (*pan* all) periacinar (or, periacinal), periacinous (*peri* around) LEADING ROOT COMPOUND: *acin*: acinitis (*itis* inflammation) *acini*: aciniform (shaped like an acinus or grape) (*forma* shape)

Element	From	Meaning	Examples
acin (cont'd)		[smallest division of a gland]	TRAILING ROOT COMPOUND: centriacinar (*kentron* point, center) tubuloacinar (composed of tubular cini, as a tubuloacinar gland) CROSS REFERENCE: aden, gland, thym[1]
acou, **acu,** **aku**	Greek *akouein* to hear	to hear, listen	SIMPLE ROOT: *acou:* acouasm (or, acousma; auditory hallucination or imaginary sound, such as that of buzzing, ringing, or hissing) [terms rarely used] acoustic, acoustics (the scientific study of sound) *acu:* acusis (the ability to perceive sound normally) PREFIXED ROOT: *acousia:* anacousia (also called *anacusis, anakusis*) (*an* privative) bradyacousia (*bradys* slow) dysacousia (also called *dysacusis*) (*dys* abnormal) hyperacousia (or, hyperacusia; an abnormally keen sense of hearing, often with pain in the ears) (*hyper* above) *acusia:* hemianacusia (*hemi* half + anacusia) hyperacusia (or, hyperacousia, hyperacusis) (*hyper* above) *acusis:* anacusis (or, anacousia, anakusis) (*an* privative) diplacusis (*diploos* double) dysacusis (or, dysacousia) (*dys* abnormal) hypacusis (or, hypacusia) (*hypo* under) paracusis (or, paracousis) (*para* abnormal) *acous:* pseudacousis (or, pseudacousma) (*pseudes* false) *akus:* anakusis (or, anacousia: total deafness) (*an* privative) LEADING ROOT COMPOUND: *acou:* acouesthesia (*esthesia* feeling) acoumeter (*metron* measure) *acouo:* acouophone, acouophonia (*phone* sound) *acousmat:* acousmatagnosis (*a* privative + *gnosis* knowledge) acousmatamnesia (*amnesia* forgetting) *acousto:* acoustogram (or, acoustigram) (*graphein* to write) TRAILING ROOT COMPOUND: *acousia:* amblyacousia (*amblys* dull) echoacousia (*echo* returned sound) presbyacousia (or, presbyacusis, presbyacusia) (*presbys* old age) *acoustic(s):* bioacoustics (*bios* life) otoacoustic (*otos* ear) statoacoustic (related to balance and hearing) (*statos* standing) stethacoustic (*stethos* chest) vibroacoustic (vibration) *acusis:* nosoacusis (hearing loss due to disease) (*nosos* disease) odynacusis (painful hearing) (*odyne* pain) osteoacusis (bone conduction of sound) (*osteon* bone) presbyacusis (or, presbyacousia) (*presbys* old age) CROSS REFERENCE: aur

Element	From	Meaning	Examples
acro	Greek *akros* topmost, extreme; *akron* extremity	highest, extreme, extremities	SIMPLE ROOT: acral (pertaining to or affecting the extremities, or peripheral parts, e.g., limbs, fingers, ears), acroteric PREFIXED ROOT: hemiacrosomia (*hemi* half + *soma* body) supracromial (or, superacromial) (*supra* above + *acromion* tip of the shoulder) See Appendix B for examples of this element used as an initial combining form. Others are placed with the root to which it is attached. CROSS REFERENCE: None
actin	Greek *aktis* ray	rays; similar to rays; of a radiated nature	SIMPLE ROOT: actinic, actinism, actinium (Ac), actinon (a radioactive, inert gaseous isotope of radon) PREFIXED ROOT: adiactinic (not transmitting the actinic rays) (*a* negative + *diactinic*) diactinism (the property of transmitting chemically active rays) {*diactinic*} (*dia* through) protoactinium (*protos* first) LEADING ROOT COMPOUND: actinobacillosis (*bakterion* little rod + *osis* condition) actinodermatitis (*derma* skin + *itis* inflammation) actinogen, actinogenesis {*actinogenic*} (*genere* to produce) actinogram, actinograph (*graphein* to write) actinology (*logos* study) actinolyte (*lyein* to loosen) actinometer (*metron* measure) actinomycoma (*mykes* fungus + *oma* tumor) actinomycosis (*mykes* fungus + *osis* condition) actinoneuritis (*neuron* nerve + *itis* inflammation) actinotherapy (*therapy* treatment) actinotoxemia (*toxikon* poison + *emia* blood condition) TRAILING ROOT COMPOUND: photoactinic (*photos* light) CROSS REFERENCE: rad[1]
ad-	Latin prefix	to, toward	See Appendix B for examples of words with this prefix. Others are listed with the roots to which it is attached. CROSS REFERENCE: pro-
aden	Greek *aden, adenos*	gland	SIMPLE ROOT: adenia (a chronic affection marked by enlargement of the lymphatic glands), adenic (or, adenous; pertaining to or resembling a gland; glandular), adenose (relating to or like a gland) PREFIXED ROOT: *adenia* gland condition: anadenia (*an* privative) hypoadenia (*hypo* under) *adenitis* gland inflammation: paradenitis (also called *periadenitis*) (*para* alongside) periadenitis (also called *paradenitis*) (*peri* around) polyadenitis (*polys* many) *adenoid*: intraadenoidal (*intra* within + *eidos* resembling) *adenoma*: macroadenoma (*makros* large + *oma* tumor) *adenopathy*: polyadenopathy (*polys* many + *pathos* disease) *adenosis* gland condition: hyperadenosis (enlargement of glands, especially of the lymph glands) (*hyper* above) polyadenosis (*polys* many) *adenous*: polyadenous (*polys* many)

Element	From	Meaning	Examples
aden (cont'd)		[gland]	LEADING ROOT COMPOUND:

aden:
adenalgia (also called *adenodynia*) (*algos* pain)
adenasthenia (*asthenia* weakness: *a* negative + *sthenos* strength)
adenectomy (*ektome* excision)
adenectopia (*ektopos* displaced)
adenemphraxis (*emphraxis* stoppage)
adenitis (*itis* inflammation)
adenodynia (also called *adenalgia*) (*odyne* pain)
adenoid, adenoidal, adenoids (*eidos* form)
adenoiditis (*eidos* form + *itis* inflammation)
adenoma (*oma* tumor)
adenoncus (also called *adenomegaly*) (*onkos* mass)
adenophthalmia (*ophthalmia* eye condition)
adenosis (*osis* condition)
adeni: adeniform (like a gland in form or shape) (*forma* shape)
adeno:
adenoacanthoma (adenocarcinoma in which some cells have under-
    gone squamous metaplasia) (*akantha* thorn + *oma* tumor)
adenoameloblastoma (*amel* enamel + *blastos* germ + *oma* tumor)
adenoblast (a proliferating embryonic cell with the potential to form
    glandular parenchyma) (*blastos* bud, shoot, germ)
adenocarcinoma (*carcinoma* malignant tumor)
adenocele (*kele* hernia)
adenocellulitis (*cella* cell + *itis* inflammation)
adenochondroma (*chondros* cartilage + *oma* tumor)
adenocystoma (cystic adenoma) (*kystis* sac + *oma* tumor)
adenocyte (*kytos* cell)
adenoepithelioma (*epi* upon + *thele* nipple + *oma* tumor)
adenofibroma (fiber + *oma* tumor)
adenogenous (*genere* to produce)
adenohypersthenia (*hyper* above + *sthenos* strength)
adenohypophysis (*hypo* under + *phyein* to grow)
adenolipoma (*lipos* fat + *oma* tumor)
adenology (*logos* study)
adenolymphitis (*lympha* liquid + *itis* inflammation)
adenolymphocele (*lympha* liquid + *kele* tumor)
adenolymphoma (*lympha* liquid + *oma* tumor)
adenomalacia (*malakos* soft)
adenomegaly (also called *adenoncus*) (*megalos* large)
adenomere (the blind terminal portion of a developing gland that will
    become the functional portion of the organ) (*meros* part)
adenomyoma (*myos* muscle + *oma* tumor)
adenomyometritis (*myos* muscle + *metra* uterus + *itis* inflammation)
adenomyosarcoma (*myos* muscle + *sarkos* flesh + *oma* tumor)
adenomyosis (*myos* muscle + *osis* condition)
adenomyxosarcoma (*myxa* mucus + *sarx* flesh + *oma* tumor)
adenopathy (*pathos* disease)
adenopharyngitis (*pharynx* throat + *itis* inflammation)
adenophlegmon (*phlegmone* acute inflammation)
adenophorous (*phorein* to bear, carry)
adenosalpingitis (*salpingos* tube + *itis* inflammation)
adenosarcoma (*sarkos* flesh + *oma* tumor)
adenosclerosis (*skleros* hard + *osis* condition)

Element	From	Meaning	Examples
aden (cont'd)		[gland]	TRAILING ROOT COMPOUND:
			aden: sialaden (*sialon* saliva)
			adenalgia: dacryoadenalgia (*dakryon* teardrop + *algos* pain)
			adenitis gland inflammation:
			blennadenitis (*blennos* mucus)
			blepharoadenitis (or, blepharadenitis) (*blepharon* eyelid)
			dacryoadenitis (*dakyryon* tear: lacrimal duct)
			gastradenitis (*gaster* stomach, belly)
			hidradenitis (*hidros* sweat)
			lymphadenitis (*lympha* water, fluid)
			maschaladenitis (*maschale* armpit)
			mastadenitis (*mastos* breast)
			myxadenitis (*myxa* mucus)
			poradenitis (also called *poradenia*) (*poros* pore)
			scleradenitis (*skleros* hard)
			sialadenitis (or, sialoadenitis) (*sialon* saliva)
			spiradenitis (*spirare* to breathe)
			tarsadenitis (*tarsus* eyelid)
			thyroadenitis (thyroid gland)
			adenosis: sialadenosis (*sialon* saliva + *osis* condition)
			CROSS REFERENCE: acin, gland, thym[1]
adip	Latin *adeps adipis*	fat	SIMPLE ROOT: adipose (as an adjective, fatty; as a noun, fat)
			PREFIXED ROOT:
			hyperadiposis (excessive fatness) (*hyper* above + *osis* condition)
			preadipocyte (*pre* before + *kytos* cell)
			LEADING ROOT COMPOUND:
			adip:
			adipectomy (also called *lipectomy*) (*ektome* excision)
			adipoid (fatlike; resembling fat; also called *lipoid*) (*eidos* form)
			adipoma (fatty tissue tumor; also called *lipoma*) (*oma* tumor)
			adiposis {adiposity; also called *obesity*} (*osis* condition)
			adipo:
			adipocele (a hernia that contains fat or fatty tissue) (*kele* hernia)
			adipocellular (composed of connective tissue and fat) (*cella* cell)
			adipocere {adipoceratous; also called *lipoceratous*} (*cera* wax)
			adipocyte (also called *fat cell*) (*kytos* cell)
			adipofibroma (*fibra* fiber + *oma* tumor)
			adipogenesis (also called *lipogenesis*) (*genere* to produce)
			adipohepatic (*hepar* liver)
			adipokinesis {adipokinetic}, adipokinin (*kinein* to move)
			adipolysis {adipolytic} (*lyein* to loosen)
			adipometer (*metron* measure)
			adiponectin (*nectere* to bind)
			adiponecrosis (*nekros* corpse + *osis* condition)
			adipopexia (or, adipopexis) {adipopectic} (*pexis* fixation)
			adipos fatty condition:
			adiposalgia (*algos* pain)
			adipositis (*itis* inflammation)
			adiposuria (also called *lipuria*) (*uria* urine condition)
			TRAILING ROOT COMPOUND:
			fibroadipose (fiber)
			granuloadipose (granule)
			scleroadipose (*skleros* hard)
			CROSS REFERENCE: ather, lip, piar, pimel, stear

Element	From	Meaning	Examples

adren	Latin
	ad to +
	ren kidney
		adrenal gland	SIMPLE ROOT: adrenal {adrenic}, adrenalin, adrenalism
			PREFIXED ROOT:
			anadrenalism (or, anadrenia) (*an* privative)
			dysadrenalism (or, adrenalism) (*dys* abnormal)
			hyperadrenalism (*hyper* over, above)
			hypoadrenalism (*hypo* below)
			isoadrenocorticism (also called *euadrenocorticism*) (*isos* equal +
			   cortex outer surface)
			LEADING ROOT COMPOUND:
			adren:
			adrenarche (*arche* beginning)
			adrenergic (*ergon* work)
			adrenitis (or, adrenalitis) (*itis* inflammation)
			adrenal:
			adrenalectomy (*ektome* excision)
			adrenalitis (or, adrenitis) (*itis* inflammation)
			adrenalinin:
			adrenalinemia (*emia* blood condition)
			adrenalinuria (*uria* urine condition)
			adrenalo: adrenalopathy (or, adrenopathy) (*pathos* suffering)
			adreno:
			adrenoceptor (also called *adrenergic receptor*) (*capere* to hold)
			adrenochrome (*chroma* color)
			adrenocortical (also called *corticoadrenal*) (*cortex* bark, rind: outer
			   covering)
			adrenogenic (*genere* to produce)
			adrenolytic (*lyein* to loosen)
			adrenomegaly (*megalos* large)
			adrenomimetic (*mimetikos* imitative)
			adrenopathy (or, adrenolopathy) (*pathos* disease)
			adrenoprival (*privare* to deprive)
			adrenotoxin (*toxikon* poison)
			adrenotropic (also called *adrenotrophic*) (*trope* a turning)
			TRAILING ROOT COMPOUND:
			corticoadrenal (also called *adrenocortical*) (*cortex* bark, rind: outer
			   covering)
			medulloadrenal (*medulla* marrow)
			sympathicoadrenal (pertaining to the sympathetic nervous system and
			   the adrenal medulla)
			CROSS REFERENCE: None

aer	Greek *aer, aeros* air	gas, air	SIMPLE ROOT: aerated, aeration aerial (pertaining to the air; growing in the air instead of in soil or water) PREFIXED ROOT: anaerobe (opposed to *aerobe*) (*an* negative + *bios* life) microaerophilic (*mikros* small + *philein* to love) LEADING ROOT COMPOUND: *aer*: aerendocardia (*endon* within + *kardia* heart) aerenterectasia (*enteron* intestine + *ektasis* dilatation) aerodontia, aerodontalgia (*odontos* tooth + *algos* pain) aerosis (*osis* condition) aerotitis (also called *barotitis*) (*otos* ear + *itis* inflammation)

A Thesaurus of Medical Word Roots

Element	From	Meaning	Examples
aer (cont'd)		[gas, air]	*aeri*:
			aeriferous (*ferre* to bear)
			aeriform (resembling air; gaseous) (*forma* shape)
			aerify {aerification} (*facere* to make)
			aero:
			aerobe {aerobic} (*bios* life)
			aerobiology (*bios* life + *logos* study)
			aerobioscope (*bios* life + *skopein* to examine)
			aerobiosis (*bios* life + *osis* condition)
			aerocele (distention of a cavity with gas) (*kele* tumor)
			aerocolpos (distention of the vagina with air) (*kolpos* vagina)
			aerocystoscopy (*kystis* bladder + *skopein* to examine)
			aerodermectasia (*derma* skin + *ektasis* dilatation)
			aerogastria (*gaster* stomach, belly)
			aerogel (*gelare* to freeze)
			aerogen {aerogenic, aerogenous} (*genere* to produce)
			aerogram (also called *pneumogram*) (*graphein* to write)
			aeropathy (the bends; decompression sickness) (*pathos* disease)
			aeroperitoneum (also called *pneumoperitoneum*) (peritoneum)
			aerophagia (or, aerophagy) (*phagein* to devour, to swallow)
			aerophil (an aerophilic organism) {aerophilic, or aerophilous; requiring air for proper growth; aerobic} (*philein* to love)
			aerophobia (morbid fear of drafts or fresh air, often connected with the idea of harmful airborne influences) (*phobia* fear)
			aeropiesotherapy (therapeutic use of air at either increased or decreased barometric pressure) (*piesis* pressure + therapy)
			aeroplethysmograph (an instrument for registering the amount of air respired) (*plethysmos* enlargement + *graphein* to write)
			aeroporotomy (*poros* passage + *tomy* incision)
			aeroscope (*skopein* to examine)
			aerosinusitis (also called *barosinusitis*) (*sinus* a hollow + *itis* inflammation)
			aerostatics (*statikos* causing to stand)
			aerotaxis (*taxis* arrangement)
			aerotherapeutics, aerotherapy (*therapy* treatment)
			aerothermotherapy (*thermos* heat + *therapy* treatment)
			aerotonometer (*tonos* tension + *metron* measure)
			aerotropic (*trope* a turning)
			aerotympanal (*tympanon* eardrum)
			aerourethroscope (urethra + *skopein* to examine)
			TRAILING ROOT COMPOUND:
			sialoaerophagy (*sialon* saliva + *phagein* to consume)
			tracheoaerocele (*trachea* windpipe + *kele* hernia)
			CROSS REFERENCE: phys, pneuma
aesthe			See esthe-.
agnos	Greek *a* privative + *gnosis* knowledge	agnosia	SIMPLE ROOT: agnosia (impairment of the ability to recognize, or comprehend the meaning of, various sensory stimuli)
			TRAILING ROOT COMPOUND:
			acousmatagnosis (*akouein* to hear: sound)
			acroagnosis (*akron* extremity—the limbs)
			amorphagnosia (*a* privative + *morphe* shape)
			apractagnosia (*a* privative + *prassein* to do, act)
			autotopoagnosia (*autos* self + *topos* place)
			baragnosis (*baros* weight)

Element	From	Meaning	Examples
agnos (cont'd)		[agnosia]	logagnosia (also called *aphasia*) (*logos* word)
			prosopagnosia (*prosopon* face)
			simultanagnosia (*simultaneous* at the same time)
			somatagnosia (*somatos* body)
			stereoagnosis (*stereos* solid)
			topagnosia (also called *atopognosis*) (*topos* place)
			CROSS REFERENCE: None
agog(ue)	Greek *agein* to lead	leading, flowing	PREFIXED ROOT: anagogy (in psychology, the spiritual, moral, or idealistic forces of the unconscious) (*ana* up)
			TRAILING ROOT COMPOUND:
			agogic: hypnagogic (*hypnos* sleep)
			agogue:
			cholagogue (*chole* bile)
			dacryagogue (*dakryon* teardrop)
			emmenagogue (*emmena* monthly—menstruation)
			galactagogue (also called *lactagogue*) (*galaktos* milk)
			helminthagogue (also called *antihelmintic*) (*helmins* tapeworm)
			hemagogue (*haima* blood)
			hormonagogue (hormone: *horman* to excite)
			hydragogue (*hydor* water)
			lactagogue (also called *galactagogue*) (*lactis* milk)
			lithagogue (a remedy that expels calculi) (*lithos* stone)
			lymphagogue (*lympha* liquid, water)
			menagogue (also called *emmenagogue*) (*mene* menstruation)
			ptyalagogue (also called *sialagogue*) (*ptyalon* saliva)
			sialagogue (also called *ptyalagogue*) (*sialon* saliva)
			succagogue (also called *secretagogue*) (*succus* juice, fluid)
			uragogue (*ouron* urine)
			CROSS REFERENCE: rrh, rrhag
agra	Greek *agra* seizure	seizure, gout (severe pain)	LEADING ROOT COMPOUND: agremia (that condition of the blood which characterizes gout) (*emia* blood condition)
			TRAILING ROOT COMPOUND:
			anconagra (also called *pechyagra*) (*ankon* elbow)
			arthragra (*arthron* joint)
			cardiagra (*kardia* heart)
			celiagra (*koilia* belly)
			cheiragra (gout of the hand, especially tophaceous gout with torsion of the fingers) (*cheir* hand) [tophaceous: hard or gritty]
			dentagra (*dens* tooth)
			glossagra (*glossa* tongue)
			gonagra (*gony* knee)
			melagra (*melos* limb)
			odontagra (a forceps for extracting teeth; also, toothache) (*odontos* tooth)
			omagra (*omos* shoulder)
			ophthalmagra (*ophthalmos* eye)
			otagra (*otos* ear)
			pechyagra (also called *anconagra*) (*pechys* forearm)
			pellagra (*pellis* skin)
			podagra (*pous* foot)
			tenontagra (tendon)
			trachelagra (*trachelos* neck)
			CROSS REFERENCE: alg, epilep, hapt, lep[2], odyn
aku			See acous-.

Element	From	Meaning	Examples
al	Latin *alere*	to nourish	SIMPLE ROOT: alible (nutritive; assimilable as a food) aliment, alimental alimentary (see Term), alimentation, alimentative altricious (slow in developing; requiring long nourishing) PREFIXED ROOT: *alesce*: coalesce (lit., to grow together, join, blend, fuse, as the halves of a broken bone; to unite or merge into a single body, group, or mass) (*com* with) *alimentation*: hyperalimentation (the ingestion of a greater than optimal amount of nutrients; also called *hypernutrition*) (*hyper* above) hypoalimentation (also called *subalimentation*) (*hypo* under) subalimentation (also called *hypoalimentation*) (*sub* under) superalimentation (also called *hyperalimentation, gavage, hypernutrition*) (*super* above) suralimentation (also called *hyperalimentation, superalimentation*) (French *sur*; from Latin *supra* above) tachyalimentation (*tachys* fast) *alimentosis*: hyperalimentosis (*hyper* above + *osis* condition) TERM: alimentary canal (consists of the mouth, pharynx, esophagus, stomach, small intestine, and large intestine; in adults, it is about 30 feet long) CROSS REFERENCE: nur, troph
album	Latin *albumin*; *albus* white	a whitish protein	SIMPLE ROOT: albumen (or, albumin; egg white), albumin {albuminous}, albuminate (albumin denatured by a base or an acid) PREFIXED ROOT: *albuminemia* albuminous blood condition: analbuminemia (*an* negative) bisalbuminemia (*bis* two) hyperalbuminemia (*hyper* above) hypoalbuminemia (*hypo* under) *albuminosis* albuminous condition: hyperalbuminosis (*hyper* above) hypoalbuminosis (*hypo* under) *albuminuria* albuminous urine condition: diploalbuminuria (the coexistence of nephritic and nonnephritic albuminuria) (*diploos* double) hemialbumosuria (also called *propeptonuria*) (*hemi* half) macroalbuminuria (also called *proteinuria*) (*makros* large) microalbuminuria (*mikros* small) *albumose*: protoalbumose (*protos* first) LEADING ROOT COMPOUND: *albumin*: albuminemia (*emia* blood condition) albuminoid (*eidos* form) albuminuria {albuminuric} (*uria* urine condition) *albuminat*: albuminaturia (the presence of an excessive amount of albuminates in the urine) (*uria* urine condition) *albumini*: albuminiferous (*ferre* to bear) albuminimeter (or, albumimeter) {albuminimetry} (*metron* measure) albuminiparous (forming albumin) (*parere* to produce)

Element	From	Meaning	Examples
album (cont'd)		[a whitish protein]	*albumino*: albuminocholia (*cholia* bile condition) albuminogenous (*genere* to produce) albuminolysis (*lyein* to loosen) albuminometer (or, albuminimeter) (*metron* measure) albuminoptysis (*ptyein* to spit) albuminorrhea (*rhein* to flow) *albumo*: albumoscope (an instrument for determining the presence of albumin in the urine) (*skopein* to examine) TRAILING ROOT COMPOUND: *albumin*: lecithalbumin (*lekithos* egg yolk) myoalbumin (*myos* muscle) parvalbumin (*parvus* small) pseudoalbinism (*pseudes* false) seralbumin (*serum* whey) *albuminuria* albuminous urine: noctalbuminuria (*nox* night) pseudalbuminuria (*pseudes* false) CROSS REFERENCE: leuk
alg	Greek *algein* to feel; *algos* pain	pain, feeling	SIMPLE ROOT: algesia (also called *algesthesia*) {algesic} PREFIXED ROOT: *alges*: analgesia, analgesic {analgetic, analgic} (*an* negative) hemianalgesia (*hemi* half + analgesia) hemihypalgesia (*hemi* half + hypalgesia) hypalgesia (or, hypoalgesia) {hypalgesic, hypalgetic} (*hypo* under) hyperalgesia (or, hyperalgia) {hyperalgesic} (*hyper* above) paralgesia {paralgesic} (*para* abnormal) para-analgesia (or, paranalgesia) (*para* alongside) *algi*: antalgic (also called *analgesic*) (*anti* against) hemialgia (pain that affects one side of the body) (*hemi* half) megalgia (severe pain, as in muscular rheumatism) (*megas* large) pantalgia (pain over the whole body) (*pantos* all) paralgia (abnormal or unusual pain) (*para* abnormal) synalgia (referred pain) {synalgic} (*syn* with, together) telalgia (pain felt at a distance from its stimulus; referred pain) (*tele* afar) LEADING ROOT COMPOUND: *alg*: algedonic (*hedone* pleasure) [h is elided] algesthesia (or, algesthesis; also called *algesia*) (*esthesia* feeling) *algesi*: algesichronometer (*chronos* time + *metron* measure) algesimeter (or, algesiometer) {algesimetry} (*metron* measure) *algesio*: algesiogenic (*genere* to produce) algesiometer (or, algesimeter) (*metron* measure) *algin*: alginuresis (painful urination) (*uresis* urine excretion) *algio*: algiomotor (also called *algiomuscular*) (*movere* to move) algiomuscular (also called *algiomotor*) (*musculus* muscle) algiovascular (or, algovascular) (*vas* blood vessel)

Element	From	Meaning	Examples
alg (cont'd)		[pain]	*algo*:

algo:

algodystrophy (*dys* abnormal + *trophein* to nourish)

algogenesia (or, algogenesis) (*genere* to produce)

algolagnia (also called *algophilia*) (*lagneia* lust)

algology (*logos* study)

algomenorrhea (painful menstruation) (*mene* month + *rhein* to flow)

algometer (in instrument for measuring sensitivity to pain) {algometry} (*metron* measure)

algophilia (or, algophily; also called *algolagnia*) (*philein* to love)

algophobia (morbid dread of experiencing or witnessing pain) (*phobia* fear)

algopsychalia (also called *psychalgia*) (*psyche* soul, mind)

algospasm (an acute, painful spasm of the muscles)

TRAILING ROOT COMPOUND:

algesia:

audioanalgesia (*audire* to hear + *an* privative)

cryalgesia (*kryos* cold)

oligoanalgesia (the use of analgesics too infrequently or at doses insufficient to relieve pain) (*oligos* little + *an* negative)

thermalgesia, thermanalgesia (absence of temperature sense; also called *thermoanesthesia*) (*therme* heat + *an* privative)

algia:

acromelalgia (also called *erythromelalgia*: a form of erythomelalgia characterized by redness, pain, and swelling of the fingers and toes, headache, and vomiting) (*akros* extremity + *melos* limb)

acrostealgia (painful inflammation of the bones of the hands and feet) (*akros* extremities + *osteon* bone)

adenalgia (*adenos* gland)

aerodontalgia (*aer* air + *odontos* tooth)

angialgia (*angeion* blood vessel)

aortalgia (aorta)

appendalgia (appendix)

arteralgia (artery)

arthralgia (also called *arthrodynia*) (*arthron* joint)

brachialgia (*brachion* arm)

cardialgia (also called *cardiodynia*) (*kardia* heart)

causalgia (intense burning pain accompanied by trophic skin changes, due to injury of nerve fibers) (*kaiein* to burn)

cephalgia (also called *cephalodynia*) (*kephale* head)

cheilalgia (*cheilos* lip)

chiralgia (*cheir* hand)

cinesalgia (pain in a muscle when it is brought into action) (*kinesis* motion)

coccyalgia (also called *coccygodynia*) (coccyx)

colonalgia (colon)

colpalgia (also called *vaginodynia*) (*kolpos* vagina)

costalgia (also called *pleurodynia*) (*costa* rib, side)

coxalgia (also called *coxodynia*) (*coxa* hip)

cystalgia (also called *cystodynia*) (*cyst* sac, bladder)

dacryoadenalgia (*dakryon* tear + *adenos* gland)

dactylalgia (also called *dactylodynia*) (*daktylos* finger, toe)

dentalgia (also called *odontalgia*) (*dens* tooth)

dermatalgia (also called *dermatodynia*) (*dermatos* skin)

Element	From	Meaning	Examples
alg (cont'd)		[pain]	desmalgia (also called *desmodynia*) (*dein* to bind: ligament)
			dorsalgia (also called *dorsodynia*) (*dorsum* back)
			encephalalgia (also called *encephalodynia*) (*enkephale* brain, head)
			enteralgia (also called *enterodynia*) (*enteron* intestine)
			esophagalgia (also called *esophodynia*) (esophagus)
			gastralgia (also called *gastrodynia*) (*gaster* stomach, belly)
			glossalgia (also called *glossodynia*) (*glossa* tongue)
			gnathalgia (also called *gnathodynia*) (*gnathos* jaw)
			gonalgia (or, gonyalgia) (*gony* knee)
			hepatalgia (also called *hepatodynia*) (*hepatos* liver)
			hysteralgia (also called *hysterodynia*) (*hystera* womb, uterus)
			iridalgia (or, iralgia) (iris of eye)
			ischialgia (also called *ischiodynia*) (*ischion* hip joint)
			keratalgia (*keratos* horn: cornea)
			kinesialgia (or, cinesalgia) (*kinein* to move)
			laryngalgia (larynx)
			mammalgia (also called *mastalgia*) (*mamma* breast, nipple)
			mastalgia (also called *mammalgia, mastodynia*) (*mastos* breast)
			melalgia (*melos* limb)
			menalgia (*mene* month: menstruation)
			meralgia (*meros* thigh)
			myalgia (or, myosalgia; also called *myodynia*) (*myos* muscle)
			myelalgia (*myelos* spinal cord)
			nephralgia {nephralgic} (*nephros* kidney)
			neuralgia (also called *neurodynia*) (*neuron* nerve)
			notalgia (now an obsolete term for *dorsalgia*) (*noton* the back)
			odontalgia (also called *odontodynia*) {odontalgic} (*odontos* tooth)
			omalgia (also called *omodynia*) (*omos* shoulder)
			oophoralgia (also called *ovarialgia*) (*oophoros* ovary passage)
			opalgia (facial neuralgia) (*ops* face)
			ophthalmalgia (also called *ophthalmodynia*) (*ophthalmos* eye)
			opsialgia (acute facial neuralgia) (*ops* face)
			orchialgia (also called *orchalgia, orchidalgia, orchodynia, testalgia*) (*orchis* testis)
			ostalgia (or, ostealgia; also called *osteodynia*) (*osteon* bone)
			otalgia (also called *earache, otodynia*) (*otos* ear)
			ovarialgia (also called *oophoralgia*) (ovary)
			pancreatalgia (pancreas)
			pectoralgia (also called *stethalgia, thoracalgia, thoracodynia*) (*pectus* chest)
			pedialgia (also called *podalgia*) (*pes* foot)
			phallalgia (also called *phallodynia*) (*phallos* penis)
			pharyngalgia (also called *pharyngodynia*) (*pharynx* throat)
			phlebalgia (*phlebos* vein)
			photalgia (also called *photodynia*) (*photos* light)
			phrenalgia (also called *diaphragmalgia, phrenodynia*) (*phrenos* diaphragm)
			plantalgia (*planta* sole of the foot)
			pleuralgia (also called *pleurodynia, costalgia*) (*pleura* rib, side)
			podalgia (also called *pedialgia, pododynia*) (*pous* foot)
			proctalgia (also called *proctodynia*) (*proktos* anus)
			prosopalgia (facial neuralgia; see *opsialgia*) (*prosopon* face)
			prostatalgia (also called *prostatodynia*) (prostate)
			psychalgia {psychalgic} (*psyche* mind)

Element	From	Meaning	Examples
alg (cont'd)		[pain]	psychroalgia (*psychros* cold)
			pternalgia (also called *calcaneodynia*) (*pterma* heel)
			pulpalgia (pain in the pulp of the tooth)
			pygalgia (*pyge* rump, buttocks)
			pyloralgia (pylorus)
			rachialgia (also called *rachiodynia*) (*rhachis* spine)
			radiculalgia (pain due to disease of the spinal nerve roots) (*radix* root)
			rectalgia (also called *proctalgia, proctodynia*) (rectum)
			rhinalgia (also called *rhinodynia*) (*rhinos* nose)
			sacralgia (also called *sacrodynia*) (sacrum: the triangular bone just below the lumbar vertebrae)
			scapulalgia (also called *scapulodynia*) (*scapula* shoulder blade)
			scelalgia (*skelos* leg)
			somatalgia (*somatos* body)
			sphincteralgia (pain in a sphincter muscle)
			splenalgia (also called *splenodynia*) (spleen)
			spondylalgia (also called *spondylodynia* (*spondylos* vertebra)
			sternalgia (also called *sternodynia*) (*sternum* chest)
			stethalgia (also called *thoracalgia, pectoralgia*) (*stethos* chest)
			stomachalgia (also called *stomachodynia, gastrodynia*)
			stomalgia (or, stomatalgia) (*stomatos* mouth)
			tarsalgia (pain in the ankle or foot) (*tarsos* ankle)
			tenalgia (also called *tenodynia*) (tendon)
			testalgia (also called *orchialgia, orchiodynia*) (*testis* testicle)
			thelalgia (*thele* nipple)
			thermalgia (a burning pain; also called *causalgia*) (*therme* heat)
			thoracalgia (also called *pectoralgia, stethalgia, thoracodynia*) (*thorakos* chest)
			tibialgia (tibia: the shin bone)
			topalgia (localized pain: seen in neurasthenia) (*topos* place)
			trachealgia (*trachea* windpipe)
			trichalgia (also called *trichodynia*) (*trichos* hair)
			ulalgia (also called *gingivalgia*) (*oulon* gum)
			ureteralgia (ureter)
			urethralgia (also called *urethrodynia*) (urethra)
			uteralgia (also called *hysteralgia, uterodynia*) (uterus)
			vasalgia (also called *angialgia*) (*vas* blood vessel)
			visceralgia (*viscera* internal organs)
			CROSS REFERENCE: odyn, path, sens
all	Greek *allos* other	other, different, mutually, another	SIMPLE ROOT:
			allaxis (change, transformation, metamorphosis)
			allele (one of two or more contrasting genes)
			PREFIXED ROOT:
			isoallele, isoallelism (*isos* equal)
			multiallelic (*multus* many)
			parallax (change of position) {parallactic}
			parallel (*para* alongside)
			See Appendix B for examples of words with this initial combining form. Others are listed with the root to which it is attached.
			CROSS REFERENCE: allotrio, heter, muta, xen
allotrio	Greek *allotrios, allos*	strange	See Appendix B for examples of words with this initial combining form. Others are listed with the root to which it is attached.
			CROSS REFERENCE: all, xen

Element	From	Meaning	Examples
alveol	Latin; from Greek *aulus* reed	trough, cavity, pit, cell	SIMPLE ROOT: alveolate (honeycombed; full of small cavities), alveolus (pl., alveoli) {alveolar}, alveus (pl., alvei) PREFIXED ROOT: interalveolar (*inter* between) LEADING ROOT COMPOUND: *alveo*: alveoalgia (pain following tooth extraction; dry socket) (*algos* pain) alveobronchiolitis (*bronchos* windpipe + *itis* inflammation) *alveol*: alveolalgia (or, alveoalgia) (*algos* pain) alveolectomy (*ektome* excision) alveolitis (*itis* inflammation) *alveolo*: alveolocapillary (pertaining to the pulmonary alveoli and capillaries) alveoloclasia (destruction of a tooth socket) (*klaein* to break) alveolodental (*dens* tooth) alveololabial (*labium* lip) alveololingual (*lingua* tongue) alveolomerotomy (*meros* part + *tomy* incision) alveoloplasty (*plassein* to form) alveoloschisis (a cleft in the alveolar process) (*schisis* cleaving) alveolotomy (*tomy* incision) TRAILING ROOT COMPOUND: bronchoalveolar (also called *bronchovesicular*) (*bronchus* windpipe) dentoalveolar (*dens* tooth) labioalveolar (*labium* lip) pseudoalveolar (*pseudes* false) CROSS REFERENCE: antr, cell, vestibul
ambi-	Latin prefix	on both sides	See Appendix B for examples of words with this prefix. Others are listed with the root to which it is attached. CROSS REFERENCE: amphi-
ambly	Greek *amblys*	dull, blunted	See Appendix B for examples of words with this initial combining form. Others are listed with the root to which it is attached. CROSS REFERENCE: None
amnio	Greek *amnion* diminutive of *amnos* lamb	inner fetal membrane	SIMPLE ROOT: amnion (the thin, transparent, silvery and tough outermost membrane of the sac enclosing the fetus, and which produces the amniotic fluid) {amnionic, amniotic} PREFIXED ROOT: anamniotic (having no amnion) (*an* privative) diamniotic (*di* two) epamniotic (*epi* upon) intra-amniotic (*intra* within) hypamnios (also called *oligohydramnios*) (*hypo* under) proamnion (*pro* before) LEADING ROOT COMPOUND: *amni*: amnioma (a tumor formed from the amnion) (*oma* tumor) *amnio*: amniocele (also called *omphalocele*) (*kele* hernia) amniocentesis (*kentein* to puncture) amniochorial (*chorion* fetal membrane) amniocyte (*kytos* cell) amniogenesis (*genere* to produce) amniography (*graphein* to write) amnioinfusion (*in* in + *fusion* a pouring)

Element	From	Meaning	Examples
amnio (cont'd)		[inner fetal membrane]	amniorrhea (*rhein* to flow) amniorrhexis (*rhexis* rupture) amnioscope, amnioscopy (*skopein* to examine) amniotome (*temnein* to cut: a cutting instrument) amniotomy (*tomy* incision) *amnion*: amnionitis (*itis* inflammation) TRAILING ROOT COMPOUND: hydramnion (also called *polyhydramnios*) (*hydor* water) oligoamnios (also called *oligohydramnios*) (*oligos* little, scant) pleuramnion (*pleura* rib, side) schizamnion (an amnion developing by the formation of a cavity within the inner cell mass) (*schizein* to split) CROSS REFERENCE: chori
amygdal	Greek *amygdale* almond	almond, tonsil	NOTE: This root originally meant "almond"; however, it is extended to mean "tonsil," because of the tonsil's shape being similar to that of an almond. SIMPLE ROOT: amygdala (used in anatomical nomenclature to designate an almond-shaped structure), amygdaline (of or like an almond or almonds; also, having to do with the tonsils) LEADING ROOT COMPOUND: *amygda*: amygdalith (*lithos* stone) *amygdal*: amygdalitis (also called *tonsillitis*) (*itis* inflammation) amygdaloid (resembling an almond, or a tonsil) (*eidos* form) *amygdalo*: amygdalopathy (or, tonsillopathy) (*pathos* disease) CROSS REFERENCE: tonsil
amyl	Greek *amylon* *a* negative + *myle* mill; thus, not ground at the mill	starch	SIMPLE ROOT: amyl {amylic}, amylaceous (of or like starch) amylase (an enzyme that helps change starch into sugar; it is found in saliva, pancreatic juices, etc.), amylum PREFIXED ROOT: endoamylase (*endon* within) hyperamylasemia (*hyper* above + *emia* blood condition) macroamylasemia (*makron* large + *emia* blood condition) paramyloidosis (*para* abnormal + *eidos* form + *osis* condition) LEADING ROOT COMPOUND: *amyl*: amylemia (*emia* blood condition) amyloid (resembling starch) (*eidos* form) amyloidoma (*eidos* form + *oma* tumor) amyloidosis (*eidos* form + *osis* condition) amyluria (*uria* urine condition) *amylas*: amylasuria (also called *diastasuria*) (*uria* urine condition) *amylo*: amylogenesis {amylogenic} (*genere* to produce) amylolysis {amylolytic} (*lyein* to loosen) amylometer (*metron* measure) amylophagia (an abnormal craving for starch) (*phagein* to devour) amyloplast (*plassein* to form) amylorrhea (*rhein* to flow) CROSS REFERENCE: None
an-	Greek prefix	negative, privative	See Appendix B for examples of words beginning with this prefix. Others are listed with the roots to which it is attached. CROSS REFERENCE: a-, ab-, de-, dis-

Element	From	Meaning	Examples
an	Latin *anus* ring	anus, ring	SIMPLE ROOT: annular (or, anular), anulus (or, annulus; a circular or ringlike structure; pl., anuli), anus {anal}, anality PREFIXED ROOT: *anal*: circumanal (also called *perianal, periproctic*) (*circum* around) perianal (also called *circumanal, periproctic*) (*peri* around, near) postanal (*post* behind, beyond) preanal (in front of the anus) (*pre* anterior) subanal (situated below the anus) (*sub* below) supraanal (or, superanal; situated superior to the anus) (*supra* above) *annular*: interannular (situated between two rings or constrictions) (*inter* between) LEADING ROOT COMPOUND: *annulo*: annuloplasty (*plassein* to form) annulorrhaphy (*rhaphe* suture) *ano*: anococcygeal (*coccyx* cuckoo: a small bone caudad to the sacrum) anoderm (*derma* skin) anogenital (relating to both the anus and the genital regions) anoperineal (perineum) anoplasty (*plassein* to form) anorectum {anorectal} anoscope, anoscopy (*skopein* to examine) anospinal (spine) anovaginal (vagina) anovesical (*vesica* bladder) *anus*: anusitis (*itis* inflammation) TRAILING ROOT COMPOUND: ileoanal (ileum) ischioanal (pertaining to the ischium and anus) (*ischion* hip) TERM: per anum (through the anus) CROSS REFERENCE: gyr, proct
ana-	Greek prefix	up, back, again	See Appendix B for examples of words with this prefix. Others are listed with the roots to which it is attached. CROSS REFERENCE: re-, retro-
ancon	Greek *ankon*	elbow	SIMPLE ROOT: ancon (the elbow), anconad (toward the elbow) anconal (pertaining to the elbow; also called *cubital*) PREFIXED ROOT: subanconeus (*sub* under) LEADING ROOT COMPOUND: anconagra (gout of the elbow) (*agra* seizure, gout) anconitis (*itis* inflammation) anconoid (*eidos* form) CROSS REFERENCE: olecran
andr	Greek *andros*	man, male	PREFIXED ROOT: anandria (the loss of virility) (*an* privative) hyperandrogenism (*hyper* above + *genere* to produce) hypoandrogenism (*hypo* under + *genere* to produce) LEADING ROOT COMPOUND: *andr*: andriatrics (also called *andrology*) (*iatrein* to heal) android (or, androidal; also called *andromorphous*) (*eidos* form)

Element	From	Meaning	Examples
andr (cont'd)		[male, man]	*andro*: androblastoma (also called *arrhenoblastoma*) (*blastos* bud, shoot, germ + *oma* tumor) androgalactozemia (*galaktos* milk + *zemia* loss) androgenesis {androgenic, androgenous} (*genere* to produce) androgynous (also called *intersexual*) (*gyne* woman, female) andrology (also called *andriatrics*) (*logos* study) andromimetic (*mimetikos* imitating) andromorphous (*morphe* form) andropathy (*pathos* disease) andropause (*pausis* cessation) androphilic (preferring humans; said of certain parasites; also called *anthropophilic*) (*philein* to love) androphobia (*phobos* fear) androsterone (a male sex hormone) (*stereos* solid) TRAILING ROOT COMPOUND: gynandrism (also called *hermaphroditism*) (*gyne* woman) holandric (the counterpart is *hologynic*) (*holos* whole, entire) CROSS REFERENCE: anthrop
anemia			See hem-.
anesthe	Greek *an* privative + *esthesia* feeling	anesthesia	SIMPLE ROOT: anesthesia (lack of feeling or sensation; artificially induced loss of ability to feel pain) {anesthetic}, anesthetist, anesthetize PREFIXED ROOT: hemianesthesia (*hemi* half) para-anesthesia (*para* alongside) postanesthesia (*post* after) LEADING ROOT COMPOUND: anesthesiology (*logos* study) TRAILING ROOT COMPOUND: acroanesthesia (*akron* extremity) bathyanesthesia (*bathys* deep) cryanesthesia (inability to perceive cold) (*kryos* cold) cryoanesthesia (also called *refrigeration anesthesia*) (*kryos* cold) gargalanesthesia (*gargalos* itching) hypnoanesthesia (*hypnos* sleep) kinanesthesia (*kinein* to move) neuroanesthesia (*neuron* nerve) pallanesthesia (also called *apallesthesia*) (*pallein* to tremble) phlebanesthesia (also called *phlebonarcosis*) (*phlebos* vein) rachianesthesia (*rhachis* spine, backbone) thermanesthesia (*therme* heat) topoanesthesia (also called *atopognosis*) (*topos* place) CROSS REFERENCE: None
aneurys	Greek *ana* up, again + *eurys* wide	widening	SIMPLE ROOT: aneurysm (also listed under eury-) {aneurysmal} PREFIXED ROOT: endoaneurysmoplasty (also called *aneurysmoplasty*) (*endon* within + *plassein* to form) endoaneurysmorrhaphy (also called *aneurysmoplasty*) (*endon* within + *rhaphe* suture) microaneurysm (*mikros* small) LEADING ROOT COMPOUND: *aneurysm*: aneurysmectomy (*ektome* excision) *aneurysmo*: aneurysmogram, aneurysmography (*graphein* to write)

A Thesaurus of Medical Word Roots

Element	From	Meaning	Examples
aneurys (cont'd)		[widening]	aneurysmoplasty (*plassein* to form) aneurysmorrhaphy (*rhaphe* suture) aneurysmotomy (*tomy* incision) TRAILING ROOT COMPOUND: osteoaneurysm (*osteon* bone) CROSS REFERENCE: eury, later
angi	Greek *angeion* vessel	blood vessel (also, lymph vessel)	PREFIXED ROOT: *angi*: anangioid (*an* privative + *eidos* form) euangiotic (well supplied with blood vessels) (*eu* well) periangioma (*peri* around + *oma* tumor) *angiitis* inflammation of a blood vessel or vessels: endangiitis (or, endangeitis) (*endon* within) panangiitis (*pan* all) periangiitis (also called *perivasculitis*) (*peri* around) polyangiitis (*polys* many) *angio*: anangioplasia (*an* privative + *plassein* to form) periangiocholitis (also, pericholangitis; inflammation of the tissues around the bile ducts, or interlobar capillaries of the liver) (*peri* around + *chole* bile + *itis* inflammation) *angium*: endangium (inner coat of a blood vessel) (*endon* within) mesangium {mesangial} (*mesos* middle) micrangium (*mikros* small) LEADING ROOT COMPOUND: *ang*: angitis (or, angiitis) (*itis* inflammation) *angi*: angialgia (also called *angiodynia, vasalgia*) (*algos* pain) angiasthenia (loss of vascular tone) (*asthenia* weakness) angiectasia (or, angiectasis) {angiectatic} (*ektasis* dilatation) angiectomy (*ektome* excision) angiectopia (also called *angioplany*) (*ektopia* displaced) angiitis (or, angitis) (*itis* inflammation) angiodynia (also called *angialgia*) (*odyne* pain) angioid (*eidos* form) angiomatosis (*oma* tumor + *osis* condition) angiosis (*osis* condition) angiosteosis (*osteon* bone + *osis* condition) angiotitis (*otos* ear + *itis* inflammation) *angio*: angioaccess (a site of entry into a blood vessel, as one maintained for recurrent hemodialysis) angioarchitecture (the arrangement and distribution of the blood vessels of any organ) angioataxia (irregular tension in the blood vessels) angioblast {angioblastic}, angioblastoma (*blastos* germ, shoot, bud + *oma* tumor) angiocardium (*kardia* heart) angiocatheter (a hollow, flexible tube inserted into a blood vessel to withdraw or instill fluids) angiocholitis (also called *cholangitis*) (*chole* bile + *itis* inflammation) angiocrine (denoting vasomotor disorders of endocrine origin) angiocyst (*kystis* bag, bladder)

Element	From	Meaning	Examples
angi (cont'd)		[blood vessel]	angiodermatitis (*dermatos* skin + *itis* inflammation)
			angiodiascopy (*dia* through + *skopein* to examine)
			angiodysplasia (*dys* abnormal + *plassein* to form)
			angiodystrophia (*dys* abnormal + *trephein* to nourish)
			angioectatic (or, angiectatic) (*ektasis* dilatation)
			angioedema {angioedematous} (*edema* swelling)
			angioendothelioma, angioendotheliomatosis (*endon* within + *thele* nipple + *oma* tumor + *osis* condition)
			angiofibroma (*fibra* fiber + *oma* tumor)
			angiofibrosis (*fibra* fiber + *osis* condition)
			angiogenesis {angiogenic} (*genere* to produce)
			angioglioma (*glia* glue + *oma* tumor)
			angiogram, angiography (*graphein* to write)
			angiohyalinosis (*hyalos* glass + *osis* condition)
			angiohypertonia (also called *vasospasm*) (*hyper* above + *tonos* tension)
			angiohypotonia (also called *vasoparalysis*) (*hypo* under + *tonos* tension)
			angiokeratoma (also called *keratoangioma*) (*keras* horn + *oma* tumor)
			angiokinetic (also called *vasomotor*) (*kinein* to move)
			angioleucitis (also called *lymphangitis*) (*leukos* white + *itis* inflammation)
			angiolipoma (*lipos* fat + *oma* tumor)
			angiolith (*lithos* stone)
			angiology (*logos* study)
			angiolupoid (*lupus* wolf + *eidos* form)
			angiolymphitis (also called *lymphangitis*) (*lympha* water, liquid + *itis* inflammation)
			angiolysis (*lyein* to loosen)
			angiomegaly (*megalos* large)
			angiomyocardiac (*myos* muscle + *kardia* heart)
			angiomyoma (*myos* muscle + *oma* tumor)
			angiomyosarcoma (*myos* muscle + *sarkos* flesh + *oma* tumor)
			angioneurectomy (*neuron* nerve + *ektome* excision)
			angioneurosis {angioneurotic} (*neuron* nerve + *osis* condition)
			angioneurotomy (*neuron* nerve + *tomy* incision)
			angionoma (ulceration of a vessel) (*noma* ulcer)
			angioparesis (also called *vasoparesis*) (*paresis* weakness)
			angiopathy, angiopathology (*pathos* disease + *logos* study)
			angioplany (also called *angiectopia*) (*planan* to wander)
			angioplasty (*plassein* to form)
			angiopoiesis (also called *angiogenesis*) (*poiein* to produce)
			angiopressure (*premere* to press)
			angiorrhaphy (*rhaphe* suture)
			angiosarcoma (*sarkos* flesh + *oma* tumor)
			angiosclerosis (*skleros* hard + *osis* condition)
			angioscope, angioscopy (*skopein* to examine)
			angiospasm {angiospastic} (*span* to contract)
			angiostenosis (*stenos* narrow + *osis* condition)
			angiosthenia (*sthenos* strength)
			angiostomy (*stoma* mouth, opening)
			angiostrophe {angiostrophy} (*strephein* to twist)
			angiotelectasis (*telos* end + *ektasis* dilatation)
			angiotome, angiotomy (*tomy* incision)

Element	From	Meaning	Examples
angi (cont'd)		[blood vessel]	angiotonia (also called *vasotonia*) {angiotonic} (*tonos* tension) angiotripsy (also called *vasotripsy*) (*tribein* to crush) angiotrophic (also called *vasotrophic*) (*trephein* to nourish) angiozyme (*zyme* ferment) TRAILING ROOT COMPOUND: *angiectasis* dilatation of vessel: hemangiectasis (*haima* blood) cholangiectasis (*chole* bile) lymphangiectasis (*lympha* water, fluid) sialoangiectasis (*sialon* saliva) telangiectasis (*telos* end) *angitis* inflammation of vessel: cholangitis (*chole* gall, bile) lymphangitis (*lympha* water, liquid) myxangitis (*myxa* mucus) thrombolympangitis (*thrombos* clot + *lymph* water, liquid) *angioma* tumor of vessel: chorioangioma (*chorion* fetal membrane) chylangioma (*chylus* gastric juice) fibroangioma (*fibra* fiber) glomangioma (*glomus* ball) hemangioma (*haima* blood) phlebangioma (a venous aneurysm) (*phlebos* vein) telangioma (*telos* end, terminal) *angiosis* vessel condition: chorioangiosis (*chorion* membrane) glomangiosis (*glomus* ball) telangiosis (also called *capillaropathy*) (*telos* end, terminal) *angium*: merosporangium (a cylindrical small sporangium containing few spores) (*meros* part + *sporos* seed) *angiuria*: lithangiuria (*lithos* stone + *uria* urine condition) CROSS REFERENCE: cell, cyt, vas
angin	Greek *anchein* to squeeze	narrow, tight	SIMPLE ROOT: angina (spasmodic, choking, or suffocative pain; now used almost exclusively to denote *angina pectoris*) {anginal} anginose (pertaining to or affected with angina, especially angina pectoris) {anginous} PREFIXED ROOT: antanginal (*anti* against) postanginal (*post* after) LEADING ROOT COMPOUND: *angin*: anginoid (resembling angina) (*eidos* form) *angini*: anginiform (also called *anginoid*) (*forma* shape) *angino*: anginophobia (irrational fear of choking) (*phobia* fear) TRAILING ROOT COMPOUND: herpangina (an inflammatory skin disease) (*herpein* to creep) staphyloangina (a mild form of sore throat) (*staphyle* uvula) SPANISH: angostura, from the town Angostura, Venezuela, lit., "the narrows" (A bitter tonic from the bark of the *angostura* tree is used as a stimulant.) CROSS REFERENCE: arct, steno
aniso	Greek *an* not + *iso* equal	unequal, dissimilar	See Appendix B for examples of words with this initial combining form. Others are placed with the roots to which it is attached. CROSS REFERENCE: all, alter, heter

Element	From	Meaning	Examples
ankyl	Greek *ankylos*	stiffness (usually of a joint)	NOTE: This element yields English *angle, ankle*. See Appendix B for examples of words with this initial combining form. Others are placed with the roots to which it is attached. CROSS REFERENCE: None
anopia	Greek *a* privative + *opia* eye condition	anopia	SIMPLE ROOT: anopia (blindness resulting from a defect in, or the absence of, one or both eyes) PREFIXED ROOT: deuteranopia (*deuteros* second) hemianopia {hemianopic} (*hemi* half) protanopia (a form of colorblindness in which the person is unable to distinguish shades of red as well as confusion of red with green or bluish green) (*protos* first) quadrantanopia (also called *tetaranopia*) (*quadrant* fourth) tetaranopia (also called *quadrantanopia*) (*tetartos* fourth) tritanopia (*tritos* third) TRAILING ROOT COMPOUND: cyanopia (or, cyanopsia) (*kyanos* blue) nyctanopia (*nyx* night) sectoranopia (loss of vision in a sector of the visual field) CROSS REFERENCE: None
ante-	Latin prefix	before	See Appendix B for examples of words with this prefix. Others are listed with the roots to which it is attached. CROSS REFERENCE: antero-, pre-, pro-
antero-	Latin prefix	before	See Appendix B for examples of words with this prefix. Others are listed with the roots to which it is attached. CROSS REFERENCE: ante-, pre-, pro-
anthrop	Greek *anthropos*	man; also mankind; human being	PREFIXED ROOT: exanthrope (a cause or source of a disease originating outside the body) {exanthropic} (*ex* out) LEADING ROOT COMPOUND: *anthrop*: anthropoid (resembling that of a man, as an *anthropoid pelvis*, or resembling a human being, as an *anthropoid ape*) (*eidos* form) *anthropo*: anthropobiology (*bios* life + *logos* study) anthropocentric (*kentron* point, center) anthropogenesis (or, anthropogeny) (*genere* to produce) anthropometer (*metron* measure) anthropophilic (preferring man; said of parasites that prefer a human host rather than other animals) (*philein* to love) anthroposomatology (*somatos* body + *logos* study) anthropotomy (also called *androtomy*) (*tomy* incision) anthropozoophilic (attracted to both human beings and animals; said of certain mosquitoes; compare *anthropophilic* and *zoophilic*) (*zoon* animal + *philein* to love) TRAILING ROOT COMPOUND: lycanthropy (mania in which patient believes himself/herself a wild beast, especially a wolf) (*lykos* wolf) misanthropy (hatred of mankind) (*misein* to hate) zoanthropy (the delusion that one has become an animal) (*zoon* animal) CROSS REFERENCE: andr
anti-	Greek prefix	against	See Appendix B for examples of words with this prefix. Others are listed with the roots to which it is attached. CROSS REFERENCE: contra-, de-, ob-

Element	From	Meaning	Examples
antr	Latin/ Greek *antron* cavern	cavity (antrum, sinus)	SIMPLE ROOT: antrum (pl., antra, antrums) PREFIXED ROOT: transantral (*trans* across) LEADING ROOT COMPOUND: *antr*: antritis (*itis* inflammation) antrodynia (*odyne* pain) *antro*: antrobuccal (*bucca* cheek) antrocele (*kele* tumor) antroduodenectomy (duodenum + *ektome* excision) antronasal (*nas* nose) antropyloric (*pylorum*) antroscope, antroscopy (*skopein* to examine) antrostomy (also called *antrotomy*) (*stoma* mouth, opening) antrotome, antrotomy (also called *antrostomy*) (*tomy* incision) antrotonia (*tonus* tone) antrotympanitis (*tympanon* eardrum + *itis* inflammation) *antron*: antronalgia (pain in the maxillary antrum) (*algos* pain) TRAILING ROOT COMPOUND: *antritis* sinus inflammation: nasoantritis (also called *rhinoantritis*) (*nasus* nose) otoantritis (inflammation of the mastoid antrum) (*otos* ear) prosopantritis (inflammation of the frontal sinuses) (*prosopon* face) rhinoantritis (also called *nasoantritis*) (*rhinos* nose) CROSS REFERENCE: alveol, atri, cell, sin, vestibul
aort	Greek *aeirein* to raise	aorta	SIMPLE ROOT: aorta (the main trunk from which the systemic arterial systems proceed; pl., aortae) {aortal, aortic} PREFIXED ROOT: *aortic*: endaortic (*endon* within) intra-aortic (*intra* within) paraaortic (or, paraortic) (*para* alongside) periaortic (*peri* around) preaortic (*pre* before) subaortic (*sub* below) transaortic (*trans* across) *aortitis* inflammation of the aorta: endaortitis (*endon* within) mesaortitis (*mesos* middle) periaortitis (*peri* around) LEADING ROOT COMPOUND: *aort*: aortalgia (*algos* pain) aortarctia (also called *aortostenosis*) (*arctare* to narrow) aortectasia (or, aortectasis) (*ektasis* dilatation) aortectomy (*ektome* excision) aortitis (*itis* inflammation) *aortico*: aorticopulmonary (also called *pulmoaortic*) (*pulmon* lung) aorticorenal (*renes* kidney) *aorto*: aortoclasia (rupture of the aorta) (*klaein* to break) aortocoronary (relating to the aorta and the coronary arteries) aortoduodenal (duodenum)

Element	From	Meaning	Examples
aort (cont'd)		[aorta]	aortoenteric (*enteron* intestine) aortogastric (*gaster* stomach) aortogram, aortography (*graphein* to write) aortopathy (*pathos* disease) aortopexy (*pexis* fixation) aortoplasty (*plassein* to form) aortoptosia (or, aortoptosis; a sinking down of the abdominal aorta in splanchoptosia) (*ptosis* a falling) aortorrhaphy (*rhaphe* suture) aortosclerosis (*skleros* hard + *osis* condition) aortostenosis (also called *aortarctia*) (*stenosis* narrow condition) aortotomy (*tomy* incision) TRAILING ROOT COMPOUND: pulmoaortic (also called *aorticopulmonary*) (*pulmon* lung) CROSS REFERENCE: None
apex, **apic**	Latin *apex,* *apicis*	apex, tip, summit	SIMPLE ROOT: *apex*: apex (pl., apexes, apices) {apical} *apic*: apicalis, apiculate, apiculus PREFIXED ROOT: *apex*: periapex {periapical} (*peri* around) *apic*: subapical (*sub* under) LEADING ROOT COMPOUND: *apex*: apexcardiograph (*kardia* heart + *graphein* to write) *apexi*: apexification (*figere* to fasten) apexigraph (*graphein* to write) *apic*: apicectomy (excision of the apex of the petrous portion of the temporal bone) (*ektome* excision) apicitis (*itis* inflammation) *apico*: apicoectomy (*ektome* excision) apicolysis (*lyein* to loosen) apicostomy (*stoma* mouth, opening) apicotomy (also called *apiceotomy*) (*tomy* incision) CROSS REFERENCE: acro
apheres	Greek *apo* away + *hairein* to take	withdrawing	SIMPLE ROOT: apheresis (infusion of a patient's own blood from which certain elements have been removed) TRAILING ROOT COMPOUND: cytapheresis (*kytos* cell) erythrocytapheresis (*erythros* red + *kytos* cell) hemapheresis (also called *aphersis*) (*haima* blood) leukapheresis (*leukos* white — leukocytes) lymphapheresis (*lympha* water, liquid) plasmapheresis (*plasma*) plateletapheresis (platelet) thrombapheresis (*thrombos* clot) thrombocytapheresis (also called *plateletpheresis*, *thrombapheresis*) (*thrombos* clot + *kytos* cell) CROSS REFERENCE: heres, priv, steres
aphia			See hapt- for *anaphia, dysaphia, hyperaphia*.
apo-	Greek prefix	away, from	See Appendix B for examples of words with this prefix. Others are listed with the root to which it is attached. CROSS REFERENCE: ab-, de-

Element	From	Meaning	Examples
apophys	Greek *apo* away + *phyein* to grow	apophysis	SIMPLE ROOT: apophysis (a natural outgrowth or process on a vertebra or other bone; pl., apophyses) PREFIXED ROOT: anapophysis (an accessory vertebral process; especially an accessory process of a dorsal or lumbar vertebra) (*ana* up, back) diapophysis (an upper transverse process of a vertebra) (*dia* across) hypapophysis (*hypo* under) hyperapophysis (*hyper* above) metapophysis (*meta* after) parapophysis (*para* alongside) postzygapophysis (a posterior zygapophysis) (*post* after, behind) LEADING ROOT COMPOUND: apophysitis (*itis* inflammation) TRAILING ROOT COMPOUND: hemapophysis (*haima* blood) neurapophysis (*neuron* nerve) pleurapophysis (*pleura* side) splanchnapophysis (*splanchnon* viscus) zygapophysis (the articular process of a vertebra) (*zygos* joined) CROSS REFERENCE: None
apoplec, **apoplex**	Greek *apo* off, from + *plessein* to strike	stroke	SIMPLE ROOT: apoplexia (or, apoplexy; apoplectic stroke; a condition caused by acute vascular lesions of the brain, such as hemorrhage, thrombosis or embolism, and marked by coma followed by paralysis) {apoplectic} PREFIXED ROOT: antapoplectic (or, antiapoplectic) (*anti* against) postapoplectic (*post* after) LEADING ROOT COMPOUND: *apoplect*: apoplectoid (resembling apoplexy) (*eidos* form) *apoplecti*: apoplectiform (resembling apoplexy) (*forma* likeness) TRAILING ROOT COMPOUND: myelapoplexy (also called *hematomyelia*) (*myelos* marrow) pseudoapoplexy (a mild condition simulating apoplexy, but not accompanied by cerebral hemorrhage) (*pseudes* false) CROSS REFERENCE: pleg
append	Latin *ad* to, toward + *pendere* to hang	hanging	SIMPLE ROOT: appendage (a thing or part appended; limb) appendicular (pertaining to the vermiform appendix) appendix (pl., appendixes, appendices) {appendical, appendiceal} PREFIXED ROOT: *appendicitis* inflammation of the appendix: endoappendicitis (*endon* within) para-appendicitis (*para* alongside) periappendicitis (*peri* around) *appendicular*: periappendicular (*peri* around) LEADING ROOT COMPOUND: *append*: appendectomy (or, appendicectomy) (*ektome* excision) *appendag*: appendagitis (inflammation of an appendage, especially of the epiploic appendages) (*itis* inflammation) *appendic*: appendicectasis (*ektasis* dilatation) appendicectomy (or, appendectomy) (*ektome* excision) appendicitis (*itis* inflammation) *appendico*: appendicocele (the vermiform appendix in a hernial sac) (*kele* hernia)

Element	From	Meaning	Examples
append (cont'd)		[hanging]	appendicolithiasis (a condition marked by concretions in the vermi-form appendix) (*lithos* stone + *iasis* condition) appendicolysis (*lysis* dissolution) appendicostomy, appendicovesicostomy (*vesica* bladder + *stoma* mouth, opening) CROSS REFERENCE: None
apse, apsis			See hapt- for *synapse, synapsis*.
arachn	Greek *arachne*	spider	SIMPLE ROOT: arachnid, arachnidism (spider poisoning) PREFIXED ROOT: intra-arachnoid (*intra* within) subarachnoid (*sub* under) LEADING ROOT COMPOUND: *arachn*: arachnitis (*itis* inflammation) arachnoiditis (*eidos* form + *itis* inflammation) *arachno*: arachnodactyly (or, arachnodactylia) (*daktylos* finger, toe) arachnogastria (spider belly) (*gaster* stomach) arachnolysin (*lyein* to dissolve) arachnomelia (*melos* limb) TRAILING ROOT COMPOUND: ventriculosubarachnoid (pertain-ing to the cerebral ventricles and subarachnoid space) CROSS REFERENCE: None
arch, **arxis**	Greek *archein* to begin, to rule	first, rule; chief, origin foremost	SIMPLE ROOT: archaic (very ancient; pertaining to early evolu-tionary stages) PREFIXED ROOT: procatarxis (lit., a first beginning, or beginning beforehand; also called *exciting cause*) (*pro* before + *kata* down) LEADING ROOT COMPOUND: *arch*: archencephalon (*enkephalon* brain) archenteron (also called *primitive gut*) (*enteron* intestine) *arche*: archegonium (*gone* seed, offspring) archespore (or, archesporium, archispore) (*sporos* seed) archetype (*typus* type) *archeo*: archeocerebellum (also called *vestibulocerebellum*) (*cerebrum* brain) archeocortex (olfactory cortex) (*cortex* bark, rind, shell) archeokinetic (*kinesis* movement) *archi*: archiblast {archiblastic} (*blastos* bud, shoot, germ) archicarp (*karpos* fruit—of fungi) archicerebellum (also called *archaecerebellum*) (*cerebrum* brain) archicortex (also called *archipallium*) (*cortex* bark, rind, shell) archikaryon (or, archicaryon) (*karyon* kernel) archinephron (the pronephros) (*nephros* kidney) archipallium (also called *archicortex*) (*pallium* cloak) archispore (or, archespore) (*sporos* seed) archistome (also called *blastopore*) (*stoma* mouth, opening) archistriatum (*striatum* striped) architectonic (*tectonic* architecture) TRAILING ROOT COMPOUND: adrenarche (a stage of development in which the adrenal glands un-dergo maturation)

Element	From	Meaning	Examples
arch (cont'd)		[first, rule]	menarche {menarchal} (*mene* menstruation) pubarche (the beginning of pubic hair growth) (*puber* adult) thelarche (*thele* nipple, breast) CROSS REFERENCE: norm, prot
arct	Latin *arctare* to press	to narrow	SIMPLE ROOT: arctation (contracture or narrowing of any canal or opening; also called *stenosis*) PREFIXED ROOT: coarct, coarctate, coarctation (*co* with) coarctectomy (*co* with + *ektome* excision) coarctotomy (*co* with + *tomy* incision) TRAILING ROOT COMPOUND: aortarctia (also called *aortostenosis*) (aorta) arteriarctia (vasoconstriction of the arteries) bronchiarctia (also called *bronchostenosis*) (*bronchos* windpipe) CROSS REFERENCE: angin, steno
arter	Greek *arteria*	artery [See Note]	NOTE: The original meaning of *arteria* may have been "windpipe," coming from *aer* air + *terein* to keep, the ancients believing that air circulated through the arteries, or from *aeirein* to lift up, to raise. Now the word designates one of the vessels carrying blood from the heart to the tissues. SIMPLE ROOT: arteria (any blood vessel carrying blood away from the heart; pl., arteriae) {arterial}, arterialization arteriola (pl., arteriolae), arteriole {arteriolar}, artery PREFIXED ROOT: *arterial*: endarterial (*endon* within) eparterial (*epi* upon) hyparterial (*hypo* under) intraarterial (*intra* within) periarterial (*peri* around) *arterectomy*: endarterectomy (*endon* within + *ektome* excision) *arteriography*: microarteriography (*mikros* small + *graphein* to write) *arteriole*: metarteriole (*meta* between) *arteriotony*: dysarteriotony (*dys* abnormal + *tonos* tension) *arteritis* inflammation of an artery: endarteritis (or, endoarteritis) (*endon* within) endoperiarteritis (also called *panarteritis*) (*endon* within + periarteritis) exarteritis (also called *periarteritis*) (*ex* out) mesarteritis (inflammation of the *tunica media*, or middle layer, of an artery) (*mesos* middle) panarteritis (also called *endoperiarteritis*) (*pan* all) periarteritis (also called *exarteritis*) (*peri* around) polyarteritis (*polys* many) *arteropathy*: endoarteropathy (*endon* within + *pathos* disease) LEADING ROOT COMPOUND: *arter*: arteritis (pl., arteritides) (*itis* inflammation) *arteri*: arteriectasia (or, arteriectasis) (*ektasis* dilatation) arteriectomy (*ektome* excision) arteriectopia (*ektopia* displacement) arteriosteogenesis (*osteon* bone + *genere* to produce)

Element	From	Meaning	Examples
arter (cont'd)		[artery]	*arterio*:
			arterioatony (an abnormally relaxed state of the arterial walls) (*a* negative + *tonos* tension)
			arteriocapillary (pertaining to the arteries and the capillaries)
			arteriogenesis (also called *angiogenesis*) (*genesis* beginning)
			arteriogram, arteriograph, arteriography (*graphein* to write)
			arteriolith (*lithos* stone, concretion)
			arteriology (*logos* study)
			arteriomalacia (*malakos* soft)
			arteriometer (*metron* measure)
			arteriomotor (*movere* to move)
			arteriomyomatosis (*myos* muscle + *oma* tumor + *osis* condition)
			arterionecrosis (*nekrosis* death)
			arteriopalmus (palpitation or throbbing of an artery or arteries)
			arteriopathy (*pathos* disease)
			arterioplania (*planan* to wander)
			arterioplasty (*plassein* to form)
			arteriopressor (an agent that increases arterial blood pressure)
			arteriorenal (*ren* kidney)
			arteriorrhaphy (*rhaphe* suture)
			arteriorrhexis (*rhexis* rupture)
			arteriosclerosis {arteriosclerotic} (*sklerosis* hardness)
			arteriospasm (*spasmos* contraction)
			arteriostenosis (*stenosis* narrow)
			arteriostrepsis (*strephein* to twist)
			arteriotomy (*tomy* incision)
			arteriotony (blood pressure) (*tonos* tension)
			arteriovenous (*vena* vein)
			arteriol: arteriolitis (*itis* inflammation)
			arteriolo:
			arteriolonecrosis {arteriolonecrotic} (*nekrosis* death)
			arteriolosclerosis (*skleros* hard + *osis* condition)
			TRAILING ROOT COMPOUND:
			arteri: phlebarteriectasia (*phlebos* vein + *ektasia* dilatation)
			arterial:
			ureteroarterial (ureter)
			venoarterial (vein)
			vertebroarterial (vertebra)
			arterio: orthoarteriotony (normal arterial pressure) (*orthos* straight, normal + *tonos* tone)
			arteritis inflammation of an artery or arteries:
			meningoarteritis (*meningos* membrane)
			myoarteritis (inflammation of the smooth muscle in the arterial wall) (*myos* muscle)
			stetharteritis (*sthethos* chest)
			thromboarteritis (*thrombos* clot)
			CROSS REFERENCE: None
arthr	Greek *arthron*	a joint; joints; connection	SIMPLE ROOT:
			arthral (or, articular; of or pertaining to a joint)
			arthritide (any skin eruption of arthritic or gouty origin), arthrous
			PREFIXED ROOT:
			arthric pertaining to a joint or joints:
			diarthric (*di* two)
			monarthric (*monos* single)

Element	From	Meaning	Examples
arthr (cont'd)		[joint, joints]	periarthric (also called *circumarticular*) (*peri* around)
			polyarthric (*polys* many)
			arthritis joint inflammation:
			acroarthritis (*akron* extremities)
			enarthritis (*en* in)
			monarthritis (*monos* single)
			oligoarthritis (*oligos* few)
			panarthritis (*pan* all)
			periarthritis (*peri* around)
			polyarthritis (*polys* many)
			arthritic pertaining to arthritis:
			antiarthritic (or, antarthritic; alleviating arthritis) (*anti* against)
			meta-arthritic (*meta* after)
			arthrosis joint condition:
			abarthrosis (*ab* away)
			amphiarthrosis (*amphi* around)
			aparthrosis (*apo* from)
			diarthrosis (any articulation, as of the hip, permitting free movement in any direction) (*dia* across)
			dysarthrosis (*dys* abnormal)
			enarthrosis (also called *ball and socket joint*) (*en* in)
			hemiarthrosis (*hemi* half)
			synarthrosis (pl., synarthroses) (*syn* with)
			LEADING ROOT COMPOUND:
			arthr:
			arthralgia (also called *arthrodynia*) {arthralgic} (*algos* pain)
			arthrectomy (*ektome* excision)
			arthrempyesis (also called *arthropyosis*) (*empyesis* suppuration)
			arthresthesia (*esthesia* feeling, sensation)
			arthritis (pl., arthritides) {arthritic} (*itis* inflammation)
			arthrodia {arthrodial} (*eidos* form)
			arthrodynia (also called *arthralgia*) {arthrodynic} (*odyne* pain)
			arthrosis (*osis* condition)
			arthrosteitis (*osteon* bone + *itis* inflammation)
			arthroncus (swelling of a joint) (*onkos* mass)
			arthri: arthrifuge (a cure for gout) (*fugere* to flee)
			arthro:
			arthrocele (a swollen joint) (*kele* tumor)
			arthrocentesis (*kentein* to puncture)
			arthrochalasis (*chalasis* relaxation)
			arthrochondritis (*chondros* cartilage + *itis* inflammation)
			arthroclasia (*klaein* to break)
			arthroconidium (arthrospore) (*konis* dust: an asexual spore)
			arthrodesis (also called *syndesis*) (*desis* a binding together)
			arthrodysplasia (*dys* abnormal + *plassein* to form)
			arthroempyesis (or, arthroempyosis) (*empyesis* suppuration)
			arthroendoscopy (also called *arthroscopy*) (*endon* within + *skopein* to examine)
			arthroereisis (or, arthrorisis) (*ereisis* a raising or propping up)
			arthrogenous (*genere* to produce)
			arthrogram, arthrography (*graphein* to write)
			arthrogryposis (*gryposis* a crooking, hooking)
			arthrokleisis (also called *ankylosis*) (*kleisis* closure)
			arthrolith, arthrolithiasis (gout) (*lithos* stone + *iasis* condition)

Element	From	Meaning	Examples
arthr (cont'd)		[joint, joints]	arthrology (*logos* study)
			arthrolysis (*lyein* to loosen)
			arthrometer (also called *goniometer*) (*metron* measure)
			arthroneuralgia (*neuron* nerve + *algos* pain)
			arthroophthalmopathy (*ophthalmos* eye + *pathos* suffering)
			arthropathia (or, arthropathy: a disease or an abnormality of a joint) {arthropathic} (*pathos* disease)
			arthrophyma (*phyma* swelling)
			arthrophyte (an abnormal growth in a joint cavity) (*phyton* growth)
			arthroplasty {arthroplastic} (*plassein* to form)
			arthropyosis (also called *arthroempyesis*) (*pyon* pus + *osis* condition)
			arthrosclerosis (*skleros* hard + *osis* condition)
			arthroscope, arthroscopy (*skopein* to examine)
			arthrospore (also called *arthroconidium*) (*sporos* seed)
			arthrostomy (*stoma* mouth, opening)
			arthrotome, arthrotomy (*tomy* incision)
			arthrotropic (*trope* a turning)
			arthroxesis (*xesis* scraping)
			TRAILING ROOT COMPOUND:
			arthritis joint inflammation:
			cheirarthritis (*cheir* hand)
			cleidarthritis (*kleidos* clavicle; collarbone)
			coxarthritis (also called *coxitis*) (*coxa* hip)
			gonarthritis (*gony* knee)
			holarthritis (*holos* entire)
			lipoarthritis (*lipos* fat)
			medulloarthritis (*medulla* marrow)
			olecranarthritis (also called *anconitis*) (*olekranon* elbow)
			omarthritis (*omos* shoulder)
			osteoarthritis (*osteon* bone)
			podarthritis (*podos* foot)
			spondylarthritis (*spondylos* vertebra)
			arthropathy joint disease:
			coxarthropathy (*coxa* hip)
			neuroarthropathy (*neuron* nerve)
			olecranarthropathy (disease of the elbow joint) (*olene* ulna)
			osteoarthropathy (*osteon* bone)
			spondyloarthropathy (*spondylos* vertebra)
			arthrosis joint condition:
			clinarthrosis (*klinein* to bend)
			coxarthrosis (*coxa* hip)
			cyclarthrosis (a joint that permits rotation) (*kyklos* circle)
			hemarthrosis (*haima* blood)
			hydrarthrosis (*hydor* water)
			nearthrosis (or, neoarthrosis; a new joint resulting from a total joint replacement operation; a pseudarthrosis arising in an ununited fracture) (*neos* new)
			osteoarthrosis (also called *osteoarthritis*) (*osteon* bone)
			peronarthrosis (*perone* fibula)
			pneumarthrosis (*pneuma* air)
			pseudoarthrosis (*pseudes* false)
			pyarthrosis (*pyon* pus)
			CROSS REFERENCE: articul

Element	From	Meaning	Examples
articul	Latin *articulus*	small joint	SIMPLE ROOT: articulate (divided into or united by joints) articulated (connected by movable joints) PREFIXED ROOT: *articular*: abarticular (*ab* away) biarticular (pertaining to or affecting two different joints; also called *diarthric, diarticular*) (*bi* two) circumarticular (*circum* around) diarticular (also called *diarthric, biarticular*) (*di* two) extraarticular (*extra* outside) interarticular (*inter* between) intraarticular (*intra* within) juxta-articular (also called *periarticular*) (*juxta* near, adjoining) monarticular (also called *uniarticular*) (*monos* single) multiarticular (*multus* many) periarticular (also called *juxta-articular*) (*peri* around) polyarticular (*polys* many) uniarticular (also called *monarticular*) (*uni* one) *articulation*: dearticulation (dislocation of a joint) (*de* negative) disarticulation (amputation or separation at a joint) (*dis* apart) exarticulation also called *dearticulation*) (*ex* out) inarticulate (not articulate in speech; unable to express oneself in words) (*in* negative) perarticulation (diarthrosis; also called *synovial joint*) (*per* intensive) TRAILING ROOT COMPOUND: osteoarticular (*osteon* bone) pauciarticular (*paucus* few) CROSS REFERENCE: arthr
asthen	Greek *a* negative + *sthenos* strength	weakness	SIMPLE ROOT: asthenia (without strength) {asthenic} PREFIXED ROOT: antasthenic (alleviating weakness, or restoring strength; an agent that alleviates weakness and restores strength) (*anti* against) panasthenia (generalized weakness or exhaustion without evidence of organic disease) (*pan* all) LEADING ROOT COMPOUND: *asthen*: asthenope, asthenopia (subjective symptoms of ocular fatigue, discomfort, lacrimation, headaches, arising from use of the eyes) {asthenopic} (*opia* vision condition) asthenoxia (lack of power to oxidize waste products) *astheno*: asthenobiosis (*bios* life + *osis* condition) asthenocoria (a condition in which the pupillary light reflex is sluggish: seen in hypoadrenia) (*kore* pupil) asthenometer (*metron* measure) asthenospermia (*sperma* seed, sperm) TRAILING ROOT COMPOUND: adenasthenia (*adenos* gland) angioasthenia (*angeion* vessel; blood vessel) encephalasthenia (*enkephalon* brain) logasthenia (a type of aphasia) (*logos* word)

31

A Thesaurus of Medical Word Roots

Element	From	Meaning	Examples
asthen (cont'd)		[weakness]	myasthenia (*myos* muscle) myxasthenia (*myxa* mucus) neurasthenia {neurasthenic} (*neuron* nerve) neuromyasthenia (*neuron* nerve + *myos* muscle) otomyasthenia {otomyasthenic} (*otos* ear + *myos* muscle) phonasthenia (*phone* sound; voice) psychasthenia (*psyche* mind) skelasthenia (*skelos* leg) somasthenia (*soma* body) thrombasthenia (or, thromboasthenia), thrombocytasthenia (*thrombos* clot + *kytos* cell) traumasthenia (*trauma* injury) CROSS REFERENCE: pares, sthen
astrag	Greek *astragalos*	ankle joint	SIMPLE ROOT: astragalus (the talus; ankle; the bone that articulates with the tibia at the ankle) {astragalar} PREFIXED ROOT: subastragalar (*sub* inferior to) LEADING ROOT COMPOUND: *astragal*: astragalectomy (*ektome* excision) astragaloid (*eidos* form, shape) *astragalo*: astragalocalcanean (relating to both the talus and the calcaneus) (*calcaneus* heel bone) astragalocrural (*crus* leg) astragalofibular (fibula) astragaloscaphoid (also called *talonavicular*) (scaphoid, or navicular bone) (*skaphe* skiff, boat) astragalotibial (*tibia* shin) CROSS REFERENCE: tal, tars[1]
atax	Greek *a* privative + *tassein* to arrange	ataxia, disorder, irregularity	SIMPLE ROOT: ataxia (total or partial inability to coordinate voluntary bodily movements, especially muscular movements) {ataxic, atactic} PREFIXED ROOT: diataxia (ataxia affecting both sides of the body) (*di* two) hemiataxia (or, hemiataxy; ataxia affecting one side of the body) (*hemi* half) parataxia (*para* alongside) preataxic (*pre* before) LEADING ROOT COMPOUND: *ataxia*: ataxiadynamia (*dynamia* power condition) ataxiagraph (also called *ataxiameter*) (*graphein* to write) ataxiaphasia (inability to form connected sentences) (*phanai* to speak) *ataxio*: ataxiophemia (*pheme* speech) TRAILING ROOT COMPOUND: acroataxia (ataxia affecting the hands, fingers, feet, and toes) (*akros* extremities) angioataxia (*angeion* blood vessel) cardiataxia (*kardia* heart) oneirotaxia (inability to distinguish between fantasy and reality) (*oneiros* dream) proximoataxia (*proximus* nearest, next to) psychataxia (*psyche* mind) CROSS REFERENCE: tax

Element	From	Meaning	Examples
atel	Greek *a* negative + *telos* end	incomplete	SIMPLE ROOT: atelia (or, ateliosis; imperfect or incomplete development) PREFIXED ROOT: microatelectasis (also called *adhesive atelectasis*) (*mikros* small + atelectasis) LEADING ROOT COMPOUND: *atel*: atelectasis (incomplete expansion of the lungs at birth; collapse of the adult lung) {atelectatic} (*ektasis* dilatation) atelencephalia (*enkephalia* brain condition) *atelo*: atelocardia (*kardia* heart) atelocephaly (*kephale* head) atelocheilia (*cheilos* lip) atelocheiria (*cheir* hand) ateloencephalia (*enkephalos* brain) ateloglossia (*glossa* tongue) atelognathia (*gnathos* jaw) atelomyelia (*myelos* spinal cord) atelopodia (*pous* foot) ateloprosopia (*prosopon* face) atelorachidia (*rhachis* spine) atelostomia (*stoma* mouth) TRAILING ROOT COMPOUND: cardiatelia (*kardia* heart) myelatelia (*myelos* spinal cord) CROSS REFERENCE: ectro, tele[1]
ather	Greek *athere* gruel	gruel; fatty degeneration	PREFIXED ROOT: antiatherogenic (*anti* against + *genere* to produce) LEADING ROOT COMPOUND: *ather*: atherectomy (*ektome* excision) atheroma (also called *atherosis*) {atheromatous} (*oma* tumor) atherosis (also called *atheroma*) (*osis* condition) *athero*: atheroembolism, atheroembolus (*embolus* plug, obstruction) atherogenesis {atherogenic} (*genere* to produce) atherosclerosis {atherosclerotic} (*sklerosis* hardening) atherothrombosis (*thrombos* clot + *osis* condition) CROSS REFERENCE: adip, lip, pimel, stear
atres, atret	Greek *a* privative + *tresis* hole	atresia, imperforation	SIMPLE ROOT: atresia (congenital absence or closure of a normal body opening or tubular structure; also called *clausura*) LEADING ROOT COMPOUND: *atret*: atretopsia (also called *atresia iridis*) (*opsia* sight condition) *atreto*: atretoblepharia (also called *symblepharon*) (*blepharon* eyelid) atretocephalus (*kephale* head) atretocormus (*kormos* trunk) atretocystia (*kystis* bladder) atretogastria (*gaster* stomach) atretolemia (*laimos* gullet, esophagus, pharynx) atretorrhinia (*rhinos* nose) atretostomia (*stoma* mouth, opening) TRAILING ROOT COMPOUND: colpatresia (also called *vaginal atresia*) (*kolpos* vagina)

Element	From	Meaning	Examples
atret (cont'd)		[imperforation]	dacryagogatresia (*dakrys* teardrop + *agein* to lead) gynatresia (*gyne* woman, female) hysteratresia (*hystera* uterus) proctatresia (also called *imperforate anus*) (*proktos* anus) urethratresia (also called *urethral atresia*) (urethra) CROSS REFERENCE: col², ethm, filt, for, tres
atri	Latin *atrium* hall	chamber (atrium of the heart)	SIMPLE ROOT: atrium (pl., atria) {atrial} PREFIXED ROOT: interatrial (*inter* between) intraatrial (within one or both atria of the heart) (*intra* within) periatrial (*peri* around, near) transatrial (*trans* across, through) LEADING ROOT COMPOUND: atriomegaly (*megas* large) atrionector (*nectere* to fasten) atrioseptoplasty (*septum* partition + *plassein* to form) atrioseptostomy (*septum* partition + *stoma* mouth, opening) atriotomy (*tomy* incision) atrioventricular (ventricle) TRAILING ROOT COMPOUND: bulboatrial (bulb) sinoatrial (or, sinuatrial) (sinus) venoatrial (*vena* vein) CROSS REFERENCE: antr, cell, thalam
atroph	Greek *a* negative + *trophein* to nourish	atrophy; wasting away	SIMPLE ROOT: atrophy (or, atrophia; a wasting away of the body or of an organ or part, as from defective nutrition or nerve damage; a diminution in the size of a cell, tissue, organ, or part) {atrophic, atrophied} PREFIXED ROOT: antatrophic (*anti* against) hemiatrophy (*hemi* half) metatrophia (atrophy from malnutrition) {metatrophic} (*meta* after) panatrophy (atrophy of all parts of a structure) (*pan* all) LEADING ROOT COMPOUND: atrophoderma (or, atrophodermia), atrophodermatosis (any skin disease having cutaneous atrophy as a prominent symptom) (*derma* skin + *osis* condition) TRAILING ROOT COMPOUND: *atrophia*: cystatrophia (*kystis* bladder) dermatrophia (*derma* skin) gastratrophia (*gaster* stomach, belly) hepatatrophia (or, hepatatrophy) (*hepatos* liver) mastatrophia (or, mastatrophy) (*mastos* breast) metratrophia (or, metratrophy) (*metra* uterus) neuratrophia (*neuron* nerve) onychatrophia (*onychos* nail) ophthalmatrophia (*ophthalmos* eye) pedatrophia (also called *marasmus*) (*pais* child) trichatrophia (*trichos* hair) ulatrophia (or, ulatrophy) (*oulon* gums) *atrophy*: encephalatrophy (*enkephalon* brain) fibroatrophy (fiber) hepatatrophy (or, hepatatrophia) (*hepatos* liver)

Element	From	Meaning	Examples
atroph (cont'd)		[wasting away]	lipoatrophy (also called *lipoatrophic diabetes*) (*lipos* fat) mastatrophy (or, mastatrophia) (*mastos* breast) metratrophy (or, metratrophia) (*metra* uterus) myatrophy (also called *muscular atrophy*) (*myos* muscle) myelatrophy (*myelos* spinal cord) onychatrophy (or, onychatrophia) (*onychos* nail) scleroatrophy (also called *sclerotylosis*) (*skleros* hard) splenatrophy (spleen) ulatrophy (or, ulatrophy) (*oule* gums) CROSS REFERENCE: phthis
aug, **aux**	Latin *augere* Greek *auxein*	to increase	SIMPLE ROOT: *aug*: augmentation (an adding on, or the resulting condition) *aux*: auxesis (increase in the size of an organism) {auxetic} PREFIXED ROOT: diauxie (two growth phases) {diauxic} (*di* two) heterauxesis (*heteros* other) isauxesis (*isos* same) monoauxotroph (*monos* single + *trophein* to nourish) polyauxotrophic (*polys* many + *trophein* to nourish) tachyauxesis (*tachys* rapid) LEADING ROOT COMPOUND: *auxano*: auxanogram, auxanography (*graphein* to write) auxanometer (*metron* measure) *auxi*: auxilytic (*lyein* to loosen) *auxilio*: auxiliomotor (*movere* to move) *auxio*: auxiometer (or, auxometer; an apparatus for measuring the magnifying powers of lenses) (*metron* measure) *auxo*: auxocardia (*kardia* heart) auxochrome (a chemical group which if introduced into a chromogen, will convert the latter into a dye) (*chroma* color) auxodrome (*dramein* to run) auxoflore (a substance which increases the intensity of fluorescence of a compound; opposed to *bathoflore*) (*fluere* to flow) auxogluc (*glykys* sweet) auxology (the study of growth) (*logos* study) auxometer (or, auxiometer) {auxometric} (*metron* measure) auxotonic (*tonos* tension) auxotox (*toxikon* poison) auxotrophic (*trephein* to nourish) TRAILING ROOT COMPOUND: *auxe*: clitoridauxe (also called *clitorism*) (clitoris) encephalauxe (hypertrophy of the brain; also called *macrencephaly*) (*enkephelon* brain) mastauxe (*mastos* breast) myelauxe (*myelos* spinal cord) nephrauxe (*nephros* kidney) prostatauxe (prostate) splenauxe (spleen) *auxesis*: bradyauxesis (a form of heterauxesis in which the part grows more slowly than the whole) (*bradys* slow)

Element	From	Meaning	Examples
aug (cont'd)		[to increase]	iridauxesis (thickening of the iris) *auxis*: onychauxis (also called *hyperonychia*) (*onychos* nail) trichauxis (excessive growth of hair) (*trichos* hair) CROSS REFERENCE: embryo, phys[1]
aur	Latin *auris* ear	ear	SIMPLE ROOT: aural (pertaining to or perceived by the ear, as an aural stimulus) auricle (the external part of the ear; pinna, or flap of the ear; an ear-like part or organ; also called *auricula*; pl., auriculae) auricular (pertaining to an auricle or to the ear) auris (the ear; pl., aures), aurist (a former name for an audiologist) PREFIXED ROOT: *aural*: binaural (pertaining to both ears; also called *binotic*) (*bin* two) endaural (also called *intraaural*) (*endon* within) interaural (*inter* between) intraaural (also called *endaural*) (*intra* within) monaural (also called *monotic, uniaural*) (*monos* single) subaural (*sub* below) uniaural (also called *monaural*) (*uni* one) *auricular*: biauricular (or, binauricular; pertaining to both auricles) (*bi* two) interauricular (also called *interatrial*) (*inter* between) intraauricular (*intra* within) periauricular (*peri* around) postauricular (also called *retroauricular*) (*post* after) preauricular (*pre* before) retroauricular (also called *postauricular*) (*retro* back, backward) subauricular (*sub* below) supraauricular (or, superauricular) (*supra* above) LEADING ROOT COMPOUND: *auri*: auriform (*forma* shape) aurinasal (*nas* nose) auriscope (also called *otoscope*) (*skopein* to examine) *auriculo*: auriculocranial (*kranion* skull) auriculotemporal (temporal region) TRAILING ROOT COMPOUND: dextraural (having better hearing in the right ear) (*dexter* right) sinistraural (having better hearing in the left ear) (*sinister* left) temporoauricular (temple) zygomaticoauricular (relating to the zygomatic bone and the auricle) CROSS REFERENCE: acou, auscul, ot
auscul	Latin *auscultare*	to listen	SIMPLE ROOT: auscultate, auscultation (the act of listening for sounds within the body with the aid of a stethoscope) PREFIXED ROOT: endoauscultation (*endo* within) LEADING ROOT COMPOUND: auscultoplectrum (an instrument for use both in auscultation and percussion) (*plectrum* anything to strike with) auscultoscope (also called *phonendoscope*) (*skopein* to examine) TRAILING ROOT COMPOUND: stereoausculation (*stereos* solid) CROSS REFERENCE: acou, aur

Element	From	Meaning	Examples
auto-	Greek pre-fix	self	EXTENDED PREFIX: autism (the condition of being dominated by subjective, self-centered trends of thought or behavior) {autistic} See Appendix B for examples of words with this prefix. Others are listed with the roots to which it is attached. CROSS REFERENCE: idi, noe
aux			See aug-.
ax	Greek *axon*; Latin *axis*	axis	SIMPLE ROOT: axial (or, axialis), axiation, axilla (the armpit, or an analogous part; pl., axillae) {axillary} axion (the brain and spinal cord), axis (pl., axes) axle, axon (or, axone) PREFIXED ROOT: *axial*: abaxial (*ab* away from) adaxial (*ad* to) coaxial (*com* with) epaxial (*epi* upon) equiaxial (*aequus* equal) extraaxial (*extra* beyond) hemiaxial (*hemi* half) heteraxial (*heteros* other) hypaxial (*hypos* under) paraxial (*para* alongside) periaxial (*peri* around) postaxial (*post* after) preaxial (*pre* before) semiaxial (*semi* half) subaxial (*sub* below) transaxial (*trans* through, across) uniaxial (*uni* one) *axillary*: bisaxillary (*bis* two, both) circumaxillary (also called *periaxillary*) (*circum* around) infra-axillary (also called *subaxillary*) (*infra* below) peraxillary (*per* through) periaxillary (surrounding or adjacent to the armpit) (*peri* around) subaxillary (also called *infra-axillary*) (*sub* inferior) supraaxillary (*supra* above) *axon*: anaxon (*an* negative) diaxon (also called *bipolar cell*) (*di* two) paraxon (*para* alongside) *axonal*: periaxonal (*peri* around) *axonic*: monaxonic (*monos* single) polyaxonic (*polys* many) LEADING ROOT COMPOUND: *axi*: axifugal (or, axofugal) (*fugere* to flee) axilemma (or, axolemma) (*lemma* husk, rind) axipetal (or, axopetal; also called *centripetal*) (*petere* to seek) *axio*: axiobuccal (pertaining to or formed by the axial and buccal walls of a tooth cavity) (*bucca* cheek)

Element	From	Meaning	Examples
ax (cont'd)		[axis]	axiocervical (*cervix* neck—of tooth)
			axiogingival (*gingiva* gums)
			axiolabial (*labium* lip)
			axiolingual (*lingua* tongue)
			axiomesal (*mesos* middle)
			axioversion (*vertere* to turn)
			axo:
			axodendritic (*dendron* tree: growth)
			axolysis (*lyein* to loosen)
			axometer (*metron* measure)
			axophage (*phagein* to devour)
			axoplasm {axoplasmic} (*plassein* to form)
			axotomy (*tomy* incision)
			axono:
			axonopathy (*pathos* disease)
			axonotmesis (*tmesis* a cutting)
			TRAILING ROOT COMPOUND:
			axial:
			organoaxial (rotation around the long axis of the organ)
			gingivoaxial (*gingivae* gums of the mouth)
			axillary: cervicoaxillary (*cervix* neck)
			axio:
			distoaxiogingival (*distans* distant + *gingivae* gums of the mouth)
			distoaxioincisal (*distans* distant + incisor)
			distoaxioocclusal (*distans* distant + occlusal)
			axis: neuraxis (*neuron* nerve)
			axon: schizaxon (*schizein* to split)
			CROSS REFERENCE: None
azo	Greek *a* negative + *zoon* life	nitrogen	SIMPLE ROOT: azoic, azote, azotized
			PREFIXED ROOT:
			azotemia: hyperazotemia (*hyper* above + *emia* blood condition)
			azoturia condition of nitrogen in the urine:
			anazoturia (deficiency or lack of nitrogenous substances, especially, urea, in the urine) (*an* privative)
			hyperazoturia (*hyper* above)
			hypoazoturia (*hypo* under)
			LEADING ROOT COMPOUND:
			azot:
			azotemia {azotemic} (*emia* blood condition)
			azoturia (*uria* urine condition)
			azoto:
			azotometer (*metron* measure)
			azotorrhea (*rhein* to flow)
			CROSS REFERENCE: zo

Element	From	Meaning	Examples
bac	Latin *baculum* little rod	an organism (rod-shaped)	SIMPLE ROOT: bacillar (or, bacillary; pertaining to bacilli or to rodlike forms), bacillin, bacillus (pl., bacilli) PREFIXED ROOT: *bacillary*: endobacillary (*endon* within) multibacillary (*multus* many) prebacillary (*pre* before) *bacillus*: diplobacillus (pl., diplobacilli) (*diploos* double) LEADING ROOT COMPOUND: *bacill*: bacillemia (*emia* blood condition) bacillosis (the state of bacillary infection) (*osis* condition) bacilluria (*uria* urine condition) *bacilli*: bacilliferous (*ferre* to bear, produce) bacilliform (*forma* shape) *baculi*: baculiform (rod-shaped) (*forma* shape) TRAILING ROOT COMPOUND: *bacillary*: coccobacillary (*kokkos* berry-shaped organism) paucibacillary (*paucus* few) *bacillin*: mycobacillin (*mykes* fungus) *bacillosis* bacillus condition: actinobacillosis (*aktis* ray) colibacillosis (pertaining to Escherichia coli; also called *coliuria*) streptobacillosis (also called *rat fever*) (*streptos* twisted) *bacillus*: coccobacillus (in microbiology, a bacterium with a shape intermediate between coccus and bacillus) lactobacillus (pl., lactobacilli) (*lactis* milk) pneumobacillus (gas-producing rods associated with urinary and respiratory problems) (*pneumon* air, gas) ANTIBIOTIC: bacitracin [from *baci*(llus) + Margaret *Trac*(y), an American girl from whose wounds the strain was isolated] CROSS REFERENCE: bacteri, rhabd
bacteri	Greek *baktron* a staff	staff, rod (single-cell microorganism)	SIMPLE ROOT: bacterinia, bacterium (pl., bacteria) {bacterial} PREFIXED ROOT: *bacterial*: abacterial (free from bacteria) (*a* privative) antibacterial (*anti* against) *bacteriophage*: probacteriophage (also called *prophage*) (*pro* before + *phagein* to consume) *bacterium*: diplobacterium (pl., diplobacteria) (*diploos* double) macrobacterium (also called *megabacterium*) (*makros* large) microbacterium (pl., microbacteria) (*mikros* small) LEADING ROOT COMPOUND: *bacter*: bacteremia (*emia* blood condition) bacteroid (*eidos* form)

Element	From	Meaning	Examples
bacteri (cont'd)		[staff, rod]	*bacteri*: bactericide (or, bacteriocide) {bactericidal} (*caedere* to kill) bacteriemia (*emia* blood condition) bacterioid (*eidos* form) bacteriosis (*osis* condition) bacteriuria (or, bacteruria) (*uria* urine condition) *bacterio*: bacteriocide (or, bactericide) (*caedere* to kill) bacterioclasis (also called *bacteriolysis*) (*klaein* to break) bacteriogenic (or, bacteriogenous) (*genere* to produce) bacteriology {bacteriologic} (*logos* study) bacteriolysin, bacteriolysis {bacteriolytic} (*lyein* to loosen) bacteriophage, bacteriophagia (*phagein* to devour, consume) bacteriophytoma (*phyton* plant: growth + *oma* tumor) bacteriospermia (*sperma* semen) bacteriostasis {bacteriostatic} (*stasis* standing) bacteriotoxic (*toxikon* poison) bacteriotropic (*trepein* to turn) TRAILING ROOT COMPOUND: mycobacterium (pl., mycobacteria) (*mykes* fungus) trichobacteria (filamentous forms of bacteria) (*trichos* hair) CROSS REFERENCE: bac, rhabd
balano	Greek *balanos* acorn, glans	glans (glans penis; glans clitoridis)	SIMPLE ROOT: balanus (the glans clitoridis or the glans penis) LEADING ROOT COMPOUND: *balan*: balanitis (inflammation of the glans penis and mucous membrane beneath it) (*itis* inflammation) *balano*: balanocele (*kele* hernia) balanoplasty (plastic surgery of the glans penis) (*plassein* to form) balanoposthitis (*posthe* prepuce + *itis* inflammation) balanoposthomycosis (*posthe* prepuce + *mykes* fungus + *osis* condition) balanopreputial (*prepuce* foreskin) balanorrhagia (balanitis with free discharge of pus) (*rhagia* bursting forth) CROSS REFERENCE: peni, phallo
ball, **bol**	Greek *ballein*	to throw	SIMPLE ROOT: ballism (or, ballismus; a condition marked by twisting, shaking, or jerking motion; also called *Parkinson's disease*) {ballistic} ballottement (tossing about) {ballotable} PREFIXED ROOT: *ball*: hemiballismus (a violent form of dyskinesia involving only one side of the body) (*hemi* half) *bole*: embole (lit., a throwing in; the reducing of a dislocated limb) {embolic} (*en* in) [see separate entry: embol-] epibole (or, epiboly; a method of gastrulation by which the smaller blastomeres at the animal pole of the fertilized ovum grow over and enclose the cells of the vegetal hemisphere) (*epi* upon) *bolia*: asymbolia (inability to comprehend words, gestures, or any type of symbol; also called *asemia*) (*a* privative + symbolia) dyssymbolia (or, dyssymboly) (*dys* abnormal + symbolia)

Element	From	Meaning	Examples
ball (cont'd)		[to throw]	symbolia (ability to identify or recognize an object by the sense of touch) (*syn* with)
			bolic:
			amphibolic (uncertain; of doubtful prognosis) (*amphi* around)
			catabolic (*kata* down)
			ecbolic (lit., a throwing out; helping to bring forth the fetus in birth, or causing abortion, by contracting the uterus; said of certain drugs; also called *oxytocic*) (*ex* out)
			bolism:
			anabolism (the synthesis in living organisms of more complex substances from simpler ones; opposed to *catabolism*) {anabolic} (*ana* again)
			catabolism (opposed to *anabolism*) (*kata* down)
			dysbolism (*dys-* + metabolism) (*dys* abnormal)
			eubolism (a condition of normal body metabolism) (*eu* well)
			metabolism (*meta* beyond)
			symbolism (*sym* with, together)
			bolite:
			anabolite (*ana* again)
			catabolite (any product of catabolism) (*kata* down)
			LEADING ROOT COMPOUND:
			ballisto:
			ballistocardiograph (an apparatus for recording the stroke volume of the heart as a means of calculating the cardiac output) (*kardia* heart + *graphein* to write)
			ballistospore (*sporos* seed)
			bolo: bolometer (an instrument for measuring minute changes in heat radiated by an object, such as a portion of the human body) (*metron* measure)
			TRAILING ROOT COMPOUND: strephosymbolia (a type of dyslexia consisting of confusion between similar but oppositely oriented letters, for example, b-d, p-q; a tendency to read backward) (*strephein* to twist)
			CROSS REFERENCE: None
bar	Greek *baros* weight *barys* heavy	heavy, weight, pressure	SIMPLE ROOT: baric, baricity, barium (Ba)
			PREFIXED ROOT:
			abarognosis (loss of ability to sense weight) (*a* negative + barognosis)
			dysbarism (*dys* abnormal)
			hyperbaric {hyperbarism} (*hyper* above)
			hypobaric, hypobaropathy (*hypo* under + *pathos* disease)
			isobar {isobaric} (*isos* equal)
			LEADING ROOT COMPOUND:
			bar:
			baragnosis (or, baroagnosis; inability to estimate weights; indicative of parietal lobe lesion; opposite of *barognosis*) (*a* privative + *gnosis* knowledge)
			baresthesia (pressure sense) (*esthesia* feeling)
			bariatrics (*iatric* healing)
			barodontalgia (*odontos* tooth + *algos* pain)
			barotitis (also called *aerotitis*) (*otos* ear + *itis* condition)
			baruria (*uria* urine condition)
			baro:
			baroceptor (or, baroreceptor) (*capere* to hold)
			barognosis (opposite of *baragnosis*) (*gnosis* knowledge)

Element	From	Meaning	Examples
bar (cont'd)		[weight]	barograph (*graphein* to write)
			barophilic (growing best under high atmospheric pressure: said of bacteria) (*philein* to love—have an affinity for)
			barosinusitis (also called *aerosinusitis*) (sinus + *itis* inflammation)
			barotaxis (also called *barotropism*) (*taxis* order)
			barotropism (reaction of living tissue to changes in pressure; also called *barotaxis*) (*tropein* to turn)
			bary:
			barylalia (indistinct, thick speech due to imperfect articulation) (*lalein* to speak)
			baryphonia (a thick, heavy quality of voice) (*phone* sound, voice)
			CROSS REFERENCE: grav
bas, **bat,** **bet**	Greek *bainein* to go, step, stand	base, step, foundation; basion; chemical base	SIMPLE ROOT:
			base {basal; of primary importance}
			basial (pertaining to the basion)
			basialis (or, basial; relating to a base or to the basion), basic
			basidium (the clublike spore-producing organ of certain of the higher fungi; pl., basidia)
			basilad (toward the basilar aspect), basilar, basilaris (situated at the base), basilic (important or prominent)
			basion, basis (base of a structure or organ; pl., bases)
			PREFIXED ROOT:
			basal:
			subbasal (*sub* beneath)
			transbasal (*trans* across)
			unibasal (having only one base) (*uni* one)
			base:
			diabase (a crossing or passing over) (*dia* across)
			prebase (that part of the dorsum of the tongue lying anterior to the base) (*pre* before)
			basia(l):
			abasia (inability to walk caused by a defect in muscular coordination) {abasic, abatic} (*a* negative)
			catabasial (denoting a skull in which the basion is lower than the opisthion) (*kata* down)
			dysbasia (difficulty in walking, especially as the result of a disorder in the nervous system) (*dys* abnormal)
			opisthiobasial (*opisthen* back, back of)
			basic:
			bibasic, dibasic (*bi, di* two)
			hexabasic [an acid which contains six hydrogen atoms (H) which can be replaced by six hydroxyl (OH) radicals] (*hex* six)
			monobasic (*monos* single)
			polybasic (*polys* many)
			tetrabasic (*tetra* four)
			tribasic (having three replaceable hydrogen atoms) (*tri* three)
			basis:
			anabasis (period of increased severity in a disease) {anabatic} (*ana* again)
			metabasis (*meta* after)
			baso: hyperbasophilic (*hyper* above + *philein* to love)
			bat: adiabatic (impassable; denoting a change in volume or pressure without loss or gain of heat) (*a* negative + *dia* across)
			bet: diabetes (*dia* across) [see separate entry: diabet-]

Element	From	Meaning	Examples
bas (cont'd)		[base, step, foundation]	LEADING ROOT COMPOUND: *basi*: basialveolar (extending from the basion to the alveolar point) basicranium {basicranial} (*kranion* skull) basifacial (*facies* face) basilateral (both lateral and basilar) (*laterus* side) basilemma (*lemma* rind) basinasial (*nas* nose) basiocciput {basioccipital} (*occipitus* back of head) basiotic (*otos* ear) basipetal (*petere* to seek) basiphobia (morbid fear of walking) (*phobia* fear) basirhinal (*rhis* nose) basisphenoid (*sphen* wedge + *eidos* form) basitemporal (temporal region) basivertebral (vertebra) *basidio*: basidiospore (a type of sexual spore that forms on a basidium) (*sporos* seed) *basio*: basioglossus (*glossa* tongue) *baso*: basocytopenia (*kytos* cell + *penia* deficiency) basocytosis (also called *basophilic leukocytosis*) (*kytos* cell + *osis* condition) basophil (or, basophile, basophilic; staining readily with basic dyes), basophilia (an abnormal increase in the blood of basophilic erythrocytes), basophilism (*philein* to love) basoplasm (the part of the cytoplasm that stains readily with basic dyes) TRAILING ROOT COMPOUND: *base*: rheobase {rheobasic} (*rheos* flow) *basia*: brachybasia (a slow, shuffling, short-stepped gait) (*brachys* short) platybasia (also called *basilar invagination*) (*platys* flat) *basilar*: occipitobasilar (*occiput* back of head: *ob* against + *caput* head) sphenobasilar (*sphen* wedge: sphenoid process) vertebrobasilar (vertebra) CROSS REFERENCE: None
bath	Greek *bathys* deep	deep, depth	See Appendix B for examples of words with this initial combining form. Others are listed with the roots to which it is attached. CROSS REFERENCE: None
bet			See bas- for *diabetes*.
bi-, **bin-**	Latin prefixes	two	See Appendix B for examples of words with these prefixes. Others are listed with the roots to which they are attached. CROSS REFERENCE: di-
bil	Latin *bilis*	gall, bile	SIMPLE ROOT: bile (a secretion of the liver) {biliary}, bilin, bilious, biliousness LEADING ROOT COMPOUND: bilicyanin (a blue pigment found in gallstones) (*kyanos* blue) bilifuscin (a brownish pigment found in gallstones) (*fuscus* brown) biligenesis {biligenetic, or biligenic} (*genere* to produce) bilihumin (*humus* earth) biliprasin (*prasinos* green) bilirachia (*rachis* spine)

Element	From	Meaning	Examples
bil (cont'd)		[gall, bile]	bilirubin, bilrubinemia (*ruber* red + *emia* blood condition)
			biliuria (*uria* urine condition)
			TRAILING ROOT COMPOUND:
			atrabiliary (*atra* black)
			enterobiliary (*enteron* intestine)
			hepatobiliary (*hepatos* liver)
			tracheobiliary (*trachea* windpipe)
			CROSS REFERENCE: chol
bin-			See bi-.
bio	Greek	life	SIMPLE ROOT:
	bios		bion (an individual living organism), biota, biotic, biotics
			biotin (a bacterial growth factor, one of the vitamin B group, found in liver, egg yolk, and yeast)
			PREFIXED ROOT:
			be: microbe {microbial, microbic} (*mikros* small)
			bi:
			abiatrophy (*a* privative + *trophein* to nourish)
			amphibious (*amphi* around, both)
			polymicrobial (*polys* many + *microbial*)
			symbion (or, symbiont), (*syn* with)
			bic: amicrobic (lacking microbes; not caused by microbes) (*a* privative + *mikros* small)
			bicide: microbicide (*mikros* small + *caedere* to kill)
			bio: abiotrophy (trophic failure; degeneration or failure of vitality; compare *abiatrophy*) (*a* privative + *trophein* to nourish)
			biogenesis beginning of life:
			abiogenesis {abiogenetic} (*a* privative)
			neobiogenesis (also called *biopoiesis*) (*neos* new)
			biology study of life:
			exobiology (*exo* outside)
			microbiology {microbiologic} (*mikros* small)
			protobiology (also called *bacteriophagology*) (*protos* first)
			symbiology (*sym* with, together)
			biosis condition of life:
			abiosis (absence or deficiency of life) {abiotic} (*a* privative)
			allobiosis (the condition of shared reactivity which an organism manifests under environmental conditions) (*allos* other)
			anabiosis (revival after apparent death) {anabiotic} (*ana* again)
			antibiosis {antibiotic; destructive of life} (*anti* against)
			apobiosis (death, especially local death of a part of the organism) (*apo* from)
			catabiosis (the normal senescence of cells) (*kata* down)
			macrobiosis (a long life) (*makron* long)
			metabiosis (the dependence of one organism upon another for its existence; also called *commensalism*) (*meta* after)
			parabiosis {parabiotic} (*para* alongside)
			probiosis {probiotic} (*pro* before)
			symbiosis {symbiotic} (*sym* with, together)
			biotic pertaining to the condition of life:
			antibiotic (*anti* against)
			endobiotic (*endon* within)
			microbiotic (*mikros* small)
			prebiotic (*pre* before)

Element	From	Meaning	Examples
bio (cont'd)		[life]	*bism*: microbism (infection with microbes) (*mikros* small) LEADING ROOT COMPOUND: *bi*: biome (*oma* mass) bionics (*bio* + *electronics*) biopsy (the process of removing tissue from patients for diagnostic examination) (*opsis* vision, sight) biosis (vitality, or life) (*osis* condition) *bio*: bioacoustics (*akouein* to hear) biocenosis (*koinos* common) biochrome (natural pigment) (*chroma* color) biocidal (*caedere* to cut, kill) biogenesis {*biogenetic*} (*genere* to produce) biokinetics (*kinein* to move) biology {*biological*} (*logos* study) biolysis {*biolytic*} (*lyein* to loosen) biomembrane {*biomembranous*} (*membrane* a thin skin) biometer {*biometrics*} (*metron* measure) biomicroscope (*mikros* small + *skopein* to examine) bionomics, bionomy (*nomos* law, custom) biophage {*biophagous*}, biophagism (*phagein* to devour) biophylaxis {*biophylactic*} (*phylaxis* protection) bioplasia, bioplasm {*bioplasmic*} (*plassein* to form) biopoiesis (*poiein* to make, produce) bioptome (a cutting instrument for taking biopsy specimens) (<u>biopsy</u> + *tome* a cutting) biopyoculture (*pyon* pus + culture) bioscopy (*skopein* to examine) biosphere (*sphaira* sphere, ball) biotaxis (also called *cytobiotaxis, cytoclesis*) (*tassein* to arrange) biotherapy (also called *biological therapy*) (*therapy* treatment) biotomy (*tomy* incision) biotope (a specific biologic habitat or site) (*topos* place) biotoxin (*toxikon* poison) TRAILING ROOT COMPOUND: aerobe, aerobic (*aer* air, gas) neobiogenesis (*neos* new + biogenesis) orthobiosis (*ortho* straight + *osis* condition) photobiotic (*photos* light) saprobe (*sapros* rotten) xenobiotic (*xenos* strange) CROSS REFERENCE: zo
blast	Greek *blastos* germ	shoot, sprout, germ, seed	SIMPLE ROOT: blast {*blastic*}, blastema {*blastemic*}, blastid (or, blastide), blastin, blastula {*blastular*}, blastulation PREFIXED ROOT: ablastemic (not concerned with germination) (*a* negative) amphiblastic, amphiblastula (*amphi* around, both) archiblast (*archein* to be first) autoblast (*autos* self) diploblastic (*diploos* two-fold) ectoblast (the ectoderm) (*ektos* outside) entoblast (the entoderm, or hypoblast) (*entos* within) epiblast {*epiblastic*} (*epi* upon)

Element	From	Meaning	Examples
blast (cont'd)		[shoot, sprout]	heteroblastic (*heteros* different)
			holoblastic (*holos* entire)
			homoblastic (*homos* same)
			hypoblast {hypoblastic} (*hypo* under)
			macroblast (*makros* large)
			megaloblast (*megalos* large)
			mesoblast {mesoblastic}, mesoblastema (*mesos* middle)
			microblast (*mikros* small)
			monoblast (*monos* single)
			panblastic (*pan* all)
			parablast {parablastic} (*para* alongside)
			periblast (*peri* around)
			promegaloblast (*pro* before + megaloblast)
			protoblast {protoblastic} (*protos* first)
			tetrablastic (*tetra* four)
			triploblastic (triple)
			LEADING ROOT COMPOUND:
			blast: blastoma (*oma* tumor)
			blasto:
			blastocele (or, blastocoele) {blastocelic} (*koilos* hollow, cavity)
			blastochyle (*chylos* juice)
			blastocyst (*kystis* bladder)
			blastocyte (*kytos* cell)
			blastoderm (or, blastoderma) {blastodermal} (*derma* skin)
			blastodisc (or, blastodisk; the small disk of protoplasm containing the egg nucleus)
			blastogenesis {blastogenetic, blastogenic} (*genere* to produce)
			blastokinin (also called *uteroglobin*) (*kinein* to move)
			blastolysis {blastolytic} (*lyein* to loosen)
			blastomere, blastomerotomy (*meros* part + *tomy* incision)
			blastomycete, blastomycosis (*mykes* fungus + *osis* condition)
			blastophyly (*phyle* tribe)
			blastopore (*poros* opening)
			blastosphere (*sphere* ball, globe)
			blastospore (also called *blastoconidium*) (*sporos* seed)
			blastotomy (also called *blastomerotomy*) (*tomy* incision)
			blastozooid (*zoon* animal + *eidos* form)
			TRAILING ROOT COMPOUND:
			blast:
			acroblast (*akron* high, extremities)
			adenoblast (*aden* gland)
			angioblast (*angeion* blood vessel)
			astroblast (*aster* star)
			chondroblast (*chondros* cartilage)
			chromoblast (*chroma* color)
			dermoblast (*derma* skin)
			erythroblast (*erythros* red)
			galactoblast (*galaktos* milk)
			ganglioblast (*ganglion* knot, swelling)
			granuloblast (granule)
			hemoblast, hemoblastosis (*haima* blood + *osis* condition)
			histioblast (*histos* web, tissue)
			inoblast (*inos* fiber)
			lecithoblast (*lekithos* egg yolk)

Element	From	Meaning	Examples
blast (cont'd)		[shoot, sprout]	lemmoblast (an immature lemmocyte) (*lemma* husk)
			leukoblast, leukoblastosis (*leukos* white + *osis* condition)
			medulloblast, medulloblast (*medulla* marrow + *osis* condition)
			melanoblast (*melanos* black, dark)
			mucinoblast (the progenitor of a mucous cell)
			myeloblast, myeloblastemia (*myelos* marrow + *emia* blood condition)
			myoblast (also called *sarcoblast*) {myoblastic} (*myos* muscle)
			nematoblast (also called *spermatid*) (*nematos* thread)
			neoblastic (*neos* new)
			neuroblast (an immature nerve cell) (*neuron* nerve)
			normoblast, normoblastosis (*norma* rule + *osis* condition)
			odontoblast, odontoblastoma (*odontos* tooth + *oma* tumor)
			ooblast (*oon* egg, ovum)
			phoroblast (also called *fibroblast*) (*phorein* to bear, carry)
			poikiloblast (*poikilos* varied, mottled)
			rubriblast (also called *proerythroblast*) (*rubeus* red)
			sarcoblast (also called *myoblast*) (*sarkos* flesh)
			spermatoblast (also called *spermatogonium*) (*spermatos* seed)
			splanchnoblast (*splanchnos* viscus)
			splenoblast (*splen* spleen)
			spongioblast, spongioblastoma (*spongia* sponge + *oma* tumor)
			sporoblast (also called *zygotomere*) (*sporos* seed)
			textoblastic (forming adult tissue) (*textus* tissue)
			trophoblast {trophoblastic} (*trophein* to nourish)
			blastema: scleroblastema (*skleros* hard)
			PREFIXED TRAILING ROOT COMPOUND:
			ectomesoblast (*ektos* outside + *mesos* middle)
			macromyeloblast (*makros* large + *myelos* marrow)
			premyeloblast (*pre* before + *myelos* marrow)
			pronormoblastosis (*pro* before + normoblastosis)
			CROSS REFERENCE: gon[1], sperm, spor
blenn	Greek *blennos* slime, mucus	mucus	PREFIXED ROOT: polyblennia (*polys* much)
			LEADING ROOT COMPOUND:
			blenn:
			blennadenitis (*adenos* gland + *itis* inflammation)
			blennemesis (vomiting of mucus) (*emein* to vomit)
			blennoid (also called *muciform*) (*eidos* form)
			blennophthalmia (also called *conjunctivitis*) (*ophthalmos* eye)
			blennuria (*uria* urine condition)
			blenno:
			blennogenous (also called *muciparous*) (*genere* to produce)
			blennorrhagic (also called *blennorrheal*) (*rhagia* bursting forth)
			blennorrheal (also called *blennorrhagic*) (*rhein* to flow)
			blennothorax (a pleural effusion containing mucus) (*thorax* chest)
			TRAILING ROOT COMPOUND:
			blennorrhea flowing of mucus:
			dacryoblennorrhea (*dacryon* tear)
			dacryocystoblennorrhea (*dacryon* tear + *kystis* sac)
			gastroblennorrhea (*gaster* stomach)
			gonoblennorrhea (*gone* seed)
			ophthalmoblennorrhea (*ophthalmos* eye)
			pyoblennorrhea (suppurative blennorrhea) (*pyon* pus)
			CROSS REFERENCE: muc, myx

A Thesaurus of Medical Word Roots

Element	From	Meaning	Examples
blephar	Greek *blepharon*	eyelid	SIMPLE ROOT: blepharal (pertaining to an eyelid; also called *palpebral*) blepharism (twitching or blinking of the eyelids; also called *palpebration*), blepharon (an eyelid; pl., blephara) PREFIXED ROOT: *blepharia*: ablepharia {ablepharous} (*a* privative) macroblepharia (*makros* large) microblepharia (*mikros* small) *blepharon*: ablepharon (also called *cryptophthalmos*), ablephary (*a* privative) epiblepharon (a congenital anomaly in which a horizontal fold of skin stretches across the border of the eyelid, pressing the lashes against the eyeball) (*epi* upon) euryblepharon (*eurys* wide) microblepharon (*mikros* small) symblepharon (an adhesion between the tarsal conjunctiva and the bulbar conjunctiva) (*syn* with) LEADING ROOT COMPOUND: *blephar*: blepharadenitis (or, blepharoadenitis) (*adenos* gland + *itis* inflammation) blepharectomy (*ektome* excision) blepharedema (*edema* swelling) blepharelosis (also called *entropion*) (*eilein* to roll) blepharitis (*itis* inflammation) blepharoncus (a tumor on the eyelid) (*onkos* bulk, mass) *blepharo*: blepharoadenoma (*aden* gland + *oma* tumor) blepharoatheroma (*athere* thick fluid + *oma* tumor) blepharochalasis (relaxation of the skin of the eyelid, due to atrophy of the intercellular tissue) (*chalasis* relaxation) blepharochromidrosis (excretion of a sweat containing pigment from the eyelids, usually of a bluish shade) (*chroma* color + *hidros* sweat + *osis* condition) [h of hidros elided] blepharoclonus (clonic spasm of orbicularis oculi muscle, appearing as an increased winking of the eye) (*clonus* turmoil) blepharoconjunctivitis (conjunctiva + *itis* inflammation) blepharodiastasis (*diastasis* separation) blepharopachynsis (*pachys* thick) blepharophimosis (*phimosis* narrowing) blepharoplasty (also called *tarsoplasia*) (*plassein* to form) blepharoplegia (paralysis of an eyelid) (*plessein* to strike) blepharoptosis (a drooping of the eyelids) (*ptein* to fall) blepharopyorrhea (also called *purulent ophthalmia*) (*pyon* pus + *rhein* to flow) blepharorrhaphy (also called *tarsorrhaphy*) (*rhaphe* suture) blepharospasm (spasmodic winking caused by involuntary contraction of an eyelid muscle) (*span* to contract) blepharosphincterectomy (*sphincter* constriction + *ektome* excision) blepharostat (also called *eye speculum*) (*stasis* standing still) blepharostenosis (also called *blepharophimosis*) (*stenosis* narrow) blepharosynechia (*synechia* a holding together) blepharotomy (*tomy* incision)

Element	From	Meaning	Examples
blephar (cont'd)		[eyelid]	TRAILING ROOT COMPOUND: *blepharic*: hygroblepharic (*hygros* moist) *blepharon*: ankyloblepharon (*ankylos* bent, fused, crooked) corneoblepharon (*cornea*) hydroblepharon (edema of the eyelids) (*hydor* water) pachyblepharon (*pachys* thick) varicoblepharon (a varicosity of the eyelid) (*varix* varicose vein) CROSS REFERENCE: cili, palpebr
brachi	Greek *brachion* arm; *brachys* short; Latin *brachium* arm	upper arm	NOTE: This root refers to the shorter upper arm, as opposed to the longer forearm. SIMPLE ROOT: brachium (the upper arm from shoulder to elbow; pl., brachia) {brachial} PREFIXED ROOT: *brachia*: abrachia (congenital absence of arms) (*a* privative) dibrachia (*di* two) macrobrachia (*makros* long, large) microbrachia (*mikros* small) monobrachia (*monos* single) tribrachia (*tri* three) *brachial*: postbrachial (*post* posterior) subbrachial (*sub* below) *brachio*: abrachiocephalus (also called *acephalobrachius*) (*a* privative + *kephale* head) *brachium*: antebrachium (also called *forearm, antibrachium*) (*ante* before) antibrachium (also called *forearm, antebrachium*) (*anti* against) *brachius*: abrachius (*a* privative) microbrachius (*mikros* small) monobrachius (*monos* single) tetrabrachius (*tetra* four) tribrachius (*tri* three) LEADING ROOT COMPOUND: *brachi*: brachialgia (neuralgia in the arm) (*algos* pain) *brachio*: brachiobasilic (pertaining to or connecting the brachial artery and the basilic vein) brachiocephalic (*kephale* head) brachiocrural (*crus* shin, leg) brachiocubital (*cubitus* forearm) brachiocyllosis (also called *brachiocyrtosis*) (*kyllosis* a crooking) brachiofaciolingual (affecting the arm, face, and tongue) brachiogram (*graphein* to write) brachiothoracoomphaloischiopagus (conjoined twins joined from the forearms and shoulder to the pelvis) TRAILING ROOT COMPOUND: cervicobrachial (*cervix* neck) faciobrachial (*facies* face) perobrachius (*peros* maimed) CROSS REFERENCE: mel[1]

Element	From	Meaning	Examples
brachy	Greek *brachys*	short	PREFIXED ROOT: acrobrachycephaly (*akros* highest + *kephale* head) hyperbrachycephalic (*hyper* above + *kephale* head) hypsibrachycephalic (*hypsos* height + *kephale* head) subbrachycephalic (*sub* under + *kephale* head) symbrachydactylia (*sym* together + *daktylos* finger, toe) ultrabrachycephalic (*ultra* beyond + *kephale* head) LEADING ROOT COMPOUND: brachybasia (a slow, shuffling, short-stepped gait, as seen in double hemiplegia) (*bainein* to walk) brachycardia (also called *bradycardia*) (*kardia* heart) brachycephaly {brachycephalic} (*kephale* head) brachycheilia (or, brachychilia) (*cheilos* lip) brachychronic (*chronos* time) brachycranial (or, brachycranic) (*kranion* skull) brachydactyly (*daktylos* finger, toe) brachyesophagus (esophagus) brachyfacial (also called *brachyprosopic*) (face) brachyglossal (*glossa* tongue) brachygnathia {brachygnathous} (*gnathos* jaw) brachykerkic (denoting a forearm relatively shorter than the upper arm) (*kerkis* radius) brachyknemic (*kneme* shin) brachymelia (*melos* limb, member) brachymorphic (also called *brachytypical*) (*morphe* form) brachyodont (*odontos* tooth) brachyonychia (*onychos* nail) brachypellic (also called *brachypelvic*) (pelvis) brachyphalangia (*phalanges* bones of the fingers or toes) brachypodous (*pous* foot) brachyprosopic (also called *brachyfacial*) (*prosopon* face) brachyrhinia (*rhinos* nose) brachyskelic (*skelos* leg) brachystaphyline (having a short, wide palate) (*staphyle* uvula) brachystasis (condition in which a muscle does not relax upon contracting but maintains its shortened state) (*stasis* standstill) brachytherapy (a type of radiotherapy) (*therapy* treatment) brachytype (also called *endomorph*), brachytypical (also called *brachymorphic*) (*typos* type) CROSS REFERENCE: ulna
brady	Greek *bradys*	slow	See Appendix B for examples of this element as an initial combining form. Others are listed with the roots to which it is attached. CROSS REFERENCE: None
brom	Greek *bromos*	stench (bromine)	SIMPLE ROOT: bromate (any salt of bromic acid) {bromated} bromide, bromine {bromic} bromism (or, brominism) bromite (also called *bromyrite*) bromization (impregnation with bromides or bromine) PREFIXED ROOT: *bromic*: antibromic (a deodorant) (*anti* against) perbromic (*per* through) *bromite*: hypobromite (a salt of hypobromous acid) (*hypo* under)

Element	From	Meaning	Examples
brom (cont'd)		[stench]	LEADING ROOT COMPOUND: *brom*: bromidrosiphobia (*hidros* sweat + *phobia* fear) [h of hidros elided] bromhidrosis (*hidros* sweat + *osis* condition) *bromo*: bromoderma (a skin eruption due to the use of bromine or bromides) (*derma* skin) bromohyperhidrosis (*hyper* above + *hidrosis* sweat condition) bromomenorrhea (menstruation characterized by an offensive odor) (*men* month: menstruation + *rhein* to flow) bromopnea (halitosis: bad breath) (*pnoia* breath) TRAILING ROOT COMPOUND: hydrobromic (also called *hydrogen bromide*) (*hydor* water) oxybromic (pertaining to, or designating certain compounds of oxygen and bromine) podobromidrosis (*podos* foot + *(h)idros* sweat + *osis* condition) CROSS REFERENCE: odor, olfact, osm[1], osphr, oz
bronch	Greek *bronchos*	windpipe	SIMPLE ROOT: bronchial (pertaining to the bronchi or bronchia) bronchiolus, bronchium (pl., bronchia) bronchiole (or, bronchiolus; pl., bronchioli) bronchismus (also called *bronchospasm*) bronchus (pl., bronchi) PREFIXED ROOT: *bronchial*: endobronchial (also called *intrabronchial*) (*endo* within) intrabronchial (also called *endobronchial*) (*intra* within) peribronchial (*peri* around) *bronchitis* inflammation of windpipe: endobronchitis (inflammation of the epithelial lining of the bronchi) (*endon* within) mesobronchitis (inflammation of the middle coat of the bronchi) (*mesos* middle) peribronchitis (inflammation of the tissues surrounding the bronchi or bronchial tubes) (*peri* around) *bronchiolitis* inflammation of bronchioles: panbronchiolitis (*pan* all) peribronchiolitis (*peri* around) *bronchiolar*: peribronchiolar (*peri* around) LEADING ROOT COMPOUND: *bronch*: bronchadenitis (*adenos* gland + *itis* inflammation) bronchitis (*itis* inflammation) *bronchi*: bronchiarctia (also called *bronchostenosis*) (*arctare* to constrict) bronchiectasis (or, bronchiectasia; a chronic dilatation of the bronchi or bronchioles marked by fetid breath and paroxysmal coughing) {bronchiectasic} (*ektasis* dilatation) bronchiloquy (*loqui* to speak) *bronchio*: bronchiocele (*kele* tumor, swelling) bronchiogenic (*genere* to produce) bronchiospasm (or, bronchospasm) (*span* to contract) bronchiostenosis (*stenos* narrow + *osis* condition)

Element	From	Meaning	Examples
bronch (cont'd)		[windpipe]	*bronchiol*: bronchiolectasia (or, bronchiolestasis) (*ektasis* a stretching) bronchiolitis (*itis* inflammation) *broncho*: bronchoadenitis (*adenos* gland + *itis* inflammation) bronchoblastomycosis (also called *pulmonary blastomycosis*) (*blastos* germ, cell + *mykes* fungus + *osis* condition) bronchocavernous (*cavus* hollow) bronchocele (*kele* tumor) bronchoedema (*edema* swelling) bronchogenic (*genere* to produce) bronchogram, bronchography (*graphein* to write) broncholith, broncholithiasis (*lithos* stone + *iasis* condition) bronchomalacia (*malakos* soft) bronchomycosis (*mykes* fungus + *osis* condition) bronchopathy (*pathos* disease) bronchophony (*phone* sound) bronchoplasty (*plassein* to form) bronchoplegia (*plessein* to strike: paralysis) bronchopleural (*pleura* side) bronchopneumonia (pneumonia) bronchopulmonary (*pulmon* lung) bronchorrhagia (*rhagia* bursting forth) bronchorrhaphy (*rhaphe* suture) bronchorrhea (*rhein* to flow) bronchorrhoncus (*rhonchos* a snoring sound) bronchoscope, bronchoscopy (*skopein* to examine) bronchosinusitis (*sinus* + *itis* inflammation) bronchospasm (or, bronchiospasm) (*span* to contract) bronchostaxis (*staxis* a dripping) bronchostenosis (or, bronchiostenosis) (*stenosis* narrow) bronchostomy (*stoma* mouth, opening) bronchotomy (*tomy* incision) bronchotracheal (also called *tracheobronchial*) (*trachea* windpipe) bronchovesicular (also called *bronchoalveolar*) (*vesica* bladder, sac) TRAILING ROOT COMPOUND: *bronchial*: esophagobronchial (esophagus) tracheobronchial (also called *bronchotracheal*) (*trachea* windpipe) vesiculobronchial (*vesica* bladder) *bronchitis* inflammation of windpipe: fibrobronchitis (also called *fibrinous bronchitis*) pleurobronchitis (*pleura* side, rib) sinobronchitis (*sinus*) tracheobronchitis (*trachea* windpipe) CROSS REFERENCE: laryng, trache
bucc	Latin *bucca*	cheek	SIMPLE ROOT: bucca (also called *mala*; pl., buccae) {buccal}, buccula (a redundant fatty fold under the chin; double chin) PREFIXED ROOT: extrabuccal (outside of the mouth or cheek) (*extra* outside) intrabuccal (*intra* within) mesiobuccal (*mesos* middle) peribuccal (surrounding the cheek) (*peri* around)

Element	From	Meaning	Examples
bucc (cont'd)		[cheek]	proximobuccal (*proximus* nearest)
			retrobuccal (pertaining to the back part of the cheek) (*retro* back)
			suprabuccal (above the buccal region) (*supra* above)
			LEADING ROOT COMPOUND:
			buccoaxial, buccoaxiocervical (*axon* axis + *cervix* neck)
			buccocervical (*cervix* neck)
			buccoclusion (*claudere* to close)
			buccodistal (*distal* distant)
			buccogingival (*gingivae* gums of the mouth)
			buccolabial (relating to the cheek and the lip; relating to the aspect of the dental arch that is in contact with the mucosa of the lip and cheek) (*labium* lip)
			buccolingual (*lingua* tongue)
			buccomaxillary (*maxilla* upper jaw)
			buccopharyngeal (*pharynx* throat)
			buccoversion (*vertere* to turn)
			TRAILING ROOT COMPOUND:
			antrobuccal (*antrum* sinus)
			cervicobuccal (also called *buccocervical*) (*cervix* neck)
			dentibuccal (*dens* tooth)
			distobuccal (*distans* distant)
			proximobuccal (*proximus* nearest, next to)
			CROSS REFERENCE: mala, mel[1]
bulb	Latin *bulbus* Greek *bolbos*	bulb	SIMPLE ROOT:
			bulb (a rounded mass, or enlargement, such as an anatomical structure of similar shape, as the head, or glans, of the penis)
			bulbar (pertaining to a bulb; often used alone to refer to the medulla oblongata)
			bulbous, bulbus (a rounded mass or enlargement; pl., bulbi)
			PREFIXED ROOT:
			circumbulbar (surrounding the eyeball) (*circum* around)
			epibulbar (upon the eyeball) (*epi* upon)
			extrabulbar (outside of or unrelated to any bulb, such as the bulb of the urethra, or the medulla oblongata) (*extra* outside)
			peribulbar (surrounding the bulb of the eye) (*peri* around)
			postbulbar (*post* posterior)
			retrobulbar (behind the eyeball) (*retro* backward)
			LEADING ROOT COMPOUND:
			bulb:
			bulbitis (inflammation of the bulb of the penis) (*itis* inflammation)
			bulboid (shaped like a bulb; also called *bulbiform*) (*eidos* form)
			bulbi: bulbiform (also called bulboid) (*forma* shape)
			bulbo:
			bulboatrial (pertaining to the bulbus cordis and atrium) [*bulbus cordis*: the foremost of the three parts of the primordial heart of the embryo]
			bulbocavernous (pertaining to the bulb of the penis or to the bulbocavernous muscle)
			bulbonuclear (relating to the nuclei of the medulla oblongata)
			bulbopontine (*pons* bridge)
			bulbospinal (also called *spinobulbar*) (spine)
			bulbospiral (*spira* coil)
			bulbourethral (pertaining to the bulb of the penis; also called *urethrobulbar*) (urethra)

A Thesaurus of Medical Word Roots

Element	From	Meaning	Examples
bulb (cont'd)		[bulb]	TRAILING ROOT COMPOUND: *bulbar*: corticobulbar (cerebral cortex) (*cortex* bark: covering) ischiobulbar (*ischion* hip) pneumobulbar (*pneumon* lung) pontobulbar (pertaining to the pons and the region of the medulla oblongata dorsal to it) (*pons* bridge) spinobulbar (also called *bulbospinal*) (spine) urethrobulbar (also called *bulbourethral*) (urethra) *bulbia*: syringobulbia (*syringos* tube, fistula) CROSS REFERENCE: tub²
burs	Latin *bursa*; Greek *brysa*	pouch, sac	SIMPLE ROOT: bursa (a sac or saclike cavity filled with a viscid fluid and situated at places in the tissues at which friction would otherwise develop; pl., bursae) {bursal} PREFIXED ROOT: peribursal (surrounding a bursa) (*peri* around) LEADING ROOT COMPOUND: *burs*: bursectomy (*ektome* excision) bursitis (*itis* inflammation) *bursa*: bursalogy (*logos* study) *burso*: bursolith (a calculus or concretion in a bursa) (*lithos* stone) bursopathy (any disease of a bursa) (*pathos* disease) bursotomy (incision of a bursa) (*tomy* incision) CROSS REFERENCE: cyst, scrot

C

Element	From	Meaning	Examples
caco-	Greek prefix *kakos*	bad, ill, abnormal	See Appendix B for examples of words with this prefix. Others are listed with the roots to which it is attached. CROSS REFERENCE: dys-, mal-
calc	Latin *calcis* lime	limestone (calcium)	SIMPLE ROOT: calcareous (pertaining to or containing lime or calcium; chalky) calcite, calcium {calcic} calculus (an abnormal concretion occurring within the animal body, and usually composed of mineral salts; pl., calculi) PREFIXED ROOTS: *calcareous*: subcalcareous (*sub* slightly) *calcemia* condition of calcium in the blood: hypercalcemia (*hyper* above) hypocalcemia {hypocalcemic} (*hypo* under) *calcia*: hypocalcia (deficiency of calcium) (*hypo* under) *calcic*: dicalcic (*di* two) monocalcic (*monos* single) tricalcic (*tri* three) *calcification* production of calcium: decalcification (*de* negative) hypocalcification (*hypo* under) microcalcification (*mikros* small) recalcification (*re* again) *calcipexy* fixation of calcium: hypercalcipexy (*hyper* above) hypocalcipexy {hypocalcipectic} (*hypo* under) *calciuria* condition of calcium in the urine: hypercalciuria (*hyper* above) hypocalciuria (*hypo* under) *calculous* pertaining to calcium: acalculous (without the presence of stones) (*a* privative) anticalculous (also called *antilithic*) (*anti* against) LEADING ROOT COMPOUND: *calc*: calcemia (also called *hypercalcemia*) (*emia* blood condition) *calcar*: calcaroid (*eidos* form, resembling) *calcari*: calcariuria (the presence of lime salts in the urine) (*uria* urine condition) *calci*: calcibilia (the presence of calcium in the bile) calcifames (calcium hunger) (*fames* hunger) calciferous (also called *calcophorous*) (*ferre* to bear) calcify {calcific, calcification} (*facere* to make) calcigerous (producing or carrying calcium salts) (*gerere* to bear) calcimeter (*metron* measure) calcipenia {calcipenic} (*penia* deficiency) calcipexis (or, calcipexy) {calcipexic, calcipectic} (*pexis* fixation) calciphilia (*philein* to love—to have an affinity for) calciphylaxis {calciphylactic} (*phylaxis* a guarding) calciprivia {calciprivic} (*privus* without)

Element	From	Meaning	Examples
calc (cont'd)		[calcium, limestone]	calcipyelitis (calculous pyelitis) (*pyelos* pelvis + *itis* inflammation)
			calciuria (*uria* urine condition)
			calcic: calcicosis (a form of pneumoconiosis from the inhalation of limestone or marble dust) (*osis* condition)
			calcin: calcinosis (*osis* condition)
			calcio:
			calciokinesis {calciokinetic} (*kinein* to move)
			calciorrhachia (*rhachis* spine)
			calco:
			calcoglobulin (*globus* ball, sphere)
			calcophorous (also called *calciferous*) (*pherein* to bear)
			calcospherite (also called *psammoma body*) (*sphaira* sphere, ball)
			calcul: calculosis (*osis* condition)
			TRAILING ROOT COMPOUND:
			fibrinocalcific (fiber + *facere* to make)
			nephrocalcinosis (*nephros* kidney + *osis* condition)
			CROSS REFERENCE: lith, petr
calcan	Latin *calcaneus*	heel bone (*os calcis*)	SIMPLE ROOT: calcaneum (pl., calcanea), calcaneus {calcaneal, calcanean}
			PREFIXED ROOT: retrocalcaneobursitis (also called *achillobursitis*) (*retro* backward, behind + bursitis)
			LEADING ROOT COMPOUND:
			calcane:
			calcaneitis (*itis* inflammation)
			calcaneodynia (pain in the heel) (*odyne* pain)
			calcaneo:
			calcaneocuboid (pertaining to the calcaneus and the cuboid bone)
			calcaneofibular (pertaining to the calcaneus and the fibula)
			calcaneonavicular (pertaining to the calcaneus and navicular bone)
			calcaneoplantar (pertaining to the calcaneus and the sole of the foot) (*planta* sole of the foot)
			TRAILING ROOT COMPOUND:
			talocalcaneal (*talus* ankle)
			tibiocalcanean (tibia)
			CROSS REFERENCE: None
camp	Greek *kamptos* bent	bent, curved	PREFIXED ROOT:
			acampsia (inflexibility of a limb) (*a* negative)
			anacamptometer (an instrument for measuring the reflexes) (*ana* back, again + *metron* measure)
			LEADING ROOT COMPOUND:
			campo: campospasm (or, camptospasm; also called *camptocormia*) (*span* to contract)
			campto:
			camptocormia (or, camptocormy; a static deformity consisting of forward flexion of the trunk; also called *camptospasm, prosternation*) (*kormos* trunk)
			camptodactylia (also called *campylodactyly*) (*daktylos* finger, toe)
			camptomelia {camptomelic} (*melos* limb, member)
			camptospasm (or, campospasm) (*span* to contract)
			campylo: campylodactyly (permanent flexion of one or more of the finger joints; also called *camptodactylia*) (*daktylos* finger)
			TRAILING ROOT COMPOUND:
			dactylocampsis (permanent flexion of the fingers) (*dactylos* finger)

Element	From	Meaning	Examples
camp (cont'd)		[bent, curved]	gonocampsis (permanent flexion of the knee) (*gony* knee) osteocampsis (or, osteocampsia; curvature or bending of a bone, as in rickets) (*osteon* bone) phallocampsis (painful downward curvature of the erect penis; also called *clubbed penis, penile curvature*) (*phallos* penis) rachiocampsis (curvature of the spinal column) (*rhachis* spine) stereocampimeter (*stereos* solid + *metron* measure) CROSS REFERENCE: None
cancr	Latin *cancer* crab	cancer	See Appendix B for examples of words with this element. Others are listed with the roots to which it is attached. CROSS REFERENCE: carcin
canth	Latin *cantus* edge; Greek *kanthus* corner of the eye	side, angle; eye corner	SIMPLE ROOT: cant, canthus (the angle at either end of the fissure between the eyelids; pl., canthi) {canthal} PREFIXED ROOT: encanthis (a tumor growing from the inner angle of the eye) (*en* in) epicanthus (the small fold of skin sometimes covering the inner corner of the eye) (*epi* upon) syncanthus (adhesion of the eyeball to the structures of the orbit) (*sym* with) telecanthus (abnormally increased distance between the medial canthi and the eyelids) (*tele* afar) LEADING ROOT COMPOUND: *canth*: canthectomy (*ektome* excision) canthitis (*itis* inflammation) *cantho*: cantholysis (*lyein* to loosen) canthopexy (*pexis* fixation) canthoplasty (*plassein* to form) canthorrhaphy (*rhaphe* suture) canthotomy (*tomy* incision) CROSS REFERENCE: cost, gon², later, pleur
capill	Latin *capillus* hair, esp. of the head	hair, capillary	NOTE: This root may be derived from *caput* head + *pilus* a hair. SIMPLE ROOT: capillarity (the action by which the surface of a liquid, as in capillary tubes, is elevated or depressed) capillary (pertaining to or resembling hair; any one of the minute vessels that connect the arterioles and venules) capillitium (a filamentous structure that interlaces among the spores in the fruiting bodies of certain bacteria) capillus (the aggregate of hair on the scalp; pl., capilli) PREFIXED ROOT: intercapillary (among or between capillaries) (*inter* between) intracapillary (*intra* within) microcapillary (*mikros* small) pericapillary (*peri* around) postcapillary (*post* after) precapillary (*pre* before) LEADING ROOT COMPOUND: *capillar*: capillarectasia (*ektasis* dilatation) capillariasis (*iasis* condition) capillaritis (also called *telangiitis*) (*itis* inflammation)

A Thesaurus of Medical Word Roots

Element	From	Meaning	Examples
capill (cont'd)		[capillary]	*capillaro*: capillaropathy (any disease of the capillaries) (*pathos* disease) capillaroscopy (*skopein* to examine) *capillo*: capillomotor (or, capillariomotor) (*movere* to move) TRAILING ROOT COMPOUND: arteriocapillary (artery) CROSS REFERENCE: trich
capit, **caput**, **ceps**, **cip**	Latin *caput*	head	SIMPLE ROOT: *capit*: capitatum (lit., having a head; the capitate bone) capitular (pertaining to the capitulum or head of a bone) capitulum (a general term for a little head, or a small eminence on a bone by which it articulates with another bone; pl., capitula) *caput*: caput (the superior extremity of the body, comprising the cranium and face, and containing the brain, the organs of special sense, and the first organs of the digestive system; pl., capita) PREFIXED ROOT: *capit*: decapitate, decapitation (the removal of the head, as of a person, a fetus, or a bone), decapitator (*de* off) *ceps*: biceps (a muscle having two heads; pl., biceps, bicepses) (*bi* two) quadriceps (a muscle with four heads or points of origin; especially the large muscle at the front of the thigh) (*quadri* four) triceps (a three-headed muscle) {tricipital} (*tri* three) uniceps (having one head or origin: said of a muscle) (*uni* one) *cip*: ancipital (having two heads or two edges) (*an* for *ambi* both) bicipital (pertaining to a biceps muscle; having two heads) (*bi* two) occipital (*ob* against) [see separate entry: occip-] sinciput (the upper half of the cranium; the forehead) (*semi* half) tricipital (three-headed, as the triceps muscle) (*tri* three) LEADING ROOT COMPOUND: capitopedal (pertaining to the head and foot) (*pes* foot) TRAILING ROOT COMPOUND: janiceps (a double fetal monster with one head and two opposite faces; also called *heteroprosopus*) (*Janus* Roman two-faced god) CROSS REFERENCE: cephal
caps	Latin *capsa* box *capsule* little box	capsule	SIMPLE ROOT: capsule PREFIXED ROOT: *capsular*: bicapsular (*bi* two) extracapsular (*extra* outside) intracapsular (*intra* within) multicapsular (*multus* many) pericapsular (*peri* around) subcapsular (*sub* beneath) *capsulation*: decapsulation (removal of the capsule, especially the removal of the renal capsule) (*de* privative) encapsulation (*en* in) LEADING ROOT COMPOUND: *capsul*: capsulectomy (*ektome* excision) capsulitis (*itis* inflammation)

Element	From	Meaning	Examples
caps (cont'd)		[capsule]	*capsulo*: capsulolenticular (lens—of eye) capsuloplasty (*plassein* to form) capsulorrhaphy (*rhaphe* suture) capsulorrhexis (*rhexis* rupture) capsulotomy (*tomy* incision) CROSS REFERENCE: None
carcin	Greek *karkinos*	crab, cancer	PREFIXED ROOT: *carcinogen* producing cancer: anticarcinogen (*anti* against) cocarcinogen (a substance that works in combination with a carcinogen in the production of cancer) (*co* with) procarcinogen (a chemical substance that becomes a carcinogen only after it is altered by metabolic processes) (*pro* before) *carcinoma*: microcarcinoma (*mikros* small + carcinoma) LEADING ROOT COMPOUND: *carcin*: carcinemia (*emia* blood condition) carcinoid (*eidos* form) carcinoma (pl., carcinomas, carcinomata) (*oma* tumor) *carcino*: carcinocythemia (*kytos* cell + *hemia* blood condition) carcinoembryonic (embryo) carcinogen, carcinogenesis {carcinogenic} (*genere* to produce) carcinolysis {carcinolytic} (*lyein* to loosen) carcinophobia (also called *cancerophobia*) (*phobia* fear) carcinosarcoma (*sarkos* flesh + *oma* tumor) carcinostatic (*statikos* standing) TRAILING ROOT COMPOUND: *carcinogen*: hepatocarcinogen (*hepatos* liver + *genere* to produce) *carcinoma* cancerous tumor: cheilocarcinoma (*cheilos* lip) choriocarcinoma (*chorion* fetal membrane) fibrocarcinoma (*fibra* fiber) hepatocarcinoma (*hepatos* liver) mastocarcinoma (*mastos* breast, nipple) melanocarcinoma (*melas* black, dark) osteocarcinoma (*osteon* bone) papillocarcinoma (*papilla* nipple-shaped projection) psammocarcinoma (*psammos* sand) syringocarcinoma (*syringos* duct, tube) ulocarcinoma (*oulon* gums) CROSS REFERENCE: cancr
cardi	Greek *kardia*	heart	SIMPLE ROOT: cardia, cardiac (pertaining to the heart; a cordial, or restorative medicine; as a noun, a person with a heart disorder) PREFIXED ROOT: *cardia*: acardia {acardiac} (*a* privative) ectocardia (also called *exocardia*) (*ektos* outside) epicardia {epicardial} (*epi* upon) exocardia (also called *ectocardia*) (*exo* outside) hemicardia (either lateral half of a normal heart) (*hemi* half) hypercardia (*hyper* above)

Element	From	Meaning	Examples
cardi (cont'd)		[heart]	macrocardia (also called *cardiomegaly*), macrocardius (a fetus with an extremely large heart) (*makros* large)
			megalocardia (or, megacardia; also called *cardiomegaly, macrocardia*) (*megalos* big, large)
			mesocardia (location of the apex of the heart in the midline of the thorax) (*mesos* middle)
			microcardia (abnormal smallness of the heart) (*mikros* small)
			polycardia (the excessive rapidity in the action of the heart; also called *tachycardia*) (*polys* many, much)
			cardiac:
			endocardiac (also called *intracardiac*) (*endon* within)
			endopericardiac (also called *intrapericardiac*) (*endon* within + pericardiac)
			infracardiac (beneath the heart; below the level of the heart) (*infra* below)
			intracardiac (also called *endocardiac*) (*intra* within)
			juxtacardiac (also called *paracardiac*) (*juxta* near, close by)
			paracardiac (near or beside the heart; also called *juxtacardiac*) (*para* alongside)
			precardiac (*pre* before)
			cardiacus: acardiacus (a parasitic twin without a heart, therefore utilizing the circulation of its twin) (*a* privative)
			cardial:
			endocardial (*endon* within)
			epicardial (*epi* upon)
			exocardial (*exo* outside)
			extracardial (*extra* outside)
			pericardial (*peri* around) [see separate entry: pericard-]
			postcardial (*post* posterior)
			subcardial (*sub* under)
			subepicardial (*sub* under + epicardial)
			supracardial (*supra* above)
			cardiectomy excision of the cardiac part of the stomach:
			epicardiectomy (*epi* upon)
			pericardiectomy (*peri* around)
			cardiography: endocardiography (*endon* within + *graphein* to write)
			cardiopathy: endocardiopathy (a disorder or disease of the endocardium) (*endon* within + *pathos* disease)
			carditis inflammation of the heart:
			endocarditis (or, encarditis) {endocarditic} (*endon* within)
			endoperimyocarditis (*endon* within + *peri* around + *myos* muscle)
			epicarditis (*epi* upon)
			pancarditis (inflamed condition involving all the structures of the heart) (*pan* all)
			pericarditis (*peri* around)
			cardium:
			antecardium (also called *precordium*) (*ante* before)
			anticardium (pit of the stomach; also called *epigastrium*) (*anti* against)
			endocardium (*endon* within)
			epicardium {epicardial} (*epi* upon)
			pericardium (the fibroserous sac that surrounds the heart) {pericardiac} (*peri* around) [see separate entry: pericard-]
			precardium (also called *precordium*) (*pre* before)
			cardius: acardius (a twin fetus without a heart) (*a* privative)

Element	From	Meaning	Examples
cardi (cont'd)		[heart]	LEADING ROOT COMPOUND:

card: carditis (*itis* inflammation)

cardi:

cardialgia (an uneasy or painful sensation in the stomach; heart burn; also called *cardiodynia*) (*algos* pain)

cardiataxia (*ataxia* disorder)

cardiatelia (*ateles* incomplete)

cardiectasia (or, cardiectasis) (*ektasis* dilatation)

cardiectomy (*ektome* excision)

cardiectopia (*ectopia* displaced)

cardiodynia (also called *cardialgia*) (*odyne* pain)

cardio:

cardioaccelerator (*ad* to + *celer* speed)

cardioactive (having an effect upon the heart) (*agere* to act)

cardioangiology (the medical specialty dealing with the heart and blood vessels) (*angeion* blood vessel + *logos* study)

cardioarterial (artery)

cardiocele (protrusion of the heart through a fissure of the diaphragm or through a wound) (*kele* hernia)

cardiocentesis (*kentein* to puncture)

cardiochalasia (relaxation or incompetence of sphincter action of the cardiac opening of the stomach) (*chalasia* relaxation)

cardioesophageal (esophagus)

cardiogenesis {cardiogenic} (*genere* to produce)

cardiogram, cardiograph {cardiographic} (*graphein* to write)

cardiohepatic (*hepatos* liver)

cardioinhibitory

cardiokinetic (*kinein* to move)

cardiokymogram, cardiokymograph (*kymo* wave + *graphein* to write)

cardiologist, cardiology (*logos* study)

cardiolysis (*lyein* to loosen)

cardiomalacia (*malakos* soft)

cardiomegaly (also called *megalocardia*) (*megas* large)

cardiomelanosis (*melanos* black + *osis* condition)

cardiometry (*metron* measure)

cardiomyoliposis (*myos* muscle + *lipos* fat + *osis* condition)

cardiomyopathy (*myos* muscle + *pathos* disease)

cardiomyoplasty (*myos* muscle + *plassein* to form)

cardiomyotomy (also called *esophagomyotomy*) (*myos* muscle + *tomy* incision)

cardionecrosis (necrosis of the myocardium) (*necrosis* death)

cardionector (*nectere* to fasten)

cardionephric (also called *cardiorenal*) (*nephros* kidney)

cardioneural, cardioneurosis (*neuron* nerve + *osis* condition)

cardioomentopexy (omentum + *pexis* fixation)

cardiopaludism (irregularity of the heart's action due to malaria) (*paludism* malaria)

cardiopathy (*pathos* disease)

cardiopericarditis (inflammation of the heart and the pericardium)

cardiophobia (irrational fear of heart disease) (*phobia* fear)

cardiophone (*phone* sound)

cardiophrenia (also called *phrenocardia*) (*phren* mind)

cardioplasty (*plassein* to form)

Element	From	Meaning	Examples
cardi (cont'd)		[heart]	cardioplegia (paralysis of the heart) {cardioplegic} (*plessein* to strike)
			cardiopneumatic (of or pertaining to the heart and respiration) (*pneuma* air, respiration)
			cardioptosia (or, cardioptosis) (*ptosis* a falling)
			cardiopulmonary (*pulmon* lung)
			cardiorenal (also called *cardionephric*) (*ren* kidney)
			cardiorrhaphy (*rhaphe* suture)
			cardiorrhexis (*rhexis* rupture)
			cardiosclerosis (fibrous induration of the heart) (*sklerosis* hardening)
			cardioscope (*skopein* to examine)
			cardiospasm (also called *achalasia*) (*span* to contract)
			cardiosphygmograph (*sphygmos* pulse + *graphein* to write)
			cardiotachometer (*tachys* swift, rapid + *metron* measure)
			cardiotherapy (*therapy* treatment)
			cardiothrombus (*thrombos* clot)
			cardiotocography (*tokos* childbirth + *graphein* to write)
			cardiotomy (*tomy* incision)
			cardiotonic (*tonos* tension)
			cardiotoxic (*toxikon* poison)
			cardiovascular (*vas* vessel—blood vessel)
			cardioversion (*vertere* to turn)
			TRAILING ROOT COMPOUND:
			cardia:
			aerendocardia (presence of undissolved air in the blood within the heart) (*aer* air + *endon* within)
			atelocardia (imperfect development of the heart) (*ateles* incomplete)
			bathycardia (a condition in which the heart is located at an abnormally low site in the thorax) (*bathys* deep, low)
			bradycardia (abnormal slowness of the heart beat) (*bradys* slow)
			dextrocardia (*dexter* right)
			diplocardia (*diploos* double)
			levocardia (location of the heart in the left hemithorax, with the apex pointing to the left) (*laevus* left)
			myocardia (*myos* muscle)
			pneumatocardia (*pneumatos* air)
			presbycardia (*presbys* old age)
			sinistrocardia (*sinister* left)
			stenocardia (also called *angina pectoris*) (*stenos* narrow)
			tachycardia (also called *polycardia*) (*tachys* swift)
			trichocardia (also called *shaggy pericardium*) (*trichos* hair)
			trochocardia (*trokhos* wheel, runner)
			cardiac:
			bradycardiac (*bradys* slow)
			lipocardiac (*lipos* fat)
			oculocardiac (*oculus* eye)
			nephrocardiac (also called *cardiorenal*) (*nephros* kidney)
			neurocardiac (*neuron* nerve)
			renicardiac (also called *cardiorenal*) (*renes* kidney)
			thyrocardiac (thyroid gland)
			cardiogram a description of the heart:
			angiocardiogram (*angeion* vessel—blood vessel)
			echocardiogram (a graphic outline of the movements of heart structures produced by ultrsonography) (echo)

Element	From	Meaning	Examples
cardi (cont'd)		[heart]	electrocardiogram (EKG, where *K* represents the original spelling: *kardia*) (*electrum* shining) kinetocardiogram (*kinein* to move) phonocardiogram (*phone* sound) radiocardiogram (radium) vectorcardiogram (vector) vibrocardiogram (vibration) *cardiopathy*: myocardiopathy (*myos* muscle + *pathos* disease) *carditis*: myocarditis (*myos* muscle + *itis* inflammation) *cardium*: myocardium (*myos* muscle) *cardius*: holoacardius (a separate, grossly defective monozygotic twin fetus in which the heart is entirely absent) (*holos* entire) CROSS REFERENCE: None
caries	Latin *caries*	rottenness	SIMPLE ROOT: caries (gradual decay and disintegration of a bone or tooth) {carious}, cariosity PREFIXED ROOT: *cariogenic* producing caries: anticariogenic (also called *anticarious*) (*anti* against) noncariogenic (*non* negative) LEADING ROOT COMPOUND: cariogenesis (conducive to caries formation) {cariogenic} (*genere* to produce) cariology (*logos* study) cariostatic (*statikos* standing, halting) CROSS REFERENCE: sapr, sep
carp	Greek *karpos*	wrist	SIMPLE ROOT: carpale (any wrist bone), carpus {carpal} PREFIXED ROOT: *carpal*: extracarpal (just outside the region of the wrist) (*extra* beyond) intercarpal (*inter* between) intracarpal (*intra* within) mediocarpal (also called *mesocarpal*, *midcarpal*) (*medius* middle) mesocarpal (also called *mediocarpal*, *midcarpal*) (*mesos* middle) metacarpal (*meta* between) midcarpal (also called *mediocarpal*, *mesocarpal*) (Old English *midd* middle) supercarpal (*super* above) *carpectomy*: metacarpectomy (*meta* after + *ektome* excision) *carpia*: polymetacarpia (*polys* many + *metacarpus*) *carpophalangeal*: metacarpophalangeal (metacarpus + phalanx) *carpus*: metacarpus (pl., metacarpi) {metacarpal} (*meta* after) LEADING ROOT COMPOUND: *carp*: carpectomy (*ektome* excision) carpitis (*itis* inflammation) *carpo*: carpocarpal (pertaining to the two parts of the carpus) carpopedal (*pes* foot) carpoptosis (wrist drop) (*ptein* to fall + *osis* condition) TRAILING ROOT COMPOUND: radiocarpal (pertaining to the radius and the carpus) ulnocarpal (*ulna* the arm) CROSS REFERENCE: None

A Thesaurus of Medical Word Roots

Element	From	Meaning	Examples
cartilag	Latin *cartilago*	gristle	SIMPLE ROOT: cartilage {cartilaginous} PREFIXED ROOT: *cartilage*: precartilage (*pre* before) *cartilaginous*: intercartilaginous (*inter* between) intracartilaginous (also called *endochondral*) (*intra* within) semicartilaginous (*semi* partly) subcartilaginous (*sub* below) LEADING ROOT COMPOUND: *cartilagin*: cartilaginoid (*eidos* form) *cartilagini*: cartilaginification (*facere* to make) *cartilago*: cartilagotropic (*tropos* a turning) TRAILING ROOT COMPOUND: *cartilage*: costicartilage (the cartilage forming the anterior continuation of a rib) (*costa* rib) neocartilage (*neos* new) *cartilaginous*: fibrocartilaginous (*fibra* fiber) membranocartilaginous (membrane) osseocartilaginous (also called *osteochondral*) (*osseo* bone) osteocartilaginous (also called *osteochondrous*) (*osteon* bone) CROSS REFERENCE: chondr
cata-	Greek prefix	down, negative	See Appendix B for examples of words with this prefix. Others are listed with the roots to which it is attached. CROSS REFERENCE: de-
caum, **caus**, **caut**	Greek *kaiein*, to burn; *kausis* burning	fever, burn	SIMPLE ROOT: *caum*: cauma (great heat, as of the body in fever) *caus*: caustic (corrosive; destructive to living tissues) causticize (to render caustic; also called *caustify*) *caut*: cauter, cauterant, cauterization, cauterize, cautery PREFIXED ROOT: encauma (an ulcer upon the cornea) (*en* in) epicauma (a superficial burn or ulcer on the eye) (*epi* upon) LEADING ROOT COMPOUND: *caum*: caumesthesia (a condition in which the patient experiences a sense of burning heat) (*esthesia* feeling) *caus*: causalgia (a burning pain, due to injury of a peripheral nerve, particularly the median nerve) (*algos* pain) *causti*: caustify (also called *causticize*) (*facere* to make) TRAILING ROOT COMPOUND: chemocautery (chemical: *chein* to pour) cryocautery (*kryos* cold) electrocautery (electricity) galvanocautery (cautery effected by a knife or needle heated by the passage of galvanic current) thermocautery (*therme* heat) CROSS REFERENCE: phleg, pyr, therm
cav	Latin *cavus*	hollow	SIMPLE ROOT: cave, caveola (pl., caveolae), cavern (or, caverna) {cavernous} cavitary, cavitas, cavitation, cavity cavum, cavus (unusually high foot arch, as though hollow)

Element	From	Meaning	Examples
cav (cont'd)		[hollow]	PREFIXED ROOT: concave {concavity}, concavoconcave (concave on both sides, as some lenses) (*com* with) excavate, excavation, excavator (*ex* out) intercavernous (*inter* between) intracavitary (*intra* within) postcava (the caudal vena cava) {postcaval} (*post* after) precava (the anterior vena cava) (*pre* before) LEADING ROOT COMPOUND: *cav*: cavitis (also called *celophlebitis*) (*itis* inflammation) *cavern*: cavernitis (or, cavernositis) (*itis* inflammation) cavernoma (*oma* tumor) *caverni*: caverniloquy (cavernous voice) (*loqui* to speak) *caverno*: cavernostomy (*stoma* mouth, opening) *cavernos*: cavernositis (or, cavernitis) (*itis* inflammation) TRAILING ROOT COMPOUND: bronchocavernous (both bronchial and cavitary) (*bronchus* wind-pipe) bulbocavernous (pertaining to the bulb of the penis or to the bulbo-cavernous muscle) ischiocavernous (relating to the ischium and the corpus cavernosum) vesiculocavernous (*vesica* bladder) CROSS REFERENCE: cel[1], colp, sin
cec	Latin *caecum* blind	blind; blind gut	SIMPLE ROOT: cecum (a cavity open at one end, as the blind end of a duct) {cecal} PREFIXED ROOT: *cecal*: centrocecal (*kentron* sharp point; center) pericecal (*peri* around) retrocecal (*retro* behind) subcecal (*sub* under) *secation*: obcecation (partial, or incomplete, blindness) (*ob* against) *cecitis*: pericecitis (*peri* around + *itis* inflammation) *cecum*: megacecum (*megas* big) mesocecum {mesocecal} (*meso* middle) LEADING ROOT COMPOUND: *cec*: cecectomy (*ektome* excision) cecitis (*itis* inflammation) *ceco*: cecocele (*kele* hernia) cecocolic, cecocolostomy (*kolon* colon + *stoma* mouth, opening) cecofixation (also called *cecopexy*) cecopexy (also called *cecofixation*) (*pexis* fixation) cecoplication (*plicare* to fold) cecorrhaphy (suture or repair of the cecum) (*rhaphe* suture) cecostomy (*stoma* mouth, opening) cecotomy (*tomy* incision) TRAILING ROOT COMPOUND: ileocecal (pertaining to the ileum and the cecum) CROSS REFERENCE: typhl

A Thesaurus of Medical Word Roots

Element	From	Meaning	Examples
cel[1], **coel**, **koil**	Greek *koilos* hollow; *koilia* belly, cavity	belly, hollow, abdomen, cavity	SIMPLE ROOT: *cel*: celiac (abdominal), celom (or, coelom) {celomic, or, coelmic} *coel*: coeliac (or, celiac; pertaining to the belly) coelarium (the membrane that lines the body cavity or coelom; also called *mesothelium*) coelom (or, coeloma; the body cavity) {coelomic} coelomate (having a coelom) PREFIXED ROOT: *cel*: acelom, acelomate (or, acelomatous) (*a* privative) dicelous (or, dicoelous; hollowed on both sides) (*di* two) encelialgia (pain in an abdominal viscus) (*en* in + *algos* pain) endoceliac (*endon* within) intracelial (within one of the body cavities) (*intra* within) parepicele (*para* beside + *epi* upon) procelia {procelous} (*pro* before) syncelom (*syn* together) *coel*: dicoelous (or, dicelous; hollowed on each of two sides) (*di* two) epicoeloma (*epi* upon + *oma* tumor) exocoelom (*exo* outside) hypocoelom (*hypo* under) metacoeloma (*meta* change + *oma* tumor) prosocoele (the foremost cavity of the brain) (*proso* before) LEADING ROOT COMPOUND: *cel*: celenteron (also called *primitive gut*) (*enteron* intestine) celitis (any abdominal inflammation) (*itis* inflammation) celonychia (or, koilonychias; spoon nail) (*onychia* nail condition) *celi*: celiagra (*agra* seizure) celiectomy (*ektome* excision) celioma (*oma* tumor) *celio*: celiocentesis (*kentein* to puncture) celiocolpotomy (*kolpos* vagina + *tomy* incision) celiohysterectomy (*hystera* uterus + *ektome* excision) celiomyalgia (*myos* muscle + *algos* pain) celiomyomectomy (*myoma* muscle tumor + *ektome* excision) celiomyositis (*myositis* muscle inflammation) celiopathy (*pathos* disease) celiorrhaphy (also called *laparorrhaphy*) (*rhaphe* suture) celiosalpingectomy (*salpingos* tube + *ektome* excision) celioscopy (also called *laparoscopy*) (*skopein* to examine) celiotomy (also called *laparotomy, ventrotomy*) (*tomy* incision) *celo*: celophlebitis (also called *cavitis*) (*phlebs* vein + *itis* inflammation) celoschisis (also called *gastroschisis*) (*schisis* fissure) celoscope, celoscopy (*skopein* to examine) celozoic (inhabiting the intestinal cavity of the body: said of parasitic protozoa) (*zoon* animal) *coelo*: coeloblastula (*blastos* bud, shoot, germ)

Element	From	Meaning	Examples
cel¹ (cont'd)		[belly, hollow, cavity]	*koil*: koilonychia (or, celonychia) (*onychia* nail condition)
			koilo:
			koilocyte, koilocytosis (*kytos* cell + *osis* condition)
			koilosternia (a congenital malformation of the chest; also called *pectus excavatum*) (*sternon* chest)
			TRAILING ROOT COMPOUND:
			cele:
			astrocele (also called *centrosphere*) (*aster* star)
			enterocele (*enteron* intestine) [another is listed under cel²]
			hemocele (*haima* blood)
			laryngocele (larynx)
			myelocele (*myelos* marrow) [another is listed under cel²]
			myocele (*myos* muscle) [another is listed under cel²]
			neurocele (*neuron* nerve)
			pharyngocele (pharynx)
			rhinocele (or, rhinocoele) (*rhinos* nose)
			syringocele (*syringos* tube, duct)
			celia: schistocelia (also called *celoschisis, gastroschisis*) (*schistos* split)
			celitis: myocelitis (*myos* muscle + *itis* inflammation)
			celous: platycelous (*platys* flat)
			coele:
			blastocoele (the cavity in the blastula of a developing embryo) (*blastos* bud, germ, shoot)
			neurocoele (the neural canal) (*neuron* nerve)
			pseudocoele (or, pseudocele) (*pseudes* false)
			rhombocoele (*rhembein* to turn)
			splanchnocoele (*splanchnos* viscus)
			CROSS REFERENCE: abdomen, colp, lapar, ventr, visc
cel², **kel**	Greek *kele*	hernia, tumor, swelling	PREFIXED ROOT: entocele (an internal hernia) (*entos* within)
			LEADING ROOT COMPOUND:
			celo: celosomia (a developmental anomaly characterized by eventration, fissure, or absence of the sternum, with hernial protrusion of the viscera), celosomus (*soma* body)
			kel: kelectome (a device for removing specimens of tissue from tumors) (*ektome* excision)
			kelo: kelotomy (also called *herniotomy*) (*tomy* incision)
			TRAILING ROOT COMPOUND:
			adenocele (also called *cystadenoma*) (*adenos* gland)
			adipocele (also called *liparocele*) (*adepos* fat)
			aerocele (distention of a cavity with gas; also called *pneumatocele, pneumocele*) (*aer* air)
			amniocele (also called *omphalocele*) (*amnion* fetal membrane)
			antrocele (*antrum* sinus)
			arthrocele (*arthron* joint)
			bronchiocele (or, bronchocele) (*bronchos* windpipe)
			bubonocele (*boubon* groin)
			cardiocele (*kardia* heart)
			cecocele (*cecum* blind gut)
			cephalocele (also called *encephalocele*) (*kephale* head)
			choriocele (*chorion* membrane)
			chylocele (*chylus* gastric juice)
			cirsocele (also called *varicocele*) (*kirsos* varix)

Element	From	Meaning	Examples
cel[2] (cont'd)		[hernia]	colpocele (also called *vaginal hernia*) (*kolpos* vagina)
			cystocele (a bladder hernia that protrudes into the vagina; also called *vesicocele*) (*kystis* bladder)
			dacryocele (also called *dacryocystocele*) (*dakryon* teardrop)
			empyocele (a suppurating hydrocele; a collection of pus in the scrotum) (*empyein* to suppurate)
			encephalocele (also called *cephalocele*) (*enkephale* brain)
			enterocele (*enteron* intestine) [another is listed under cel[1]]
			epiplocele (also called *omental hernia*) (*epiploon* omentum)
			esophagocele (esophagus)
			femorocele (also called *femoral hernia*) (femur)
			galactocele (also called *lactocele*) (*galaktos* milk)
			gastrocele (*gaster* stomach)
			glossocele (*glossa* tongue)
			gonyocele (synovitis of the femorotibial part) (*gony* knee)
			hepatocele (*hepatos* liver)
			hydrocele (*hydor* water)
			hysterocele (*hystera* womb, uterus)
			iridocele (*iridos* rainbow; iris)
			ischiocele (sciatic hernia) (*ischion* hip joint)
			keratocele (*keratos* horn: cornea)
			lactocele (also called *galactocele*) (*lactis* milk)
			laparocele (also called *abdominal hernia*) (*lapara* flank)
			lienocele (also called *splenocele*) (*lien* spleen)
			liparocele, lipocele (also called *adipocele*) (*lipos* fat)
			lymphocele (*lymph* liquid, water)
			meningocele (*meningos* membrane)
			metrocele (also called *hysterocele*) (*metra* womb)
			mucocele (a mucous cyst) (mucus)
			myelocele (*myelos* marrow) [another is listed under cel[1]]
			myocele (*myos* muscle) [another is listed under cel[1]]
			nephrocele (*nephros* kidney)
			omphalocele (*omphalos* navel)
			ophthalmocele (also called *exophthalmos*) (*ophthalmos* eye)
			orchiocele (scrotal hernia; also, a tumor of the testis) (*orchis* testis)
			oscheocele (a swelling or tumor in the scrotum) (*osche* scrotum)
			ovariocele (ovary)
			perineocele (perineum)
			phacocele (*phakos* lens of the eye)
			physocele (*physa* air)
			pleurocele (*pleura* rib, side)
			pneumatocele, pneumocele (*pneumatos* breath)
			pneumonocele (*pneumon* lung)
			proctocele (also called *rectocele*) (*proktos* anus, rectum)
			pseudocephalocele (*pseudes* false + *kephale* head)
			ptyalocele (a cystic tumor containing saliva) (*ptyalon* saliva)
			pyocele (*pyon* pus)
			rectocele (also called *proctocele*) (rectum)
			salpingocele (*salpingos* tube)
			sarcocele (*sarkos* flesh)
			scrotocele (also called *scrotal hernia*) (*scrotum* bag: testicle pouch)
			sialocele (a salivary cyst) (*sialon* saliva)
			spermatocele (*spermatos* seed)
			splanchnocele (*splanchnos* viscus)

Element	From	Meaning	Examples
cel² (cont'd)		[hernia]	splenocele (also called *lienocele*) (*splen* spleen)
			steatocele (*steatos* fat)
			syringocele (*syringos* tube, duct)
			typhlocele (*typhlon* blind gut)
			thyrocele (also called *goiter*) (thyroid gland)
			tracheocele (*trachea* windpipe)
			ureterocele (ureter)
			urethrocele (urethra)
			urocele (*ouron* urine)
			vaginocele (also called *vaginal hernia*) (vagina)
			varicocele (*varix* varicose vein)
			vesicocele (also called *cystocele*) (*vesica* bladder)
			CROSS REFERENCE: edema, gangli, onc, phyma, tub²
cell	Latin *cella*	room, cell, chamber	SIMPLE ROOT: cell {cellular}, cellula (pl., cellulae)
			PREFIXED ROOT:
			cellular:
			acellular (*a* privative)
			bicellular (*bi* two)
			endocellular (*endon* within)
			extracellular (*extra* outward)
			heterocellular (*heteros* other)
			hypercellular (*hyper* above)
			hypocellular (*hypo* under)
			intercellular (*inter* between)
			intracellular (*intra* within)
			isocellular (*isos* equal)
			magnocellular (or, magnicellular) (*magnus* large)
			multicellular (also called *polycellular*) (*multus* many)
			noncellular (also called *subcellular*) (*non* negative)
			pericellular (*peri* around)
			polycellular (also called *multicellular*) (*polys* many)
			subcellular (also called *noncellular*) (*sub* under)
			tricellular (*tri* three)
			unicellular (*uni* one)
			cellulose: hemicellulose (*hemi* half, partly)
			LEADING ROOT COMPOUND:
			celli:
			cellicolous (inhabiting cells) (*colere* to dwell)
			celliferous (also called *cytogenic*) (*ferre* to bear)
			cellifugal (or, cellulifugal) (*fugere* to flee)
			cellipetal (or, cellulipetal) (*petere* to seek)
			cellul:
			cellulitis (*itis* inflammation)
			cellulose (*ose* carbohydrate)
			celluli:
			cellulicidal (destructive to cells) (*caedere* to kill)
			cellulifugal (or, cellifugal) (*fugere* to flee)
			cellulipetal (or, cellipetal) (*petere* to seek)
			TRAILING ROOT COMPOUND:
			cellular:
			adipocellular (*adipos* fat)
			cholangiocellular (*chole* bile + *angeion* vessel)
			fibrinocellular (fibrin)

Element	From	Meaning	Examples
cell (cont'd)		[room, cell, chamber]	fibrocellular (fiber) fusocellular (*fusus* spindle) hepatocellular (*hepatos* liver) parvocellular (*parvus* small) spinocellular (spine) squamocellular (*squama* scale, plate) *cellulitis* inflammation of a cell or cells: adenocellulitis (*adenos* gland) dermatocellulitis (*dermatos* skin) myocellulitis (*myos* muscle) pelvicellulitis (*pyelos* pelvis) CROSS REFERENCE: cyt, vestibul
cen	Greek *koinos*	common, shared	PREFIXED ROOT: acenesthesia (absence of the normal sensation of physical existence) (*a* privative + *esthesia* feeling) paracenesthesia (any abnormality of the general sense of well-being) (*para* abnormal + *esthesia* feeling) LEADING ROOT COMPOUND: *cen*: cenesthesia (also called *somatognosis*) {cenesthesic, cenesthetic} (*esthesia* sensation) cenesthopathy (a general feeling of discomfort not referable to any particular part of the body) (*esthesia* sensation + *pathos* feeling) *ceno*: cenobium (living in communion with others) (*bios* life) cenocyte (or, coenocyte) {cenocytic} (*kytos* cell) cenosite (or, coinosite; a free or unfixed commensal organism) (*sitos* food) cenotrope (*tropein* to turn) cenotype (the original type from which all forms have arisen) TRAILING ROOT COMPOUND: biocenosis (the relation of diverse organisms that live in association) (*bios* life + *osis* condition) CROSS REFERENCE: hom
cente	Greek *kentein* to prick	puncture	SIMPLE ROOT: centesis (surgical puncture of a cavity; can also refer to perforation or tapping, as with an aspirator, trocar, or needle) PREFIXED ROOT: paracentesis (puncture of a cavity with removal of fluid, as in pleural effusion; also called *keratocentesis, tapping*) {paracentetic} (*para* alongside) pericardiocentesis (*peri* around + *kardia* heart: pericardium) TRAILING ROOT COMPOUND: abdominocentesis (also called *celiocentesis*) (abdomen) amniocentesis (*amnion* membrane) aqueocentesis (*aqua* water) arthrocentesis (*arthron* joint) cardiocentesis (*kardia* heart) celiocentesis (also called *abdominocentesis*) (*koilia* belly) cephalocentesis (*kephale* head) colocentesis (also called *colopuncture*) (colon) cordocentesis (*chorda* string, cord) culdocentesis (*cul de sac* a blind pouch or cecum)

Element	From	Meaning	Examples
cente (cont'd)		[puncture]	enterocentesis (*enteron* intestine)
			keratocentesis (also called *keratonyxis*) (*keratos* horn: cornea)
			laryngocentesis (larynx)
			mastoideocentesis (mastoid process)
			ovariocentesis (ovary)
			peritoneocentesis (peritoneum)
			pleurocentesis (also called *thoracentesis*) (*pleura* rib, side)
			pneumocentesis (or, pneumonocentesis) (*pneumon* lung)
			rachiocentesis (also called *lumbar puncture*) (*rhachis* spine)
			thoracocentesis (also called *pleurocentesis*) (*thorax* chest)
			tympanocentesis (*tympanon* eardrum)
			CROSS REFERENCE: nyx, punct
centr	Greek *kentron*; Latin *centrum*	point, center	SIMPLE ROOT:
			centrad (toward the center or a center)
			centrage (the condition in which the centers of the various refracting surfaces of the eye are in the same straight line)
			central, centralis, centration
			centric, centricity, centrist, centriole
			centrum (the central portion of the body of a vertebra; pl., centra)
			PREFIXED ROOT:
			center: isocenter (*isos* equal)
			centr:
			concentrate (to bring to a common center), concentration, concentric (*con* with)
			decentration (*de* negative)
			central:
			epicentral (*epi* upon)
			intercentral (*inter* between)
			paracentral (near the center) (*para* alongside)
			pericentral (*peri* around)
			postcentral (*post* posterior)
			precentral (*pre* before)
			subcentral (*sub* below)
			supercentral (*super* above, over)
			unicentral (or, unicentric) (*uni* one)
			centri: ultracentrifuge (a high-speed centrifuge, up to 100,000 rpm) (*ultra* more, beyond + *fugere* to flee)
			centric:
			acentric (having no center; off center) (*a* privative)
			allocentric (also called *heterocentric*) (*allos* other)
			amphicentric (beginning and ending in the same vessel, as a branch of a rete mirabile) (*amphi* around, both) [rete mirabile: a vascular network]
			concentric (having a common center) (*con* with)
			dicentric (*di* two)
			eccentric (or, excentric; lit., away from the center) (*ek* out)
			heterocentric (also called *allocentric*) (*heteros* different, other)
			homocentric (having the same center or focus) (*homos* same)
			metacentric (*meta* after)
			multicentricity (also called *polycentricity*) (*multus* many)
			polycentric, polycentricity (also called *multicentricity*) (*polys* many)
			submetacentric (*sub* under + metacentric)
			centriole: procentriole (the early phase in development of centrioles of basal bodies from the centrosphere) (*pro* before)

Element	From	Meaning	Examples
centr (cont'd)		[point, center]	*centro*:
			eccentrochondroplasia (*ek* out + *chondros* cartilage + *plassein* to form)
			eccentropiesis (*ek* out + *piesis* pressure)
			centrum:
			hemicentrum (*hemi* half)
			microcentrum (also called *cytocentrum*) (*mikros* small)
			LEADING ROOT COMPOUND:
			centr: centrencephalic (*enkephalon* brain)
			centri:
			centriciput (the part of the head situated between the occiput and the sinciput; the midhead) (*caput* head) [occiput: back of the head]
			centrifugal, centrifugation, centrifuge (*fugere* to flee)
			centrilobular (or, centrolobular) (*lobus* lobe)
			centripetal (*petere* to seek)
			centro:
			centroblast (*blastos* germ, bud, shoot)
			centrocecal (also called *cecocentral*) (*caecus* blind—blind spot)
			centrocyte {centrocytic} (*kytos* cell)
			centrodesmose (or, centrodesmus) (*desmos* a band)
			centrokinesia {centrokinetic} (*kinein* to move)
			centrolecithal (*lekithos* egg yolk)
			centromere {centromeric} (*meros* part)
			centronucleus (also called *amphinucleus*) (nucleus)
			centro-osteosclerosis (also called *centrosclerosis*) (*osteon* bone + *sclerosis* hardening)
			centrophose (*phos* light)
			centroplasm, centroplast (*plassein* to form)
			centrosclerosis (shortening of *centro-osteosclerosis*; the filling of the marrow cavity with osseous, or bony, material) (*skleros* hard + *osis* condition)
			centrosome (*soma* body)
			centrosphere (the portion of the centrosome surrounding the centriole) (*sphere* ball)
			TRAILING ROOT COMPOUND:
			central: neurocentral (*neuron* nerve)
			centration: hemocentration (*haima* blood)
			centric:
			acrocentric (pertaining to a chromosome in which the centromere is located near one end) (*akron* extremity)
			angiocentric (also called *angiogenic*) (*angeion* vessel)
			egocentric (*ego* self, I)
			telocentric (*teleos* end, complete)
			centrum:
			cytocentrum (also called *microcentrum*) (*kytos* cell)
			neurocentrum (*neuron* nerve)
			pleurocentrum (*pleura* side, rib)
			CROSS REFERENCE: cente, foc, punct, scolop, spic
cephal	Greek *kephale*	head	SIMPLE ROOT: cephalic, cephalization
			PREFIXED ROOT:
			cephalgia: hemicephalalgia (also called *hemicrania*) (*hemi* half + *algos* pain)
			cephalgic: anticephalalgic (*anti* against + *algos* pain)

Element	From	Meaning	Examples
cephal (cont'd)		[head]	*cephalia*: acephalia (congenital absence of the head) (*a* privative) dyscephalia (or, dyscephaly) (*dys* abnormal) hemicephalia (*hemi* half) megacephalia (*mega* big) microcephalia {microcephalic} (*mikros* small) *cephalic*: encephalic (pertaining to the encephalon; within the skull) (*en* in, on) [see separate entry: encephal-] eurycephalic (*eurys* broad, wide) holocephalic (*holos* entire) intracephalic (within the head, or within the brain) (*intra* within) megacephalic (*mega* big, large) mesocephalic (or, mesocephalous; also called *normocephalic*) (*mesos* middle) pericephalic (*peri* around, near) procephalic (*pro* before, anterior) *cephalous*: acephalous (headless) (*a* privative) bicephalous (also called *dicephalous*) (*bi* two) dicephalous (also called *bicephalous*) (*di* two) megacephalous (*mega* big, large) *cephalus*: bicephalus (also called *dicephalus*) (*bi* two) diplocephalus (*diploos* double) heterocephalus (*heteros* other) hemicephalus (*hemi* half) monocephalus (also called *syncephalus*) (*monos* single) paracephalus (*para* alongside) peracephalus (a fetus or individual with a malformed head) (*per* completely + *acephalus*) syncephalus (also called *monocephalus*) (*syn* together) tricephalus (a fetal monster with three heads) (*tri* three) *cephaly*: acephaly (congenital absence of the head) (*a* privative) dicephaly (also called *diplocephaly*) {dicephalous} (*di* two) diplocephaly (also called *dicephaly*) (*diploos* double) dyscephaly (or, dyscephalia) (*dys* abnormal) macrocephaly {macrocephalic} (*makros* long, large) megacephaly (*mega* big, large) megalocephaly (also called *macrocephaly*) (*megalos* large) microcephaly {microcephalic} (*mikros* small) LEADING ROOT COMPOUND: *cephal*: cephalad (proceeding toward the head) (*ad* to) cephalalgia (headache; also called *cephalodynia*) (*algos* pain) cephaledema (*edema* swelling) cephalemia (*emia* blood condition) cephalhematocele (*haima* blood + *kele* tumor) cephalhematoma (*haima* blood + *oma* tumor) cephalhydrocele (*hydor* water + *kele* tumor) cephalodynia (headache; also called *cephalalgia*) (*odyne* pain) *cephalo*: cephalocaudal (from head to tail) (*cauda* tail)

Element	From	Meaning	Examples
cephal (cont'd)		[head]	cephalocele (protrusion of the brain from the cranial cavity; also called *encephalocele*) (*kele* hernia)
			cephalocentesis (*kentein* to puncture)
			cephalochord (*chorde* cord)
			cephalodactyly (malformation of the head and digits) (*daktylos* finger, toe)
			cephalodidymus (*didymos* twin)
			cephalodiprosopus (*di* twice + *prosopus* face)
			cephalodymus {cephalodymia} (*didymos* twin)
			cephalogenesis (*genere* produce)
			cephalogram, cephalograph (*graphein* to write)
			cephalogyric (*gyros* a turn)
			cephalohemometer (*haima* blood + *metron* measure)
			cephalomegaly (*megalos* great)
			cephalomelus (*melos* a limb)
			cephalomenia (*men* month: menstruation)
			cephalometer (also called *craniometer*) {cephalometry} (*metron* measure)
			cephalopagus (also called *craniopagus*) (*pagos* fixation)
			cephalopathy (*pathos* disease)
			cephalopelvic, cephalopelvimetry (pelvis + *metron* measure)
			cephaloplegia (*plessein* to strike)
			cephalorhachidian (*rhachis* spine)
			cephalothoracopagus (*thorax* chest + *pagos* fixation)
			cephalotome, cephalotomy (*tomy* incision)
			cephalotribe (*tribein* to crush)
			TRAILING ROOT COMPOUND:
			cephalalgia: faciocephalalgia (*facies* face + *algos* pain)
			cephalia:
			acrocephalia (also called *oxycephaly*) (*akron* extremity)
			oxycephalia (or, oxycephaly; also called *acrocephalia*) (*oxys* sharp)
			pachycephalia (*pachys* thick)
			trochocephalia (*trokhos* wheel, runner)
			cephalic:
			acrocephalic (*akron* extremity)
			cymbocephalic (also called *scaphocephalic*) (*kymbe* boat)
			cynocephalic (*kynos* dog)
			dolichocephalic (or, dolichocephalous) (*dolichos* long)
			hydrocephalic (*hydor* water)
			hypsibrachycephalic (*hypsos* high + *brachys* broad, wide)
			hypsocephalic (*hypsos* high)
			medicephalic (*medius* middle)
			normocephalic (also called *mesocephalic*)
			orthocephalic (*orthos* straight)
			oxycephalic (*oxys* sharp)
			pachycephalic (*pachys* thick)
			cephalitis: meningocephalitis (*menix* membrane + *itis* inflammation)
			cephalous:
			acrocephalous (*akron* extremity)
			atelocephalous (*ateles* incomplete)
			cephalus:
			homalocephalus (*homalos* flat)
			ethmocephalus (*ethmos* sieve)
			omocephalus (*omos* shoulder)

Element	From	Meaning	Examples
cephal (cont'd)		[head]	opocephalus (*ops* face) pseudacephalus (*pseudes* false + *a* privative) pyocephalus (brain abscess; also called *pyoencephalus*) (*pyon* pus) schistocephalus (*schistos* split) *cephaly*: acrocephaly (*akron* extremity) brachycephaly {brachycephalic} (*brachys* short) leptocephaly {leptocephalic} (*leptos* slender) otocephaly (*otos* ear) oxycephaly (also called *acrocephalia*) (*oxys* sharp) pelvicephalography (*pyelos* pelvis + *graphein* to write) perocephalus (also called *strophocephalus*) (*peros* maimed) plagiocephaly {plagiocephalic} (*plagios* oblique) platycephaly {platycephalic} (*platys* flat) pneumatocephalus (*pneumatos* air) rhinocephaly (*rhinos* nose) scaphocephaly {scaphocephalic} (*scaphe* boat) sphenocephaly (*sphenos* wedge) stenocephaly (*stenos* narrow) tapeinocephaly {tapeinocephalic} (*tapeinos* low-lying) tectocephaly (also called *scaphocephaly*) {tectocephalic} (*tectum* roof) PREFIXED TRAILING ROOT COMPOUND: subscaphocephaly (*sub* under + *skaphe* skiff) ultrabrachycephalic (*ultra* beyond + *brachys* short) ultradolichocephalic (*ultra* beyond + *dolichos* long) CROSS REFERENCE: capit, cran
ceps			See capit- for *biceps, triceps*.
cerat			See kerat- for *ceratocricoid*.
cereb	Latin *cerebrum*	brain	SIMPLE ROOT: cerebellum (diminutive of *cerebrum*; pl., cerebella) {cerebellar} cerebron (a crystalline cerebroside from brain tissue) cerebrum (the largest part of the brain consisting of two hemispheres separated by a deep longitudinal fissure) {cerebral} PREFIXED ROOT: *cerebellar*: intracerebellar (*intra* within) paracerebellar (*para* alongside) supracerebellar (*supra* above) *cerebr*: decerebrate, decerebration, decerebrize (*de* removal) *cerebral*: infracerebral (*infra* below) intercerebral (*inter* between) intracerebral (*intra* within) supracerebral (*supra* above) *cerebrum*: hemicerebrum {hemicerebral} (*hemi* half) LEADING ROOT COMPOUND: *cerebell*: cerebellitis (*itis* inflammation) *cerebelli*: cerebellifugal (*fugere* to flee) cerebellipetal (*petere* to seek) *cerebello*: cerebellofugal (or, cerebellifugal) (*fugere* to flee)

Element	From	Meaning	Examples
cereb (cont'd)		[brain]	cerebellolental (lens—of eye)
			cerebellomedullary (*medulla* marrow)
			cerebellopontine (*pons* bridge)
			cerebellorubrial (*ruber* red)
			cerebellospinal (spine)
			cerebr:
			cerebritis (*itis* inflammation)
			cerebroid (resembling the cerebral substance) (*eidos* form)
			cerebroma (also called *encephaloma*) (*oma* tumor)
			cerebrosis (any disorder of the cerebrum; also called *encephalosis*) (*osis* condition)
			cerebri:
			cerebriform (*forma* shape)
			cerebrifugal (*fugere* to flee)
			cerebripetal (*petere* to seek)
			cerebro:
			cerebrocerebellar (pertaining to the cerebrum and the cerebellum)
			cerebrocortical (*cortex* rind—the outer portion of an organ)
			cerebromacular (also called *maculocerebral*) (*macula* spot)
			cerebromalacia (abnormal softness of the substance of the cerebrum; also called *encephalomalacia*) (*malakos* soft)
			cerebromeningitis (*meningos* membrane + *itis* inflammation)
			cerebropathia (or, cerebropathy) (*pathos* disease)
			cerebropontile (pertaining to the cerebrum and pons) (*pontis* bridge) [pons: any bridgelike formation connecting two more or less disjointed parts of the same structure]
			cerebrorachidian (also called *cerebrospinal*) (*rhachis* spine)
			cerebrosclerosis (morbid hardening of the substance of the cerebrum) (*skleros* hard + *osis* condition)
			cerebrospinal (also called *cerebrorachidian*)
			cerebrotomy (incision of the brain substance; anatomy or dissection of the brain) (*tomy* incision)
			cerebrotonia (personality pattern) (*tonos* tone) [term rarely used]
			cerebrovascular (pertaining to the blood vessels and blood supply of the brain) (*vas* vessel)
			TRAILING ROOT COMPOUND:
			cerebellar:
			cerebrocerebellar (*cerebrum* brain)
			spinocerebellar (spine)
			cerebellum:
			neocerebellum (*neos* new)
			paleocerebellum (*palaios* old, ancient)
			vestibulocerebellum (vestibule)
			cerebral:
			craniocerebral (*kranion* skull)
			dextrocerebral (*dexter* right)
			maculocerebral (pertaining to the macula retinae and the brain; also called *cerebromacular*) (*macula* spot)
			sinistrocerebral (located in the left cerebral hemisphere) (*sinister* left)
			cerebritis brain inflammation:
			meningocerebritis (*meningos* membrane)
			otocerebritis (*otos* ear)
			CROSS REFERENCE: encephal, ment, phren[2], psych, thym[2]
ceros			See kerat- for *megaloceros*.

Element	From	Meaning	Examples
cervi	Latin *cervix* neck	neck neck of an organ; neck of a tooth	SIMPLE ROOT: cervix (designates the lower front portion of the part connecting the head and trunk, or a constricted part of an organ; pl., cervixes, cervices) {cervical, or cervicalis}

SIMPLE ROOT: cervix (designates the lower front portion of the part connecting the head and trunk, or a constricted part of an organ; pl., cervixes, cervices) {cervical, or cervicalis}
PREFIXED ROOT:
cervical:
ectocervical (*ektos* outside)
endocervical (*endon* within)
intracervical (*intra* within)
mesiocervical (also called *mesiogingival*) (*mesos* middle)
paracervical (*para* alongside)
retrocervical (back of the cervix uteri) (*retro* behind)
cervix:
ectocervix (or, exocervix) (*ektos* outside)
endocervix (*endon* within)
exocervix (or, ectocervix) (*exo* outside, outward)
paracervix (*para* alongside)
LEADING ROOT COMPOUND:
cervi: cervimeter (*metron* measure)
cervic:
cervicectomy (removal of the cervix uteri) (*ektome* excision)
cervicitis (*itis* inflammation)
cervicodynia (*odyne* pain)
cervico:
cervicoaxillary (pertaining to the neck and the axilla) (*axilla* the fossa axillaris: a small hollow underneath the arm)
cervicobrachial, cervicobrachialgia (*brachion* arm + *algos* pain)
cervicocolpitis (also called *cervicovaginitis*) (*kolpos* vagina + *itis* inflammation)
cervicodorsal (*dorsum* back)
cervicofacial (*facies* face)
cervicolabial (*labium* lip—lip side of the neck of an incisor or a canine tooth)
cervicolingual (*lingua* tongue)
cervicooccipital (*occiput* back of head)
cervicopexy (*pexis* fixation)
cervicoplasty (*plassein* to form)
cervicoscapular (*scapula* shoulder blade)
cervicoscopy (*skopein* to examine)
cervicothoracic (thorax)
cervicotomy (incision of the neck; incision of the uterine cervix) (*tomy* incision)
cervicouterine (uterus)
cervicovaginal, cervicovaginitis (also called *cervicocolpitis*) (vagina + *itis* inflammation)
cervicovesical (also called *vesicocervical*) (*vesica* bladder)
TRAILING ROOT COMPOUND:
buccocervical (*bucca* cheek)
costicervical (*costa* side, rib)
craniocervical (*kranion* skull)
distocervical (*distans* distant)
faciocervical (*facies* face)
labiocervical (also called *labiogingival*) (*labium* lip)
linguocervical (also called *linguogingival*) (*lingua* tongue)
occipitocervical (*occiput* back of head: *ob* against + *caput* head)

Element	From	Meaning	Examples
cervi (cont'd)		[neck; neck of an organ or tooth]	occlusocervical (pertaining to the occlusal surface and neck of a tooth) thyrocervical (relating to the thyroid gland and the neck; denoting an arterial trunk) ureterocervical (ureter) uterocervical (pertaining to the uterus and the cervix uteri) vesicocervical (*vesica* bladder) TERM: cervix uteri (the neck of the uterus) CROSS REFERENCE: trachel
chalas, calat	Greek *chalao* to abate, release	relaxation, loosening	SIMPLE ROOT: chalasia (or, chalasis; relaxation of a bodily opening) PREFIXED ROOT: *calation:* excalation (absence, suppression, or failure of development of one in a series of structures, e.g., a digit, vertebra) (*ex* from) *chalasia:* achalasia (also called *cardiospasm*) (*a* negative) TRAILING ROOT COMPOUND: *chalasin:* cytochalasin (*kytos* cell) *chalasis:* arthrochalasis (*arthron* joint) blepharochalasis (*blepharon* eyelid) cardiochalasia (*kardia* heart) dermatochalasis (a tissue disorder in which the skin hangs in loose pendulous folds; also called *cutis laxa*) (*dermatos* skin) CROSS REFERENCE: pares
chancr			See cancr- for *chancriform.*
cheil, chil	Greek *cheilos* lip	lip, edge, brim	PREFIXED ROOT: *cheilia:* acheilia {acheilous} (*a* privative) dicheilia (the appearance of a double lip) (*di* two) macrocheilia (or, macrochilia) (*makros* large) microcheilia (or, microchilia; abnormal smallness of the lips) (*mikros* small) procheilia (or, prochilia; protruding lips) (*pro* before) syncheilia (or, synchilia; congenital adhesion of the lips or atresia of the mouth) (*sym* together) LEADING ROOT COMPOUND: *cheil:* cheilalgia (or, chilalgia) (*algos* pain) cheilectomy (excision of a lip; the operation of chiseling off the irregular bony edges of a joint cavity which interfere with motion) (*ektome* excision) cheilectropion (eversion of the lip) (*ektrope* a turning aside) cheilitis (*itis* inflammation) cheilosis (a particular disorder of the lips) (*osis* condition) *cheilo:* cheiloangioscopy (*angeion* blood vessel + *skopein* to examine) cheilocarcinoma (*karkinos* crab, cancer + *oma* tumor) cheilognathoglossoschisis (*gnathos* jaw + *glossa* tongue + *schisis* fissure) cheilognathopalatoschisis (*gnathos* jaw + *palate* roof of mouth + *schisis* fissure) cheilognathoprosoposchisis (*gnathos* jaw + *prosopon* face + *schisis* fissure)

Element	From	Meaning	Examples
cheil (cont'd)		[lip, edge]	cheilophagia (biting of the lips) (*phagein* to devour)
			cheiloplasty (plastic operation upon the lips; also called *labioplasty*) (*plassein* to form)
			cheilorrhaphy (*rhaphe* suture)
			cheiloschisis (harelip) (*schisis* fissure)
			cheilostomatoplasty (*stoma* mouth + *plassein* to form)
			cheilotomy (*tomy* incision)
			chil:
			chilalgia (or, cheilalgia) (*algos* pain)
			chilectomy (or, cheilectomy) (*ektome* excision)
			chilitis (or, cheilitis) (*itis* inflammation)
			chilosis (or, cheilosis) (*osis* condition)
			TRAILING ROOT COMPOUND:
			ankylocheilia (*ankylos* fused)
			atelocheilia (*atelos* incomplete: *a* negative + *telos* end)
			brachycheilia (or, brachychilia) (*brachys* short)
			opisthocheilia (recession of the lips) (*opisthen* behind)
			pachycheilia (thickening of the lips) (*pachys* thick)
			rhinocheiloplasty (*rhinos* nose + *plassein* to form)
			CROSS REFERENCE: labi[1]
cheir			See chir-.
chem	Greek *chein*	to pour	SIMPLE ROOT: chemical, chemist, chemistry
			LEADING ROOT COMPOUND:
			chem: chemurgy (chemistry applied to the industrial use of raw organic products, especially agricultural products) (*ergon* work)
			chemi:
			chemiluminescence (luminescence produced by direct transformation of chemical energy into light energy) (*luminare* to shine)
			chemisorption (or, chemosorption) (*sorbere* to suck in)
			chemico: chemicocautery (or, chemocautery; also called *chemical cautery*)
			chemo:
			chemobiotic (the combination of a chemotherapeutic agent and an antibiotic) (*bios* life)
			chemocautery (*kalein* to burn)
			chemoceptor (*capere* to hold, take)
			chemodectoma (a relatively rare, usually benign tumor originating in chemoreceptor tissue; also called *aortic-body tumor, glomus jugulare tumor*) (*dektikos* receptive + *oma* tumor)
			chemohormonal (hormone)
			chemokinesis (chemokinetic} (*kinein* to move)
			chemolysis (chemical decomposition) (*lyein* to loosen)
			chemomorphosis (*morphe* form + *osis* condition)
			chemosorption (or, chemisorption) (*sorbere* to suck in)
			chemotaxis {chemotactic} (*tassein* to arrange)
			chemotherapy (*therapy* treatment)
			chemotropic (elicited by chemical stimulation) (*trope* a turning)
			TRAILING ROOT COMPOUND:
			cytochemistry (*kytos* cell)
			histochemistry (*histos* web, tissue)
			iatrochemistry (*iatrien* to heal)
			neurochemistry (*neuron* nerve)
			pharmacochemistry (*pharmakon* medicine, drug)

Element	From	Meaning	Examples
chem (cont'd)		[to pour]	physiochemistry (*physis* nature) psychochemistry (*psyche* mind) radiochemistry (radium) zymochemistry (*zyme* leaven, fermentation) CROSS REFERENCE: None
chez	Greek *chezein*	to defecate	PREFIXED ROOT: allochezia (the discharge of nonfecal matter by the anus, or the discharge of fecal matter by an abnormal passage) (*allos* other) dyschezia (or, dyschesia; difficult or painful evacuation of feces from the rectum) (*dys* abnormal) TRAILING ROOT COMPOUND: hematochezia (the passage of bloody feces) (*hematos* blood) pyochezia (presence of pus in the stools; also called *pyofecia*) (*pyon* pus) urochezia (or, urochesia; the discharge of urine in the feces) (*ouron* urine) CROSS REFERENCE: copr, sterc
chir, **cheir**	Greek *cheir*	hand	SIMPLE ROOT: chiral, chirality (the property of handedness) PREFIXED ROOT: *cheiria*: acheiria (congenital absence of one or both hands) (*a* privative) dicheiria (also called *diplocheiria*) (*di* two) diplocheiria (also called *dicheiria*) (*diploos* two-fold) dyscheiria (or, dychiria) {dyscheirial, dychirial} (*dys* abnormal) macrocheiria (or, macrochiria; long-handedness; also called *megalocheiria*) (*makros* large) megalocheiria (also called *macrocheiria*) (*megalos* large) microcheiria (*mikros* small) polycheiria (or, polychiria; the condition of having more than two hands) (*polys* many) syncheiria (or, synchiria) (*syn* with, together) tricheiria (a developmental anomaly characterized by tripling of a hand) (*tri* three) *chiral*: heterochiral (reversed as regards right and left, but otherwise the same in form and size) (*heteros* other) *chiria*: allochiria (or, allocheiria) (*allos* other) dyschiria (derangement of the power to tell which side of the body has been touched) (*dys* abnormal) synchiria (or, syncheiria) (*sym* with) *chiro*: acheiropody (a developmental anomaly characterized by absence of hands and feet) (*a* privative + *pous* foot) *chirus*: tetrachirus (*tetra* four) LEADING ROOT COMPOUND: *cheir*: cheiragra (gout in the hand) (*agra* seizure) cheiralgia (*algos* pain) cheirarthritis (*arthron* joint + *itis* inflammation) *cheiro*: cheirology (signing; also called *dactylology*) (*logos* word) cheiromegaly (or, chiromegaly) (*megalos* large) cheiroplasty (or, chiroplasty) (*plassein* to form) cheiropodalgia (*pous* foot + *algos* pain)

Element	From	Meaning	Examples
chir (cont'd)		[hand]	cheiroscope (*skopein* to examine)
			cheirospasm (*spasmos* contraction)
			chiro:
			chirognostic (having the ability to distinguish the right from the left, as of the hands or of which side of the body is touched) (*gnosis* knowledge)
			chirokinesthesia {chirokinesthetic} (*kinein* to move + *esthesia* perception)
			cheirology (also called *dactylology*) (*logos* word)
			chiromegaly (also called *megalocheiria*) (*megalos* large)
			chiroplasty (or, cheiroplasty) (*plassein* to form)
			chiropodist (podiatrist), chiropody (treatment of minor disorders of the foot; also called *podiatry*) (*pous* foot)
			chiropractic (or, chiropraxis; the manipulation of joints, especially of the spine), chiropractor (*prassein* to do)
			chirospasm (or, cheirospasm) (*spasmos* contraction)
			TRAILING ROOT COMPOUND:
			acephalochiria, acephalochirus (*a* privative + *kephale* head)
			ectrochiry (or, ectrocheiry) (*ektrosis* absence)
			perochirus (a fetus with malformed hands) (*peros* maimed)
			DISGUISED ROOT: surgeon, surgery (from *cheirourgia*, lit., a working with the hands; handicraft; skill)
			CROSS REFERENCE: dactyl
chlor	Greek *chloros*	green	SIMPLE ROOT:
			chloral (an oily liquid having a bitter taste; chloral hydrate)
			chlorate (a salt of chloric acid)
			chloride, chlorinated, chlorine, chlorite (a salt of chlorous acid: used as a disinfectant and bleaching agent)
			chlorous (derived from or containing trivalent chlorine)
			PREFIXED ROOT:
			achlorhydria (a stomach disorder in which the stomach fails to secrete hydrochloric acid) (*a* negative + *hydor* water)
			bichloride (*bi* two)
			dechloridation (or, dechlorination) (*de* opposite)
			hyperchloremia (excess of chloride in the blood; also called *chloremia*) (*hyper* above + chloremia)
			hyperchloruria (*hyper* above + chloruria)
			hypochloremia (also called *chloroprivic*) {hypochloremic} (*hypo* under + chloremia)
			hypochloruria (*hypo* under + chloruria)
			polychloruria (*polys* many, much + chloruria)
			subchloride (*sub* under)
			LEADING ROOT COMPOUND:
			chlor:
			chloremia (also called *hyperchloremia, chlorosis*) (*emia* blood condition)
			chloroma (a malignant green-colored tumor) (*oma* tumor)
			chloropia (or, chloropsia; a vision defect in which all things appear green) (*opia* vision condition)
			chlorosis (also called *chloremia, hyperchloremia*) {chlorotic} (*osis* condition)
			chloruresis (also called *chloriduria*) (*uresis* passage of urine)
			chloruria (*uria* urine condition)

Element	From	Meaning	Examples
chlor (cont'd)		[green]	*chlorid*: chloriduria (excess of chlorides in the urine; also called *chloruresis*) (*uria* urine condition)
			chloridi: chloridimeter {chloridimetry} (*metron* measure)
			chlorido: chloridometer (*meter* measure)
			chloro:
			chloroform, chloroformism (the habitual use of chloroform for its narcotic effect) (*formica* ant)
			chloroleukemia (also called *chloroma*) (*leukos* white + *emia* blood condition)
			chloropenia (*penia* deficiency)
			chlorophane (a green-yellow pigment in the retina) (*phainein* to show)
			chlorophyll (the green coloring matter of plants) (*phyllon* leaf)
			chloroplast (*plassein* to form)
			chloroprivic (also called *hypochloremic*) (*privare* to deprive)
			CROSS REFERENCE: None
chol	Greek *chole*	gall, bile	SIMPLE ROOT: cholera {choleraic}, choleric (hot-tempered; bilious), cholic (or, choleic)
			PREFIXED ROOT:
			chol:
			anticholinesterase (action that opposes the action of cholinesterase) (*anti* against)
			pericholangitis (*peri* around + *angeion* vessel + *itis* inflammation)
			chole:
			anticholelithogenic (serving to prevent the formation of gallstones) (*anti* against + *lithos* stone + *genere* to produce)
			isocholesterol (*isos* equal + *stereos* solid + *ol* oil)
			cholera: paracholera (*para* resembling)
			cholia:
			acholia (lack or absence of the secretion of bile) (*a* privative)
			dyscholia (a disordered condition of the bile) (*dys* abnormal)
			eucholia (normal condition of the bile) (*eu* well)
			hypercholia (*hyper* above, over)
			polycholia (excessive flow or secretion of bile) (*polys* much)
			syncholia (*syn* together)
			cholic: acholic (free from bile) (*a* privative)
			choluria bile condition in the urine:
			acholuria (absence of bile pigments in the urine) (*a* privative)
			hypocholuria (*hypo* below)
			LEADING ROOT COMPOUND:
			chol:
			cholagogic, cholagogue (*agein* to lead)
			cholangium [see separate entry: cholang-]
			cholanopoiesis {cholanopoietic} (*ano* upward + *poiein* to make)
			cholemesis (*emein* to vomit)
			cholemia {cholemic} (*emia* blood condition)
			cholemimetry (*haima* blood + *metron* measure) [h of haima elided]
			choleresis {choleretic} (*hairesis* a taking) [h of hairesis is elided]
			choluria (*uria* urine condition)
			chole:
			cholechromopoesis (*chroma* color + *poiein* to make, produce)
			cholecyst (*kystis* bladder) [see separate entry: cholecyst-]
			choledochus [see separate entry: choledoch-]

Element	From	Meaning	Examples
chol (cont'd)		[gall, bile]	cholelithiasis (*lithos* stone + *iasis* condition)
			cholepathia (*pathia* disease)
			choleperitoneum (the presence of bile in the peritoneum; also called *biliary peritonitis, choleperitonitis*)
			cholepoiesis {cholepoietic} (*poiein* to make, produce)
			cholerrhagia {cholerrhagic} (*rhagia* bursting forth)
			cholestasis (or, cholestasia) {cholestatic} (*stasis* standing still)
			cholesterol (*stereos* solid + *ole* oil) [see separate entry: cholester-]
			choletherapy (*therapy* treatment)
			choleuria (*uria* urine condition)
			choler: choleroid (also called *choleriform*) (*eidos* form)
			cholera:
			choleragen (*genere* to produce)
			choleraphage (*phagein* to consume)
			choli: cholicele (*kele* tumor)
			cholo:
			cholochrome (any biliary pigment) (*chroma* color)
			cholocyanin (also called *bilicyanin*) (*kyanos* blue)
			chologenetic (also called *cholepoietic*) (*genere* to produce)
			cholohemothorax (presence of bile and blood in the thorax)
			chololithiasis (*lithos* stone + *iasis* condition)
			choloplania (*planan* to wander)
			cholopoiesis (or, cholepoiesis) (*poiein* to produce)
			cholothorax (*thorax* chest)
			TRAILING ROOT COMPOUND:
			albuminocholia (the presence of albumin in the bile)
			bactericholia (bacteria in the bile)
			melancholia (or, melancholy; severe depression) {melancholic} (*melos* dark)
			oligocholia (a deficient secretion of bile) (*oligos* scant)
			pachycholia (*pachys* thick)
			uricocholia (the presence of uric acid in the bile) (*ouron* urine)
			PREFIXED TRAILING ROOT COMPOUND: hypomelancholia (mild depression) (*hypo* under + *melanos* dark)
			CROSS REFERENCE: bil
cholang	Greek *chole* bile + *angeion* vessel	bile vessel	SIMPLE ROOT: cholangiole (a small bile duct)
			PREFIXED ROOT: pericholangitis (*peri* around + cholangitis)
			LEADING ROOT COMPOUND:
			cholang: cholangitis (or, choleangitis) (*itis* inflammation)
			cholangi:
			cholangiectasis (*ektasis* dilatation)
			cholangioma (*oma* tumor)
			cholangio:
			cholangioadenoma (*adenos* gland + *oma* tumor)
			cholangiocarcinoma (*carcinoma* cancerous tumor)
			cholangiocyte (*kytos* cell)
			cholangioenterostomy (*enteron* intestine + *stoma* opening)
			cholangiofibrosis (fibrosis of the bile ducts)
			cholangiogastrostomy (*gaster* belly + *stoma* mouth, opening)
			cholangiogram, cholangiography (*graphein* to write)
			cholangiohepatoma (*hepatoma* liver tumor)
			cholangioscopy (*skopein* to examine)
			cholangiostomy (*stoma* mouth, opening)

Element	From	Meaning	Examples
cholang (cont'd)		[bile vessel]	cholangiotomy (*tomy* incision) *cholangiol*: cholangiolitis (*itis* inflammation) TRAILING ROOT COMPOUND: duodenocholangeitis (duodenum + *itis* inflammation) hepatocholangeitis (*hepar* liver + *itis* inflammation) CROSS REFERENCE: None
cholecyst	Greek *chole* bile + *kystis* bladder	gall bladder	SIMPLE ROOT: cholecyst (gall bladder) {cholecystic} LEADING ROOT COMPOUND: *cholecys*: cholecystomy (*tomy* incision) *cholecyst*: cholecystagogue (*agein* to lead) cholecystatony (*atony* lack of tone) cholecystectasia (*ektasis* dilation, distention) cholecystectomy (*ektome* excision) cholecystenterostomy (*enteron* intestine + *stoma* mouth) cholecystenterotomy (*enteron* intestine + *tomy* incision) cholecystitis (*itis* inflammation) cholecystosis (*osis* condition) *cholecysto*: cholecystocolotomy (colon + *tomy* incision) cholecystoduodenostomy (duodenum + *stoma* mouth, opening) cholecystoenterotomy (*enteron* intestine + *tomy* incision) cholecystogastric (*gaster* stomach, belly) cholecystogram, cholecystography (*graphein* to write) cholecystoileostomy (ileum + *stoma* mouth, opening) cholecystointestinal (also called *cholecystenteric*) cholecystojejunostomy (jejunum + *stoma* mouth, opening) cholecystokinetic (*kinein* to move) cholecystolithotripsy (*lithos* stone + *tribein* to rub, crush) cholecystopathy (*pathos* disease) cholecystopexy (*pexis* fixation) cholecystoptosis (*ptosis* a falling) cholecystorrhaphy (*rhaphe* suture) cholecystostomy (*stoma* mouth, opening) cholecystotomy (or, cholecystomy) (*tomy* incision) TRAILING ROOT COMPOUND: *cholecystitis* inflammation of the gall bladder: hemocholecystitis (*haima* blood) pleurocholecystitis (*pleura* rib, side) pseudocholecystitis (*pseudes* false) CROSS REFERENCE: None
choledoch	Greek *chole* bile + *dochus* receptacle	bile duct	SIMPLE ROOT: choledochus (common bile duct) {choledochal} PREFIXED ROOT: megacholedochus (*megas* large) LEADING ROOT COMPOUND: *choledoch*: choledochectomy (*ektome* excision) choledochendysis (also called *choledochotomy*) (*endysis* an entering in) choledochitis (*itis* inflammation) *choledocho*: choledochocele (*kele* hernia) choledochoduodenostomy (duodenum + *stoma* mouth, opening) choledochoenterostomy (*enteron* intestine + *stoma* mouth, opening)

A Thesaurus of Medical Word Roots

Element	From	Meaning	Examples
choledoch (cont'd)		[bile duct]	choledochogastrostomy (*gaster* stomach, belly + *stoma* opening) choledochogram, choledochography (*graphein* to write) choledochohepatostomy (*hepatos* liver + *stoma* opening) choledochoileostomy (ileum + *stoma* mouth, opening) choledochojejunostomy (jejunum + *stoma* mouth, opening) choledocholithiasis (*lithos* stone + *iasis* condition) choledocholithotomy (*lithos* stone + *tomy* incision) choledocholithotripsy (*lithos* stone + *tribein* to rub, crush) choledochoplasty (*plassein* to form) choledochorrhaphy (*rhaphe* suture) choledochoscope (*skopein* to examine) choledochostomy (*stoma* mouth, opening) choledochotomy (*tomy* incision) CROSS REFERENCE: None
cholester	Greek *chole* bile + *stereos* solid	cholesterol	SIMPLE ROOT: cholesterol (so called, because the substance was first found in the gall bladder) (*ole* oil, fat) PREFIXED ROOT: hypercholesterolemia (*hyper* above + *emia* blood condition) hypocholesterolemia (*hypo* below + *emia* blood condition) LEADING ROOT COMPOUND: *cholester*: cholesterosis (or, cholesterolosis) (*osis* condition) *cholesterol*: cholesterolemia (*emia* blood condition) cholesterolosis (*osis* condition) cholesteroluria (*uria* urine condition) *cholesterolo*: cholesterologenesis (*genere* to produce) cholesterolopoiesis (*poiein* to make, produce) CROSS REFERENCE: None
chondr	Greek *chondros* grain	cartilage	SIMPLE ROOT: chondral, chondric PREFIXED ROOT: dyschondrogenesis (*dys* abnormal + *genere* to produce) dyschondroplasia (*dys* abnormal + *plassein* to form) dyschondrosteosis (*dys* abnormal + *osteon* bone + *osis* condition) ecchondroma (also called *echondrosis*) (*ek* from + *oma* tumor) ecchondrotome (*ek* from + *tome* a cutting instrument) enchondroma (also called *intracartilaginous*) {enchondromatous} (*en* in + *oma* tumor) endochondral (also called *intrachondral*) (*endon* within) entochondrostosis (*entos* inside + *ostosis* bone condition) hypochondrium (*hypo* under) interchondral (also called *intercartilaginous*) (*inter* between) intrachondral (or, intrachondrial; also called *endochondral*) (*intra* within) perichondrium {perichondral, perichondrial}, perichondritis (*peri* around + *itis* inflammation) perichondroma (*peri* around + *oma* tumor) polychondritis (*polys* many + *itis* inflammation) polychondropathia (relapsing polychondritis) (*polys* many + *pathia* disease) prochondral (occurring previous to the formation of cartilage) (*pro* before) subchondral (also called *subcartilaginous*) (*sub* under)

A Thesaurus of Medical Word Roots

Element	From	Meaning	Examples
chondr (cont'd)		[cartilage]	synchondrectomy (*syn* with + *ektome* excision)
			synchondrosis (*syn* with + *osis* condition)
			synchondrotomy (*syn* with + *tomy* incision)
			LEADING ROOT COMPOUND:
			chondr:
			chondralgia (also called *chondrodynia*) (*algos* pain)
			chondralloplasia (also called *dyschondroplasia*) (*allos* other + *plassein* to form)
			chondrectomy (*ektome* excision)
			chondritis (*itis* inflammation)
			chondrodynia (also called *chondralgia*) (*odyne* pain)
			chondroid (*eidos* form)
			chondroma {chondromatous}, chondromatosis (*oma* tumor + *osis* condition)
			chondrosteoma (*osteoma* bone tumor)
			chondri: chondrification, chondrify (*facere* to make)
			chondrio: chondriosome (*soma* body)
			chondro:
			chondroangioma (*angeion* blood vessel + *oma* tumor)
			chondroblast, chondroblastoma (*blastos* germ + *oma* tumor)
			chondrocalcinosis (calcium + *osis* condition)
			chondrocarcinoma (*karkinos* cancer + *oma* tumor)
			chondroclast (*klaein* to break)
			chondrocostal (*costa* rib, side)
			chondrocranial (*kranion* skull)
			chondrocyte (*kytos* cell)
			chondrodermatitis (*derma* skin + *itis* inflammation)
			chondrodysplasia (also called *dyschondroplasia*) (*dys* abnormal + *plassein* to form)
			chondrodystrophia (or, chondrodystrophy) (*dys* abnormal + *trophein* to nourish)
			chondroectodermal (*ektos* outside + *derma* skin)
			chondrofibroma (a mixed tumor of chondroma and fibroma; also called *fibrochondroma*) (*fibra* fiber + *oma* tumor)
			chondrogenesis {chondrogenic} (*genere* to produce)
			chondroglossus (*glossa* tongue)
			chondrolipoma (also called *lipochondroma*) (*lipos* fat + *oma* tumor)
			chondrology (*logos* study)
			chondrolysis (*lyein* to loosen)
			chondromalacia (*malakos* soft)
			chondromere (*meros* part)
			chondromyxoma (*myxa* mucus + *oma* tumor)
			chondromyxosarcoma (*myxa* mucus + *sarkos* flesh + *oma* tumor)
			chondroosseous (*ossa* bone)
			chondropathy (*pathy* disease)
			chondrophyte (*phyton* plant: growth)
			chondroplasia, chondroplast (also called *chondroblast*), chondroplasty (*plassein* to form)
			chondroporosis (*porosis* pore condition)
			chondrosarcoma (*sarkos* flesh + *oma* tumor)
			chondrosternoplasty (*sternon* chest + *plassein* to form)
			chondrotome, chondrotomy (*tomy* incision)
			chondrotrophic (*trophein* to nourish)
			chondroxiphoid (*xiphos* sword + *eidos* appearance)

Element	From	Meaning	Examples
chondr (cont'd)		[cartilage]	TRAILING ROOT COMPOUND: *chondral* pertaining to cartilage: costochondral (*costa* rib, side) osteochondral (*osteon* bone) vertebrochondral (vertebra) *chondrion*: mitochondrion (pl., mitochondria) (*mitos* thread) *chondritis* inflammation of cartilage: arthrochondritis (*arthron* joint) costochondritis (*costa* rib, side) fibrochondritis (also called *inochondritis*) (fiber) inochondritis (also called *fibrochondritis*) (*inos* fiber) osteochondritis (*osteon* bone) *chondroma* cartilaginous tumor: adenochondroma (also called *pulmonary hamartoma*; pl., adeno-chondromas, adenochondromata (*adenos* gland) fibrochondroma (also called *chondrofibroma*) (*fibra* fiber) lipochondroma (also called *chondrolipoma*) (*lipos* fat) myxochondroma (*myxa* mucus) osteochondroma (*osteon* bone) rhabdomyochondroma (*rhabdos* rod + *myos* muscle) *chondrium*: protochondrium (*protos* first) *chondrodystrophy*: osteochondrodystrophy (*osteon* bone + dystrophy) *chondropathy*: osteochondropathy (*osteon* bone + *pathos* disease) CROSS REFERENCE: cartilag
chord, **cord**	Greek *chorde*	cord, string	SIMPLE ROOT: *cord*: cord (any long, rounded flexible body or organ) cordal (pertaining to a cord; used specifically in referring to the vocal cord) *chord*: chord (or, cord), chorda (any cord or sinew; pl., chordae) chordal (pertaining to any chorda; chiefly used of the notochord) chordate (any of a phylum of animals having a notochord, gill slits, and a dorsal tubular nerve cord) chordee (downward bowing of the penis as a result of a congenital anomaly or a urethral infection) PREFIXED ROOT: *chordal*: epichordal (*epi* upon) hypochordal (*hypo* under) intrachordal (*intra* within) parachordal (*para* alongside) perichordal (*peri* around) prechordal (also called *prochordal*) (*pre* before) subchordal (*sub* below) *cord*: mesocord (*mesos* middle) LEADING ROOT COMPOUND: *chord*: chordectomy (or, cordectomy; excision of a cord, as a vocal cord or spinal cord) (*ektome* excision) chorditis (*itis* inflammation) chordoid (resembling the notochord) (*eidos* form)

Element	From	Meaning	Examples
chord (cont'd)		[cord, string]	chordoma (also called *chordosarcoma*) (*oma* tumor)
			chordo:
			chordoblastoma (*blastos* germ, sprout + *oma* tumor)
			chordocarcinoma (also called *chordoma*) (*karkinos* cancer + *oma* tumor)
			chordosarcoma (also called *chordoma*) (*sarkos* flesh + *oma* tumor)
			chordotomy (*tomy* incision)
			cord:
			cordectomy (or, chordectomy) (*ektome* excision)
			corditis (inflammation of the spermatic cord) (*itis* inflammation)
			cordo:
			cordocentesis (also called *percutaneous umbilical blood sampling*) (*kentesis* puncture)
			cordopexy (*pexis* fixation)
			TRAILING ROOT COMPOUND:
			cephalochord (*kephale* head)
			notochord (*noton* back)
			CROSS REFERENCE: funi
chori	Greek *chorion*	membrane	SIMPLE ROOT: chorion (the outermost envelope of the growing zygote or fertilized ovum which serves as a protective and nutritive covering) {chorionic}
			PREFIXED ROOT:
			chorial:
			dichorial (or, dichorionic) (*di* two)
			monochorial (or, monochorionic) (*monos* single)
			synchorial (sharing a common placenta) (*syn* together)
			chorion:
			endochorion (the inner chorionic layer) (*endon* within)
			epichorion (the portion of the uterine mucosa which encloses the implanted conceptus) (*epi* upon)
			exochorion (the part of the chorion which is derived from the ectoderm) (*exo* outside)
			chorionic pertaining to the chorion:
			dichorionic (or, dichorial) (*di* two)
			monochorionic (or, monochorial) (*monos* single)
			subchorionic (or, subchoroidal) (*sub* below)
			choroid like a membrane:
			perichoroidal (surrounding the choroid coat of the eye) (*peri* around)
			suprachoroid (on the outer side of the choroid of the eye)
			choroido:
			choroidocyclitis (*kyklos* circle + *itis* inflammation)
			choroidopathy (*pathos* disease)
			choroidea:
			entochoroidea (*entos* within)
			suprachoroidea (also called *suprachoroid lamina of sclera*) (*supra* above)
			LEADING ROOT COMPOUND:
			chor: choroid, choroideremia (*eidos* form + *eremia* destitution)
			chorio:
			chorioadenoma (*adenos* gland + *oma* tumor)
			chorioangioma (*angeion* blood vessel + *oma* tumor)
			chorioblastoma (also called *choriocarcinoma*) (*blastos* germ + *oma* tumor)

Element	From	Meaning	Examples
chori (cont'd)		[membrane]	choriocarcinoma (also called *chorioblastoma*) (*karkinos* cancer + *oma* tumor) choriocele (*kele* tumor) choriogenesis (*genere* to produce) choriomeningitis (*meningos* membrane + *itis* inflammation) chorioplacental (placenta) chorioretinal, chorioretinitis (retina + *itis* inflammation) TRAILING ROOT COMPOUND: allantochorion (a compound membrane formed by fusion of the allantois and chorion) (*allantos* sausage) omphalochorion (the structure formed by fusion of the yolk sac with the chorion) (*omphalos* navel) sclerochoroiditis (*skleros* hard + *itis* inflammation) syndesmochorial (*syndesis* bound together) tapetochoroidal (*tapetum* membranous covering) CROSS REFERENCE: amnio, ependym, hymen, membran, mening, myring, pia, tympan
chrom, **chro**	Greek *chroma*	color; orig., the color of skin	SIMPLE ROOT: chromate (a salt of chromic acid) chromatic (of color, or having color or colors; readily stained; pertaining to chromatin) chromatics (the scientific study of color in reference to hues and saturation), chromaticity, chromatid, chromatin, chromatism chromium (Cr) {chromic} PREFIXED ROOT: *chroia*: dyschroia (or, dyschroa; discoloration of the skin) (*dys* abnormal) *chroic*: amphichroic (or, amphichromatic; exhibiting two colors; affecting both red and blue litmus) (*amphi* both) monochroic (or, monochromatic) (*monos* single) trichroic (*tri* three) *chroous*: isochroous (or, isochromatic) (*isos* equal) *chroism*: allochroism (*allos* other) dichroism {dichroic} (*di* two) trichroism {trichroic} (*tri* three) *chroma*: parachroma (abnormal coloration of the skin) (*para* abnormal) *chromasia*: achromasia (also called *hypopigmentation, achromatosis*) (*a* privative) allochromasia (*allos* other) anisochromasia (*aniso* unequal, dissimilar: *an* negative + *isos* equal) hyperchromasia (*hyper* above) hypochromasia (also called *hypochromia*) (*hypo* under) metachromasia (*meta* after) polychromasia (also called *polychromatophilia*) (*polys* many) *chromas*: dichromasy {dichromatic, dichromic} (*di* two) polychromasia (also called *polychromatophilia*) (*polys* many) *chrom(at)*: achroma, achromatin, achromatize, achromatous (*a* privative)

Element	From	Meaning	Examples
chrom (cont'd)		[color]	achromaturia (the excretion of colorless urine) (*a* privative + *uria* urine condition)
			apochromat (an apochromatic objective) (*apo* from)
			dyschromatopsia (*dys* abnormal + *opsia* vision condition)
			dyschromatosis (*dys* abnormal + *osis* condition)
			hemiachromatopsia (*hemi* half + *a* privative + *opsia* vision condition)
			chromatic pertaining to color:
			achromatic (*a* privative)
			amphichromatic (*amphi* both)
			apochromatic (free from chromatic and spherical aberration) (*apo* from)
			euchromatic (also called *orthochromatic*) (*eu* good, well)
			heterochromatic (*heteros* other)
			hyperchromatic (*hyper* above)
			hypochromatic (*hypo* under)
			isochromatic (*isos* equal)
			metachromatic (*meta* after)
			monochromatic (or, monochroic; one color; also, of or producing light of one wavelength) (*monos* single)
			orthochromatic (also called *euchromatic*) (*orthos* straight)
			pachychromatic (*pachys* thick)
			panchromatic (*pan* all)
			polychromatic (*polys* many)
			trichromatic (*tri* three)
			chromatin:
			euchromatin (*eu* good)
			parachromatin (*para* alongside)
			chromatism:
			achromatism (*a* privative)
			dichromatism (also called *dichromatopsia*) (*di* two)
			hyperchromatism (or, hyperchomasia) (*hyper* above)
			hypochromatism (or, hypochromia) (*hypo* under)
			metachromatism (*meta* after)
			monochromatism (*monos* single)
			pleochromatism (*pleon* more)
			chromato:
			amphochromatophil (or, amphochromophil; both also called *amphophilic*) (*ampho* both + *philein* to love)
			monochromatophil (*monos* single + *philein* to love)
			chrome:
			endochrome (*endon* within)
			hemichrome (*hemi* half)
			perichrome (*peri* around)
			chromemia colored condition of the blood:
			hypochromemia (*hypo* under)
			polychromemia (*polys* many, much)
			chromia:
			achromia {achromic} (*a* privative)
			anisochromia (*aniso* unequal: *an* negative + *isos* equal)
			dyschromia (also called *dyschroia, dyschroa*) (*dys* abnormal)
			heterochromia {heterochromic} (*heteros* other)
			hypochromia (or, hypochromatism, hypochromasia) {hypochromic} (*hypo* below)

Element	From	Meaning	Examples
chrom (cont'd)		[color]	panchromia (the condition of staining with various dyes) (*pan* all)
			chromic:
			dichromic (*di* two)
			heptachromic (*hepta* seven)
			hypochromic (*hypo* under)
			monochromic (*monos* one, single)
			tetrachromic (*tetra* four)
			trichromic (*tri* three)
			chroming:
			postchroming (also called *afterchroming*) (*post* after)
			prechroming (*pre* before)
			chromo:
			dichromophile (*di* two + *philein* to love—an affinity for)
			extrachromosomal (*extra* outside + *soma* body)
			chromous: heterochromous (*heteros* other)
			chrosis color condition:
			hypochrosis (*hypo* under)
			metachrosis (*meta* change)
			LEADING ROOT COMPOUND:
			chrom:
			chromesthesia (*esthesia* feeling)
			chromhidrosis (*hidrosis* sweat condition)
			chromonychia (*onychia* nail condition)
			chromopsia (*opsia* vision condition)
			chroma: chromaphil (also called *chromaffin*) (*philein* to love)
			chromat:
			chromatoid (*eidos* form)
			chromatopsia (*opsia* vision condition)
			chromaturia (*uria* urine condition)
			chromato:
			chromatoblast (*blastos* bud, shoot, germ)
			chromatogenous (*genere* to produce)
			chromatogram, chromatography (*graphein* to write)
			chromatokinesis (*kinesis* movement)
			chromatolysis {chromatolytic} (*lyein* to loosen)
			chromatometer (*metron* measure)
			chromatopexis (*pexis* fixation)
			chromatophagus (destroying pigments) (*phagein* to devour)
			chromatophilic (or, chromatophilous) (*philein* to love)
			chromatophore (*pherein* to bear)
			chromatoplasm (*plassein* to form)
			chromatoscope, chromatoscopy (*skopein* to examine)
			chromatoskiameter (*skia* shadow + *metron* measure)
			chromatotaxis (*taxis* arrangement)
			chromatotropism (*tropein* to turn)
			chromo:
			chromoblast, chromoblastomycosis (*blastos* germ + *mykes* fungus + *osis* condition)
			chromocyte (*kytos* cell)
			chromodiagnosis (diagnosis by change of color)
			chromogenesis {chromogenic} (*genere* to produce)
			chromolipoid (*lipos* fat + *eidos* form)
			chromomere (*meros* part)
			chromometer (also called *colorimeter*) (*metron* measure)

A Thesaurus of Medical Word Roots

Element	From	Meaning	Examples
chrom (cont'd)		[color]	chromomycosis (*mykes* fungus + *osis* condition) chromonema (pl., chromonemata) {chromonemal} (*nema* thread) chromoparic (*parere* to produce) chromopexy {chromopectic} (*pexy* fixation) chromophage (*phagein* to devour, consume) chromophil {chromophilic} (*philein* to love—have an affinity for) chromophobe {chromophobia} (*phobos* fear) chromophore {chromophoric} (*phorein* to bear) chromophose (*phos* light) chromoplast (*plassein* to form) chromorhinorrhea (*rhin* nose + *rhein* to flow) chromoscope, chromoscopy (*skopein* to examine) chromosome (*soma* body) chromospermism (unusual coloration of the sperm) chromotherapy (*therapy* treatment) chromotoxic (*toxikon* poison) chromotrichia (coloration of the hair) (*trichia* hair condition) chromotropic (*tropein* to turn) TRAILING ROOT COMPOUND: *chromasia*: amblychromasia (the condition of staining faintly or having little chromatin) (*amblys* dull) *chromatic*: amblychromatic (*amblys* dull) leptochromatic (*leptos* slender) photochromatic (*photos* light) trachychromatic (*trachys* rough) *chrome*: auxochrome (*auxein* to increase) cholochrome (*chole* gall, bile) cytochrome (*kytos* cell) echinochrome (*echinos* sea urchin: prickly, spiny) gyrochrome (*gyros* circle, ring) hemachrome (*haima* blood) hypsochrome (*hypsos* height) proteinochrome (protein) somatochrome (*somatos* body) urochrome (*ouron* urine) *chromatic*: orthochromatic (also called *euchromatic*) (*orthos* straight) oxychromatic (staining with acid dyes) (*oxys* sharp: acid) trachychromatic (strongly or deeply staining) (*trachys* rough) *chromatosis*: hemochromatosis (*haima* blood + *osis* condition) *chromemia*: oligochromemia (*oligos* scant + *emia* blood condition) *chromia*: erythrochromia (*erythros* red) normochromia (also called *orthochromia*) (*norma* normal) orthochromia (also called *normochromia*) (*orthos* straight) *chromic*: bathochromic (*bathos* deep) xanthochromic (*xanthos* yellow) *chromosome*: idiochromosome (sex chromosome) (*idios* one's own + *soma* body) *chrosis*: thermochrosis (*therme* heat) CROSS REFERENCE: None

Element	From	Meaning	Examples
chron	Greek *chronos*	time	SIMPLE ROOT: chronic (persisting over a long period of time) {chronicity} PREFIXED ROOT: *chronation*: dischronation (a disturbance in the consciousness of time) (*dis* separation) *chronia*: heterochronia {heterochronous} (*heteros* different) isochronia (or, isochronism) (*isos* equal) synchronia (or, synchronism) (*syn* with, together) *chronic*: diachronic (*dia* across, through) isochronic (or, isochronous; performed in equal times: said of vibrations occurring at the same time) (*isos* equal) subchronic (between chronic and subacute) (*sub* under) synchronic (*syn* with, together) *chronism*: dyschronism (separate in time; disturbance of any time relation) (*dys* abnormal) *chronobiology* study of time on living organisms: anachronobiology (the study of the constructive effects of time on a living organism) (*ana* again) catachronobiology (the study of the deleterious effects of time on a living organism) (*kata* down) *chronous*: homochronous (also called *synchronous*) (*homos* same) metachronous (*meta* different) synchronous (occurring at the same time; also called *homochronous*) (*syn* with, together) *chrony*: asynchrony (*a* negative + synchrony) desynchrony (jet lag, for instance) (*de* reversal + synchrony) synchrony (*syn* with, together) LEADING ROOT COMPOUND: *chron*: chronaxy (or, chronaxie; the time required for the excitation of a nervous element by a definite stimulus) (*axios* fit) *chrono*: chronobiology (the scientific study of the effect of time on living organisms; compare *anachronobiology, catachronobiology*) (*bios* life + *logos* study) chronognosis (*gnosis* knowledge) chronograph (*graphein* to write) chronometry (*metron* measure) chronophotograph (*photos* light + *graphein* to write) chronoscope (*skopein* to examine) chronotaraxis (*taraxis* confusion) chronotherapy (*therapy* treatment) chronotropic (affecting the time or rate), chronotropism (*tropein* to turn) chronotype (a person's preference for daytime versus nighttime activities) TRAILING ROOT COMPOUND: gastrochronorrhea (*gaster* stomach + *rhein* to flow) mychronoscope (*myos* muscle + *skopein* to examine) CROSS REFERENCE: temp

Element	From	Meaning	Examples
chyl	Greek *chylus* juice	gastric juice	SIMPLE ROOT: chyle (the milky fluid taken up by the lacteals from the food in the intestine after digestion) {chylous} PREFIXED ROOT: achylia, achylous (*a* privative) dyschylia (disorder of the chyle) (*dys* abnormal) euchylia (normal condition of the chyle) (*eu* well) heterochylia (the sudden varying of the gastric secretion from normal acidity to hyperacidity or anacidity) (*heteros* other) hyperchylia (*hyper* over, excessive) polychylia (*polys* much) LEADING ROOT COMPOUND: *chyl*: chylangioma (a mass made up of prominent, dilating lacteals and larger intestinal lymphatic vessels) (*angeion* vessel + *oma* tumor) chylaqueous (both chylous and watery) (*aqua* water) chylectasia (dilatation of a chylous vessel) (*ektasis* dilatation) chylemia (*emia* blood condition) chylidrosis (chylous perspiration) (*hidros* sweat) [h of hidros elided] chyloid (*eidos* form) chylosis (*osis* condition) chyluria (*uria* urine condition) *chyli*: chylifacient, chylifaction (also called *chylopoiesis*), chylifactive (also called *chylopoietic*) (*facere* to make) chyliferous (forming chyle; conveying chyle) (*ferre* to bear) chyliform (resembling chyle) (*forma* shape, form) *chylo*: chylocele (a chylous effusion into the tunica vaginalis of the testis) (*kele* tumor) [tunica vaginalis testis: the serous membrane covering the front and sides of the testis and epididymis] chylocyst (*kystis* bladder) chyloderma (elephantiasis) (*derma* skin) chylopericardium (pericardium: *peri* around + *kardia* heart) chyloperitoneum (also called *chyliform ascites*) (peritoneum) chylophoric (*phorein* to bear, carry) chylopleura (also called *chylothorax*) (*pleura* rib, side) chylopoiesis (also called *chylifaction*) (*poiein* to produce) chylorrhea (*rhein* to flow) chylothorax (*thorax* chest) TRAILING ROOT COMPOUND: oligochylia (*oligos* little, scant) pseudochylous (resembling chyle) (*pseudes* false) CROSS REFERENCE: chym
chym	Greek *chymos*	juice	SIMPLE ROOT: chyme (also, chymus; the semifluid, homogeneous, creamy, or gruel-like material produced by gastric digestion of food) {chymous}, chymosin (rennin) PREFIXED ROOT: achymia (*a* privative) ecchymosis (pl., ecchymoses) {ecchymotic} (*ek* out + *osis* condition) enchyma (*en* in) parenchyma {parenchymatous} (*para* alongside + enchyma) parenchymatitis (*para* alongside + enchyma + *itis* inflammation) LEADING ROOT COMPOUND: *chymi*: chymification (also called *chymopoiesis*) (*facere* to make)

Element	From	Meaning	Examples
chym (cont'd)		[juice]	*chymo*: chymopoiesis (the production of chyme: the physical state of semi-fluid food brought about by digestion in the stomach; also called *chymification*) (*poiein* to produce) chymorrhea (*rhein* to flow) TRAILING ROOT COMPOUND: ischochymia (*ischein* to suppress) mesenchyme, mesenchymoma (*mesos* middle + *oma* tumor) oligochymia (*oligos* deficiency) pachychymia (inspissation of the chyme) (*pachys* thick) CROSS REFERENCE: chyl
chys	Greek *chein*	to pour	PREFIXED ROOT: synchysis (lit., a mixing together; fluid state of the vitreous body of the eye) (*sym* with) TRAILING ROOT COMPOUND: cirsenchysis (sclerotherapy for treatment of varicose veins) (*kirsos* varix) ophthalmosynchysis (effusion into the eye) (*ophthalmos* eye + synchysis) pyecchysis (the effusion of purulent matter) (*pyon* pus + *ek* out) rachiochysis (the effusion of a fluid within the vertebral canal) (*rhachis* spine) rhinenchysis (a washing out the nasal cavities) (*rhis* nose) CROSS REFERENCE: chem, fund
cide, cis	Latin *caedere*	to cut, kill	PREFIXED ROOT: *cisal*: mesoincisal (*mesos* middle) *cision*: circumcision (the removal of all or a part of the prepuce, or foreskin) (*circum* around) contraincision (*contra* against + incision) excision (an act of cutting away or taking out) (*ex* out) incision (a cut, or wound produced by cutting) (*in* in) introcision (*intro* within) microincision (*mikros* small + incision) *cisor*: incisor (a tooth for cutting or gnawing) (*in* in) *cisura*: incisura (or, incisure; a cut, notch, or incision; pl., incisurae) (*in* in) TRAILING ROOT COMPOUND: acaricide (*akarus* tick, mite) amebicide (*ameba*) cytocide (*kytos* cell, vessel) febricide (*febris* fever) fungicide (*fungus*) gametocide (*gamete*) larvicide (*larva* ghost, specter) menticide (brainwashing) (*mentis* mind) spermatocide (*sperma* sperm, seed) sporicide (*sporos* seed) CROSS REFERENCE: sex, tom
cili	Latin *cilium* eyelash	eyelash; also, hairlike outgrowth	NOTE: This root can also designate a minute vibratile, hairlike process attached to a free surface of a cell. SIMPLE ROOT: ciliate (or, ciliated; possessing cilia), cilium (pl., cilia: hairlike outgrowths of certain cells which help produce locomotion) {ciliary}

A Thesaurus of Medical Word Roots

Element	From	Meaning	Examples
cili (cont'd)		[eyelash]	PREFIXED ROOT: biciliate (*bi* two) infraciliature (*infra* below) intercilium (*inter* between) supercilia, superciliary (or, supraciliary; pertaining to the eyebrow), supercilium (*super* over) LEADING ROOT COMPOUND: *cili*: ciliectomy (excision of a portion of the ciliary body or ciliary border of the eyelid) (*ektome* excision) *ciliari*: ciliariscope (*skopein* to examine) *ciliaro*: ciliarotomy (*tomy* incision) *cilio*: ciliogenesis (*genere* to originate, produce) cilioretinal (retina) cilioscleral (*skleros* hard) ciliospinal (spine) ciliotomy (*tomy* incision) *cill*: cillosis (spasmodic twitching of the eyelids; also called *cillo*) (French *ciller* to wink + *osis* condition) TRAILING ROOT COMPOUND: *cil*: cnidocil (*knide* a nettle) *ciliary*: iridociliary (*iridos* rainbow: iris) mucociliary (mucus) nasociliary (*nasus* nose) opticociliary (*optokos* sight) *cilium*: kinocilium (*kinein* to move) stereocilium (*stereos* solid) *cillium*: Penicillium (a genus of fungi, some species of which yield several antibiotic substances and biologics) (*penis* tail) CROSS REFERENCE: blephar, palpebr
cin, kin	Greek *kinein* to move	movement	SIMPLE ROOT: *cin*: cinematics (or, kinematics) *kin*: kinase, kinematics (science of motion), kinesia (also called *kinetosis, motion sickness*), kinesics, kinesin, kinesis kinetic, kinetics, kineticist, kinetid, kinetin, kinetism, kinety kinin, kininase PREFIXED ROOT: *cinesia*: acinesia (or, akinesia) (*a* privative) hyperanacinesia (hyperactivity) (*hyper* above + *ana* again) hypocinesia (or, hypokinesia) (*hypo* under) paracinesia (or, parakinesia) (*para* abnormal) *cinesis*: autocinesis (or, autokinesis) (*autos* self) syncinesis (or, synkinesis) (*syn* with) *kine*: monokine (*monos* single) *kinemia*: hyperkinemia (*hyper* over + *emia* blood condition) *kinesia*: akinesia (or, acinesia; complete or partial loss of muscle movement) (*a* privative)

Element	From	Meaning	Examples
cin (cont'd)		[movement]	dyskinesia (or, dyscinesia) {dyskinetic} (*dys* abnormal)
			eukinesia (or, eukinesis) {eukinetic} (*eu* well)
			heterokinesia (or, heterokinesis) (*heteros* other)
			hyperkinesia (or, hyperkinesis: hyperactivity) {hyperkinetic} (*hyper* above, beyond)
			hypokinesia (or, hypokinesis) {hypokinetic} (*hypo* under)
			palikinesia (or, palicinesia) (*palin* backward)
			parakinesia (or, parakinesis) {parakinetic} (*para* abnormal)
			kinesis:
			allokinesis (passive or reflex movement; nonvoluntary movement) (*allos* other)
			autokinesis {autokinetic} (*autos* self)
			diakinesis (*dia* across)
			hyperkinesis {hyperkinetic} (*hyper* above)
			hypsokinesis (*hypso* high, aloft)
			interkinesis (*inter* between)
			metakinesis (or, metakinesia) (*meta* after)
			synkinesis (or, syncinesis; an involuntary movement of one part occurring simultaneously with reflex or voluntary movement of another part) {synkinetic} (*syn* with)
			telekinesis (the power claimed by certain persons of moving objects without contact with the object moved; also motion produced without contact with a moving object) (*tele* afar)
			thrombokinesis (*thrombos* a clot)
			kinemia blood movement condition:
			hyperkinemia {hyperkinemic} (*hyper* above)
			hypokinemia (*hypo* under)
			kinesi: myokinesimeter (*myos* muscle + *metron* measure)
			kinetic:
			akinetic (*a* privative)
			isokinetic (*isos* equal)
			telekinetic (*tele* afar)
			kinety: polykinety (*polys* many)
			LEADING ROOT COMPOUND:
			cin: cineplasty (or, kineplasty) (*plassein* to form)
			kin:
			kinanesthesia (also called *akinesthesia*) (*an* privative + *esthesia* feeling)
			kinesthesia {kinesthetic}, kinesthesiometer (*esthesia* feeling + *metron* measure)
			kine:
			kineplasty (or, cineplasty) (*plassein* to form)
			kinescope (*skopein* to examine)
			kinemo: kinemometer (*metron* measure)
			kines:
			kinesalgia (or, kinesialgia) (*algos* pain)
			kinesiatrics (*iatrein* to heal)
			kinesi:
			kinesigenic (*genere* to produce)
			kinesimeter (or, kinesiometer) (*metron* measure)
			kinesitherapy (*therapy* treatment)
			kinesio:
			kinesiology (*logos* study)

Element	From	Meaning	Examples
cin (cont'd)		[movement]	kinesioneurosis (*neurosis* nerve condition) *kineso*: kinesophobia (or, kinetophobia) (*phobia* fear) *kinet*: kinetosis (any disorder caused by unaccustomed motion) (*osis* condition) *kineto*: kinetocardiogram, kinetocardiograph (*kardia* heart + *graphein* to write) kinetochore (a proteinaceous structure beside the centromere and to which the spindle fibers are attached) (*chora* space) kinetodesma (pl., kinetodesmata) (*desmos* band) kinetogenic (also called *kinetoplast*) (*genere* to produce) kinetonucleus (also called *kinetoplast*) (*nux* kernel: nucleus) kinetophobia (or, kinesophobia) (*phobia* fear) kinetoplasm (or, kinoplasm), kinetoplast (*plassein* to form) kinetoscope, kinetoscopy (*skopein* to examine) kinetosome (basal body) (*soma* body) *kinino*: kininogen (*genere* to produce) *kino*: kinocentrum (also called *centrosome*) (*kentron* center) kinocilium (*cilium* small hair: filament) kinology (*logos* study) kinoplasm (or, kinetoplasm) {kinoplasmic} (*plassein* to form) kinosphere (also called *aster*) (*sphaira* ball, globe: sphere) *kinomo*: kinomometer (also called *goniometer*, an instrument for measuring angles) (*metron* measure) TRAILING ROOT COMPOUND: *cinesia*: allocinesia (*allos* other) bradycinesia (or, bradykinesia) (*bradys* slow) oxycinesia (also called *kinesialgia*) (*oxys* sharp) *cinesis*: acrocinesis {acrocinetic} (*akron* extremities) *kinesia*: acrokinesia (*akros* extremities) bradykinesia (abnormally slow movement) (*bradys* slow) planotopokinesia (*planan* to wander + *topos* place) *kinesis*: adipokinesis {adipokinetic} (*adeps* fat) angiokinesis {angiokinetic} (*angeion* blood vessel) calciokinesis {calciokinetic} (*calx* lime, calcium) cytokinesis (*kytos* cell) echokinesis (also called *echopraxia*) (*echo* a returned sound) dictyokinesis (the migration and distribution of the dictyosomes to the daughter cells in mitosis) (*diktyon* net) hemokinesis (also called *circulation*) {hemokinetic; also called *circulatory*} (*haima* blood) karyokinesis {karyokinetic} (*karyon* nucleus) leukokinesis {leukokinetic} (*leukos* white—blood cells) lymphokinesis (or, lymphocinesis) (*lympha* water, liquid) myokinesis {myokinetic} (*myos* muscle) ookinesis {ookinetic} (*oon* egg, ovum) photokinesis (*photos* light) psychokinesis (*psyche* mind) schizokinesis (*schizein* to divide) stathmokinesis (*stathmos* standing place)

Element	From	Meaning	Examples
cin (cont'd)		[movement]	*kinetic(s)*: adrenokinetic (*adren* pertaining to the kidney) angiokinetic (also called *vasomotor*) (*angeion* vessel) astrokinetic (*aster* star) cardiokinetic (*kardia* heart) enterokinetic (*enteron* intestine) hydrokinetic (*hydor* water) myokinetic (*myos* muscle) neokinetic (*neos* new) optokinetic (*optokos* sight) orthokinetics (*orthos* straight) photokinetic (*photos* light) thymokinetic (*thymus*) toxicokinetics (*toxikon* poison) PREFIXED TRAILING ROOT COMPOUND: adiadochokinesis (inability to make rapid alternating movements) (*a* negative + *diadochus* successive) anesthekinesia (or, anesthecinesia) (*an* not + *esthesia* feeling) diadochokinesia (the function of arresting one motor impulse and substituting for it one that is diametrically opposite) {diadochokinetic} (*dia* across + *docho* succeeding) CROSS REFERENCE: mot
circum-	Latin *circum*	around, encircling	See Appendix B for examples of words with this prefix. Others are placed with the roots to which it is attached. CROSS REFERENCE: peri-
cirrh	Greek *kirrhos* orange-yellow, tawny	orange-yellow	PREFIXED ROOT: precirrhosis (the early stages of cirrhosis of the liver) (*pre* before) LEADING ROOT COMPOUND: *cirrh*: cirrhosis (a chronic disease of the liver; so named because of the orange-yellow appearance of the diseased liver) {cirrhotic} (*osis* condition) *cirrho*: cirrhogenous (or, cirrhogenic) (*genere* to produce) TRAILING ROOT COMPOUND: *cirrhosis* diseased liver condition: cardiocirrhosis (also called *cardiac cirrhosis*) (*kardia* heart) hepatocirrhosis (cirrhosis of the liver) (*hepatos* liver) pseudocirrhosis (also called *cardiac cirrhosis*) (*pseudes* false) CROSS REFERENCE: lut, xanth
cirs	Greek *kirsos*	varix (varicose vein)	LEADING ROOT COMPOUND: *cirs*: cirsenchysis (treatment of varicose veins by injection of a sclerosing solution) (*enchysis* injection) cirsoid (also called *variciform, varicoid*) (*eidos* form) cirsomphalos (*omphalos* navel) cirsophthalmia (*ophthalmos* eye) *cirso*: cirsocele (a variocele) (*kele* tumor) CROSS REFERENCE: vari
cis			See cide- for *circumcision, incision*.
clas	Greek *klaein* to break	breakage, division, destroy	SIMPLE ROOT: clastic (causing or undergoing a division into parts; separable into parts) PREFIXED ROOT: *clasis*: aclasis (or, aclasia) (*a* negative)

Element	From	Meaning	Examples
clas (cont'd)		[breakage, division, destroy]	anaclasis (reflection or refraction of light) (*ana* up, back)
			autoclasis (or, autoclasia) (*autos* self)
			diaclasis (or, diaclasia; also called *osteoclasis*) (*dia* through)
			clast: disdiaclast (lit., broken through twice; any one of the doubly refracting elements of the contractile substance of muscle) (*dis* twice + *dia* across)
			LEADING ROOT COMPOUND:
			clasmat: clasmatosis (the breaking off of parts of a cell) (*osis* condition)
			clasto:
			clastogenic (giving rise to or inducing disruption or breakages, as of chromosomes) (*genere* to produce)
			clastothrix (splitting of the hair) (*thrix* hair)
			TRAILING ROOT COMPOUND:
			clasia:
			alveoloclasia (destruction of a tooth socket) (*alveus* hollow)
			arthroclasia (the breaking down of an ankylosis in order to secure free movement of a joint) (*arthron* joint)
			clasis:
			cytoclasis (also called *cytolysis*) (*kytos* cell)
			hemoclasis (also called *hemolysis*) {hemoclastic} (*haima* blood)
			mucoclasis (destruction of the mucous lining of any organ, e.g., the gallbladder with thermocautery) (mucus)
			myelinoclasis (myelin)
			onychoclasis (breaking of the nails) (*onychos* nail)
			osteoclasis (also called *diaclasis*) (*osteon* bone)
			tarsoclasis (*tarsus* ankle)
			thromboclasis (*thrombos* clot)
			trichoclasis (also called *trichorrhexis*) (*trichos* hair)
			clast:
			chondroclast (*chondros* cartilage)
			cranioclast (*kranion* skull)
			erythroclast {erythroclastic} (*erythryos* red)
			lithoclast (also called *lithotrite*) (*lithos* stone)
			myeloclast (*myelos* marrow)
			odontoclast (also called *cementoclast*) (*odontos* tooth)
			osteoclast {osteoclastic} (*osteon* bone)
			clastic:
			cytoclastic (also called *cytolytic*) (*kytos* cell, vessel)
			hemoclastic (also called *hemolytic*) (*haima* blood)
			histoclastic (*histos* web, tissue)
			polioclastic (*polios* gray matter)
			proteoclastic (protein)
			CROSS REFERENCE: lys
clavi	Latin *clavis* key	clavicle	SIMPLE ROOT: clavicle (or, clavicula; a bone, resembling a key, that articulates with the sternum and scapula; also called *collarbone*; pl., claviculae) {clavicular}
			PREFIXED ROOT:
			clave:
			autoclave (a self-locking, strong, pressurized, steam-heated vessel, as for laboratory experiments, sterilization, and cooking) (*autos* self)
			enclave (an enclosure) (*en* in)

Element	From	Meaning	Examples
clavi (cont'd)		[clavicle]	*clavicular*: infraclavicular (*infra* below) interclavicular (*inter* between) postclavicular (*post* after) subclavicular (or, subclavian) (*sub* under) supraclavicular (*supra* over) LEADING ROOT COMPOUND: *clavi*: clavipectoral (*pectus* chest) *clavico*: clavicotomy (the operation of cutting or dividing the clavicle) (*tomy* incision) *clavicul*: claviculectomy (*ektome* excision) TRAILING ROOT COMPOUND: acromioclavicular (of or relating to the acromion and the clavicle, or to the articulation between the clavicle and the scapula and its ligaments) (*acromion* tip of the shoulder) coracoclavicular (relating to the coracoid process and the clavicle) [coracoid: shaped like a crow's beak; denoting a process of the scapula] costoclavicular (*costa* rib) omoclavicular (*omos* shoulder) scapuloclavicular (*scapula* shoulder blade) sternoclavicular (*sternum*) CROSS REFERENCE: cleid, scapul
cleid, **cleis**	Greek *kleis* closure; *kleistos* closed	collarbone, clavicle; closure	NOTE: Greek *kleis* refers to the collarbone (the clavicle), and is so named because it locks the neck and breast together. *Clavicle* literally means "small key," which the collarbone resembles. (See clavi.) SIMPLE ROOT: cleidal (pertaining to or affecting the clavicle) cleidoic (isolated from the environment, as the ova of birds) LEADING ROOT COMPOUND: *cleid*: cleidagra (gouty pain in the clavicle) (*agra* seizure) cleidarthritis (*arthron* joint + *itis* inflammation) *cleido*: cleidocostal (*costa* rib) cleidocranial (*kranion* skull, head) cleidomastoid (mastoid process) cleidotomy (*tomy* incision) TRAILING ROOT COMPOUND: *cleidal*: sternocleidal (also called *sternoclavicular*) (*sternon* chest) *cleisis*: colpocleisis (operation of occluding the vagina) (*kolpos* vagina) enterocleisis (*enteron* intestine) hysterocleisis (*hystera* uterus) iridencleisis (surgical incarceration of a slip of the iris within a corneal or limbal incision to act as a wick for aqueous drainage in glaucoma) (iris + *en* in) neurosarcocleisis (an operation for the relief of neuralgia) (*neuron* nerve + *sarkos* flesh) otocleisis (*otos* ear) proctencleisis (a rectal stricture) (*proktos* anus + *en* in) rhinocleisis (also called *rhinostenosis*) (*rhis* nose) splenocleisis (*splen* spleen) CROSS REFERENCE: clavi, scapul

Element	From	Meaning	Examples
clep			See klept- for *amnioclepsis*.
clon, **klon**	Greek *klonos*	turmoil, spasm	SIMPLE ROOT: clonism (or, clonismus; a succession of clonic spasms) clonus (spasm in which rigidity and relaxation alternate in rapid succession) {clonic, clonicity} PREFIXED ROOT: polyclonia (myoclonus multiplex) (*polys* many) synclonus (muscular tremor) (*syn* with) LEADING ROOT COMPOUND: *clonico*: clonicotonic (both clonic and tonic, as some forms of muscle spasms) (*tonus* tone) *clono*: clonograph (an instrument for recording spasmodic movements of parts and tendon reflexes) (*graphein* to write) clonospasm (clonic spasm) (*span* to contract) TRAILING ROOT COMPOUND: *clonia*: logoclonia (also called *logospasm, logoklony*) (*logos* word) *clonic*: myoclonic (showing myclonus) (*myos* muscle) neuroclonic (marked by nervous spasm) (*neuron* nerve) tonoclonic (*tonos* tension) *clonus*: blepharoclonus (*blepharon* eyelid) myoclonus {myoclonic} (*myos* muscle) opsoclonus (*ops* eye) phonomyoclonus (*phone* sound + *myos* muscle) pseudoclonus (*pseudes* false) *klony*: logoklony (spasmodic repetition of the end syllables of a word; also called *logoclonia*) (*logos* word) CROSS REFERENCE: spas, tetan
clys	Greek *klysis* a drenching; *klyster* a syringe	a syringe	SIMPLE ROOT: clysis (an infusion of fluid for therapeutic purposes) clysma (a cluster), clyster (an injection into the rectum) [both old terms for *enema*] clysterize (to treat with enemas, or with injections into the rectum) TRAILING ROOT COMPOUND: *clysis*: coloclysis (irrigation of the colon) (*kolon* colon) enteroclysis (the injection of a nutrient or medicinal fluid into the bowel) (*enteron* intestine) peritoneoclysis (irrigation of the peritoneal, or abdominal, cavity) (peritoneum) phleboclysis (also called *venoclysis*) (*phlebos* vein) pleuroclysis (*pleura* side, rib) proctoclysis (also called *rectoclysis*) (*proktos* anus) rectoclysis (also called *proctoclysis*) (rectum) venoclysis (also called *phleboclysis*) (*vena* vein) vesicoclysis (*vesica* bladder) *clyster*: coloclyster (an enema injected into the colon through the rectum) (*kolon* colon) PREFIXED TRAILING ROOT COMPOUND: hypodermoclysis (subcutaneous infusion) (*hypo* under + *derma* skin) CROSS REFERENCE: None

Element	From	Meaning	Examples
co-	Latin prefix	with, together	See Appendix B (com-) for examples of words with this prefix. Others are listed with the roots to which it is attached. CROSS REFERENCE: com-, syn-
coagul	Latin *co* together + *agere* to drive	to clot	SIMPLE ROOT: coagulant (or, coagulative), coagulase coagulate {coagulable} coagulum (a blood clot; pl., coagula) PREFIXED ROOT: *coagulable*: hypercoagulable (*hyper* above) hypocoagulable (*hypo* under) *coagulant*: anticoagulant (*anti* against) procoagulant (*pro* before) *coagulation*: anticoagulation (*anti* against) LEADING ROOT COMPOUND: coagulogram (*graphein* to write) coagulopathy (*pathos* disease) CROSS REFERENCE: thromb
cocc	Greek *kokkos* berry	a bacterium (berry- shaped)	SIMPLE ROOT: coccidium (pl., coccidia) {coccidial} coccus (a berry-shaped bacterium; pl., cocci) {coccal} PREFIXED ROOT: diplococcus (a spherical bacterium occurring predominantly in pairs) (*diploos* two-fold) macrococcus (also called *megacoccus*; pl., megacocci) (*makron* large) megacoccus (also called *macrococcus*) (*mega* big, large) micrococcus (pl., micrococci) (*mikros* small) monococcus (*monos* single) LEADING ROOT COMPOUND: *cocc*: coccoid (*eidos* form, resembling) *cocci*: coccigenic (caused by cocci) (*genere* to produce) *coccidi*: coccidioidomycosis (*eidos* form + *mykosis* fungal condition) coccidiosis (also called *coccidioidomycosis*) (*osis* condition) *cocco*: coccobacillus (pl., coccobacilli) (*bacillus* rod-shaped bacterium) coccobacteria (*bakterion* rod: bacterium) coccogenous (or, coccigenic) (*genere* to produce) TRAILING ROOT COMPOUND: ascococcus (*askos* wineskin, bladder) Cryptococcus (any of a genus of yeastlike fungi commonly occurring in the soil and including certain pathogenic species) (*kryptos* hidden, concealed) echinococcus (*echinos* hedgehog: spiny, thorny) enterococcus (*enteron* intestine) gonococcus (causative agent of gonorrhea) (*gone* seed) meningococcus (*meningos* membrane) pyococcus (*pyon* pus) staphylococcus (*staphyle* bunch of grapes: uvula) streptococcus (*strephein* to twist) CROSS REFERENCE: None

Element	From	Meaning	Examples
coccy	Greek *kokkyx* cuckoo (see Note)	caudal triangular bone	NOTE: This bone is said to resemble the beak of the cuckoo. SIMPLE ROOT: coccyx [the small bone below the sacrum in man, formed by union of four (sometimes five or three) rudimentary vertebrae, and forming the caudal extremity of the vertebral column; pl., coccyges] {coccygeal} PREFIXED ROOT: intercoccygeal (*inter* between) LEADING ROOT COMPOUND: *coccy*: coccycephaly (*kephale* head) coccyodynia (or, coccygodynia) (*odyne* pain) *coccyg*: coccygectomy (*ektome* excision) coccygodynia (or, coccyodynia) (*odyne* pain) *coccygo*: coccygotomy (incision of the coccyx) (*tomy* incision) TRAILING ROOT COMPOUND: proctococcypexia (suture of rectum to the coccyx; also called *rectococcypexy*) (*proktos* anus + *pexis* fixation) rectococcypexy (also called *proctococcypexy*) (rectum + *pexis* fixation) sacrococcyx (the sacrum and the coccyx regarded as one bone) CROSS REFERENCE: spondyl, vertebr
cochl	Latin *cochlea* snail shell	spiral form, spoon; spoonful	SIMPLE ROOT: cochlea (anything of a spiral form; the essential organ of hearing; a spirally wound tube, resembling a snail shell; pl., cochleae) cochlear (pertaining to the cochlea) cochleare (spoon or spoonful), cochleate (coiled like a snail shell) PREFIXED ROOT: retrocochlear (*retro* behind) LEADING ROOT COMPOUND: *cochel*: cochleitis (*itis* inflammation) *cochleari*: cochleariform (shaped like a spoon) (*forma* shape) *cochleo*: cochleotopic (relating to the organization of the auditory pathways and auditory area of the brain) (*topos* place) cochleovestibular (vestibule—of ear) TRAILING ROOT COMPOUND: olivocochlear (a bundle of fibers that originates from the periolivary nuclei bilaterally; also called *bundle of Rasmussen*) vestibulocochlear (vestibule) CROSS REFERENCE: helix, spir
coel			See cel[1] for *coeloblastula*.
col-	Latin prefix	with, together	See Appendix B (com-) for examples of words with this prefix. Others are listed with the roots to which it is attached. CROSS REFERENCE: com-, syn-
col	Greek *kolon*	colon	SIMPLE ROOT: colic (or, colica; spasm in any hollow or tubular soft organ accompanied by pain; pertaining to the colon) colon (the lower end of the large intestine) {colonic} PREFIXED ROOT: *colectomy* excision of the colon: hemicolectomy (*hemi* half) pancolectomy (*pan* all) *colic*: intracolic (*intra* within)

Element	From	Meaning	Examples
col (cont'd)		[colon]	juxtacolic (*juxta* near)
			pericolic (*peri* around)
			retrocolic (*retro* behind)
			colitis inflammation of the colon:
			endocolitis (*endon* within)
			exocolitis (*exo* outer)
			microcolitis (*mikros* small)
			pancolitis (*pan* all)
			paracolitis (*para* alongside, near)
			pericolitis (also, pericolonitis; inflammation around the colon, especially of the peritoneal coat of the colon) (*peri* around)
			colon:
			ectocolon (dilatation of the colon) (from *ectasia* dilatation)
			macrocolon (*makros* large)
			megacolon (also called *giant colon*) (*mega* large, dilated)
			mesocolon, mesocolopexy (*mesos* middle + *pexis* fixation)
			microcolon (*mikros* small)
			LEADING ROOT COMPOUND:
			col:
			colectasia (*ektasis* stretching)
			colectomy (*ektome* excision)
			colitis (or, colonitis) (*itis* inflammation)
			coli: colipuncture (also called *colocentesis*) (*pungere* to pierce)
			colico: colicoplegia (*plessein* to strike)
			colo:
			colocentesis (also called *colipuncture*) (*kentein* to puncture)
			colocholecystostomy (establishment of communication between the gall bladder and the colon) (*chole* bile + *kystis* bladder + *stoma* mouth, opening)
			coloclysis, coloclyster (*klysis* a drenching)
			colocolostomy (surgical formation of an anastomosis between two portions of the colon) (*stoma* mouth, opening)
			colocutaneous (*cutis* skin)
			colocystoplasty (*kystis* bladder, sac + *plassein* to form)
			coloenteritis (also called *enterocolitis*) (*enteron* intestine + *itis* inflammation)
			colofixation (also called *colopexy*) (*figere* to fasten)
			colohepatopexy (*hepatos* liver + *pexy* fixation)
			cololysis (*lysis* loosening)
			colopathy (or, colonopathy) (*pathos* disease)
			colopexotomy (*pexis* fixation + *tomy* incision)
			colopexy (also called *colofixation*) (*pexis* fixation)
			coloplication (or, coliplication) (*plicare* to fold)
			coloproctectomy (also called *proctocolectomy*) (*proktos* anus + *ektome* excision)
			coloproctitis (also called *proctocolitis, colorectitis*) (*proktos* anus + *itis* inflammation)
			coloptosis (or, coloptosia) (*ptein* to fall; prolapse)
			colopuncture (also called *colocentesis*) (*pungere* to pierce)
			colorectal, colorectitis (also called *coloproctitis, proctocolitis*) (rectum + *itis* inflammation)
			colorrhaphy (suture or repair of the colon) (*rhaphe* suture)
			colorrhea (*rhein* to flow)
			coloscope, coloscopy (*skopein* to examine)

Element	From	Meaning	Examples
col (cont'd)		[colon]	colosigmoidostomy (sigmoid + *stoma* mouth, opening)
			colostomy (*stoma* mouth, opening)
			colotomy (*tomy* incision)
			colovaginal (vagina)
			colovesical (also called *vesicocolonic*) (*vesica* sac, bladder)
			colon: colonitis (or, colitis) (*itis* inflammation)
			colono:
			colonogram, colonography (*graphein* to write)
			colonopathy (or, colopathy) (*pathos* disease)
			colonorrhagia (*rhagia* bursting forth)
			colonoscope, colonoscopy (*skopein* to examine)
			TRAILING ROOT COMPOUND:
			colic:
			duodenocolic (duodenum)
			gastrocolic (*gaster* stomach belly)
			hepatocolic (*hepatos* liver)
			ileocolic (ileum)
			phrenocolic (*phren* diaphragm)
			splenocolic (spleen)
			vesicocolic (or, vesicocolonic) (*vesica* bladder)
			colitis colon inflammation:
			enterocolitis (also called *coloenteritis*) (*enteron* intestine)
			gastrocolitis (*gaster* stomach, belly)
			ileocolitis (ileum)
			mucocolitis (mucus)
			proctocolitis (also called *coloproctitis*) (*proktos* anus)
			rectocolitis (also called *proctocolitis*) (rectum)
			typhlocolitis (*typhlos* cecum: blind gut)
			colon:
			dolichocolon (*dolichos* long)
			pneumocolon (*pneumon* air)
			colostomy colon opening:
			enterocolostomy (*enteron* intestine)
			gastrocolostomy (*gaster* stomach)
			colotomy: gastrocolotomy (*gaster* stomach, belly + *tomy* incision)
			CROSS REFERENCE: None
colla	Greek *kolla*	glue	SIMPLE ROOT: collodion (or, collodium)
			PREFIXED ROOT:
			precollagenous (*pre* before + *genere* to produce)
			procollagen (*pro* before + *genere* to produce)
			LEADING ROOT COMPOUND:
			coll: colloid {colloidal} (*eidos* form, resembling)
			colla:
			collagen (a fibrous insoluble protein found in the connective tissue), collagenation (or, collagenization)
			collagenic (also called *collagenous, collagenogenic*) (*genere* to produce)
			collagen: collagenosis (collagen disease) (*osis* condition)
			collageno producing collagen:
			collagenoblast (a cell that differentiates from a fibroblast and functions in the formation of collagen) (*blastos* cell, shoot, germ)
			collagenocyte (*kytos* cell)
			collagenolysis {collagenolytic} (*lyein* to dissolve)

A Thesaurus of Medical Word Roots

Element	From	Meaning	Examples
colla (cont'd)		[glue]	TRAILING ROOT COMPOUND: *col*: protocol (a clinical report from notes first taken; minutes of a meeting; description of steps to be taken in an experiment (*protos* first) [orig., from the first leaf glued to a manuscript, describing its contents] *colla*: ichthyocolla (a form of gelatin prepared from the swimming bladders of the Russian sturgeon; used as a clarifying agent; also called *isinglass*) (*ichthys* fish) *collagenous*: fibrocollagenous (fiber) *colloid*: pseudocolloid (*pseudes* false + *eidos* form) FRENCH: décollement (lit., ungluing; rarely used term for the operation of separating an organ from the adjoining tissue to which it normally adheres) (*de* away) CROSS REFERENCE: gli, glut[2]
colp	Greek *kolpos* a fold, or bosomlike hollow	hollow; vagina; womb	PREFIXED ROOT: encolpism (medication administered via the vagina) (*en* in) endocolpitis (inflammation of the vaginal mucosa) (*endon* within + colpitis) paracolpium, paracolpitis (*para* alongside + colpitis) pericolpitis (*peri* around + colpitis) LEADING ROOT COMPOUND: *colp*: colpalgia (also called *colpodynia, vaginodynia*) (*algos* pain) colpatresia (also called *vaginal atresia*) (*atresia* imperforate) colpectasis (or, colpectasia) (*ektasis* stretching, dilatation) colpectomy (also called *vaginectomy*) (*ektome* excision) colpeurysis (operative dilatation of the vagina) (*eurynein* to dilate) colpitis (*itis* inflammation) colpodynia (also called *colpalgia, vaginodynia*) (*odyne* pain) *colpo*: colpocele (also called *vaginal hernia*) (*kele* hernia) colpoceliocentesis (*koilia* cavity + *kentesis* puncture) colpoceliotomy (*koilia* cavity + *tomy* incision) colpocleisis (surgical closure of the vaginal canal) (*kleisis* closure) colpocystitis (*kytis* bladder + *itis* inflammation) colpocystoplasty (*kystis* bladder + *plassein* to form) colpocystocele (*kystis* bladder + *kele* hernia) colpocystotomy (*kystis* bladder + *tomy* incision) colpocytology (*kytos* cell + *logy* study) colpohyperplasia (*hyper* above + *plassein* to form) colpohysterectomy (*hyster* uterus + *ektome* excision) colpohysteropexy (*hyster* uterus + *pexy* fixation) colpohysterotomy (*hyster* uterus + *tomy* incision) colpomicroscope (*mikros* small + *skopein* to examine) colpomycosis (also called *vaginomycosis*) (*mykes* fungus + *osis* condition) colpomyomectomy (*myoma* muscle tumor + *ektome* excision) colpoperineoplasty (perineum + *plassein* to form) colpoperineorrhaphy (perineum + *rhaphe* suture) colpopexy (also called *vaginofixation*) (*pexis* fixation) colpoplasty (also called *vaginoplasty*) (*plassein* to form) colpopoiesis (the creation of a vagina by plastic surgery) (*poiein* to make, produce) colpoptosis (or, colpoptosia) (*ptosis* a falling)

Element	From	Meaning	Examples
colp (cont'd)		[vagina]	colporectopexy (rectum + *pexy* fixation)
			colporrhagia (*rhagia* bursting forth)
			colporrhaphy (*rhaphe* suture)
			colporrhexis (also called *vaginal laceration*) (*rhexis* rupture)
			colposcope, colposcopy (*skopein* to examine)
			colpospasm (also called *vaginal spasm*) (*spasmos* contraction)
			colpostat (appliance for use in the vagina for treatment of cancer in the cervix) (*statos* standing)
			colpostenosis (*stenosis* narrow condition)
			colpostenotomy (surgical correction of a colpostenosis) (*stenos* narrow + *tomy* incision)
			colpotomy (also called *coleotomy*, *vaginotomy*) (*tomy* incision)
			colpoureterotomy (ureter + *tomy* incision)
			colpoxerosis (*xerosis* dry condition)
			TRAILING ROOT COMPOUND:
			colpitis inflammation of vagina:
			cervicocolpitis (cervix)
			myocolpitis (*myos* muscle)
			colpos:
			aerocolpos (distention of the vagina with air) (*aer* air)
			ankylocolpos (*ankylos* bent, fused)
			hematocolpos (*hematos* blood)
			hydrocolpos (*hydor* water)
			hydrometrocolpos (*hydor* water + *metra* uterus)
			lochiocolpos (*lochia* vaginal discharge)
			mucocolpos (accumulation of mucus in the vaginal canal)
			pyocolpos (*pyon* pus)
			CROSS REFERENCE: cav, lemma, sin, uter
com-	Latin prefix	with, together	See Appendix B for examples of words with this prefix. Others are listed with the roots to which it is attached.
			CROSS REFERENCE: con-, syn-
con-	Latin prefix	with, together	See Appendix B (com-) for examples of words with this prefix. Others are listed with the roots to which it is attached.
			CROSS REFERENCE: com-, syn-
con	Latin *conus* Greek *konos*	cone	SIMPLE ROOT:
			conarium (also called *pineal body*)
			cone (a solid figure or body with a circular base tapering to a point: specifically one of the conelike bodies of the retina) {conic, conical, conular}
			conization (excision of a cone of tissue, as of the mucous membrane of the cervix)
			conus (a structure resembling a cone; posterior staphyloma of the myopic eye; pl., coni)
			PREFIXED ROOT:
			entocone (*entos* within)
			hypocone, hypoconid, hypoconule, hypoconulid (*hypo* under)
			metacone, metaconid, metaconule (*meta* after)
			paracone (the mesiobuccal cusp of an upper molar tooth), paraconid (*para* alongside)
			protocone (*protos* first)
			LEADING ROOT COMPOUND:
			con: conoid (shaped like a cone; conical) (*eidos* form)
			cono: conomyoidin (*myos* muscle + *eidos* form)

Element	From	Meaning	Examples
con (cont'd)		[cone]	TRAILING ROOT COMPOUND: keratoconus (a conical protrusion of the central part of the cornea) (*keratos* horn: cornea) lenticonus (conical protrusion of the anterior or posterior surfaces of the lens) (*lens* lentil) CROSS REFERENCE: cune, pine
condyl	Greek *kondylos* knuckle	rounded projection on a bone	SIMPLE ROOT: condylion, condyloma (knuckle, knob; pl., condylomata) {condylo-matous} condylus (or, condyle; pl., condyli) {condylar, condylicus} PREFIXED ROOT: *condylar*: hypocondylar (*hypo* under) epicondylar (*epi* upon) intercondylar (or, intercondylic, intercondyloid) (*inter* between) postcondylare (the highest point of the curvature posterior to the occipital condyle) (*post* after) supraepicondylar (*supra* above + epicondylar) transcondylar (*trans* across, through) *condyle*: ectocondyle (*ektos* external) epicondyle {epicondylic} (*epi* upon) *condyloid*: supracondyloid (*supra* above + condyloid) LEADING ROOT COMPOUND: *condyl*: condylarthrosis (*arthrosis* bone condition) condylectomy (*ektome* excision) condyloid (*eidos* form; similar to) *condylo*: condylotomy (*tomy* incision) PREFIXED LEADING ROOT COMPOUND: epicondylitis (*epi* upon + *itis* inflammation) CROSS REFERENCE: None
coni, koni	Greek *konis*	dust, spore	SIMPLE ROOT: conidium (a small asexual spore; also called *exo-spore*; pl., conidia) {conidial} PREFIXED ROOT: macroconidium (pl., macroconidia) (*makros* large) microconidium (pl., microconidia) (*mikros* small) LEADING ROOT COMPOUND: *coni*: coniosis (a disease state caused by the inhalation of dust) (*osis* condition) *conidio*: conidiophore (*phorein* to bear) conidiospore (conidium) (*sporos* seed) *conio*: coniofibrosis (*fibra* fiber + *osis* condition) coniology (or, koniology; the science of atmospheric dust, its influence, and its effects) (*logos* study) coniolymphstasis (*lymph* water, liquid + *stasis* a standing still) coniometer (or, koniometer, konometer) (*metron* measure) coniophage (also called *alveolar microphage*) (*phagein* to consume) coniophobia (*phobia* fear of) coniotomy (also called *cricothyrotomy*) (*tomy* incision) coniotoxicosis (*toxikon* poison + *osis* condition)

Element	From	Meaning	Examples
coni (cont'd)		[dust, spore]	*konio*: koniocortex (the granular cortex of sensory areas) TRAILING ROOT COMPOUND: deuteroconidium (*deuteros* second) hemoconia, hemoconiosis (*haima* blood + *osis* condition) pneumonoultramicroscopicsilicovolcano<u>coni</u>osis (a diseased lung condition caused by ultramicroscopic volcanic silicon dust; or "black lung disease," a particular disease of miners) (*pneumono* lung + *ultra* beyond + *microscopic* small-looking + *silico* silicon + *volcano* volcanic + *coni* dust + *osis* condition) statoconium (pl., statoconia; minute calciferous granules within the gelatinous statoconic membrane surmounting the maculae; also called *otoconia*) (*statos* standing) CROSS REFERENCE: None
contra-	Latin prefix	against	EXTENDED PREFIX: contrast See Appendix B for examples of words with this prefix. Others are listed with the roots to which it is attached. CROSS REFERENCE: anti-, ob-
copr	Greek *kopros*	dung, feces	PREFIXED ROOT: acoprosis (absence of fecal matter in the intestine) {acoprous} (*a* privative + *osis* condition) encopresis (incontinence of feces not due to organic defect or illness) (*en* negative) LEADING ROOT COMPOUND: *copr*: copracrasia (fecal incontinence) (*akrasia* lack of self-control) copragogue (cathartic) (*agein* to lead) copremesis (vomiting of fecal matter) (*emein* to vomit) coproma (*oma* tumor) *copra*: copraemia (or, copremia) (*emia* blood condition) *copro*: coproantibodies (antibodies found in the feces) coprolagnia (*lagneia* lust) coprolalia (involuntary utterances of vulgar or obscene words; also called *coprophrasia*) (*lalein* to speak) coprolith (also called *fecalith*) (*lithos* stone) coprology (study and analysis of feces, as for diagnosis; an obsession with excrement or excretory functions; also called *scatology*) (*logos* study) coprophagy (also called *scatophagy*) {coprophagous} (*phagein* to devour) coprophilia (attraction of microorganisms to fecal matter; also called *mysophilia*), coprophilous (*philein* to love) coprophobia (*phobia* fear) coprophrasia (also called *coprolalia*) (*phrazein* to speak) coproplanesia (escape of feces from the bowel through a wound or fistula) (*planan* to wander) copropraxia (obscene gesturing) (*praxis* action, behavior) coprostasis (impaction of the feces in the intestine) (*stasis* stoppage) CROSS REFERENCE: chez, sterc
cor-	Latin prefix	with, together	See Appendix B (com-) for examples of words with this prefix. Others are listed with the roots to which it is attached. CROSS REFERENCE: com-, syn-
cord			See chord- for *cordectomy, corditis*.

Element	From	Meaning	Examples
corm	Greek *kormos* trunk	trunk, torso	PREFIXED ROOT: acormus {acormia} (*a* privative) TRAILING ROOT COMPOUND: *cormia*: camptocormia (also called *prosternation*) (*kamptos* bent) nanocormia (*nanos* dwarf) schistocormia (also called *schistosomia*) (*schistos* split) *cormus*: atretocormus (*atretos* imperforate, closed) perocormus (also called *perosomus*) (*peros* maimed) schistocormus (also called *schistosomus*) (*schistos* split) CROSS REFERENCE: corp, som
corn	Latin *cornu* horn	horn; cornea; projecting point	SIMPLE ROOT: corn, cornea {corneal}, corneous, corneum corniculate (shaped like a small horn), corniculum cornu (any projection resembling a horn; pl., cornua) {cornual, cornuate} PREFIXED ROOT: *corn*: bicornate (or, bicornuate), bicornis (*bi* two) tricorn (*tri* three) unicorn (or, unicornous; having only one cornu) (*uni* one) *cornea*: ectocornea (*ektos* outside) entocornea (*enton* within) macrocornea (also called *megalocornea*) (*makros* large) megalocornea (also called *macrocornea*) (*megalos* large) mesocornea (*mesos* middle) microcornea (*mikros* small) *corneal*: circumcorneal (*circum* around) pericorneal (also called *perikeratic*) (*peri* around) precorneal (anterior to or outside the cornea) (*pre* before) subcorneal (*sub* beneath) *cornu(te)*: antecornu (the anterior cornu of a lateral ventricle of the brain) (*ante* before) medicornu (the middle or inferior horn of each lateral ventricle of the brain) (*medius* middle) postcornu (the posterior horn of each lateral ventricle of the brain) tricornute (having three horns, cornua, or processes) (*tri* three) LEADING ROOT COMPOUND: *corn*: cornoid (resembling horn) (*eidos* form) *corne*: corneitis (also called *keratitis*) (*itis* inflammation) *corni*: cornification, cornified (*facere* to make) *corneo*: corneoblepharon (*blepharon* eyelid) corneocyte (*kytos* cell) corneoiritis (iris + *itis* inflammation) corneosclera {corneoscleral} (*skleros* hard) TRAILING ROOT COMPOUND: iridocorneal (iris) sclerocornea {sclerocorneal} (*skleros* hard) CROSS REFERENCE: cerat

A Thesaurus of Medical Word Roots

Element	From	Meaning	Examples
corp	Latin *corpus*	body	SIMPLE ROOT: corporal (or, corporeal; pertaining to the body) corporic (affecting the body, or corpus, of an organ) corps (an organized body, or group of individuals; corpus) corpse (a dead body; used to refer specifically to a human body in the early period after death) corpulency (fatness of the body), corpulent (fat; obese) corpus (a discrete mass of material, as of specialized tissue; the entire body of the organism, or the main portion of an anatomical part, structure, or organ; pl., corpora) corpuscle (any small mass or body) {corpuscular}, corpusculum (pl., corpuscula) PREFIXED ROOT: *corpor:* bicorporate (having two bodies) (*bi* two) extracorporeal (*extra* outside) hemicorporectomy (the amputation of most of a person's body, essentially everything below the lumbar vertebrae; also called *translumbar amputation*) (*hemi* half + *ektome* excision) intracorporal (or, intracorporeal) (*intra* within) *corpuscular:* endocorpuscular (*endon* within) extracorpuscular (*extra* outside) intracorpuscular (also called *endoglobular*) (*intra* within) LEADING ROOT COMPOUND: corpectomy (the removal of a vertebral body) (*ektome* excision) CROSS REFERENCE: som
cort	Latin *cortex* bark, rind	external layer, cortex	SIMPLE ROOT: cortex (pl., cortices) {cortical}, corticalization (also called *encephalization*), corticate PREFIXED ROOT: *cortex:* isocortex (*isos* equal) paracortex (*para* alongside) subcortex (*sub* below) *cortical:* infracortical (*infra* below) subcortical (*sub* under) transcortical (*trans* across) *cortication:* decortication (*de* off, from) hemidecortication (*hemi* half + decortication) *corticism:* dyscorticism (*dys* abnormal) hypercorticism (*hyper* over) hypocorticism (*hypo* under) LEADING ROOT COMPOUND: *cortic:* corticectomy (also called *topectomy*) (*ektome* excision) corticoid (also called *corticosteroid*) (*eidos* form) *cortici:* corticifugal (or, corticofugal) (*fugere* to flee) corticipetal (or, corticopetal: proceeding, conducting, or moving toward the cortex; also called *corticoafferent*) (*petere* to seek)

Element	From	Meaning	Examples
cort (cont'd)		[external layer, cortex]	*cortico*: corticoadrenal (also called *adrenocortical*) (*ad* to + *ren* kidney) corticoafferent (also called *corticipetal*) (*ad* to + *ferre* to bear) corticodiencephalic (*dienkephalon* innerbrain) corticoefferent (also called *corticifugal*) (*ef* out + *ferre* to bear) corticomedullary (*medulla* marrow) corticomesencephalic (mesencephalon) corticopeduncular (peduncles of the brain) corticopleuritis (also called *pulmonary pleurisy*) (*pleura* side + *itis* inflammation) corticopontine (*pons* bridge) corticospinal (spine) corticosteroid (*stereos* solid + *eidos* form) corticothalamic (thalamus) corticotroph {corticotrophic} (*trophein* to nourish) corticotropic (*trope* a turning) TRAILING ROOT COMPOUND: *cortex*: archicortex (the cortex forming the hippocampus) (*archein* to begin) neocortex (*neos* new) *cortical*: cerebrocortical (*cerebrum* brain) meningocortical (*meningos* membrane) psychocortical (*psyche* mind) renocortical (*ren* kidney) spinocortical (also called *corticospinal*) thalamocortical (thalamus) CROSS REFERENCE: lam
cost	Latin *costa*	rib, side	SIMPLE ROOT: costa (pl., costae), costal (pertaining to a rib or ribs) costalis (costal; used in anatomical nomenclature to denote relationship to a rib) PREFIXED ROOT: epicostal (*epi* upon) infracostal (*infra* below) intercostal (*inter* between) intracostal (on the inner surface of the rib) (*intra* within) postcostal (*post* behind) precostal (*pre* before) subcostal, subcostalgia (*sub* below + *algos* pain) subcostosternal (*sub* below + *sternum* chest) supracostal (*supra* over, above) LEADING ROOT COMPOUND: *cost*: costalgia (*algos* pain) costectomy (*ektome* excision) *costi*: costicartilage (the cartilage of a rib) costiferous (*ferre* to bear) costiform (*forma* shape) costispinal (spine) *costo*: costocentral (*kentron* point, center)

Element	From	Meaning	Examples
cost (cont'd)		[rib, side]	costochondral, costochondritis (*chondros* cartilage + *itis* inflammation)
			costoclavicular (clavicle)
			costogenic (*genere* to produce)
			costophrenic (*phren* diaphragm)
			costopleural (*pleura* rib, side)
			costoscapular (*scapula* shoulder blade)
			costosternal, costosternoplasty (*sternum* breastbone + *plassein* to form)
			costotome, costotomy (*tomy* incision)
			costovertebral (vertebra)
			costoxiphoid (xiphoid process)
			TRAILING ROOT COMPOUND:
			chondrocostal (*chondros* cartilage)
			cleidocostal (*kleidos* clavicle)
			iliocostal (ileum)
			lumbocostal (*lumbus* loin)
			sternocostal (*sternon* chest)
			vertebrocostal (vertebra)
			xiphocostal (*xiphos* sword: xiphoid process)
			CROSS REFERENCE: canth, later, pleur
couch			See loc- for *accouchement*.
cox	Latin *coxa*	hip	SIMPLE ROOT: coxa (the hip or hip joint; pl. coxae)
			PREFIXED ROOT:
			paracoxalgia (*para* similar to + coxalgia)
			pericoxitis (*peri* around + coxitis)
			LEADING ROOT COMPOUND:
			cox:
			coxalgia (hip joint disease; also called *coxodynia*) (*algos* pain)
			coxarthria, coxarthritis (or, coxitis) (*arthron* joint + *itis* inflammation)
			coxitis (also called *coxarthritis*) (*itis* inflammation)
			coxodynia (also called *coxalgia*) (*odyne* pain)
			coxo:
			coxofemoral (relating to the hip and the thigh) (femur)
			coxotuberculosis (tuberculous condition of the hip joint)
			TRAILING ROOT COMPOUND:
			pseudocoxalgia (*pseudes* false + coxalgia)
			sacrocoxalgia (sacrum + coxalgia)
			sacrocoxitis (sacrum + *itis* inflammation)
			NB: *Coxsackie virus* is derived from Coxsackie, New York, where the virus was first identified.
			CROSS REFERENCE: ischi
cran	Greek *kranion* Latin *cranium*	skull	SIMPLE ROOT: craniad (in a cranial direction; toward the head end of the body; also called *cephalad*) {cranial}, cranium (pl., crania)
			PREFIXED ROOT:
			crania:
			acrania (partial or complete congenital absence of the cranium) {acranial} (*a* privative)
			amphicrania (pain in both sides of the head) (*amphi* around)
			hemicrania (pain in one side of the head; incomplete anencephaly) (*hemi* half) [see Disguised Root]
			macrocrania (*makros* large)

Element	From	Meaning	Examples
cran (cont'd)		[skull]	microcrania (*mikros* small)
			cranial:
			acranial (*a* privative)
			encranial (*en* in)
			endocranial (or, entocranial) (*endon* within)
			extracranial (*extra* outside)
			eurycranial (*eurys* wide)
			intracranial (*intra* within)
			pericranial (*peri* around)
			postcranial (*post* behind)
			subcranial (*sub* below)
			supracranial (*supra* above)
			transcranial (*trans* across, through)
			cranitis inflammation of the skull:
			endocranitis (*endon* within)
			pericranitis (*peri* around)
			cranium:
			endocranium (or, entocranium) (*endon* within)
			epicranium (the integument, aponeurosis, and muscular expansions of the scalp) {epicranial} (*epi* upon)
			macrocranium (*makros* large)
			pericranium {pericranial} (*peri* around)
			cranius:
			acranius (a fetus in which the cranium is absent or rudimentary) (*a* privative)
			encranius (in conjoined twins, a form of fetal inclusion in which the smaller parasite lies partly or wholly within the cranial cavity of the larger autosite) (*en* in)
			monocranius (also called *syncephalus*) (*monos* single)
			LEADING ROOT COMPOUND:
			crani:
			craniad (toward the cranium; opposite of *caudad*) (*ad* to)
			craniamphitomy (division of the entire circumference of the skull for securing decompression) (*amphi* around + *tomy* incision)
			craniectomy (*ektome* excision)
			craniostosis (*osteon* bone + *osis* condition)
			cranio:
			cranioacromial (*acromion* tip of the shoulder)
			cranioaural (*auris* ear)
			craniobuccal (*bucca* cheek, mouth)
			craniocele (a protrusion of any part of the cranial contents through a defect in the skull; also called *encephalocele*) (*kele* hernia)
			craniocerebral (*cerebrum* portion of the brain)
			craniocervical (*cervix* neck)
			cranioclasia (or, cranioclasis), cranioclast (*klaein* to break)
			craniodidymus (*didymos* twin)
			craniofacial (face)
			craniofenestria (also called *craniolacunia*) (*fenestra* opening)
			craniognomy (*gnomon* judge)
			craniograph, craniography (*graphein* to write)
			craniolacunia (also called *craniofenestria*) (*lacuna* a hollow)
			craniology (*logos* study)
			craniomalacia (abnormal softness of the skull) (*malakos* soft)
			craniomeningocele (*meningos* membrane + *kele* hernia)

Element	From	Meaning	Examples
cran (cont'd)		[skull]	craniometer, craniometry {craniometric} (*metron* measure)
			craniopagus (*pagos* thing fixed)
			craniopathy (*pathos* disease)
			craniopharyngeal, craniopharyngioma (*pharynx* throat + *oma* tumor)
			craniophore (*phoros* bearing)
			cranioplasty (*plassein* to form)
			craniopuncture (also called *cephalocentesis*) (*pungere* to pierce)
			craniorhachidian (also called *craniospinal*) (*rhachis* spine)
			craniosacral (*sacrum*)
			cranioschisis (cranium bifidum) (*schisis* fissure)
			craniosclerosis (*skleros* hard + *osis* condition)
			cranioscopy (*skopein* to examine)
			craniospinal (also called *craniorhachidian*) (spine)
			craniostenosis (*stenosis* narrowing)
			craniosynostosis (*syn* together + *osteon* bone + *osis* condition)
			craniotabes (*tabes* wasting away)
			craniotome, craniotomy (*tomy* incision)
			craniotonoscopy (*tonos* tone + *skopein* to examine)
			craniotrypesis (*trypesis* trephination, boring)
			craniotympanic (*tympanom* eardrum)
			TRAILING ROOT COMPOUND:
			cranial:
			auriculocranial (auricle of ear)
			basicranial (pertaining to the base of the skull)
			brachycranial (*brachys* short)
			cleidocranial (or, clidocranial) (*kleidos* clavicle)
			dolichocranial (*dolichos* long)
			opisthocranial (*opisthen* back, behind)
			otocranial (*otos* ear)
			platycranial (*platys* flat)
			rhaebocrania (also called *torticollis, wry neck*) (*rhaibos* crooked)
			cranium:
			neurocranium (*neuron* nerve)
			splanchnocranium (*splanchnos* viscus)
			viscerocranium (*viscera* internal organs)
			DISGUISED ROOT: migraine (a migraine headache, usually affecting only one side of the head; also called *megrim*) (*hemi* half)
			CROSS REFERENCE: cephal
cras, crat	Greek *krasis* mixture	mixing, temperament	PREFIXED ROOT:
			dyscrasia (orig., bad temperament; also called *disease, pathologic condition*) {dyscrasic, dyscratic} (*dys* abnormal)
			eucrasia (*eu* well)
			TRAILING ROOT COMPOUND:
			crasia:
			galactacrasia (*galaktos* milk + *a* negative)
			hemodyscrasia (*haima* blood + *dys* abnormal)
			spermacrasia (*sperma* seed, semen + *a* privative)
			uracrasia (*ouron* urine + *a* privative)
			crasy: idiosyncrasy (*idios* one's own + *syn* with)
			cratia: uracratia (*a* privative + *ouron* urine)
			DISGUISED ROOT: crater (lit., mixing bowl; a circular area of depression surrounded by an elevated margin)
			CROSS REFERENCE: misc

Element	From	Meaning	Examples
creat, **creas**	Greek *kreas*	flesh, meat	SIMPLE ROOT: creatinase, creatine, creatinine PREFIXED COMPOUND: pancreas (lit., all flesh; a long, soft, ir-regularly shaped gland lying behind the stomach, and secreting a digestive juice) (*pan* all) [see separate entry: pancrea-] LEADING ROOT COMPOUND: *crea*: creatoxicon (also called *kreotoxicon*) (*toxikon* poison) *creatin*: creatinemia (*emia* blood condition) creatinuria (*uria* urine condition) *creato*: creatorrhea (the presence of undigested muscle fibers in the feces) (*rhein* to flow) creatotoxism (meat poisoning) (*toxikon* poison) *creo*: creophagy (the eating of flesh, or meat) (*phagein* to eat) CROSS REFERENCE: sarc
crin, **cris,** **crit,** **crem**	Greek *krinein*	to separate, distinguish, judge	SIMPLE ROOT: crisis (pl., crises) criterion (pl., criteria), critical PREFIXED ROOT: *crem*: recrement (secretion, such as the saliva or part of the bile, hav-ing performed its function, is reabsorbed by the body) (*re* back) *crin*: apocrine, apocrinitis (*apo* from + *itis* inflammation) autocrine (*autos* self) eccrine (the flow of sweat glands; also called *exocrine*), eccrinology (*ec* out + *logos* study) diacrinous (*dia* through) ectocrine (*ektos* outside) endocrine (*endon* within) exocrine (secreting outwardly, via a duct; also called *eccrine*), exo-crinology, exocrinosity (*exo* outer + *logos* study) heterocrine (*heteros* other) holocrine (*holos* whole) intercrines (also called *chemokines*) (*inter* between) intracrine (*intra* within) juxtacrine (*juxta* near) paracrine (*para* alongside) *crisia*: hypereccrisia {hypereccritic} (*hyper* above + eccrisis) hypoeccrisia (or, hypoeccrisis; abnormally diminished excretion) {hypoeccritic} (*hypo* under + eccrisis) *crisis*: diacrisis (also called *diagnosis*) (*dia* through) eccrisis (the removal of waste products) (*ek* out) epicrisis (a second or supplementary crisis) (*epi* upon) heterocrisis (*heteros* other) metasyncrisis (the elimination of waste or morbid matter, particu-larly through the pores of the skin) (*meta* after + *syn* with) paraeccrisis (*para* alongside + eccrisis) *crit*: acritical (not marked by a crisis) (*a* negative) acritochromacy (color blindness) (*a* negative + *chroma* color) diacritic (diagnostic; said of symptoms) (*dia* across)

Element	From	Meaning	Examples
crin (cont'd)		[to separate]	epicritic (*epi* upon)
			intercritical (*inter* between)
			precritical (*pre* before)
			LEADING ROOT COMPOUND:
			crinogenic (stimulating secretion) (*genere* to produce)
			crinophagy (disposal of excess secretory granules by lysosomes) (*phagein* to devour)
			TRAILING ROOT COMPOUND:
			crin:
			angiocrine, angiocrinosis (*angeion* blood vessel + *osis* condition)
			merocrine (partly secreting) (*meros* part)
			cris: pseudocrisis (*pseudes* false)
			crit:
			cryocrit (*kryos* cold)
			hematocrit (*hematos* blood)
			lipocrit (*lipos* fat)
			lactocrit (*lactis* milk)
			plasmacrit (plasma)
			CROSS REFERENCE: None
cris, crit			See crin- for *crisis, critical*.
crot	Greek *krotos* stroke	stroke, beat, pulse	PREFIXED ROOT:
			crotic:
			acrotic (pertaining to extreme weakness or absence of the pulse)
			acrotism (absent or imperceptible pulse) (*a* privative)
			anacrotic (*ana* again)
			anadicrotic (pertaining to a pulse with more than one artery expansion) (*ana* again + dicrotic)
			anatricrotic (*ana* again + tricrotic)
			bradycrotic (pertaining to slowness of pulse) (*bradys* slow)
			catacrotic (indicating the downstroke of pulse tracing interrupted by an upstroke) (*kata* down)
			catadicrotic (*kata* down + dicrotic)
			dicrotic (*di* two)
			hyperdicrotic (*hyper* above + dicrotic)
			monocrotic (*monos* single)
			polycrotic (*polys* many)
			postdicrotic (*post* after + dicrotic)
			predicrotic (*pre* before + dicrotic)
			superdicrotic (*super* above + dicrotic)
			tachycrotic (*tachys* rapid)
			tetracrotic (*tetra* four)
			tricrotic (or, tricrotous) (*tri* three)
			crotism:
			anacrotism (an anomaly of the pulse evidenced by appearance of a small additional wave or notch in the ascending limb of the pulse tracing) (*ana* again)
			anadicrotism (*ana* again + dicrotism)
			anatricrotism (*ana* again + tricrotism)
			catacrotism (*kata* down)
			catadicrotism (*kata* down + dicrotism)
			catatricrotism (*kata* down + tricrotism)
			dicrotism (*di* two)
			hyperdicrotism (*hyper* above + dicrotism)

Element	From	Meaning	Examples
crot (cont'd)		[stroke, beat, pulse]	monocrotism (*monos* single) polycrotism (*polys* many) tricrotism (*tri* three) CROSS REFERENCE: ict, palp, pleg, puls, sphygmo
crur, crus	Latin *crus*	shin, leg; also, leglike part; see crurotomy]	SIMPLE ROOT: crus (the part of the lower limb from the knee to the ankle; anatomic nomenclature for a leglike part; pl., crura) {crural, e.g., crural arch, crural hernia, crural nerve} PREFIXED ROOT: intercrural (between two crura, e.g., the crus cerebri or the cerebral peduncles, of the brain) (*inter* between) intracrureus (*intra* within) retrocrural (*retro* backward, posterior) subcruralis, subcrureus (*sub* under) LEADING ROOT COMPOUND: crurotomy [surgical cutting of a crus of the stapes (of the ear), usually the anterior crus] (*tomy* incision) TRAILING ROOT COMPOUND: brachiocrural (pertaining to the upper limb and the lower limb) (*brachion* arm) genitocrural (pertaining to the genitalia, or the reproductive organs, and the thigh) inguinocrural (*inguen* groin) lumbocrural (*lumbus* loin) talocrural (*talus* ankle) vulvocrural (*vulva* the external genitalia of the female) CROSS REFERENCE: scel
cry	Greek *kryos* cold; *krymos* frost	cold	PREFIXED ROOT: *hypercry* excessive cold: hypercryalgesia (also called *hypercryesthesia*) (*algesia* pain) hypercryesthesia (also called *hypercryalgesia*) (*esthesia* feeling) LEADING ROOT COMPOUND: *cry*: cryalgesia (pain from the application of cold) (*algesia* pain) cryanesthesia (loss of sense of cold) (*an* privative + *esthesia* feeling) cryesthesia (abnormal sensitiveness to cold) (*esthesia* feeling) *crym*: crymodynia (pain from cold) (*odyne* pain) *crymo*: crymophilic (also called *cryophilic, psychrophilic*) (*philein* to love) crymophylactic (or, cryophylactic; resistant to cold) (*phylaxis* a guarding) crymotherapy (or, cryotherapy) (*therapy* treatment) *cryo*: cryoablation (*ablation* separation, detachment) cryoanalgesia (*an* negative + *algesia* pain) cryobank (a facility for cryopreservation of tissue, organs, embryos, sperm, or other substances, such as while waiting for transplantation) cryobiology (*bios* life + *logos* study) cryocardioplegia (*kardia* heart + *plegia* stroke) cryocautery (cauterization by freezing; also called *cold cautery*) cryodamage (damage to tissues, cells, or other biological substrates as a result of exposure to cold) cryoextraction, cryoextractor (*ex* out + *trahere* to pull, draw)

A Thesaurus of Medical Word Roots

Element	From	Meaning	Examples
cry (cont'd)		[cold]	cryogen (a substance for lowering temperatures) {cryogenic} (*genere* to produce)
			cryoglobulin, cryoglobulinemia (*globus* sphere + *emia* blood condition)
			cryohydrate (*hydor* water)
			cryolysis (*lysis* dissolution)
			cryometer (*metron* measure)
			cryopathy (*pathos* disease)
			cryopexy (*pexis* fixation)
			cryophile (also called *psychrophile*) {cryophilic, or crymophilic} (*philein* to love)
			cryophylactic (or, crymophylactic) (*phylaxis* a guarding)
			cryoscope, cryoscopy {cryoscopical} (*skopein* to examine)
			cryospasm (*spasmos* convulsion)
			cryostat (a freezing chamber) (*histanai* to stand)
			cryosurgery (the destruction of tissue by application of extreme cold)
			cryotherapy (also called *crymotherapy*) (*therapy* treatment)
			TRAILING ROOT COMPOUND:
			hemocryoscopy (the determination of the freezing point of blood) (*haima* blood + *skopein* to examine)
			urinocryoscopy (cryoscopy of the urine) (urine + *skopein* to examine)
			CROSS REFERENCE: None
crypt	Greek *kryptein* to hide	hidden, concealed	SIMPLE ROOT:
			crypt (a small sac or cavity extending into an epithelial surface)
			crypta (a minute tubelike depression opening on a free surface; pl., cryptae)
			cryptic (having a hidden meaning; tending to hide or disguise)
			PREFIXED ROOT: metacryptozoite (*meta* after + *zoon* animal)
			LEADING ROOT COMPOUND:
			crypt:
			cryptanamnesia (or, cryptomnesia; subconscious memory) (*an* privative + *amnesia* forgetfulness)
			cryptesthesia (subconscious appreciation or perception of occurrences not ordinarily perceptible to the senses; clairvoyance) (*esthesia* feeling)
			cryptitis (inflammation of a crypt or follicle, especially an anal crypt) (*itis* inflammation)
			cryptophthalmos (*ophthalmos* eye)
			cryptorchid (or, cryptorchis; an individual whose testicles have not descended into the scrotum), cryptorchidism (*orchis* testis)
			cryptotia (*otia* ear condition)
			crypto:
			cryptocephalus (a fetus with an inconspicuous head) (*kephale* head)
			cryptococcoma (*kokkos* berry-shaped bacterial cell + *oma* tumor)
			cryptocrystalline (composed of crystals of microscopic size)
			cryptodeterminant (a hidden determinant)
			cryptodidymus (a congenital anomaly in which one fetus is concealed within another; also called *endadelphos*) (*didymos* twin)
			cryptoempyema (*empyema* accumulation of pus)
			cryptogam {cryptogamic} (*gamos* reproduction)
			cryptogenic (or, cryptogenetic; of unknown or indeterminate origin) (*genere* to produce)

Element	From	Meaning	Examples
crypt (cont'd)		[hidden]	cryptoglandular (pertaining to or arising from an anal gland or an anal crypt)
			cryptolith (a concretion in a glandular follicle) (*lithos* stone)
			cryptomenorrhea (*men* month: menstruation + *rhein* to flow)
			cryptomere (a cystic or saclike condition) (*meros* part)
			cryptomnesia {cryptomnesic} (*mnesia* memory)
			cryptoneurous (*neuron* nerve)
			cryptoplasmic (*plassein* to form)
			cryptopodia (swelling of the lower leg and foot, covering all but the sole of the foot) (*pous* foot)
			cryptopyic (*pyon* pus)
			cryptoscope (fluoroscope), cryptoscopy (*skopein* to examine)
			cryptotoxic (*toxic* poisonous)
			cryptozygous (*zygon* yoke)
			TRAILING ROOT COMPOUND:
			onychocryptosis (*onychos* nail + *osis* condition)
			phallocrypsis (retraction of the penis) (*phallos* penis)
			trichocryptosis (*trichos* hair + *osis* condition)
			CROSS REFERENCE: None
cune	Latin *cuneus* wedge, peak	wedge	SIMPLE ROOT: cuneus (pl., cunei) {cuneate}
			PREFIXED ROOT:
			cuneal: precuneal (*pre* anterior)
			cuneiform wedge-shaped:
			ectocuneiform (the outermost one of the three cuneiform bones of the distal row of tarsal bones; the ectocuneiform or ectosphenoid bones of the foot) (*ektos* external)
			entocuneiform (*entos* inside)
			mesocuneiform (*mesos* middle)
			cuneus: precuneus {precuneate} (*pre* before)
			LEADING ROOT COMPOUND:
			cunei: cuneiform (shaped like a wedge) (*forma* shape)
			cuneo:
			cuneocuboid (*kubos* cube + *eidos* form)
			cuneonavicular (also called *cuneoscaphoid*) (*navicula* boat)
			cuneoscaphoid (also called *cuneonavicular*) (*scaphe* skiff, boat)
			CROSS REFERENCE: embol, sphen
cuss	Latin *quatere*	to shake, strike	PREFIXED ROOT:
			concussion (a violent jar or shock; loss of function either partial or complete as that resulting from a blow or fall) (*com* with)
			discussive (or, discutient; as an adjective, scattering; causing a disappearance) (*dis* apart)
			percuss (to subject to percussion)
			percussible (discoverable on percussion)
			percussion (the act of striking a part with short, sharp blows)
			percussor (a vibrator that produces relatively coarse movements) (*per* intensive)
			repercussion {repercussive} (*re* back + percussion)
			succuss, succussion (shaking of the body to detect the presence of fluid in a body cavity by listening for a splashing sound, especially in the thorax) (*sub* under)
			FRENCH: percuteur (an instrument for therapeutic or diagnostic percussion)
			CROSS REFERENCE: pact

Element	From	Meaning	Examples
cut	Latin *cutis*	skin	SIMPLE ROOT: cutaneous, cuticle, cuticula (pl., cuticulae), cutis PREFIXED ROOT: *cutaneous*: epicutaneous (*epi* upon) intracutaneous (also called *intradermal*) (*intra* within) percutaneous (also called *transcutaneous*) (*per* through) subcutaneous (*sub* under) transcutaneous (also called *transdermal*) (*trans* through, across) *cutaneo*: intercutaneomucous (*inter* between + mucus) LEADING ROOT COMPOUND: cutaneomucosal (also called *mucocutaneous*) (mucus) TRAILING ROOT COMPOUND: colocutaneous (*kolon* colon) enterocutaneous (*enteron* intestine) gastrocutaneous (*gaster* stomach, belly) mucocutaneous (also called *cutaneomucosal*) (mucus) musculocutaneous (also called *myocutaneous*) (muscle) myocutaneous (also called *musculocutaneous*) (*myos* muscle) nephrocutaneous (also called *renocutaneous*) (*nephros* kidney) neurocutaneous (*neuron* nerve) oculocutaneous (*oculus* eye) photocutaneous (*photos* light) pleurocutaneous (*pleura* rib, side) psychocutaneous (*psyche* mind) pulmocutaneous (*pulmo* lung) pyelocutaneous (*pyelos* pelvis) rectocutaneous (rectum) renocutaneous (also called *nephrocutaneous*) (*ren* kidney) urethrocutaneous (urethra) vaginocutaneous (vagina) TERM: per cutem (through the skin) CROSS REFERENCE: chori, derm
cycl	Greek *kuklos* circle	wheel, circle	SIMPLE ROOT: cyclase, cycle {cyclic} PREFIXED ROOT: *cyclic*: acyclic (not cyclic; in chemistry, having the structure of an open chain rather than a closed ring) (*a* negative) endocyclic (*endon* within) exocyclic (pertaining to cyclic chemical compounds having their double bond in the side chain) (*exo* outside) heterocyclic (*heteros* other, different) homocyclic (also called *isocyclic*) (*homos* same) isocyclic (also called *homocyclic*) (*isos* equal) monocyclic (containing one ring of atoms in the molecule) (*monos* single, one) polycyclic (containing more than one ring or cycle) (*polys* many) tetracyclic (*tetra* four) tricyclic (*tri* three) *cyclo*: incycloduction (a cycloduction in which the upper pole of the cornea is rotated inward, or medially) (*in* in + *ducere* to lead) incyclophoria (also called *minus cyclophoria*) (*in* in + *phorein* to bear)

Element	From	Meaning	Examples
cycl (cont'd)		[circle, wheel]	incyclotropia (*in* in + *tropein* to turn) *cycloidal*: hypocycloidal (*hypo* under + *eidos* form) *cyclosis*: hypocyclosis (*hypo* under + *osis* condition) LEADING ROOT COMPOUND: *cycl*: cyclarthrosis {cyclarthrodial} (*arthrosis* a jointing) cyclectomy (*ektome* excision) cyclencephaly (*enkephalon* brain) cyclitis (inflammation of the ciliary body) (*itis* inflammation) cycloid (*eidos* form, resembling) cyclopia (*opia* vision condition) cyclops (a fetal malformation with only one eye) (*ops* eye) cyclosis (movement of the protoplasm within a cell, without deformation of the cell wall; also called *cytoplasmic*) (*osis* condition) *cyclico*: cyclicotomy (or, cyclotomy) (*tomy* incision) *cyclo*: cyclocephalus (also called *cyclops*) (*kephale* head) cycloceratitis (inflammation of cornea and ciliary body; also called *cyclokeratitis*) (*keras* cornea + *itis* inflammation) cyclochoroiditis (*choroid* skinlike + *itis* inflammation) cyclocryotherapy (transscleral freezing of the ciliary body in the treatment of glaucoma) (*kryos* cold + *therapy* treatment) cyclodamia (subdued or suppressed accommodation of the eyes) (*damazein* to subdue) cyclodialysis (dialysis: *dia* through + *lyein* to loosen) cyclodiathermy (diathermy: *dia* through + *therme* heat) cycloduction (also called *cyclotorsion*) (*ducere* to lead) cyclogeny (the developmental cycle of a microorganism) (*genere* to produce) cyclokeratitis (*keras* horn: cornea + *itis* inflammation) cyclomastopathy (*mastos* breast + *pathos* disease) cyclophoria (a strabismus in which the eye or eyes rotate inward or outward) (*phorein* to bear) cyclophorometer (*phorein* to bear + *metron* measure) cycloplegia {cycloplegic} (*plessein* to strike: paralysis) cyclorotation {cyclorotary} (*rotare* to turn) cyclospasm (spasm of accommodation of the eyes) cyclothyme (a person with a cyclothymic disorder) cyclothymia {cyclothymic, cyclothymiac} (*thymos* mind) cyclotome, cyclotomy (*tomy* incision) cyclotorsion (also called *cycloduction*) (*torquere* to twist) cyclotropia (*tropia* turning) CROSS REFERENCE: gyr, orb, spir
cyes	Greek *kyesis*	pregnancy	SIMPLE ROOT: cyesis (obsolete term for *pregnancy*), cyestein (a skinlike formation sometimes seen on the surface of urine of a pregnant woman) PREFIXED ROOT: eccyesis (ectopic pregnancy) (*ec* out) encyesis (normal uterine pregnancy) (*en* in) hypercyesis (superfetation) (*hyper* above, beyond) metacyesis (extrauterine gestation) (*meta* after) paracyesis (also called *ectopic pregnancy*) (*para* alongside) polycyesis (multiple pregnancy) (*polys* many)

A Thesaurus of Medical Word Roots

Element	From	Meaning	Examples
cyes (cont'd)		[pregnancy]	TRAILING ROOT COMPOUND: oocyesis (an ectopic ovarian pregnancy) (*oon* egg, ovum) ovariocyesis (ovarian pregnancy) (*ovum* egg) pseudocyesis (*pseudes* false) salpingocyesis (*salpingos* tube) CROSS REFERENCE: grav
cyst	Greek *kystis*	sac, bladder	SIMPLE ROOT: cyst {cystic, cystous} cystine, cystis (pl., cystides), cystose (cystoid) PREFIXED ROOT: *cyst*: ectocyst (the exterior coat of a dermoid cyst) (*ektos* outside) endocyst (*endon* within) macrocyst (*makros* large, long) microcyst (*mikros* small) pseudocyst (*pseudes* false) *cystation*: encystation (*en* in) excystation (*ex* out) *cysted*: encysted (enclosed in a sac, bladder, or cyst), encystment (*en* in) *cystia*: acystia (congenital absence of a bladder) (*a* privative) *cystic*: extracystic (*extra* outside) intracystic (*intra* within) multicystic (also called *polycystic*) (*multus* many) paracystic (*para* alongside) pericystic (*peri* around) polycystic (also called *multicystic*) (*polys* many) *cystis*: megalocystis (*megalos* large) *cystitis* bladder inflammation: endocystitis (*endon* within) epicystitis (*epi* upon) paracystitis (*para* alongside) pericystitis (*peri* around) *cystium*: paracystium (*para* alongside) pericystium (*peri* around) *cystotomy*: epicystotomy (*epi* upon + *tomy* incision) LEADING ROOT COMPOUND: *cyst*: cystacanth (*akantha* thorn, spine) cystadenoma (*aden* gland + *oma* tumor) cystalgia (also called *cystodynia*) (*algos* pain) cystatrophia (atrophy of the urinary bladder) (*a* negative + *trophein* to nourish) cystectomy (*ektome* excision) cystelcosis (*helcosis* ulceration) [h of helcosis elided] cystitis (*itis* inflammation) cystodynia (also called *cystalgia*) (*odyne* pain) cystoid (*eidos* form, resembling) cystoma (*oma* tumor) *cysti*: cystiferous (also called *cystogenous*) (*ferre* to bear)

A Thesaurus of Medical Word Roots

Element	From	Meaning	Examples
cyst (cont'd)		[sac, bladder]	cystiform (*forma* shape)
			cystigerous (containing cysts) (*gerere* to bear)
			cystistaxis (*staxis* a dripping)
			cystitome, cystitomy (*tomy* incision)
			cystico:
			cysticolithectomy (removal of a calculus from the cystic duct) (*lithos* stone + *ektome* excision)
			cysticolithotripsy (*lithos* stone + *tripsy* a crushing)
			cysticorrhaphy (*rhaphe* suture)
			cysticotomy (*tomy* incision)
			cystin:
			cystinemia (*emia* blood condition)
			cystinosis (*osis* condition)
			cystinuria {cystinuric} (*uria* urine condition)
			cysto:
			cystoblast (*blastos* bud, shoot, germ)
			cystocele (*kele* hernia)
			cystoenterocele (also called *enterocystocele*) (*enteron* intestine + *kele* hernia)
			cystoenterostomy (*enteron* intestine + *stoma* mouth, opening)
			cystoepiplocele (*epiloon* omentum + *kele* hernia)
			cystofibroma (*fibroma* fibrous tumor)
			cystogastrostomy (*gaster* stomach + *stoma* mouth, opening)
			cystogenesis, cystogenous (*genere* to produce)
			cystogram, cystography (*graphein* to write)
			cystolith, cystolithectomy (*lithos* stone + *ektome* excision)
			cystolithiasis (*lithos* stone + *iasis* condition)
			cystolithotomy (incision of the urinary bladder for removal of a calculus) (*lithos* stone + *tomy* incision)
			cystometer, cystometry (*metron* measure)
			cystomorphous (*morphe* shape)
			cystomyoma (*myos* muscle + *oma* tumor)
			cystomyxoma (*mykes* mucus + *oma* tumor)
			cystonephrosis (also called *nephrocystosis*) (*nephros* kidney + *osis* condition)
			cystoparalysis (also called *cystoplegia, cystoparesis*)
			cystoparesis (also called *cystoparalysis, cystoplegia*) (*paresis* slight or incomplete paralysis)
			cystopexy (*pexy* fixation)
			cystophorous (*phorein* to bear)
			cystoplasty (*plassein* to form)
			cystoplegia (also called *cystoparalysis, cystoparesis*) (*plege* a blow, stroke)
			cystoprostatectomy (prostate + *ektome* excision)
			cystoptosis (*ptosis* a falling)
			cystopyelitis (also called *pyelocystitis*) (*pyelos* pelvis + *itis* inflammation)
			cystorrhagia (*rhagia* bursting forth)
			cystorrhaphy (*rhaphein* to suture)
			cystorrhea (*rhein* to flow)
			cystosarcoma (a sarcoma in which cysts have formed; also called *phyllodes tumor*) (*sarkos* flesh + *oma* tumor)
			cystoschisis (*schisis* fissure)
			cystosclerosis (*sklerosis* hardening)

Element	From	Meaning	Examples
cyst (cont'd)		[sac, bladder]	cystoscope {cystoscopic}, cystoscopy (*skopein* to examine)
			cystospasm (*span* to contract)
			cystostomy (also called *vesicostomy*) (*stoma* mouth, opening)
			cystotome, cystotomy (also called *vesicotomy*) (*tomy* incision)
			cystotrachelotomy (also called *bladder neck incision*) (*trachelos* neck + *tomy* incision)
			cystoureteritis (ureter + *itis* inflammation)
			cystoureterogram (ureter + *graphein* to write)
			cystourethritis (also called *urethrocystitis*) (urethra + *itis* inflammation)
			cystourethrocele (prolapse of the urethra and bladder) (urethra + *kele* hernia)
			cystourethrogram, cystourethrography (urethra + *graphein* to write)
			cystourethropexy (also called *bladder neck suspension*) (urethra + *pexy* fixation)
			cystourethroscope, cystourethroscopy (urethra + *skopein* to examine)
			TRAILING ROOT COMPOUND:
			cyst:
			blastocyst (*blastos* bud, shoot, germ)
			dacryocyst (*dakryon* teardrop)
			dermatocyst (*dermatos* skin)
			enterocyst, enterocystoma (*enteron* intestine + *oma* tumor)
			gonecyst (*gone* seed)
			hematocyst (*hematos* blood)
			hydrocyst (a cyst with watery contents) (*hydor* water)
			hypnocyst (*hypnos* sleep)
			lymphocyst (also called *lymphocele*) (*lympha* fluid, water)
			mucocyst (mucus)
			myelocyst (a cyst developed from rudimentary medullary canals) (*myelos* marrow)
			nematocyst (*nematos* thread)
			oocyst (*oon* egg, ovum)
			otocyst (*otos* ear)
			phacocyst, phacocystitis (*phakos* lens of eye + *itis* inflammation)
			pseudocyst (*pseudes* false)
			pyocyst (*pyon* pus)
			spermatocyst (*spermatos* seed, sperm)
			sporocyst (*sporos* seed)
			statocyst (*statos* standing)
			toxicyst (*toxikon* poison)
			trichocyst (*trichos* hair)
			tubulocyst (*tubus* tube)
			cystectomy excision of bladder (or sac):
			dacryocystectomy (*dakryon* tear)
			laparocystectomy (*lapara* loin, flank)
			oophorocystectomy (*oophoron* ovary duct)
			phacocystectomy (*phakos* lens—of eye)
			cystia: atretocystia (*atretos* imperforate)
			cystic:
			fibrocystic (fiber)
			hepatocystic (*hepatos* liver)
			myelocystic (*myelos* marrow)
			oligocystic (*oligos* scant, few)

Element	From	Meaning	Examples
cyst (cont'd)		[sac, bladder]	pilocystic (*pilus* hair)
			serocystic (*serum* whey)
			cystis:
			cholecystis (gallbladder) (*chole* bile)
			gonecystis (seminal gland) (*gone* seed)
			pyocystis (*pyon* pus)
			schistocystis (*schistos* split)
			cystitis bladder inflammation:
			cholecystitis (*chole* bile)
			dacryocystitis (*dakryon* tear: lacrimal sac or duct)
			nephrocystitis (*nephros* kidney)
			myxocystitis (*myxa* mucus)
			nephrocystitis (*nephros* kidney)
			phacocystitis (*phakos* lens of eye)
			pyelocystitis (also called *cystopyelitis*) (*pyelos* pelvis)
			spermatocystitis (*spermatos* seed, sperm)
			cysto: myelocystocele (*myelos* marrow + *kele* tumor)
			cystoplasty cell formation:
			colocystoplasty (colon)
			colpocystoplasty (*kolpos* vagina)
			enterocystoplasty (*enteron* intestine)
			gastrocystoplasty (*gaster* stomach)
			proctocystoplasty (*proktos* anus)
			cystostomy bladder or sac opening:
			cholecystostomy (*chole* bile)
			dacryocystostomy (*dakryon* tear, teardrop)
			duodenocystostomy (duodenum)
			ileocystostomy (ileum)
			neocystostomy (also called *ureteroneocystostomy*) (*neos* new)
			ureterocystostomy (also called *ureterneocystostomy*) (ureter)
			cystotomy incision of bladder or sac:
			cholecystotomy (*chole* bile)
			colpocystotomy (*kolpos* vagina)
			dacryocystotomy (*dakryon* tear, teardrop)
			laparocystotomy (*laparos* flank, loin)
			lithocystotomy (*lithos* stone)
			proctocystotomy (also called *rectocystotomy*) (*proktos* anus, rectum)
			prostatocystotomy (prostate)
			rectocystotomy (also called *proctocystotomy*) (rectum)
			cystosis bladder or sac condition:
			metrocystosis (formation of cysts in the uterus) (*metra* uterus)
			nephrocystosis (*nephros* kidney)
			oophorocystosis (*oophoron* ovary duct)
			pneumocystosis (also called *pneumocystis pneumonia*)
			sarcocystosis (*sarkos* flesh)
			CROSS REFERENCE: bursa, vesic
cyt	Greek *kytos* a hollow vessel	cell, vessel	SIMPLE ROOT: cyton (also called *perikaryon*)
			PREFIXED ROOT:
			cyte:
			amphicyte (*amphi* around)
			amphocyte (an amphophilic cell) (*ampho* both)
			endocyte, endodyocyte (*endon* within + *dys* two)
			entocyte (*entos* inside)

Element	From	Meaning	Examples
cyt (cont'd)		[cell, vessel]	epicyte (*epi* upon)
			macrocyte (*makros* large)
			macromonocyte (*makros* large + monocyte)
			megalocyte (*megalos* large)
			microcyte (*mikros* small)
			monocyte (*monos* single)
			pericyte {pericytial; also called *pericellular*} (*peri* around)
			platycyte (*platys* flat)
			polycyte (*polys* many)
			promonocyte (*pro* before + monocyte)
			cythemia blood cell condition:
			carcinocythemia (*karkinos* cancer)
			hypercythemia (also called *polycythemia*) (*hyper* above)
			hypocythemia (also called *erythropenia*) (*hypo* under)
			macrocythemia (also called *macrocytosis*) (*makros* large)
			microcythemia (*mikros* small)
			megalocythemia (*megalos* large)
			polycythemia (also called *erythrocythemia*) (*polys* many)
			cytic:
			ectocytic (*ektos* outside)
			endocytic (*endon* within)
			paracytic (*para* alongside)
			cyto:
			anticytolysin (*anti* against + *lyein* to loosen)
			anticytotoxin (*anti* against + *toxin* poison)
			autocytolysin, autocytolysis (*autos* self + *lyein* to loosen)
			heterocytotropic (*heteros* other + *tropos* a turning)
			hypercytochromia (*hyper* above + *chromia* color condition)
			intracytoplasmic (within the cytoplasm of a cell) (*intra* within + *plassein* to form)
			cytopenia cell deficiency:
			monocytopenia (*monos* single)
			pancytopenia (*pan* all)
			cytosis cell condition:
			anisocytosis (*aniso* unequal: *an* negative + *isos* equal)
			endocytosis (*endon* within)
			exocytosis (*exo* out)
			hypercytosis (*hyper* above)
			hyperorthocytosis (*hyper* above + *orthos* straight)
			hypocytosis (also called *cytopenia*) (*hypo* under)
			isocytosis (*isos* equal)
			macrocytosis (also called *macrocythemia*) (*makros* large)
			megalocytosis (*megalos* large)
			microcytosis (*mikros* small)
			monocytosis (*monos* single)
			transcytosis (*trans* across)
			LEADING ROOT COMPOUND:
			cyt:
			cytapheresis (*apheresis* removal)
			cytarme (*arme* union; not to be confused with Latin *arm* shield)
			cytode, cytoid (*eidos* form)
			cytoma (*oma* tumor)
			cytosis (a condition where there is an excess number of cells) (*osis* condition)

Element	From	Meaning	Examples
cyt (cont'd)		[cell, vessel]	cyturia (*uria* urine condition)
			cyto:
			cytoanalyzer (an electronic optical apparatus for the detection of malignant cells in smears)
			cytoarchitectonic (architecture)
			cytobiology (*bios* life + *logos* study)
			cytobiotaxis (*bios* life + *tassein* to arrange)
			cytocentrum (also called *centrosphere, microcentrum*) (*kentron* point, center)
			cytocerastic (or, cytokerastic) (*kerastos* mixed)
			cytochalasins (*chalasis* relaxing)
			cytochemism (chemical activity of cells), cytochemistry
			cytochrome (*chroma* color)
			cytochylema (also called *hyaloplasm*) (*chylos* juice)
			cytocide {cytocidal} (*caedere* to cut, kill)
			cytocinesis (or, cytokinesis) (*kinein* to move)
			cytoclasis (also called *cytolysis*) {cytoclastic; also called *cytolytic*} (*klaein* to break)
			cytoclesis (the influence of one cell on another) {cytocletic} (*klesis* a call)
			cytodendrite (also called *dendrite*) (*dendron* tree: growth)
			cytodesma (*desma* band)
			cytodiagnosis
			cytodieresis (cell division; also called *cytokinesis*) (*dieresis* a taking)
			cytodifferentiation
			cytodistal (*distal* remote)
			cytogene (also called *plasmagene*), cytogenesis {cytogenic}, cytogenous, cytogeny (*genere* to produce)
			cytoglucopenia (also called *cytoglycopenia*) (*glykys* sweet + *penia* deficiency)
			cytogony (also called *cytogenic reproduction*) (*gone* seed)
			cytohistogenesis (*histos* web, tissue + *genere* to produce)
			cytohormone (a cell hormone)
			cytohyaloplasm (the clear substance of cytoplasm) (*hyalos* glass + *plassein* to form)
			cytokalipenia (*kalium* potassium + *penia* deficiency)
			cytokerastic (or, cytocerastic) (*kerastos* mixed)
			cytokine, cytokinesis (also called *cytodieresis*) (*kinein* to move)
			cytolemma (also called *cell membrane*) (*lemma* husk)
			cytology {cytologic} (*logos* study)
			cytolysin, cytolysis {cytolytic} (*lyein* to loosen)
			cytomegaly {cytomegalic} (*megalos* large)
			cytomembrane (also called *cell membrane*) (*membrane* a thin skin)
			cytomere (*meros* part)
			cytometer, cytometry (*metron* measure)
			cytomorphology (*morphe* form + *logos* study)
			cytomorphosis (*morphosis* a shaping, forming)
			cytonecrosis (*necrosis* death)
			cytopathic, cytopathogenesis {cytopathogenetic} (*pathos* disease + *genesis* origin)
			cytopathology, cytopathy (*pathos* disease + *logos* study)
			cytopenia (*penia* deficiency)
			cytophagy {cytophagous} (*phagein* to devour)
			cytophil {cytophilic} (*philein* to love)

A Thesaurus of Medical Word Roots

Element	From	Meaning	Examples
cyt (cont'd)		[cell, vessel]	cytophotometry (*photos* light + *metron* measure)
			cytophylaxis {cytophylactic} (*phylaxis* a guarding)
			cytophyletic (*phyletic* genealogy)
			cytophysiology (the physiology of the cell)
			cytopipette (a pipette for taking cytological smears)
			cytoplasm {cytoplasmic}, cytoplast (*plassein* to form)
			cytopoiesis (*poiein* to produce)
			cytoproct (also called *cytopyge*) (*proktos* anus)
			cytoproximal (*proximal* nearer)
			cytopyge (also called *cytoproct*) (*pyge* rump)
			cytosome (*soma* body)
			cytospongium (also called *spongioplasm*) (*spongos* sponge)
			cytostasis {cytostatic} (*stasis* stoppage)
			cytostome (*stoma* mouth, opening)
			cytotaxis {cytotactic} (*tassein* to arrange)
			cytothesis (the restitution of injured cells to their normal condition) (*thesis* a placing)
			cytotoxic {cytotoxicity}, cytotoxin (*toxikon* poison)
			cytotrophoblast {cytotrophoblastic} (*trophein* to nourish + *blastos* germ)
			cytotropic, cytotropism (*tropos* a turning)
			cytozoic (living within or attached to cells; said of parasites) (*zoa* animal)
			TRAILING ROOT COMPOUND:
			acanthocyte (*akantha* thorn)
			adipocyte (*adipos* fat)
			blastocyte (*blastos* bud, shoot, germ)
			chondrocyte (*chondros* cartilage)
			chromocyte (*chroma* color)
			desmocyte (*desme* ligament)
			eosinocyte (*eos* dawn: rose-colored)
			erythrocyte (*erythros* red)
			fibrocyte, fibrocytogenesis (also called *fibroblast*) (fiber + *genere* to produce)
			gametocyte (*gamos* marriage: reproduction)
			gangliocyte (*ganglion* knot, swelling)
			gliacyte (or, gliocyte; a cell of the neuroglia) (*glia* glue)
			gonocyte (also called *primordial germ cell*) (*gone* seed)
			granulocyte (also called *granular leukocyte*) (*granum* grain)
			hemocyte (also called *blood cell*) (*haima* blood)
			hepatocyte (alsos called *hepatic cell*) (*hepatos* liver)
			histocyte (*histos* web, tissue)
			inocyte (*inos* fiber)
			lemmocyte (*lemma* husk)
			leptocyte (*leptos* slender)
			leukocyte (*leukos* white)
			lipocyte (also called *fat cell*) (*lipos* fat)
			lymphocyte (*lympha* water, fluid)
			mastocyte (*mastos* breast, nipple)
			melanocyte (also called *melanodendrocyte*) (*melanos* dark)
			meningocyte (*meningos* membrane)
			myelocyte (*myelos* marrow)
			myocyte (*myos* muscle)
			myxocyte (*myxa* mucus)

Element	From	Meaning	Examples
cyt (cont'd)		[cell, vessel]	neocyte (*neos* new)
			neurocyte (also called *neuron*) (*neuron* nerve)
			normocyte, normocytosis (*norma* right + *osis* condition)
			oligocythemia (*oligos* scant + *emia* blood condition)
			oocyte (*oon* egg, ovum)
			opsonocytophagic (opsonin + *phagein* to consume)
			osteocyte (*osteon* bone)
			ovocyte (*ovum* egg)
			phagocyte (*phagein* to consume)
			pilocytic (composed of fiber-shaped cells) (*pilus* hair)
			pinocyte (*pinein* to drink; fluid)
			pituicyte (*pituitia* phlegm, rheum)
			planocyte (a wandering cell) (*planan* to wander)
			plasmacyte (*plassein* to form)
			poikilocyte (*poikilos* varied, mottled)
			pyknocyte (*pyknos* thick)
			reticulocyte (*rete* net)
			schistocyte (also called *schizocyte*) (*schistos* split)
			siderocyte (*sideros* iron)
			spermatocyte (*sperma* seed, sperm)
			spherocyte (*sphaira* sphere, ball, globe)
			spongiocyte (sponge)
			stomatocyte (*stomatos* mouth)
			synoviocyte (synovial: *syn* with + *oon* egg)
			teknocyte (*teknon* newborn)
			thymocyte (thymus)
			trephocyte (or, trophocyte) (*trephein* to nourish)
			tricholeukocyte (*trichos* hair + *leukos* white)
			cythemia cell blood condition:
			erythrocythemia (also called *polycythemia*) (*erythros* red)
			myelocythemia (*myelos* marrow)
			thrombocythemia (also called *thrombocytosis*) (*thrombos* clot)
			cyto:
			leukocytoplania (*leukos* white + *planan* to wander)
			lymphocytopenia (*lympha* water, fluid + *penia* deficiency)
			cytolysis cell dissolution:
			myocytolysis (*myos* muscle)
			neurocytolysis (*neuron* nerve)
			phagocytolysis (*phagein* to consume)
			cytopenia cell deficiency:
			erythrocytopenia (*erythros* red)
			granulocytopenia (*granulum* small grain)
			leukocytopenia (*leukos* white)
			thrombocytopenia (*thrombos* clot)
			cytosis cell condition:
			acanthocytosis (*akantha* thorn)
			anisocytosis (*aniso* unequal: *an* negative + *isos* equal)
			astrocytosis (*astron* star)
			athrocytosis (*athro* gathered together)
			basocytosis (base)
			crenocytosis (*crena* a notch)
			erythrocytosis (*erythrys* red)
			granulocytosis (*granule* small grain)
			histiocytosis (*histion* web, tissue)

Element	From	Meaning	Examples
cyt (cont'd)		[cell, vessel]	hydrocytosis (also called *stomatocytosis*) (*hydor* water)
			leptocytosis (*leptos* slender)
			leukocytosis (*leukos* white—blood cell)
			lymphocytosis (*lympha* fluid, water)
			mastocytosis (*mastos* breast)
			melanocytosis (*melanos* black, dark)
			myelocytosis (*myelos* marrow)
			necrocytosis (*nekros* corpse, death)
			neocytosis (*neos* new)
			normocytosis (*norma* rule, normal)
			orthocytosis (*orthos* straight)
			phagocytosis (*phagein* to consume)
			phorocytosis (*phorein* to bear)
			plasmacytosis (*plasma*)
			pleocytosis (*pleon* more)
			poikilocytosis (*poikilos* many colors, varied)
			pyknocytosis (*pyknos* thick, compact)
			reticulocytosis (*reticulum* a small net)
			schistocytosis (*schistos* split)
			spherocytosis (*sphaira* globe)
			stomatocytosis (also called *hydrocytosis*) (*stomatos* mouth)
			PREFIXED TRAILING ROOT COMPOUND:
			cyte:
			agranulocyte (also called *nongranular leukocyte*) (*a* negative + *granum* grain)
			polykaryocyte (*polys* many + *karyon* nucleus)
			premyelocyte (or, promyelocyte) (*pre* before + *myelos* marrow)
			progranulocyte (also called *promyelocyte*) (*pro* before + *granum* grain)
			proplasmacyte (*pro* before + *plassein* to form)
			protoleukocyte (*protos* first + *leukos* white)
			cytic:
			intraerythrocytic (*intra* within + *erythros* red)
			intraleukocytic (*intra* within + *leukos* white)
			cytosis cell condition:
			agranulocytosis (*a* negative + *granum* grain)
			aleukocytosis (*a* privative + *leukos* white)
			alymphocytosis (*a* privative + *lympha* water, fluid)
			dysphagocytosis (*dys* abnormal + *phagein* to consume)
			hyperleukocytosis (*hyper* above + *leukos* white)
			hyperneocytosis (*hyper* above + *neos* new)
			hyperorthocytosis (*hyper* above + *orthos* straight, normal)
			hypogranulocytosis (also called *granulocytopenia*) (*hypo* under + *granulum* small grain)
			hyponeocytosis (also called *hyposkeocytosis*) (*hypo* under + *neos* new)
			hyposkeocytosis (also called *hyponeocytosis*) (*hypo* under + *skaios* left)
			megakaryocytosis (*megas* large + *karyon* nucleus)
			micropinocytosis (also called *pinocytosis*) (*mikros* small + *pinea* to drink)
			CROSS REFERENCE: angi, cell, vas

$\mathcal{D}$

Element	From	Meaning	Examples
dacry	Greek *dakryon*	tear, as in teardrop	See Appendix B for examples of words with this initial combining form. Others are listed with the roots to which it is attached. CROSS REFERENCE: lacri
dactyl	Greek *daktylos* finger	finger, toe	SIMPLE ROOT: dactylus (a digit; a finger or toe; pl., dactyli) PREFIXED ROOT: *dactyl:* pentadactyl (also called *quinquedigitate*) (*penta* five) syndactyl (or, syndactyle; also called *syndactylous*) (*syn* with) *dactylia:* adactylia (*a* privative) bidactylia (*bi* two) heptadactylia (*hepta* seven) hyperdactylia (the presence of more than the normal number of fingers or toes; also called *polydactyly*) (*hyper* above) hypodactylia (or, hypodactylism) (*hypo* under) microdactylia (or, microdactyly) {microdactylous} (*mikros* small) polydactylia (or, polydactylism, polydactyly) (*polys* many) syndactylia (or, syndactylism) (*syn* with, together) *dactylism:* didactylism (*di* two) hexadactylism (or, hexadactyly) (*hexa* six) isodactylism (*isos* equal) monodactylism (or, monodactyly) (*monos* one) polydactylism (or, polydactyly) (*polys* many) syndactylism (or, syndactyly; a fusion of two or more fingers or toes) {syndactylous} (*sym* with, together) tridactylism (*tri* three) *dactylous:* adactylous (congenitally lacking fingers or toes, or both) (*a* privative) anisodactylous (*aniso* unequal: *an* negative + *isos* equal) didactylous (*di* two) tridactylous (also called *tridigitate*) (*tri* three) *dactyly:* adactyly (*a* privative) heptadactyly (*hepta* seven) hypodactyly (also called *oligodactyly*) (*hypo* under) macrodactyly (also called *megalodactyly*) (*makros* large) megalodactyly {megalodactylous} (*megalos* large, great) megalosyndactyly (a condition in which the digits are very large and more or less completely grown together) (*megalos* large + syndactyly) microdactyly (or, microdactylia) (*mikros* small) monodactyly (or, monodactylism) (*monos* single) polydactyly (also called *hyperdactylia*) (*polys* many) polysyndactyly (syndactyly of several fingers or toes) (*polys* many + syndactyly) syndactyly (*syn* with, together) synpolydactyly (*syn* with + polydactyly) tetradactyly (also called *quadridigitate*) (*tetra* four)

Element	From	Meaning	Examples
dactyl (cont'd)		[finger, toe]	LEADING ROOT COMPOUND: *dactyl*: dactylalgia (also called *dactylodynia*) (*algos* pain) dactylitis (*itis* inflammation) dactylodynia (also called *dactylalgia*) (*odyne* pain) *dactylo*: dactylocampsis, dactylocampsodynia (*kampsis* bending + *odyne* pain) dactylogram, dactylography (the scientific classification of finger-prints) (*graphein* to write) dactylogryposis (*gryposis* hooking) dactylology (sign language, that of using fingers and hands; also called *cheirology, chirology*) (*logos* word) dactylolysis (loss or amputation of a finger) (*lysis* a loosening) dactylomegaly (also called *megalodactyly*) (*megalos* large) dactyloscopy (*skopein* to examine) dactylospasm (*spasmos* contraction) TRAILING ROOT COMPOUND: ankylodactyly (fusion or adhesion of fingers or toes to one another) (*ankylos* bent, crooked) arachnodactyly (also called *dolichostenomelia, acromacria, spider finger*) (*arachne* spider) brachydactyly (*brachys* short) camptodactyly (*kamptos* bent) clinodactyly (*klinein* to bend) ectrodactyly (*ektrosis* congenitally absent) leptodactyly {*leptodactylous*} (*leptos* slender) oligodactyly (also called *hypodactyly*) (*oligos* few) pachydactyly (also called *megalodactyly*) (*pachys* thick) perodactyly (or, perodactylia) (*peros* maimed) sclerodactyly (scleroderma of the fingers and toes) (*skleros* hard) symphysodactyly (*symphysis* growing together) zygodactyly (*zygon* yoke) PREFIXED TRAILING ROOT COMPOUND: symbrachydactylia (*sym* with, together + *brachys* short) CROSS REFERENCE: chir
de-	Latin prefix	away from, down from	See Appendix B for examples of words with this prefix. Others are listed with the roots to which it is attached. CROSS REFERENCE: cata-
dent	Latin *dens*	tooth, teeth (see *dentate* under *Simple Root*)	SIMPLE ROOT: dens (pl., dentes) dental (relating to the teeth) dentata (the second vertebra or axis, so called from its toothlike process) dentate (having teeth, or projections like saw teeth on the edges) dentatum (the nucleus dentatus) dentia (the process of tooth development or eruption; also serves to denote a relationship to the teeth) denticle, denticulate (or, denticulated) dentin (or, dentinum; the chief substance or tissue of the teeth) {*dentinal*}, dentist, dentition dentulous (possessing natural teeth) denture (a set of natural or artificial teeth, but usually artificial; also called *artificial dentition*), denturism, denturist

Element	From	Meaning	Examples
dent (cont'd)		[tooth]	PREFIXED ROOT:

dens:

mesiodens (*mesos* middle)

peridens (*peri* around)

dental:

bidental (having, pertaining to, or affecting two teeth) (*bi* two)

interdental (*inter* between)

paradental (also called *periodontal*) (*para* beside)

peridental (also called *periodontal*) (*peri* around)

subdental (beneath the roots of the teeth) (*sub* below)

dentale:

infradentale (also called *lower alveolar point*) (*infra* below)

interdentale (*inter* between)

dentate:

bidentate (having two teeth) (*bi* two)

edentate (or, edentulous; having no teeth) (*e* out)

indentation (the act of notching or pitting; a notch) (*in* in)

multidentate (*multus* many)

tridentate (or, trident; having three prongs) (*tri* three)

dentia: polydentia (the presence of supernumerary teeth; also called
    polyodontia) (*polys* many)

dentitis tooth inflammation:

paradentitis (also called *periodontitis*) (*para* alongside)

peridentitis (now referred to *periodontitis*) (*peri* around)

dentium: interdentium (the interval between two contiguous teeth)
    (*inter* between)

LEADING ROOT COMPOUND:

dent:

dentagra (a forceps or key for extracting teeth; also, odontalgia, or
    toothache) (*agra* seizure)

dentalgia (toothache) (*algos* pain)

dentoid (also called *odontoid*) (*eidos* form)

dentoma (or, dentinoma) (*oma* tumor)

dentonomy (also called *odontonomy*) (*onoma* name)

denti:

dentibuccal (*bucca* cheek)

dentification (*facere* to make)

dentiform (*forma* shape)

dentifrice (*fricare* to rub)

dentigerous (bearing teeth) (*gerere* to bear)

dentilabial (*labium* lip)

dentilingual (*lingua* tongue)

dentimeter (*metron* measure)

dentiparous (*parere* to produce)

dentin:

dentinalgia (pain in the dentin) (*algos* pain)

dentinoid (*eidos* form)

dentinoma (*oma* tumor)

dentinosteoid (a tumor composed of dentin and bone; also called *os-
    teodentinoma*) (*osteon* bone + *eidos* form)

dentino:

dentinoblast (a cell that forms dentin) (*blastos* bud, shoot)

dentinocemental (also called *cementodentinal*)

dentinoenamel (also called *amelodentinal*)

Element	From	Meaning	Examples
dent (cont'd)		[tooth]	dentinogenesis {dentinogenic} (*genere* to produce) *dento*: dentoalveolar (pertaining to a tooth and its alveolus, or dental socket) (*alveolus* hollow: a small saclike dilatation) dentoalveolitis (*alveolus* hollow + *itis* inflammation) dentofacial (of or pertaining to the teeth and alveolar process and the face) dentography (also called *odontography*) (*graphein* to write) dentophobia (fear of dentists) (*phobia* fear) dentotropic (having an affinity for tissues composing the teeth) (*trepein* to turn) TRAILING ROOT COMPOUND: *dental*: alveolodental (*alveolus* hollow) labiodental (*labium* lip) linguodental (*lingua* tongue) maxillodental (*maxilla* upper jaw) *dentosis*: poikilodentosis (mottling of enamel due to excessive fluoride in the water supply) (*poikilos* mottled + *osis* condition) TERM: alveolodental membrane (periodontium, or peridontium; also called *odontoperiosteum, paradentium*; the tissues that invest or help to invest and support the teeth, including the periodontal ligament, gingivae, cementum, and alveolar and supporting bone) CROSS REFERENCE: odont
derm	Greek *derma, dermatos*	skin	SIMPLE ROOT: derma {dermal, dermic; also called *cutaneous*}, dermis PREFIXED ROOT: *derm*: ectoderm {ectodermal, ectodermic} (*ektos* outside) endoderm (or, entoderm; also called *endoblast, entoblast*) {endodermal} (*endon* within) entoderm (or, endoderm) {entodermal, entodermic } (*entos* within) epiderm (or, epiderma) (epidermal, epidermatic} (*epi* upon) hypoderm (also called *subcutaneous tissue*) {hypodermal} (*hypo* under) mesectoderm (*mesos* middle + ectoderm) mesoderm (*mesos* middle) paraderm (*para* alongside) periderm (or, periderma) {peridermal, peridermic} (*peri* around) protoderm (the undifferentiated cells of very young embryos) (*protos* first) *dermal*: intradermal (also called *intracutaneous, intradermic*) (*intra* within) intraepidermal (*intra* within + epidermal) peridermal (or, peridermic) (*peri* around) transdermal (also called *transcutaneous*) (*trans* across) *dermatomy*: hypodermatomy (*hypo* under + *tomy* incision) *dermatosis* skin condition: ectodermatosis (*ektos* outside) hypodermatosis (*hypo* under) *dermia*: adermia (*a* privative) *dermic*: autodermic (*autos* self) endermic (or, endermatic) (*en* in)

A Thesaurus of Medical Word Roots

Element	From	Meaning	Examples
derm (cont'd)		[skin]	heterodermic (*heteros* other)
			hypodermic (also called *subcutaneous*) (*hypo* under)
			transdermic (also called *percutaneous*) (*trans* across, through)
			tridermic (derived from all three germ layers: ectoderm, endoderm, and mesoderm) (*tri* three)
			dermis:
			epidermis (*epi* upon)
			hypodermis (*hypo* under)
			dermoclysis: hypodermoclysis (*hypo* under + *klysis* a washing out)
			dermoid: epidermoid (composed of or resembling epidermal tissue)
			dermoma: tridermoma (*tri* three + *oma* tumor)
			dermosis skin condition:
			ectodermosis (*ektos* outside)
			endermosis (*en* in)
			epidermosis (*epi* upon)
			LEADING ROOT COMPOUND:
			derm: dermoid (resembling skin; dermoid cyst), dermoidectomy (*eidos* form + *ektome* excision)
			derma: dermatome {dermatomic} (*tome* a cutting instrument)
			dermat:
			dermatalgia (also called *dermatodynia*) (*algos* pain)
			dermatitis (pl., dermatitides) (*itis* inflammation)
			dermatodynia (also called *dermatalgia*) (*odyne* pain)
			dermatoid (*eidos* form)
			dermatoma (*oma* tumor)
			dermatosis (also called *dermopathy*) (*osis* condition)
			dermato:
			dermatoarthritis (*arthron* joint + *itis* inflammation)
			dermatoautoplasty (*autos* self + *plassein* to form)
			dermatocellulitis (*cellula* little cell + *itis* inflammation)
			dermatochalasis (also called *cutis laxa*) (*chalasis* relaxation)
			dermatoconiosis (*konis* dust + *osis* condition)
			dermatocyst (*kystis* sac, bladder)
			dermatodysplasia (*dys* abnormal + *plassein* to form)
			dermatofibroma (*fibra* fiber + *oma* tumor)
			dermatoglyphics (*glyphein* to carve)
			dermatographism {dermatographic} (*graphein* to write)
			dermatology {dermatologic} (*logos* study)
			dermatolysis (also called *dermatochalasis*) (*lyein* to loosen)
			dermatomegaly (*megalos* large)
			dermatomere (any part of the embryonic integument) (*meros* part)
			dermatomycosis (*mykes* fungus + *osis* condition)
			deermatomyoma (also called *leiomyoma cutis*) (*myoma* muscle tumor)
			dermatomyositis (*myositis* muscle inflammation)
			dermatoneurology (*neuron* nerve + *logos* study)
			dermatoneurosis (*neuron* nerve + *osis* condition)
			dermatonosology (*nosos* disease + *logos* study)
			dermatopathy (also called *dermatosis*) (*pathos* disease)
			dermatophylaxis (*phylaxis* protection)
			dermatophyte, dermatophytosis (*phyton* growth + *osis* condition)
			dermatoplasty {dermatoplastic} (*plassein* to mold)
			dermatorrhagia (discharge of blood into or from the skin) (*rhagia* bursting forth)

Element	From	Meaning	Examples
derm (cont'd)		[skin]	dermatorrhea (*rhein* to flow)

derm (cont'd) [skin]

dermatorrhea (*rhein* to flow)
dermatorrhexis (*rhexis* rupture)
dermatoscopy (*skopein* to examine)
dermatosclerosis (also called *scleroderma*) (*sklerosis* hardening)
dermatosparaxis (also called *cutaneous asthenia*) (*sparaxis* a tearing)
dermatotherapy (*therapy* treatment)
dermatotropic (*tropein* to turn)
dermatozoon (*zoon* animal)
dermo:
dermoblast (*blastos* bud, shoot, germ)
dermocyma (also called *endadelphos*) (*kyma* fetus)
dermohygrometer (*hygros* moisture + *metron* measure)
dermolipectomy (*lipos* fat + *ektome* excision)
dermolipoma (*lipos* fat + *oma* tumor)
dermometer, dermometry (*metron* measure)
dermonecrosis {dermonecrotic} (*nekrosis* death)
dermopathy {dermopathic} (*pathos* disease)
dermophlebitis (*phlebos* vein + *itis* inflammation)
dermophyte (or, dermatophyte) (*phyton* plant: growth)
dermoreaction (also called *cutaneous reaction*)
dermoskeleton (also called *exoskeleton*)
dermostenosis (*stenosis* narrow condition)
dermotoxin (*toxin* poison)
dermotropic (or, dermatotropic) (*trepein* to turn)
dermovascular (*vas* blood vessel)
TRAILING ROOT COMPOUND:
derm:
echinoderm (*echinos* prickly)
somatoderm (*somatos* body)
splanchnoderm (also called *splanchnopleure*) (*splanchnos* viscus)
trophoderm (*trophe* nourishment)
derma:
acropachyderma (*akron* extremity + *pachys* thick)
acroscleroderma (also called *acrosclerosis*) (*akron* extremity + *skleros* hard)
anetoderma (atrophy of the skin with soft fibromas forming large pendulous masses) (*anetos* slack)
atrophoderma (*atrophia* lack of nourishment)
chyloderma (also called *elephantiasis*) (*chylus* gastric juice)
erythroderma (or, erythrodermia) (*erythros* red)
geroderma (*geras* old age)
haloderma (*hals* salt)
leukoderma (or, leukodermia) (*leukos* white)
melanoderma, melanodermatitis (*melanos* dark + *itis* inflammation)
melanoleukoderma (a mottled appearance of the skin, as in chronic arsenic poisoning) (*melanos* dark + *leukos* white)
mycoderma (*mykes* fungus)
myoderma (*myos* muscle)
pachyderma (unusual thickness of skin) (*pachys* thick)
phrynoderma (a papular dry skin eruption) (*phryne* toad)
pneumoderma (*pneuma* air)
poikiloderma (*poikilos* varied, mottled)
pyoderma (any purulent or pyogenic skin disease) (*pyon* pus)

Element	From	Meaning	Examples
derm (cont'd)		[skin]	scleroderma (also called *dermatosclerosis*) (*skleros* hard)
			sideroderma (*sideros* iron)
			sphaceloderma (*sphakelos* gangrenous*)*
			xanthoderma (*xanthos* yellow)
			xeroderma (or, xerodermia) {xerodermatic} (*xeros* dry)
			dermatitis skin inflammation:
			acarodermatitis (*acarus* mite)
			acrodermatitis (*akros* extremity)
			actinodermatitis (*aktis* ray)
			angiodermatitis (*angeion* blood vessel)
			chondrodermatitis (*chondros* cartilage)
			haplodermatitis (*haplos* single)
			melanodermatitis (*melanos* dark)
			mycodermatitis (also called *dermatomycosis*) (*mykes* fungus)
			myringodermatitis (*myringa* membrane)
			neurodermatitis (*neuron* nerve)
			photodermatitis (*photos* light)
			toxicodermatitis (*toxikon* poison)
			ulodermatitis (*oule* scar)
			dermatology study of skin:
			genodermatology (*genos* birth: genes)
			immunodermatology (immune)
			dermatoneurosis: trophodermatoneurosis (trophic changes to the skin due to neural inflammation) (*trophe* nourishment + neurosis)
			dermatosis skin condition:
			acrodermatosis (*akron* extremities)
			genodermatosis (genetic)
			pachydermatosis (*pachys* thick)
			photodermatosis (*photos* light)
			dermia:
			carotenodermia (*carotene* yellowish red)
			gerodermia (or, geroderma) (*geras* old age)
			keratodermia (any horny superficial growth) (*keras* horn)
			leiodermia (*leios* smooth)
			ochrodermia (*ochros* pale yellow)
			osteodermia (a condition in which skeletal changes occur in the skin, such as a bony tumor of the skin; also called *osteoma cutis*) (*osteon* bone)
			pachydermia (*pachys* thick)
			pyodermia (or, pyoderma; any suppurative skin disease) (*pyon* pus)
			xanthoerythrodermia (*xanthos* yellow + *erythros* red)
			dermoid similar to skin:
			tubulodermoid (*tubus* tube)
			xerodermoid (*xeros* dry)
			dermoplasty: septodermoplasty (*septum* partition + *plassein* to form)
			PREFIXED TRAILING ROOT COMPOUND: achromoderma (also called *leukoderma*) (*a* privative + *chroma* color)
			CROSS REFERENCE: cut
desm, **det**, **-desis**	Greek *dein* to bind; *desmios* binding	ligament, band	SIMPLE ROOT: desmid, desmin, desmose
			PREFIXED ROOT:
			dein: syndein (also called *ankyrin*) (*syn* with, together)
			desis: syndesis (*syn* with) [see separate entry: syndes-]
			desmitis: peridesmitis (*peri* around + *itis* inflammation)
			desmium: peridesmium {peridesmic} (*peri* around)

Element	From	Meaning	Examples
desm (cont'd)		[ligament, band]	*desmosome*: hemidesmosome (*hemi* half + desmosome)
			desmotic:
			heterodesmotic (*heteros* other)
			homodesmotic (*homos* same)
			LEADING ROOT COMPOUND:
			desm:
			desmalgia (also called *desmodynia*) (*algos* pain)
			desmectasis (the stretching of a ligament) (*ektasis* dilatation)
			desmepithelium (the covering of internal and external surfaces of the body, including the lining of vessels and other small cavities) (*epi* upon + *thele* nipple)
			desmitis (*itis* inflammation)
			desmodontium (also called *desmodentium, periodontal ligament*) (*odontos* tooth)
			desmodynia (also called *desmalgia*) (*odyne* pain)
			desmoid (*eidos* form)
			desmoma (also called *desmoid tumor*) (*oma* tumor)
			desmosis (*osis* condition)
			desmio: desmiognathus (a fetal monster with a parasitic head attached to the lower jaw or neck) (*gnathos* jaw)
			desmo:
			desmocranium (*kranion* skull)
			desmocyte (also called *fibroblast*), desmocytoma (also called *fibroma*) (*kytos* cell + *oma* tumor)
			desmogenous (of ligamentous origin) (*genere* to produce)
			desmography (a description of the ligaments) (*graphein* to write)
			desmohemoblast (also called *mesenchyme*) (*haima* blood + *blastos* bud, shoot, germ)
			desmology (*logos* study)
			desmopathy (any disease of the ligaments) (*pathos* disease)
			desmoplasia {desmoplastic} (*plassein* to form)
			desmorrhexis (*rhexis* rupture)
			desmosome (a bridge corpuscle; a small thickening at the middle of an intercellular bridge) (*soma* body)
			desmotomy (*tomy* incision)
			TRAILING ROOT COMPOUND:
			desis:
			arthrodesis (the surgical immobilization of a joint) (*arthron* joint)
			epiphysiodesis (premature union of the epiphysis with the diaphysis, resulting in cessation of growth) (*epiphysis* long bone)
			fasciodesis (a surgical procedure in which a fascia is attached to another fascia or to a tendon) (*fascia* band)
			iridesis (or, iridodesis; ligature of a portion of the iris brought out through an incision in the cornea) (*iridos* rainbow: iris)
			pleurodesis (the surgical creation of a fibrous adhesion between the visceral and parietal layers of the pleura) (*pleura* rib, side)
			spondylosyndesis (*spondylos* vertebra + syndesis)
			tenodesis (tendon fixation) (*tenon* tendon)
			desmitis: ophthalmodesmitis (*ophthalmos* eye + *itis* inflammation)
			desmosis: osteodesmosis (*osteon* bone + *osis* condition)
			CROSS REFERENCE: fasci, lig, syndes
deuter	Greek *deuteros*	second	See Appendix B for examples of words with this element. Others are placed with the roots to which it is attached.
			CROSS REFERENCE: None

Element	From	Meaning	Examples
dextr	Latin *dexter*	right, right-hand	SIMPLE ROOT: dextral, dextrality, dextrin PREFIXED ROOT: ambidexterity (the ability to perform acts requiring manual skill with either hand) (*ambi* both) LEADING ROOT COMPOUND: *dexio*: dexiotropic (wound in a spiral from left to right) (*trepein* to turn) *dextr*: dextrad (*ad* to, toward) dextraural (*auris* ear) dextrocular, dextrocularity (*oculus* eye) *dextrin*: dextrinosis (*osis* condition) dextrinuria (*uria* urine condition) *dextro*: dextroaorta (dextropositioned aorta) dextrocardia, dextrocardiogram (*kardia* heart + *graphein* to write) dextrocerebral (pertaining to or situated in the right cerebral hemisphere) (*cerebrum* brain) dextroclination (also called *dextrotorsion*) (*clinare* to bend) dextrocycloduction (also called *dextroclination*) (*kyklos* circle + *ducere* to lead) dextroduction (*ducere* to lead) dextrogastria (*gaster* stomach, belly) dextroglucose (also called *dextrose*) (*gleukos* sweetness) dextrogyral (also called *dextrorotatory*) (*gyrare* to turn) dextromanual (right-handed) (*manus* hand) dextroposition (displacement to the right) (*ponere* to place) dextrorotatory (also called *dextrogyral*) (*rotare* to turn) dextroscoliosis (*skoliosis* curvature) dextrosinistral (extending from right to left) (*sinister* left) dextrotorsion (also called *dextroclination*) (*torquere* to twist) dextrotropic (turning to the right) (*tropein* to turn) dextroversion, dextroverted (*vertere* to turn) CROSS REFERENCE: orth, rect
di-	Greek prefix	two	See Appendix B for examples of words with this prefix. Others are listed with the roots to which it is attached. CROSS REFERENCE: bi-
dia-	Greek prefix	across, through	See Appendix B for examples of words with this prefix. Others are listed with the roots to which it is attached. CROSS REFERENCE: per-, trans-
diabet	Greek *dia* across + *bainein* to go	a urine deficiency	SIMPLE ROOT: diabetes (a deficiency condition marked by habitual discharge of an excessive quantity of urine) {diabetic} diabetid (a cutaneous manifestation of diabetes) PREFIXED ROOT: antidiabetic (*anti* against) prediabetes (*pre* before) LEADING ROOT COMPOUND: diabetogenous {diabetogenic} (*genere* to produce) diabetograph (in urinalysis, a graduated scale to show the proportion of glucose content) (*graphein* to write) diabetology (*logos* study) diabetometer (*metron* measure) CROSS REFERENCE: None

Element	From	Meaning	Examples
dialys	Greek *dia* across + *lysis* a loosening	separation	SIMPLE ROOT: dialysis (a form of filtration to separate crystalloid from colloid substances) PREFIXED ROOT: microdialysis (*mikros* small) TRAILING ROOT COMPOUND: cyclodialysis (a treatment for glaucoma) (*kyklos* circle) encephalodialysis (*enkephalon* brain) electrodialysis (electricity) gastrodialysis (*gaster* stomach, belly) hemodialysis (*haima* blood) histodialysis (*histion* web, tissue) iridodialysis (iris—of eye) lithodialysis (*lithos* stone, calculus) staphylodialysis (also called *uvuloptosis*) (*staphyle* uvula) urodialysis (*ouron* urine) vividialysis (*vivus* alive) CROSS REFERENCE: None
diaphragm	Greek *dia* across + *phrassein* to enclose	wall, partition, diaphragm	SIMPLE ROOT: diaphragm (the partition of muscles and tendons between the chest cavity and the abdominal cavity) {diaphragmatic} diaphragma (or, diaphragm; used in anatomical nomenclature in the names of other separating structures; pl., diaphragmata) {diaphragmatic} PREFIXED ROOT: hemidiaphragm (*hemi* half) hypodiaphragmatic (also called *subphrenic*) (*hypo* under) infradiaphragmatic (also called *subdiaphragmatic*) (*infra* beneath) subdiaphragmatic (also called *infradiaphragmatic, subphrenic*) (*sub* beneath) supradiaphragmatic (*supra* above) transdiaphragmatic (*trans* across) LEADING ROOT COMPOUND: *diaphragm*: diaphragmalgia (also called *diaphragmodynia*) (*algos* pain) *diaphragmat*: diaphragmatitis (*itis* inflammation) *diaphragmato*: diaphragmatocele (also called *diaphragmatic hernia*) (*kele* hernia) TRAILING ROOT COMPOUND: cardiodiaphragmatic (*kardia* heart) costodiaphragmatic (movement of the ribs in breathing) (*costa* rib) hepatodiaphragmatic (*hepatos* liver) hernia-diaphragmatic (congenital hernia of the diaphragm) CROSS REFERENCE: parie, phren[1], sept[1]
diastas	Greek *dia* through + *stasis* standing	separation	SIMPLE ROOT: diastasis (a simple separation of normally joined parts) {diastatic} TRAILING ROOT COMPOUND: adenodiastasis (*adenos* gland) blepharodiastasis (*blepharon* eyelid) corediastasis (dilatation of the pupil) (*kore* pupil—of eye) iridodiastasis (iris—of eye) myelodiastasis (*myelos* spinal cord) myodiastasis (*myos* muscle) osteodiastasis (*osteon* bone) splanchnodiastasis (*splanchnos* viscus) CROSS REFERENCE: None

Element	From	Meaning	Examples
diastol	Greek *dia* across + *stalsis* contraction	contraction	SIMPLE ROOT: diastole (the dilatation, or period of dilatation, of the heart, especially that of the ventricles) {diastolic} (*dia* across) PREFIXED ROOT: holodiastolic (pertaining to the entire diastole) (*holos* whole) mesodiastolic (also called *middiastolic*) (*mesos* middle) postdiastolic (*post* after) prediastolic (*pre* before) protodiastolic (*protos* first) LEADING ROOT COMPOUND: diastology (*logos* study) TRAILING ROOT COMPOUND: bradydiastolic (*bradys* slow) merodiastolic (*meros* part) pseudodiastolic (*pseudes* false) CROSS REFERENCE: peristol, systol
didym	Greek *didymos*	twin, double; testicle, testis	SIMPLE ROOT: didymous (occurring in pairs), didymus (a testis) PREFIXED ROOT: *didymis:* epididymis (the elongated cordlike structure along the posterior border of the testis; pl., epididymides) {epididymal} paradidymis {paradidymal} (*para* alongside) perididymis, perididymitis (also called *periorchitis*) (*peri* around + *itis* inflammation) *didymus:* anadidymus (conjoined twins that are divided below but single toward the cephalic pole) (*ana* again, back, up) catadidymus (a type of conjoined twins) (*kata* down) anakatadidymus (conjoined twins that are separate above and below, but united in the middle) (*ana* again + *kata* down) heterodidymus (or, heterodymus; a fetus with a second head, neck, and thorax attached to the thorax) (*heteros* other) katadidymus (*kata* down) miodidymus (or, miodymus) (*meion* smaller) LEADING ROOT COMPOUND: didymalgia (also called *orchialgia*) (*algos* pain) didymitis (also called *orchiditis, orchitis*) (*itis* inflammation) didymodynia (also called *didymalgia, orchialgia*) (*odyne* pain) TRAILING ROOT COMPOUND: *didymus* a conjoined twin: cephalodidymus (*kephale* head) craniodidymus (a fetus with two heads) (*kranion* skull) cryptodidymus (also called *endadelphos*) (*kryptos* hidden) derodidymus (also called *dicephalus*) (*dere* neck) gastrodidymus (also called *omphalodidymus*) (*gaster* stomach) iniodymus (also called *iniopagus*) (*inion* occiput: back of head) ischiodidymus (*ischion* hip joint) melodidymus (*melos* limb) omphalodidymus (also called *gastrodidymus*) (*omphalos* navel) opodidymus (conjoined twins with a single body having two heads fused in the back) (*ops* face) pygodidymus (*pyge* rump, buttocks) somatodidymus (*somatos* body) vertebrodidymus (or, vertebrodymus) (*vertebra*) xiphodidymus (also called *xiphopagus*) (*xiphos* sword) CROSS REFERENCE: diplo, orchi, osche, test

Element	From	Meaning	Examples

diplo	Greek
	di two +
	ploos fold
		two-fold,
		twin, double
			SIMPLE ROOT: diploë (spongy tissue between the two layers of
			    compact bone of the skull) {diploic}
			PREFIXED ROOT:
			amphodiplopia (*ampho* both + *opia* vision condition)
			hyperdiploid (*hyper* above + *eidos* form)
			hypodiploid (*hypo* under + *eidos* form)
			monodiplopia (*monos* one, single + *opia* vision condition)
			See Appendix B for examples of words with this initial combining
			    form. Others are listed with the roots to which it is attached.
			CROSS REFERENCE: adelph, didym, gem, ploos

dis-	Latin prefix	apart, away, out	See Appendix B for examples of words with this prefix. Others are listed with the roots to which it is attached. CROSS REFERENCE: ab-, de-, ex-

dist	Latin
	distans
		distant,
		remote
			NOTE: This root comprises *dis* apart + *stare* to stand.
			SIMPLE ROOT:
			distad (in a distal direction)
			distal (farthest from the center, from a medial line, or from the
			    trunk; opposed to *proximal*), distalis, distally, distance
			See Appendix C for examples of words with this element. Others
			    are placed with the roots to which it is attached.
			CROSS REFERENCE: tele[2]

divertic	Latin *dis* away + *vertere* to turn	diverticulum	SIMPLE ROOT: diverticulum (lit., turned aside; a sac or pouch in the walls of a canal or organ; pl., diverticula) PREFIXED ROOT: peridiverticulitis (*peri* around + diverticulitis) LEADING ROOT COMPOUND: diverticulectomy (*ektome* excision) diverticulitis (*itis* inflammation) diverticuloma (*oma* tumor) diverticulosis (*osis* condition) CROSS REFERENCE: None
dolicho	Greek *dolikhos*	long	See Appendix B for examples of words with this element. Others are placed with the roots to which it is attached. CROSS REFERENCE: macr

dors	Latin
	dorsum
		the back	SIMPLE ROOT: dorsal (or, dorsel), dorsalis (denoting a position
			    closer to the back surface), dorsum (pl., dorsa)
			PREFIXED ROOT:
			mediodorsal (*medius* middle)
			predorsal (*pre* before)
			subdorsal (*sub* below)
			LEADING ROOT COMPOUND:
			dors:
			dorsabdominal (abdomen)
			dorsad (toward the back or dorsal aspect) (*ad* to, toward)
			dorsalgia (also called *dorsodynia*) (*algos* pain)
			dorsi:
			dorsiduct (to draw backward or toward the back) (*ducere* to lead)
			dorsiflexion (upward movement or extension of the foot or toes or
			    of the hands or fingers) (*flectere* to bend)
			dorsimesal (or, dorsomesial) (*mesos* middle)
			dorsiscapular (*scapula* collarbone)
			dorsispinal (*spina* spine)
			dorso:
			dorsoanterior (*anterior* front)
			dorsocephalad (*kephale* head)

Element	From	Meaning	Examples
dors (cont'd)		[the back]	dorsointercostal (*inter* between + *costa* rib)
			dorsolateral (*latus* side)
			dorsolumbar (*lumbar* loins)
			dorsomesial (*mesos* middle)
			dorsonasal (*nas* nose)
			dorsonuchal (*nucha* back of the neck)
			dorsoradial (pertaining to the radial or lateral side of the back of the forearm or hand)
			dorsoventral (*venter* belly)
			TRAILING ROOT COMPOUND: ventrodorsad, ventrodorsal (*venter* belly, abdomen)
			CROSS REFERENCE: noto, opist, rachi, spin
drom	Greek *dromos* course; *dramein* to run	to run; a course	PREFIXED ROOT:
			drome:
			hemisyndrome (*hemi* half + syndrome)
			prodrome (or, prodroma; the initial stage of a disease) {prodromal, prodromic} (*pro* forward)
			syndrome (a group of signs and symptoms that collectively "run together" to characterize or indicate a particular disease or abnormal condition) (*syn* with, together)
			[Note: There are hundreds of medical terms ending with syndrome.]
			dromia:
			adromia (absence of conduction in a nerve of a muscle) (*a* privative)
			palindromia (the recurrence of a disease) {palindromic} (*palin* again, back)
			dromic:
			antidromic (*anti* against)
			prodromic (*pro* forward)
			syndromic (*syn* with)
			dromology: syndromology (*syn* with + *logos* study)
			dromous:
			heterodromous (*heteros* other)
			homodromous (*homos* same)
			LEADING ROOT COMPOUND:
			dromograph (*graphein* to write)
			dromomania (*mania* madness)
			dromotropic (pertaining to supposed fibers in cardiac nerves which influence conductivity of muscles) (*trepein* to turn)
			TRAILING ROOT COMPOUND:
			hemadromometer (*haima* blood + *metron* measure)
			orthodromic (*orthos* straight)
			toxidrome (*toxikon* poison)
			CROSS REFERENCE: rhe
duoden	Latin *duo* two + *den* ten	twelve; duodenum (see Note)	NOTE: The duodenum was originally thought to be the length of the breadth of twelve fingers.
			SIMPLE ROOT: duodenum (the first part of the small intestine, connecting with the pylorus of the stomach and extending to the jejunum; pl., duodena) {duodenal}
			PREFIXED ROOT:
			duodenal: intraduodenal (*intra* within)
			duodenitis: periduodenitis (*peri* around + *itis* inflammation)
			duodenum:
			megaduodenum (*mega* large)
			mesoduodenum (*mesos* middle)

Element	From	Meaning	Examples
duoden (cont'd)		[duodenum]	metaduodenum (*meta* after)
			protoduodenum (*protos* first)
			LEADING ROOT COMPOUND:
			duoden:
			duodenectomy (*ektome* excision)
			duodenitis (*itis* inflammation)
			duodeno:
			duodenocolic (*kolon* colon)
			duodenocystostomy (*kystis* bladder + *stoma* mouth, opening)
			duodenoenterostomy (*enteron* intestine + *stoma* mouth, opening)
			duodenogastric (also called *gastroduodenal*) (*gaster* belly)
			duodenogram, duodenography (*graphein* to write)
			duodenohepatic (*hepatos* liver)
			duodenoileostomy (ileum + *stoma* mouth, opening)
			duodenojejunal (jejunum)
			duodenolysis (*lysis* loosening)
			duodenopancreatectomy (pancreas + *ektome* excision)
			duodenorrhaphy (*rhaphe* suture)
			duodenoscope, duodenoscopy (*skopein* to examine)
			duodenostomy (*stoma* mouth, opening)
			duodenotomy (*tomy* incision)
			TRAILING ROOT COMPOUND:
			esophagoduodenostomy (esophagus + *stoma* mouth, opening)
			gastroduodenal, gastroduodenitis (*gaster* stomach + *itis* inflammation)
			pyloroduodenitis (pylorus + *itis* inflammation)
			ureteroduodenal (ureter)
			CROSS REFERENCE: None
dynam	Greek *dynamis* power, strength	power, force	SIMPLE ROOT:
			dynamic (pertaining to vital force or inherent power; opposed to *static*)
			dynamics (the science of bodies in motion and their forces)
			dyne (a unit of force)
			dynein (a large protein playing several key roles)
			PREFIXED ROOT:
			adynamia (also called *asthenia*) {adynamic} (*a* privative)
			hyperdynamia (hyperactivity) {hyperdynamic} (*hyper* above)
			hypodynamia (diminished power) {hypodynamic} (*hypo* under)
			isodynamic, isodynamogenic (*isos* equal + *genere* to produce)
			megadyne (a unit of force equal to one million dynes) (*megas* large)
			LEADING ROOT COMPOUND:
			dynamogenesis (or, dynamogeny; the development of energy or force, as in muscle or nerves) (*genere* to produce)
			dynamograph (a self-registering dynamometer) (*graphein* to write)
			dynamophore (food or any substance that supplies energy to the body) (*phorein* to bear)
			dynamoscope, dynamoscopy (*skopein* to examine)
			TRAILING ROOT COMPOUND:
			aerodynamics (science of air or gases in motion) (*aer* air)
			cardiodynamics (*kardia* heart)
			hemodynamics (*haima* blood)
			hydrodynamics (that branch of the science of mechanics which treats of the movement of fluids and of solids contained in cells) (*hydor* water)

Element	From	Meaning	Examples
dynam (cont'd)		[power]	myodynamics (*myos* muscle) neurodynamic (*neuron* nerve) oligodynamic (*oligos* little, scant) ophthalmodynamometer (*ophthalmos* eye + *metron* measure) pedodynamometer (*pes* foot + *metron* measure) pharmacodynamics (*pharmakon* medicine, drugs) phlebodynamics (*phlebos* vein) pneumodynamics (*pneuma* breath) psychodynamics (*psyche* mind) trophodynamics (*trophe* nourishment) urodynamics (*ouron* urine) CROSS REFERENCE: erg, sthen
dys-	Greek prefix	bad, abnormal	See Appendix B for examples of words with this prefix. Others are listed with the roots to which it is attached. CROSS REFERENCE: cac-, mal-
dysplas	Greek *dys* abnormal + *plassein* to form	dysplasia	SIMPLE ROOT: dysplasia (abnormal tissue formation or develop- ment) PREFIXED ROOT: adysplasia (severe dysplasia) (*a* intensive) polydysplasia (*polys* many) TRAILING ROOT COMPOUND: angiodysplasia (*angeion* vessel) arthrodysplasia (*arthron* joint) chondrodysplasia (*chondros* cartilage) dermatodysplasia (*dermatos* skin) epidermodysplasia (*epidermis* outer layer of skin) fibrodysplasia (fiber) myelodysplasia (also called *myelodyspoiesis*) (*myelos* spinal cord) myodysplasia (*myos* muscle) odontodysplasia (*odontos* tooth) osteodysplaia (*osteon* bone) CROSS REFERENCE: None
dystroph	Greek *dys* abnormal + *trophein* to nourish	dystrophy	SIMPLE ROOT: dystrophy (or, dystrophia; progressive changes that may result from defective nutrition of a tissue or organ) PREFIXED ROOT: hemidystrophy (*hemi* half) polydystrophy {polydystrophic} (*polys* many) TRAILING ROOT COMPOUND: algodystrophy (or, algesidystrophy) (*algos* pain) algoneurodystrophy (*algos* pain + *neuron* nerve) angiodystrophy (*angeion* vessel) chondrodystrophy (*chondros* cartilage) chondro-osteodystrophy (*chondros* cartilage + *osteon* bone) hemodystrophy (*haima* blood) leukodystrophy (*leukos* white) lipodystrophy (*lipos* fat) myodystrophy (also called *muscular dystrophy*) (*myos* muscle) odontodystrophy (*odontos* tooth) onychodystrophy (*onychos* nail) osteodystrophy (*osteon* bone) poliodystrophy (*polios* gray matter) trichodystrophy (*trichos* hair) CROSS REFERENCE: None

Element	From	Meaning	Examples
e-	Latin prefix	out, away	See Appendix B for examples of words with this prefix. Others are listed with the roots to which it is attached. CROSS REFERENCE: ab-, dis-, ex-
ec-	Latin/ Greek prefix	out of	See Appendix B for examples of words with this prefix. Others are listed with the roots to which it is attached. CROSS REFERENCE: ab-, exo-
ectas			See ten[1] for words ending with *ectasia, ectasis*.
ecto-	Greek prefix	outside	See Appendix B for examples of words with this prefix. Others are listed with the roots to which it is attached. CROSS REFERENCE: ex-, exo-, extra-
-ectomy			See tom-.
ectop	Greek *ek* out + *topos* place	out of place; displaced	SIMPLE ROOT: ectopia (malposition of a body part or organ, espe- cially if congenital) {ectopic; also called *atopic*} TRAILING ROOT COMPOUND: adenectopia (*adenos* gland) angiectopia (*angeion* blood vessel) arteriectopia (*arteria* artery) cardiectopia (*kardia* heart) corectopia (*core* pupil) metrectopia (*metra* uterus) myectopia (*myos* muscle) neurectopia (*neuron* nerve) osteectopia (*osteon* bone) phlebectopia (*phlebos* vein) splanchnectopia (*splanchnos* viscus) splenectopia (*splen* spleen) tarsectopia (*tarsos* instep of the foot) CROSS REFERENCE: None
ectro	Greek *ektrosis*	congenitally absent; miscarriage	SIMPLE ROOT: ectrosis (abortion) {ectrotic} PREFIXED ROOT: hemiectromelia (*hemi* half + ectromelia) LEADING ROOT COMPOUND: ectrocheiry (or, ectrochiry) (*cheir* hand) ectrodactyly (*daktylos* finger, toe) ectrogeny {ectrogenic} (*genere* to produce) ectromelia {ectromelic} (*melos* limb) ectrometacarpia (metacarpal bone) ectrometatarsia (metatarsal bone) ectrophalangia (*phalange* bone of finger or toe) ectropody (*podos* foot) ectrosyndactyly (a condition in which some of the digits are missing and those that remain are cohesive) (*syn* with + *daktylos* finger, toe) CROSS REFERENCE: atel
eczema			See zein.
edema (alternate spelling: **oedema**)	Greek *oidein* to swell	swelling	SIMPLE ROOT: edema (the presence of abnormally large amounts of fluid in the intercellular tissue spaces of the body; usually ap- plied to demonstrable accumulation of excessive fluid in the sub- cutaneous tissues) {edematous}, edematization LEADING ROOT COMPOUND: edematigenous (*genere* to pro- duce)

Element	From	Meaning	Examples
edema (cont'd)		[swelling]	TRAILING ROOT COMPOUND: acroedema (*akros* extremities) angioedema (also called *angioneurotic edema*) (*angeion* vessel) blepharedema (*blepharon* eyelid) bronchoedema (*bronchos* windpipe) cephaledema (*kephale* head) dactyledema (*daktylos* finger, toe) erythroedema (*erythros* red) leukoedema (*leukos* white) lipedema (*lipos* fat) lymphedema (see *trophedema*) (*lympha* water, fluid) melanedema (also called *anthracosis*) (*melanos* black, dark) myoedema (also called *mounding*) (*myos* muscle) myxedema (*myxa* mucus) nephredema (also called *nephremia*) (*nephros* kidney) papilledema (also called *choked disk*) (*papilla* projection: optic disk) periosteoedema (periosteum) podedema (*podos* foot) pseudoedema (a puffy state resembling edema) (*pseudes* false) rhinedema (*rhis* nose) scleredema (*skleros* hard) staphyloedema (or, staphyledema) (*staphyle* uvula) trophedema (also called *hereditary lymphedema*) (*trophe* nourishment) uroedema (or, uredema) (*ouron* urine) CROSS REFERENCE: cel^2, gangli, onc, tub^2, tum
ef-	Latin prefix	out	See Appendix B (ex-) for examples of words with this prefix. Others are listed with the roots to which it is attached. CROSS REFERENCE: ex-
eid, **-oid**	Greek *eidos*	image, form; resembling	SIMPLE ROOT: eidetic (relating to or having the ability of total visual recall of anything previously seen) PREFIXED ROOT: apeidosis (progressive disappearance of characteristic form in either the histologic or clinical aspect of a disease) (*apo* from + *osis* condition) LEADING ROOT COMPOUND: *eid*: eidoptometry (measurement of the acuteness of vision for the perception of form) (*optos* vision + *metron* measure) *eido*: eidogen (*genere* to produce) TRAILING ROOT COMPOUND: acanthoid (*akantha* thorn) acaroid (*akari* mite) adenoid (*adenos* gland) adipoid (*adeps* fat) ameboid (ameba) amyloid (*amylon* starch) anconoid (*ankon* elbow) angioid (*angeion* vessel) anthracoid (*anthrax* charcoal, carbuncle) belonoid (*belone* needle) blennoid (muciform) (*blenna* mucus) cancroid (cancer) choroid (the thin, highly vascular membrane covering most of the posterior of the eye between the retina and the sclera) (*chorion* membrane)

Element	From	Meaning	Examples
eid, oid (cont'd)		[resembling]	chromatoid (*chromatos* color) cricoid (having a ring shape, e.g., the cricoid cartilage) (*krikos* ring) cystoid (*kystis* sac, bladder) dermoid (*derma* skin) desmoid (*desmos* band, ligament) embryoid (*embryein* to swell) lymphoid (*lympha* water, liquid) myeloid (*myelos* marrow) toxoid (*toxikon* poison) typhoid (*typhus* fever) CROSS REFERENCE: form, ide, morph, plas
elcosis			See helc- for *enterelcosis*, for example.
em-	Greek prefix	in	See Appendix B (en-) for examples of words with this prefix. Others are listed with the roots to which it is attached. CROSS REFERENCE: en-, in-
embol	Greek *en* in + *ballein* to throw; thus, to insert	plug, wedge	SIMPLE ROOT: embole (or, embolia, emboly; the reducing of a dislocated limb) embolism (the sudden blocking of an artery or vein by a clot or obstruction which has been brought to its place by the blood current), embolization embolus (pl., emboli) {embolic}, emboly (the invagination of the blastula by which the gastrula is formed) PREFIXED ROOT: microembolus (*mikros* small) LEADING ROOT COMPOUND: *embol*: embolectomy (*ektome* excision) embolemia (*emia* blood condition) *emboli*: emboliform (*forma* shape) *embolo*: embololalia (or, embolalia; the interpolation of meaningless words into speech; also called *embolophrasia*) (*lalein* to speak) embolomycotic (pertaining to or marked by an infective embolism) (*mykes* fungus + *osis* condition) embolophrasia (also called *embololalia*) (*phrazein* to speak) embolotherapy (embolization) (*therapy* treatment) TRAILING ROOT COMPOUND: aeroembolism (obstruction of a blood vessel by air or gas) (*aer* air) atheroembolism (embolism due to blockage of a blood vessel by an atheroembolus) (*athere* gruel) thromboembolism (*thrombos* clot) CROSS REFERENCE: cune, emphrax, sphen
embryo	Greek *embryon*; *en* in + *bryein* to swell, to be full	to grow (embryo)	SIMPLE ROOT: embryo {embryonal, embryonic}, embryoism, embryonate embryonism, embryonization PREFIXED ROOT: *embryo*: preembryo (*pre* before) *embryonic*: abembryonic (*ab* away, from) extraembryonic (*extra* external) intraembryonic (*intra* within) postembryonic (*post* after) preembryonic (*pre* before) *embryoma* embryonic tumor: dysembryoma (teratoma) (*dys* abnormal)

Element	From	Meaning	Examples
embryo (cont'd)		[to grow]	polyembryoma (*polys* many) *embryony*: diembryony (*di* two) polyembryony (*polys* many) *embryoplasia*: dysembryoplasia (*dys* abnormal + *plassein* to form) LEADING ROOT COMPOUND: *embry*: embryectomy (*ektome* excision) embryoid (*eidos* form) embryoma (*oma* tumor) embryulcus (*elkein* to draw) *embryo*: embryoblast (*blastos* bud, shoot, germ) embryocardia (*kardia* heart) embryoctony (*kteinein* to kill) embryogenesis {embryogenic} (*genere* to produce) embryograph {embryography} (*graphein* to write) embryology (*logos* study) embryomorphous (*morphe* form) embryopathology, embryopathy (*pathos* disease + *logos* study) embryophore (*phorein* to bear) embryoplastic (*plassein* to form) embryoscope (*skopein* to examine) embryotome, embryotomy (*tomy* incision) embryotroph, embryotrophy (*trophein* to nourish) TRAILING ROOT COMPOUND: carcinoembryonic (*karkinos* cancer) pseudoembryonic (*pseudes* false) CROSS REFERENCE: aug, creat, phys[1]
emes, **emet**	Greek *emein*	to vomit	SIMPLE ROOT: emesis (vomiting) {emetic} PREFIXED ROOT: antiemetic (*anti* against) autemesia (functional or idiopathic vomiting) (*autos* self) hyperemesis {hyperemetic} (*hyper* over, beyond) LEADING ROOT COMPOUND: emetocathartic (both emetic and cathartic; an agent that causes vomiting and purging of the lower intestines) (*katharsis* a cleansing) emetogenic (having the capacity to induce vomiting, a common property of anticancer agents, narcotics, and amorphine), emetogenicity (*genere* to produce) emetology (or, emeticology) (*logos* study) emetophobia (*phobia* fear) TRAILING ROOT COMPOUND: blennemesis (*blenna* mucus) cholemesis (*chole* bile) copremesis (*kopros* dung, excrement) helminthemesis (*helminth* worm) hematemesis (*haima* blood) melanemesis (*melanos* black, dark) pyemesis (*pyon* pus) sialemesis (*sialon* saliva) tyremesis (*tyros* cheese) CROSS REFERENCE: None

Element	From	Meaning	Examples
emia			See hemo- for *anemia*, for example.
emphrax, **emphrac**	Greek *emphraxis*	stoppage, obstruction	SIMPLE ROOT: *emphrac*: emphractic (tending to obstruct the pores; an agent that closes the pores of the skin) *emphrax*: emphraxis (a stoppage, obstruction, or infarction) TRAILING ROOT COMPOUND: adenemphraxis (*aden* gland) laryngemphraxis (larynx) pancreatemphraxis (pancreas) pharyngemphraxis (pharynx) phlebemphraxis (*phlebos* vein) phrenemphraxis (*phren* diaphragm: phrenic nerve) pylemphraxis (*pyle* gate) salpingemphraxis (obstruction of the auditory tube) (*salpingos* tube) spermatemphraxis (*sperma* seed, sperm) splenemphraxis (*splen* spleen) urethremphraxis (urethra) CROSS REFERENCE: embol
en-	Greek prefix	in	See Appendix B for examples of words with this prefix. Others are listed with the roots to which it is attached. CROSS REFERENCE: in-[1] [another *in-* is a negative]
encephal	Greek *en* in, on + *kephale* head	brain	SIMPLE ROOT: encephalon (pl., encephala) {encephalic, pertaining to the encephalon; also, within the cranium} PREFIXED ROOT: *encephalia*: anencephalia (or, anencephaly) {anencephalic}, anencephalus (congenital absence of the brain and spinal cord) (*an* privative) dysencephalia (*dys* abnormal) exencephalia (or, exencephaly) (*ex* out) macrencephalia (*makros* large) micrencephalia (*mikros* small) parencephalia (congenital defect of the brain) {parencephalous} (*para* abnormal) *encephalitis* inflammation of the brain: mesencephalitis (*mesos* middle) panencephalitis (*pan* all) parencephalitis (inflammation of the cerebellum) (*para* alongside) periencephalitis (*peri* around) *encephalitic*: postencephalitic (following encephalitis) (*post* after) *encephalocele* brain hernia: exencephalocele (*ex* out) parencephalocele (*para* alongside) synencephalocele (*syn* with) *encephalon*: deutencephalon (also called *diencephalon*) (*deuteros* second) diencephalon {diencephalic} (*dia* across, through) hypencephalon (*hypo* under) macroencephalon (also called *megaloencephahlon*) (*makros* large) megaloencephalon (also called *macroencephalon*) (*megalos* large) mesencephalon (*mesos* middle) metencephalon {metencephalic} (*meta* after) microencephalon {microencephalous} (*mikros* small) myelencephalon (also called *medulla oblongata*) (*myelos* marrow) oligoencephalon (also called *micrencephalon*) (*oligos* little, small)

Element	From	Meaning	Examples
encephal (cont'd)		[brain]	prosencephalon (or, proencephalon) (*proso* before)
			encephalo: mesencephalotomy (*mesos* middle + *tomy* incision)
			encephalus:
			hemiencephalus (*hemi* half)
			pseudoencephalus (a malformed fetus with a tumor in place of the brain) (*pseudes* false)
			encephaly:
			exencephaly (or, exencephalia) (*ex* out)
			hemianencephaly (*hemi* half + anencephaly)
			holoprosencephaly (*holos* whole + *proso* forward)
			hyperencephaly (*hyper* above)
			macroencephaly (or, macrencephaly) (*makros* large)
			megaloencephaly (*megalos* large)
			microencephaly (or, micrencephaly) (*mikros* small)
			LEADING ROOT COMPOUND:
			encephal:
			encephalalgia (headache; also called *encephalodynia*) (*algos* pain)
			encephalemia (also called *brain congestion*) (*emia* blood condition)
			encephalitis (pl., encephalitides) {encephalitic} (*itis* inflammation)
			encephalodynia (also called *encephalalgia*) (*odyne* pain)
			encephaloid (*eidos* form)
			encephaloma (*oma* tumor)
			encephalopsy (a condition in which the patient associates certain colors with certain visual phenomena) (*opsis* vision)
			encephalosis (also called *encephalopathy*) (*osis* condition)
			encephalo:
			encephalocele (*kele* hernia)
			encephaloclastic (*klastos* broken)
			encephalodysplasia (*dysplasia* ill-formed, badly formed)
			encephalogram, encephalography (EEG, for both) (*graphein* to write)
			encephalolith (*lithos* stone)
			encephalology (*logos* study)
			encephalomalacia (*malakos* soft)
			encephalomeningitis (also called *meningoencephalitis*) (*meningos* membrane + *itis* inflammation)
			encephalomeningocele (*meningos* membrane + *kele* hernia)
			encephalomeningopathy (also called *meningoencephalopathy*) (*meningos* membrane + *pathos* disease)
			encephalomere (also called *neuromere*) (*meros* part)
			encephalometer (*metron* measure)
			encephalomyelitis (*myelos* spinal cord + *itis* inflammation)
			encephalomyelocele (*myelos* spinal cord + *kele* hernia)
			encephalomyeloneuropathy (*myelos* spinal cord + *neuron* nerve + *pathos* disease)
			encephalomyelopathy (*myelos* spinal cord + *pathos* disease)
			encephalomyocarditis (*myocarditis* heart muscle inflammation)
			encephalonarcosis (stupor due to brain disease)
			encephalopathy (also called *encephalosis*) (*pathos* disease)
			encephalopuncture (*pungere* to pierce)
			encephalopyosis (*pyosis* suppuration)
			encephaloradiculitis (*radix* root + *itis* inflammation)
			encephalorachidian (also called *cerebrospinal*) (*rhachis* spine)
			encephalorrhagia (*rhagia* bursting forth)

Element	From	Meaning	Examples
encephal (cont'd)		[brain]	encephaloschisis (*schisis* fissure) encephalosclerosis (*skleros* hard + *osis* condition) encephaloscope, encephaloscopy (*skopein* to examine) encephalospinal (also called *cerebrospinal*) encephalotomy (also called *cerebrotomy*) (*tomy* incision) TRAILING ROOT COMPOUND: *encephalia* brain condition: sclerencephalia (*skleros* hard) syringoencephalia (*syringos* duct, tube) *encephalitis* inflammation of the brain: leukoencephalitis (*leukos* white) meningoencephalitis (*meningos* membrane) myelencephalitis (also called *encephalomyelitis*) (*myelos* marrow) otoencephalitis (*otos* ear) polioencephalitis, poliomyeloencephalitis (*polios* grey + *myelos* marrow) porencephalitis (*poros* pore) *encephalocele*: hydroencephalocele (*hydor* water + *kele* tumor) *encephalo*: neuroencephalomyelopathy (*neuron* nerve + *myelos* spinal cord + *pathos* disease) *encephalon*: hematencephalon (also called *cerebral hemorrhage*) (*haima* blood) neencephalon (*neos* new) ophthalmencephalon (*ophthalmos* eye) rhombencephalon (*rhembein* to turn) telencephalon (*telos* the end) *encephalus*: cyclencephalus (*kyklos* circle) cystencephalus (*kystis* sac) derencephalus (*dere* neck) hydrencephalus (*hydor* water) iniencephalus (*inion* occiput: back of the head) necrencephalus (also called *encephalomalacia*) (*nekros* dead) nosencephalus (a fetus with defective cranium and brain) (*nosos* disease) notencephalus (*noton* back) podencephalus (*pous* foot; in this word, pedicle) pyencephalus (also called *brain abscess*) (*pyon* pus) thlipsencephalus (*thlipsis* pressure) *encephaly*: iniencephaly (*inion* occiput: back of head) lissencephaly (also called *agyria*) (*lissos* smooth) meroanencephaly (*meros* part + *anencephaly*) perencephaly (a condition marked by one or more cerebral cysts) (*pera* a purse, wallet) platystencephaly (*platys* flat, broad) porencephaly (*porus* pore, opening) rhinoencephaly (*rhinos* nose) schizencephaly (*schizein* to divide) sclerencephaly (*skleros* hard) CROSS REFERENCE: cerebr, phren[2]
endo-	Greek prefix	within	See Appendix B for examples of words with this prefix. Others are placed with the root to which it is attached. CROSS REFERENCE: intra-

A Thesaurus of Medical Word Roots

Element	From	Meaning	Examples
endothel	Greek *endon* within + *thele* nipple	cell layer	SIMPLE ROOT: endothelium (the layer of epithelial cells that lines the cavities of the heart and of the blood and lymph vessels, and the serous cavities of the body; pl., endothelia) {endothelial} PREFIXED ROOT: subendothelium {subendothelial} (*sub* under) LEADING ROOT COMPOUND: *endotheli*: endotheliitis (*itis* inflammation) endothelioid (*eidos* form, resembling) endothelioma, endotheliomatosis (*oma* tumor + *osis* condition) endotheliosis (*osis* condition) *endothelio*: endothelioblastoma (*blastos* bud, shoot, germ + *oma* tumor) endotheliochorial (*chorion* membrane) endotheliocyte (*kytos* cell) endotheliolytic (*lysis* loosening) endotheliosarcoma (*sarkos* flesh + *oma* tumor) endotheliotoxin (*toxin* poison) CROSS REFERENCE: None
enter	Greek *enteron*	intestine, bowel	SIMPLE ROOT: enteron {enteral, enteric}, entrails PREFIXED ROOT: *enteral*: parenteral (*para* alongside) *enteration*: exenteration (also called *evisceration*) (*ex* out) *enteric*: circumenteric (also called *circumintestinal*) (*circum* around) *enteritis* inflammation of intestines: endoenteritis (*endon* within) exenteritis (*exo* outside) mesenteritis (*mesos* middle) perienteritis (*peri* around) *enteron*: megaloenteron (also called *enteromegaly, enteromegalia*) (*megalos* large) mesenteron (midgut) (*mesos* middle) perienteron {perienteric}, perienteritis (*peri* around + *itis* inflammation) *enterous*: anenterous (*an* privative) *entery*: dysentery (an inflammatory disorder of the lower intestinal tract, resulting in pain, fever, and severe diarrhea) (*dys* abnormal) mesentery (*mesos* middle) LEADING ROOT COMPOUND: *enter*: enteradenitis (*aden* gland + *itis* inflammation) enteralgia (also called *enterodynia*) (*algos* pain) enterectasis (*ektasis* dilatation) enterectomy (*ektome* excision) enteritis (*itis* inflammation) enterodynia (also called *enteralgia*) (*odyne* pain) enteruria (*uria* urine condition) *entero*: enteroadherent (adhering to the intestinal mucosa) enteroaggregative (adhering to, and forming colonies on, the intestinal mucosa) enterobiliary (bile) enteroblastic (*blastos* germ)

Element	From	Meaning	Examples
enter (cont'd)		[intestine]	enterocele (*kele* hernia)
			enterocentesis (*kentein* to puncture)
			enterocholecystostomy (*chole* bile + *kystis* bladder + *stoma* opening)
			enterocholecystotomy (*chole* bile + *kystis* bladder + *tomy* incision)
			enterocidal (an agent that kills parasites in the gastrointestinal tract)
			enterocinesia (also called *peristalsis*) (*kinein* to move)
			enterocleisis (*kleisis* closure)
			enteroclysis (*klysis* a drenching)
			enterococcus (pl., enterococci) (*kokkos* berry-shaped bacterium)
			enterocoele (the abdominal cavity) (*koilia* belly)
			enterocolitis (*kolon* colon + *itis* inflammation)
			enterocolostomy (*kolon* colon + *stoma* opening)
			enterocutaneous (*cutis* skin)
			enterocyst (a cyst in the wall of the intestines; also called *enterocystoma*) (*kystis* sac, bladder)
			enteroepiplocele (or, enterepiplocele) (*epiploon* omentum + *kele* hernia)
			enterogastric (also called *gastrointestinal*), enterogastritis (also called *gastroenteritis*) (*gaster* stomach + *itis* inflammation)
			enterogenous (*genere* to produce)
			enterogram, enterograph (*graphein* to write)
			enterohepatitis (*hepatos* liver + *itis* inflammation)
			enterohepatocele (*hepatos* liver + *kele* hernia)
			enterohydrocele (*hydor* water + *kele* hernia)
			enteroidea (*eidos* resemblance)
			enterokinesis {enterokinetic} (*kinesis* movement)
			enterolith, enterolithiasis (*lithos* stone + *iasis* condition)
			enterology (*logos* study)
			enterolysis (*lysis* dissolution)
			enteromegalia (or, enteromegaly) (*megalos* large)
			enteromenia (*mene* month: menstruation)
			enteromere (*meros* part)
			enteromycosis (*mykes* fungus + *osis* condition)
			enteroneuritis (*neuron* nerve + *itis* inflammation)
			enteroparesis (*paresis* relaxation)
			enteropathy (*pathos* illness, disease)
			enteropexy (*pexis* fixation)
			enteroplasty (*plassein* to form)
			enteroplegia (also called *adynamic ileus*) (*plege* stroke)
			enteroptosis {enteroptotic} (*ptosis* a falling)
			enterorenal (also called *renointestinal*) (*ren* kidney)
			enterorrhagia (*rhagia* bursting forth)
			enterorrhaphy (*rhaphe* suture)
			enterorrhexis (*rhexein* to rupture)
			enteroscope (*skopein* to examine)
			enterosepsis (*sepsis* putrefaction)
			enterospasm (*span* to contract)
			enterostasis (also called *intestinal stasis*) (*stasis* obstruction)
			enterostaxis (*staxis* dripping: slow hemorrhage)
			enterostenosis (*stenosis* a narrowing)
			enterostomy {enterostomal} (*stoma* mouth, opening)
			enterotome, enterotomy (*tomy* incision)
			enterotoxication, enterotoxin, autotoxism (*toxin* poison)
			enterotropic (*tropein* to turn)

Element	From	Meaning	Examples
enter (cont'd)		[intestine]	enterovaginal (vagina)
			enterovenous (*vena* vein)
			enterovesical (also called *vesicoenteric, vesicointestinal*) (*vesica* bladder)
			enterovirus {enteroviral} (*virus* poison)
			enterozoon {enterozoic} (*zoon* animal; parasite)
			TRAILING ROOT COMPOUND:
			enteralgia: gastroenteralgia (*gaster* stomach + *algos* pain)
			enteric:
			gastroenteric (*gaster* belly, stomach)
			hepatoenteric (*hepatos* liver)
			neurenteric (*neuron* nerve)
			omphaloenteric (*omphalos* umbilicus, navel)
			pneumatoenteric (also called *celomic bay*) (*pnematos* air)
			ureteroenteric (ureter)
			vesicoenteric (also called *vesicointestinal, enterovesical*) (*vesica* bladder)
			enteritis inflammation of the intestines:
			coloenteritis (colon)
			gastroenteritis (*gaster* stomach, belly)
			lymphenteritis (*lymph* water, fluid)
			mucoenteritis (mucus)
			pneumoenteritis (*pneumon* lung)
			psorenteritis (also called *psorenteria*) (*psoros* scabby, itchy)
			seroenteritis (*serum* whey; serous coat)
			typhlenteritis (*typhlon* blind gut)
			enterocele intestinal hernia:
			cystoenterocele (*kystis* bladder)
			epiploenterocele (*epiploon* omentum)
			enterocolitis: gastroenterocolitis (*gaster* stomach + colon + *itis* inflammation)
			enteron:
			archenteron (the primitive enteron or undifferentiated sac of a gastrula or other embryo) (*archein* to be first)
			celenteron (or, coelenteron; also called *archenteron, gastrovascular cavity, primitive gut*) (*koilia* cavity)
			myenteron {myenteric} (*myos* muscle)
			PREFIXED TRAILING ROOT COMPOUND: synechtenterotomy (division of an intestinal adhesion) (*syn* together + *echein* to hold + *tomy* incision)
			CROSS REFERENCE: ile, intestine, visc
ento-	Greek prefix	inside	See Appendix B for examples of words with this prefix. Others are listed with the roots to which it is attached.
			CROSS REFERENCE: endo-, intra-
enzym	Greek *en* in + *zyme* leaven	enzyme	SIMPLE ROOT: enzyme (an organic catalyst produced by living cells but capable of acting independently) {enzymatic, enzymic}
			PREFIXED ROOT:
			enzyme:
			antienzyme (a protein or polypeptide that inhibits or destroys an enzyme) (*anti* against)
			apoenzyme (an enzyme without its cofactor) (*apo* away)
			coenzyme (a substance needed by enzymes to produce many of the reactions in energy and protein metabolism in the body) (*com* with, together)

A Thesaurus of Medical Word Roots

Element	From	Meaning	Examples
enzym (cont'd)		[enzyme]	ectoenzyme (an extracellular enzyme; an enzyme situated on the outer surface of a cell's membrane) (*ektos* outside) endoenzyme (*endon* within) exoenzyme (*exo* outside) holoenzyme (*holos* entire) isoenzyme (or, isozyme) (*isos* equal) multienzyme (*multus* many) proenzyme (*pro* before) *enzymia*: anenzymia (congenital absence of an enzyme) (*an* privative) LEADING ROOT COMPOUND: enzymology (*logos* study) enzymolysis (*lyein* to loosen) enzymopathy (*pathos* disease) TRAILING ROOT COMPOUND: holoenzyme (*holos* whole, complete) lyoenzyme (*lyein* to dissolve) flavoenzyme (an enzyme that possesses a flavin nucleotide as coenzyme) (*flavus* yellow) molybdoenzyme (*molybdos* lead) CROSS REFERENCE: None
ependym	Greek *epi* upon + *en* on + *dyein* to put on; upper garment	membrane lining	SIMPLE ROOT: ependyma (the lining membrane of the ventricles of the brain and of the central canal of the spinal cord; also called *endyma*) {ependymal} PREFIXED ROOT: periependymal (*peri* around) subependymal (*sub* under) subependymoma (*sub* under + *oma* tumor) LEADING ROOT COMPOUND: *ependym*: ependymitis (*itis* inflammation) ependymoma (also called *ependymocytoma*) (*oma* tumor) *ependymo*: ependymoblast, ependymoblastoma (*blastos* germ + *oma* tumor) ependymocyte, ependymocytoma (*kytos* cell + *oma* tumor) ependymopathy (*pathos* disease) CROSS REFERENCE: amnio, membran
epi-	Greek prefix	upon, on	See Appendix B for examples of words with this prefix. Others are listed with the roots to which it is attached. CROSS REFERENCE: None
epilep	Greek *epi* upon + *lambanein* to seize	seizure	SIMPLE ROOT: epilepsy (or, epilepsia; any of a group of syndromes characterized by paroxysmal transient disturbances of the brain function) {epileptic} PREFIXED ROOT: *epileptic*: antiepileptic (also called *anticonvulsant*) (*anti* against) postepileptic (*post* after) *epilepsy*: hemiepilepsy (*hemi* half) paraepilepsy (*para* alongside, similar to) LEADING ROOT COMPOUND: *epilept*: epileptoid (also called *epileptiform*) (*eidos* form, shape) *epilepti*: epileptiform (resembling epilepsy or its manifestations; also called *epileptoid*) (*forma* shape)

Element	From	Meaning	Examples
epilep (cont'd)		[seizure]	*epilepto*: epileptogenous {epileptogenic} (*genere* to produce) epileptologist, epileptology (*logos* study) TRAILING ROOT COMPOUND: pseudoepilepsy (*pseudes* false) CROSS REFERENCE: agra, hapt, lep[2]
epiphys	Greek *epi* upon + *physis* growth	bone excrescence	SIMPLE ROOT: epiphysis (the expanded articular end of a long bone; pl., epiphyses) {epiphyseal, epiphysial} PREFIXED ROOT: extraepiphysial (not relating to, or connected with an epiphysis) (*extra* outside—not related) intraepiphysial (within the epiphysis of a long bone) (*intra* within) juxtaepiphysial (close to or adjoining the epiphysis) (*juxta* near) LEADING ROOT COMPOUND: *epiphys*: epiphysitis (*itis* inflammation) *epiphysi*: epiphysioid (*eidos* form) *epiphysio*: epiphysiodesis (*desis* binding) epiphysiolysis (*lysis* loosening) epiphysiometer (*metron* measure) epiphysiopathy (*pathos* disease) CROSS REFERENCE: condyl
epiplo	Greek *epiploon*	omentum (see Note)	NOTE: The omentum is a fold of peritoneum extending from the stomach to adjacent organs in the abdominal cavity. SIMPLE ROOT: epiploon (the omentum, especially the greater omentum) {epiploic; also called *omental*} PREFIXED ROOT: anepiploic (devoid of omentum) (*an* privative) LEADING ROOT COMPOUND: *epipl*: epiplomphalocele (*omphalos* navel + *kele* hernia) epiploscheocele (*osche* scrotum + *kele* hernia) *epiplo*: epiplocele (omental hernia) (*kele* hernia) epiploectomy (also called *omentectomy*) (*ektome* excision) epiploenterocele (hernia consisting of omentum and intestine) (*enteron* intestine + *kele* hernia) epiploitis (also called *omentitis*) (*itis* inflammation) epiplomerocele (*meros* thigh + *kele* hernia) epiplopexy (also called *omentopexy*) (*pexis* fixation) epiploplasty (*plassein* to form) CROSS REFERENCE: oment
episio	Greek *epision*	pubic region; vulva	See Appendix B for examples of words with this combining form. Others are placed with the roots to which it is attached. CROSS REFERENCE: labi[1], vulv
epithel	Greek *epi* upon + *thele* nipple	epithelium	SIMPLE ROOT: epithelium (the covering of internal and external surfaces of the body, including the lining of vessels and other small cavities; pl., epithelia) {epithelial}, epithelialization PREFIXED ROOT: *epithelial*: antiepithelial (*anti* against) intraepithelial (*intra* within) subepithelial (*sub* under) *epithelium*: mesepithelium (or, mesothelium) (*mesos* middle) subepithelium {subepithelial} (*sub* beneath)

Element	From	Meaning	Examples
epithel (cont'd)		[epithelium]	LEADING ROOT COMPOUND:
			epith: epithalaxia (desquamation of epithelium) (*allaxis* exchange)
			epitheli:
			epitheliitis (*itis* inflammation)
			epithelioid (*eidos* form)
			epithelioma {epitheliomatous}, epitheliomatosis (*oma* tumor + *osis* condition)
			epitheliosis (*osis* condition)
			epithelio:
			epitheliochorial (*chorion* membrane)
			epitheliocyte (*kytos* cell)
			epitheliofibril (*fibra* fiber)
			epitheliogenetic, epitheliogenic (*genere* to produce)
			epithelioglandular
			epitheliolysis {epitheliolytic} (*lyein* to dissolve)
			epitheliomuscular
			epitheliotoxin (*toxikon* poison)
			epitheliotropic (*tropic* turning; having an affinity for)
			TRAILING ROOT COMPOUND:
			epithelio: keratoepithelioplasty (*keratos* cornea + *plassein* to form)
			epithelium:
			desmepithelium (the endothelial lining of blood vessels, lymphatics, and synovial membranes) (*dein* to bind: ligament)
			myoepithelium (*myos* muscle)
			neurepithelium (*neuron* nerve)
			pioepithelium (*pion* fat)
			epithelioma tumorous epithelium:
			chordoepithelioma (also called *chordoma*) (*chord* cord, sinew)
			chorioepithelioma (*chorion* membrane)
			cystoepithelioma (*kystis* cyst, sac)
			fibroepithelioma (fiber)
			lymphoepithelioma (*lymph* water, fluid)
			medulloepithelioma (*medulla* marrow)
			myoepithelioma (*myos* muscle)
			neuroepithelioma (*neuron* nerve)
			trichoepithelioma (*trichos* hair)
			CROSS REFERENCE: None
epulis			See oulo-.
eresis			See heres- for *apheresis, syneresis*.
erg, **urg**	Greek *ergon* work	work, deed	SIMPLE ROOT: erg (the amount of work done when a force of 1 dyne acts through a distance of 1 cm), ergasia
			PREFIXED ROOT:
			ergasis: metergasis (change of function) (*meta* change)
			ergetic:
			energetics (*en* in)
			isoenergetic (exhibiting equal energy) (*isos* equal + energetic)
			synergetic (or, synergistic; acting together) (*syn* with)
			ergia:
			asynergia (or, asynergy) {asynergic} (*a* negative + synergia)
			dysergia (motor incoordination due to effect of efferent nerve impulse) (*dys* abnormal)
			dyssynergia (*dys* abnormal + synergia)
			hemiasynergia (*hemi* half + asynergia)
			hemidysergia (*hemi* half + dysergia)

Element	From	Meaning	Examples
erg (cont'd)		[work]	hyperenergia (hyperactivity), hyperergia (*hyper* above)
			hypoergia (or, hypoergy) (*hypo* under)
			synergia (or, synergy, synergism) (*syn* with, together)
			ergic:
			anallergic (*an* negative + allergic)
			antienergic (*anti* against + energy)
			endoergic (also called *endergonic, endothermic*) (*endon* within)
			exoergic (*exo* outside)
			heterergic (*heteros* other)
			hypoergic (*hypo* under)
			polyergic (*polys* many)
			synergic (*syn* with)
			ergism: synergism (or, synergia, synergy) (*syn* with, together)
			ergometer: energometer (energy + *metron* measure)
			ergonic:
			endergonic (also called *endoergic*) (*endon* within)
			exergonic (*exo* outside)
			ergy:
			allergy (altered energy, or reaction) {allergic} (*allos* other)
			anergy (or, anergia) {anergic} (*an* privative)
			energy (*en* in)
			parallergy (*para* alongside + allergy)
			synergy (or, synergism) (*syn* with, together)
			urg: micrurgical (*mikros* small)
			LEADING ROOT COMPOUND:
			ergasio: ergasiophobia (aversion to work of any kind) (*phobia* fear)
			ergo:
			ergodynamograph (*dynamis* force + *graphein* to write)
			ergoesthesiograph (*esthesia* feeling + *graphein* to write)
			ergogenic (*genere* to produce)
			ergogram, ergograph {ergographic} (*graphein* to write)
			ergometer (also called *dynamometer*) (*metron* measure)
			ergonomics (*nomos* law)
			ergoplasm (*plassein* to form)
			ergotherapy (*therapy* treatment)
			ergotropic (*tropic* turning)
			TRAILING ROOT COMPOUND:
			bioenergetics (a system of exercises based on the concept that natural healing will be enhanced by bringing the patient's body rhythms and the natural environment into harmony) (*bios* life)
			pathergy (*pathos* disease)
			peptidergic (peptide)
			DISGUISED ROOT: surgery (*cheiros* hand + *ergon*)
			CROSS REFERENCE: dynam, sthen
erythr	Greek *erythros* red	red	SIMPLE ROOT:
			erythema (redness due to capillary dilation) {erythematous}
			erythrism (redness of the hair and beard and a ruddy complexion) {erythristic; also called *rufous*}
			erythron (the circulating erythrocytes in the blood)
			PREFIXED ROOT:
			anerythroplasia (*an* privative + *plassein* to form)
			anerythropoiesis (*an* privative + *poiein* to make, produce)
			dyserythropoiesis (defective development of erythrocytes) (*dys* abnormal + *poiein* to make, produce)

Element	From	Meaning	Examples
erythr (cont'd)		[red]	hypererythrocythemia (also called *polycythemia*) (*hyper* above + erythrocyte + *hemia* blood condition)
			intraerythrocytic (*intra* within + *kytos* cell)
			macroerythroblast (*makros* large + *blastos* germ)
			macroerythrocyte (*makros* large + *kytos* cell)
			microerythrocyte (*mikros* small + *kytos* cell)
			proerythroblast (also called *pronormoblast*) (*pro* before + *blastos* germ)
			proerythrocyte (*pro* before + *kytos* cell)
			protoerythrocyte (*protos* first + *kytos* cell)
			LEADING ROOT COMPOUND:
			erysi: erysipelas, erysipeloid (*pella* skin + *eidos* form)
			erythemo: erythemogenic (*genere* to produce)
			erythr:
			erythralgia (also called *erythromelalgia*) (*algos* pain)
			erythremia (polycythemia vera) (*emia* blood condition)
			erythrodontia (*odontia* tooth condition)
			erythroid (*eidos* form, likeness)
			erythropia (or, erythropsia) (*opia* vision condition)
			erythrosis (a reddish-purple discoloration of the skin and mucous membranes in polycythemia) (*osis* condition)
			erythruria (the passing of red urine) (*uria* urine condition)
			erythro:
			erythroblastoma (*blastos* germ + *oma* tumor)
			erythrocatalysis (phagocytosis of the red blood cells) (*katalysis* dissolution)
			erythrochromia (hemorrhagic pigmentation of the spinal fluid, giving it a red color) (*chromia* color condition)
			erythroclasis, erythroclast {erythroclastic} (*klasis* a breaking)
			erythrocuprein (also called *cytocuprein*) (*cuprum* copper)
			erythrocyanosis (*kyanos* the color blue + *osis* condition)
			erythrocyte (*kytos* cell)
			erythrodegenerative (*de* opposite + *genere* to produce)
			erythroderma (also called *erythrodermatitis*) (*dermia* skin condition)
			erythrogenesis {erythrogenic} (*genere* to produce)
			erythrokinetics (*kinein* to move)
			erythroleukemia (*leukos* white + *emia* blood condition)
			erythroleukosis (*leukos* white + *osis* condition)
			erythrolysis (also called *hemolysis*) (*lyein* to loosen)
			erythromelalgia (also called *erythermalgia*) (*melos* limb + *algos* pain)
			erythromelia (*melos* limb)
			erythrometer {erythrometry} (*metron* measure)
			erythromycin (*mykes* fungus)
			erythromyeloblastosis (*myelos* marrow + *blastos* germ, cell + *osis* condition)
			erythroneocytosis (*neos* new + *kytos* cell + *osis* condition)
			erythropenia (also called *erythrocytopenia*) (*penia* deficiency)
			erythrophagia, erythrophagocytosis (*phagein* to devour + *kytos* cell + *osis* condition)
			erythrophil {erythrophilous} (*philein* to love—have an affinity for)
			erythrophobia (*phobia* fear)
			erythrophore (*phorein* to bear)
			erythrophose (*phos* light)

Element	From	Meaning	Examples
erythr (cont'd)		[red]	erythroplakia (a red patch in the mouth, often a sign of oral cancer) (*plax* plate)
			erythroplasia (erythema and dysplasia of the epithelium) (*plassein* to form)
			erythropoiesis (the formation of red blood vessels; also called *erythrocytopoiesis, erythrogenesis*} {*erythropoietic*} (*poiein* to produce)
			erythroprosopalgia (a neuropathy characterized by redness and pain in the face) (*prosopon* face + *algos* pain)
			erythropyknosis (*pyknosis* density)
			erythrorrhexis (also called *erythrocytorrhexis*) (*rhexis* rupture)
			erythrostasis (*stasis* stoppage)
			TRAILING ROOT COMPOUND:
			photoerythema (erythema due to exposure to light) (*phos* light)
			ulerythema (*oule* scar)
			CROSS REFERENCE: rub(r)
eso-	Greek prefix	inward, inside	See Appendix B for examples of words with this prefix. Others are listed with the roots to which it is attached.
			CROSS REFERENCE: intra-
esophag	Greek *oisein* to carry + *phagema* food; from *phagein* to devour	alimentary canal	SIMPLE ROOT:
			esophagism (esophageal spasm causing dysphagia; also called *dysphagia nervosa, nervous dysphagia*)
			esophagus (the musculomembranous passage extending from the pharynx to the stomach; also called *gullet;* pl., esophagi) {*esophageal*}
			PREFIXED ROOT:
			esophageal:
			intraesophageal (*intra* within)
			juxtaesophageal (*juxta* near)
			paraesophageal (*para* alongside)
			periesophageal (*peri* around)
			postesophageal (*post* behind)
			retroesophageal (*retro* posterior)
			transesophageal (*trans* across)
			esophagus:
			megaesophagus (or, megalo-esophagus) (*megas* large)
			mesoesophagus (the transitory mesentery of the embryonic esophagus) (*mesos* middle)
			LEADING ROOT COMPOUND:
			esophag:
			esophagalgia (also called *esophagodynia*) (*algos* pain)
			esophagectasia (or, esophagectasis) (*ektasis* dilatation)
			esophagectomy (*ektome* excision)
			esophagitis (*itis* inflammation)
			esophagodynia (also called *esophagalgia*) (*odyne* pain)
			esophago:
			esophagobronchial (also called *bronchoesophageal*) (*bronchos* windpipe)
			esophagocardioplasty (*kardia* heart + *plassein* to form)
			esophagocardiomyotomy (*kardia* heart + *myos* muscle + *tomy* incision)
			esophagocele (*kele* hernia)
			esophagocologastrostomy (colon + *gaster* stomach + *stoma* opening)
			esophagocoloplasty (colon + *plassein* to form)
			esophagoduodenostomy (duodenum + *stoma* mouth, opening)

Element	From	Meaning	Examples
esophag (cont'd)		[alimentary canal]	esophagoenterostomy (*enteron* intestine + *stoma* mouth, opening) esophagoesophagostomy (*stoma* mouth, opening) esophagofundopexy (*fundus*—of the stomach + *pexis* fixation) esophagogram, esophagography (*graphein* to write) esophagology (*logos* study) esophagomalacia (*malakos* soft) esophagomycosis (*mykes* fungus + *osis* condition) esophagomyotomy (*myos* muscle + *tomy* incision) esophagoplasty (*plassein* to form) esophagoptosis (or, esophagoptosia) (*ptosis* prolapse; a falling) esophagoscope, esophagoscopy (*skopein* to examine) esophagospasm (*span* to contract) esophagostenosis (*stenosis* stricture) esophagostoma (or, esophagostomy) (*stoma* mouth, opening) esophagotome, esophagotomy (*tomy* incision) esophagotracheal (also called *tracheoesophageal*) (*trachea* windpipe) TRAILING ROOT COMPOUND: aortoesophageal (aorta) bronchoesophageal (*bronchos* windpipe) cardioesophageal (*kardia* heart) gastroesophageal, gastroesophagitis (*gaster* stomach + *itis* inflammation) pharyngoesophageal (*pharynx* the throat) pleuroesophageal (*pleura* rib, side) tracheoesophageal (also called *esophagotracheal*) (*trachea* windpipe) CROSS REFERENCE: None
esthes (also spelled **aesthes**)	Greek *aisthesis*	feeling, perception	SIMPLE ROOT: esthesia (or, aesthesia) {esthesic, or aesthesic; or, esthetic} esthete (or, aesthete), esthetic (or, aesthetic) PREFIXED ROOT: *esthecinesia*: anesthecinesia (combined sensory and motor paralysis) (*an* privative + *kinesis* movement) *esthesia*: alloesthesia (or, allesthesia; a referred pain or other sensation that is perceived at a remote site on the same or other side of the body that is remote from the point that was stimulated) (*allos* other) anacatesthesia (a hovering feeling or perception) (*ana* again + *kata* down) anesthesia (*an* privative) [see separate entry: anesthe-] cacesthesia (disordered sensibility) (*kakos* bad, abnormal) dysesthesia {dysesthetic} (*dys* abnormal, painful) hemianesthesia (*hemi* half + anesthesia) hemidysesthesia (*hemi* half + dysesthesia) hemihyperesthesia (*hemi* half + hyperesthesia) hemihypesthesia (or, hemihypoesthesia) (*hemi* half + hypesthesia) heteresthesia (*heteros* other, different) hyperesthesia {hyperesthetic} (*hyper* above) hypoesthesia (or, hypesthesia) {hypoesthetic} (*hypo* under) macroesthesia (a state in which objects seen or felt appear greatly magnified) (*makros* large) monoparesthesia (*monos* single + paresthesia) panesthesia {panesthetic} (*pan* all) paresthesia {paresthetic} (*para* abnormal)

Element	From	Meaning	Examples
esthes (cont'd)		[feeling]	polyesthesia (*polys* many)
			synesthesia (a sensation in one area from a stimulus applied in another area), synesthesialgia (*syn* with + *algos* pain)
			telesthesia (*tele* afar)
			LEADING ROOT COMPOUND:
			esthesi: esthesiodic (or, estheodic) (*hodos* way) [h of hodos elided]
			esthesio:
			esthesiogenesis {esthesiogenic} (*genere* to produce)
			esthesiography (*graphein* to write)
			esthesiology (*logos* study)
			esthesiometer, esthesiometry (*metron* measure)
			esthesioneuroblastoma (*neuron* nerve + blastoma)
			esthesioneurocytoma (*neuron* nerve + cytoma)
			esthesiophysiology (the physiology of sensation and the sense organs)
			esthesioscopy (*skopein* to examine)
			TRAILING ROOT COMPOUND:
			acanthesthesia (*akantha* thorn, sharp point)
			acmesthesia (sensitivity to pinprick; a cutaneous sensation of a sharp point) (*acme* point)
			acroesthesia (increased sensitiveness in the extremities), acroparesthesia (*akros* extremities + paresthesia)
			arthesthesia (joint sensibility; the perception of joint motions) (*arthron* joint)
			baresthesia (or, baryesthesia: pressure sense) (*baros* weight)
			baresthesiometer (*baros* weight + *metron* measure)
			bathyesthesia (or, bathesthesia; deep sensibility of deep structures of the body) (*bathys* deep)
			bathyhyperesthesia (*bathys* deep + *hyper* beyond)
			bathyhypesthesia (*bathys* deep + *hypo* below)
			bradyesthesia (*bradys* slow)
			caumesthesia (*kauma* burning)
			cenesthesia (also called *somatognosis*) (*koinos* common)
			cheirokinesthesia (*cheiros* hand + *kinein* to move)
			chromesthesia (a condition in which another sensation, such as taste or smell, is stimulated by the perception of color) (*chroma* color)
			cryesthesia (*kryos* cold)
			cryptesthesia (also called *clairvoyance*) (*kryptos* hidden)
			gargalesthesia (*gargalos* itching)
			graphesthesia (*graphein* to write)
			kinesthesia (movement sense) {kinesthetic} (*kinein* to move)
			myoesthesia (also called *kinesthetic sense*) (*myos* muscle)
			osmesthesia (*osme* smell, odor)
			piesesthesia (*piesis* pressure)
			pseudoesthesia (also called *paraphia, phantom limb*) (*pseudes* false)
			psychroesthesia (*psychros* cold)
			somesthesia (also called *somatognosis*) (*soma* body)
			splanchnesthesia (*splanchnos* viscus)
			strangalesthesia (also called *zonesthesia*) (*strangalizein* to choke, strangle)
			thermoesthesia (*therme* heat)
			topesthesia (*topos* place)
			trichoesthesia (*trichos* hair)
			zonesthesia (*zona* girdle: encircling region)

Element	From	Meaning	Examples
esthes (cont'd)		[feeling]	PREFIXED TRAILING ROOT COMPOUND: acenesthesia (*a* privative + *koinos* common) akinesthesia (*a* privative + *kinein* to move) amyoesthesia (*a* privative + *myos* muscle) apallesthesia (*a* privative + *pallein* to tremble) aphotesthesia (*a* privative + *photos* light) CROSS REFERENCE: path, sens
ethm	Greek *ethein* to strain; *ethmos* sieve	sieve, strainer	PREFIXED ROOT: ectethmoid (also called *ethmoidal labyrinth*) (*ektos* outside) esoethmoiditis (also called *ethmoid sinusitis*) (*eso* within + *itis* inflammation) transethmoidal (*trans* across) LEADING ROOT COMPOUND: *ethm*: ethmoid {ethmoidal: of or pertaining to the ethmoid bone, the sievelike bone that forms a roof for the nasal fossae and part of the floor of the anterior fossa of the skull} (*eidos* form) *ethmo*: ethmocephalus (*kephale* head) ethmocranial (*kranion* skull) ethmofrontal (pertaining to the ethmoid and frontal bones) ethmolacrimal (*lacrima* teardrop) ethmomaxillary (*maxilla* upper jaw) ethmonasal (*nas* nose) ethmopalatal (*palate* roof of mouth) ethmosphenoid (pertaining to the ethmoid and sphenoid bones) ethmoturbinal (pertaining to the superior and middle nasal conchae) ethmovomerine (relating to the ethmoid bone and the vomer) (*vomer* plowshare) [vomer: a flat trapezoid bone forming the inferior and posterior portion of the nasal septum] *ethmoid* similar to a sieve: ethmoidectomy (removal of all or part of the mucosal lining and bony partitions between the ethmoid tissues) (*ektome* excision) ethmoiditis (*itis* inflammation) *ethmoido*: ethmoidotomy (*tomy* incision) TRAILING ROOT COMPOUND: sphenoethmoid (*sphenos* wedge) CROSS REFERENCE: for, tres
eu-	Greek prefix	well	See Appendix B for examples of words with this prefix. Others are listed with the roots to which it is attached. CROSS REFERENCE: None
eury	Greek *eurynein* to widen, to stretch	broad, wide	SIMPLE ROOT: euryon (the point at either end of the greatest transverse diameter of the skull) PREFIXED ROOT: aneurysm (a widening; localized abnormal dilation of a blood vessel) {aneurysmal} (*ana* up) [see separate entry: aneurys-] LEADING ROOT COMPOUND: euryblepharon (*blepharon* eyelid) eurycephalic (or, eurycephalous; broad-headed) (*kephale* head) eurycranial (also called *eurycephalic*) (*kranion* skull) eurygnathism (broad-jawed) {eurygnathic, eurygnathous} (*gnathos* jaw) euryopia (abnormally wide opening of the eyes) {euryopic} (*opia* vision condition) eurysomatic (*somatos* body) eurythermal {eurythermic} (*therme* heat)

Element	From	Meaning	Examples
eury (cont'd)		[broad, wide]	TRAILING ROOT COMPOUND: *eurysis*: colpeurysis (operative dilatation of the vagina) (*kolpos* vagina) hystereurysis (dilation of the ostium uteri) (*hystera* uterus) [ostium uteri: the external opening of the uteri cervix into the vagina] *eurynter*: metreurynter (an inflatable bag for dilating the cervical canal of the uterus) (*metra* uterus) procteurynter (a baglike device used in dilating the rectum) (*proktos* rectum, anus) CROSS REFERENCE: platy, later
ex-	Latin prefix	out, away, from	See Appendix B for examples of words with this prefix. Others are listed with the root to which it is attached. CROSS REFERENCE: ab-, de-, dis-
exo-	Gree prefix	outside, outer	EXTENDED PREFIX: exoteric (of external origin) See Appendix B for examples of words with this prefix. Others are listed with the root to which it is attached. CROSS REFERENCE: extero-
extero-	Latin prefix	on the outside	EXTENDED PREFIX: exterior, extern, external See Appendix B for examples of words with this prefix. Others are listed with the root to which it is attached. CROSS REFERENCE: exo-
extra- **extro-**	Latin prefix	beyond	EXTENDED PREFIX: extraneous (outside the organism and not belonging to it), extreme {extremital}, extremity See Appendix B for examples of words with this prefix. Others are listed with the root to which it is attached. CROSS REFERENCE: meta-, super-

A Thesaurus of Medical Word Roots

$\mathcal{F}$

Element	From	Meaning	Examples
fac, **fec,** **fic,** **fy**	Latin *facere*	to make, do, cause	TRAILING ROOT COMPOUND: *facient:* abortifacient (causing abortion; also called *abortient*) absorbefacient (also called *sorbefacient*) (absorb) algefacient (*algos* cold) calefacient, calorifacient (*calor* heat) chylifacient (*chylus* gastric juice) delirifacient (delirium) dormifacient (*dormire* to sleep) febrifacient (*febris* fever) hemafacient (also called *hematopoietic*) (*haima* blood) immunifacient (*immunis* exempt, immune) liquefacient (*liquere* to flow) motofacient (*movere* to move) parturifacient (inducing or facilitating childbirth; an agent that in- duces or facilitates childbirth) (*parere* to bear young) putrifacient (causing or promoting bacterial putrefaction) (*putrere* to rot) rubefacient (*ruber* red) sanguifacient (also called *hematopoietic*) (*sanguis* blood) somnifacient (*somnus* sleep) stupefacient (*stupere* to be dazed) tumefacient (*tumere* to swell) *faction:* liquefaction {liquefactive} (*liquere* to flow) putrefaction {putrefactive} (*putrere* to rot) tumefaction (*tumere* to swell) *fic:* acidific (acid) dolorific (*dolor* pain) febrific (*febris* fever) morbific (disease-causing; also called *pathogenic*) (*morbus* sickness) prolific (fruitful; reproductive) (*proles* offspring) somnific (also called *hypnotic*) (*somnus* sleep) soporific (*sopor* deep sleep) sudorific (*sudor* perspiration, sweat) *fication:* amelification (Middle English *amel* enamel) ammonification (ammonia) apexification (apex—of a tooth) calcification (calcium) cementification (also called *cementogenesis*) (*cementum*—of a tooth) chondrification (*chondros* cartilage) chymification (*chymos* juice) cornification (conversion into keratin, or horn) (*cornu* horn) dentification (*dens* tooth) detoxification (*de* reversal + *toxikon* poison) etherification (*aither* upper and purer air) gelatification (*gelare* to freeze, set) hornification (also called *cornification*)

Element	From	Meaning	Examples
fac (cont'd)		[to make, do]	mortification (gangrene or sphacelus; molar death) (*mors* death) opsonification (opsonin) ossification (*os* bone) purification (pure) sanguification (also called *hemopoiesis*) (*sanguis* blood) tabification (*tabescere* to waste away) *fice*: orifice (any foramen, meatus, or opening) (*os* mouth) *fy*: acetify (*acetum* vinegar) acidify (acid) calcify (calcium) chondrify (*chondros* cartilage) clarify (*clarus* clear) putrefy (*putrere* to rot) CROSS REFERENCE: gen, par, poie
faci, **fic**	Latin *facies*	face, surface of a body structure	SIMPLE ROOT: face {facial}, facet, facies (pl., also, facies) LEADING ROOT COMPOUND: *facet*: facetectomy (*ektome* excision) *facial*: facialplasty (also called *rhytidectomy, facelift*) (*plassein* to form) *facio*: faciobrachial (*brachium* upper arm) faciocephalalgia (*kephale* head + *algos* pain) faciocervical (*cervix* neck) faciodigitogenital (pertaining to or affecting the face, digits, and genitalia) faciolingual (*lingua* tongue) facioplasty (plastic surgery on the face) (*plassein* to form) facioplegia (facial paralysis) (*plessein* to strike) facioscapulohumeral (pertaining to the face, scapula, and arm) faciostenosis (failure of the midface to grow) (*stenosis* narrow) TRAILING ROOT COMPOUND: basifacial (pertaining to the inferior part of the face) (base) brachyfacial (also called *brachyprosopic*) (*brachys* short) cervicofacial (*cervix* neck) craniofacial (*kranion* skull) dentofacial (*dens* tooth) dolichofacial (also called *dolichoprosopic*) (*dolichos* long) genufacial (genufacial position: a position in which the patient is supported on the knees and face) (*genu* knee) linguofacial (*lingua* tongue) mandibulofacial (*mandible* lower jaw) maxillofacial (*maxilla* upper jaw) occipitofacial (*occiput* back of the head) oculofacial (*oculus* eye) orodigitofacial (*oris* mouth + *digit* finger) temporofacial (temple) zygomaticofacial (zygon yoke: zygomatic process) CROSS REFERENCE: opo, prosop
fasci	Latin *fascia*	band, fillet	SIMPLE ROOT: fascia (pl., fasciae, fascias) {fascial}, fascicle, fascicular, fasciculate (or, fasciculated), fasciculation, fasciculus (pl., fasciculi) fasciola (a small band or striplike structure; pl., fasciolae) {fasciolar}

Element	From	Meaning	Examples
fasci (cont'd)		[band, fillet]	PREFIXED ROOT: *fascial*: epifascial (*epi* upon) subfascial (*sub* below) *fascicular*: bifasicular (*bi* two) interfascicular (*inter* between) intrafascicular (*intra* within) perifascicular (*peri* around) LEADING ROOT COMPOUND: *fasci*: fasciectomy (*ektome* excision) fasciitis (or, fascitis) (*itis* inflammation) fasciosis (*osis* condition) *fascio*: fasciodesis (*dein* to bind, attach) fascioplasty (*plassein* to form) fasciorrhaphy (*rhaphein* to suture) fasciotomy (*tomy* incision) *fasciol*: fascioliasis (*iasis* condition; infection) fasciolopsiasis (*opsis* appearance + *iasis* condition) fasciorrhaphy (*rhaphe* suture) fasciotomy (*tomy* incision) TRAILING ROOT COMPOUND: myofascial, myofascitis (*myos* muscle + *itis* inflammation) CROSS REFERENCE: desm, lig, syndes
femor, **femur**	Latin *femur, femoris*	thigh bone	SIMPLE ROOT: femoral (pertaining to the thigh, or to the femur) femur (the thigh bone; pl., femora) PREFIXED ROOT: interfemoral (*inter* between) transfemoral (*trans* across) LEADING ROOT COMPOUND: femorocele (*kele* hernia) femorofemoral (pertaining to both the right and left femoral arteries) femoroiliac (ilium) femorotibial (tibia) TRAILING ROOT COMPOUND: aortofemoral (aorta) axillofemoral (axillary: pertaining to the armpit) coxofemoral (*coxa* hip) femorofemoral (pertaining to both the right and left femoral arteries) genitofemoral (also called *genitocrural*) (genitals) gluteofemoral (*gloutos* buttock) iliofemoral (ilium) ischiofemoral (ischium) patellofemoral (patella—kneecap) pelvifemoral (pelvis) pubofemoral (os pubis: pubic bone) saphenofemoral (*saphena* a type of vein) tibiofemoral (tibia) vertebrofemoral (vertebra) CROSS REFERENCE: None

Element	From	Meaning	Examples

fer	Latin
	ferre
	to bear;
	latus
	borne
		to bear, carry,
		produce
			SIMPLE ROOT: fertile, fertility, fertilization
			TRAILING ROOT COMPOUND:
			ferate: proliferate (to grow by the reproduction of similar cells)
			    (*proles* offspring)
			ferous:
			acidiferous (acid)
			aeriferous (conveying air) (*aer* air)
			albuminiferous (albumin)
			calciferous (calcium)
			chyliferous (forming or conveying chyle) (*chylus* gastric juice)
			costiferous (bearing a rib, as the thoracic vertebrae of man) (*costa* rib,
			    side)
			cystiferous (also called *cystigerous*) (*kystis* sac)
			lactiferous (*lac* milk)
			lipoferous (carrying fat) (*lipos* fat)
			melaniferous (*melanos* black, dark)
			odoriferous (*odor* smell)
			ossiferous (*ossis* bone)
			oviferous (*ovum* egg)
			proliferous (or, proliferative) (*proles* offspring)
			sanguiferous (also called *circulatory*) (*sanguis* blood)
			somniferous (*somnus* sleep)
			soporiferous (*sopor* deep sleep)
			sporiferous (*sporos* seed)
			sudoriferous (*sudor* perspiration, sweat)
			toxiferous (also called *toxicogenic*) (*toxikon* poison)
			TERM: referred pain (pain felt in a part removed from its point of
			    origin; also called *synalgia*) (*re* back)
			CROSS REFERENCE: gen, ger[1], phor, poie

ferr	Latin
	ferrum
		iron	SIMPLE ROOT: ferric, ferrous, ferrugination, ferruginous (contain-
			    ing iron or iron rust; of the color of iron rust)
			PREFIXED ROOT:
			ferremia condition of iron in the blood:
			hyperferremia {hyperferremic} (*hyper* above)
			hypoferremia {hypoferremic} (*hypo* under)
			LEADING ROOT COMPOUND:
			ferri: ferri-albuminic (containing iron and albumin)
			ferro:
			ferroflocculation (a flocculation test for malaria, performed with a
			    fine-grained antigen) (*floccus* flock of wool)
			ferrokinetics {ferrokinetic} (*kinein* to move)
			ferroproteins [proteins containing iron in a prosthetic group, e.g.,
			    heme (short for *hematin*), cytochromes] (protein)
			ferrotherapy (*therapy* treatment)
			TRAILING ROOT COMPOUND: organoferric (containing iron and
			    some organic compound)
			CROSS REFERENCE: sider

fibr, **fiber**	Latin *fibra*	fiber	SIMPLE ROOT: *fiber*: fiber (an elongated, threadlike structure) *fibr*: fibrate, fibrates (also called *fibric acids*) fibrose, fibrous *fibra*: fibra (pl., fibrae) *fibril*: fibril, fibrilla (pl., fibrillae), fibrillar (or, fibrillary), fibrillate, fibrillated, fibrillation *fibrin*: fibrin {fibrinous}

A Thesaurus of Medical Word Roots

Element	From	Meaning	Examples
fibr (cont'd)		[fiber]	PREFIXED ROOT: *fibril*: microfibril (*mikros* small) protofibril (*protos* first) *fibrill*: afibrillar (not containing fibrils) (*a* negative) antifibrillatory (*anti* against) defibrillation, defibrillator (termination of atrial or ventricular fibrillation, usually by electroshock) (*de* negative) interfibrillar (or, interfibrillary) (*inter* between) *fibrino*: antifibrinolysin {antifibrinolytic} (*anti* against + *lyein* to loosen) hyperfibrinogenemia (also called *fibrinogenemia*) (*hyper* above + *genere* to produce + *emia* blood condition) hypofibrinogenemia (*hypo* under + *genere* to produce + *emia* blood condition hyperfibrinolysis (*hyper* above + *lyein* to dissolve) *fibrotic*: antifibrotic (inhibiting fibrosis) (*anti* against) *fibrous*: interfibrous (*inter* between) LEADING ROOT COMPOUND: *fiber*: fiberoptics {fiberoptic} (*optikos* optical) fiberscope (also called *flexible endoscope*) (*skopein* to examine) *fibr*: fibroid, fibroidectomy (*eidos* form + *ektome* excision) fibroma (also called *fibroid, fibroid tumor*) {fibromatous} (*oma* tumor) fibrosis {fibrotic}, fibrositis (*osis* condition + *itis* inflammation) *fibrillo*: fibrilloblast (also called *odontoblast*) (*blastos* bud, germ) fibrillogenesis (*genere* to produce) fibrillolysis {fibrillolytic} (*lyein* to loosen) *fibrin*: fibrinoid (*eidos* form) fibrinuria (*uria* urine condition) *fibrino*: fibrinocellular fibrinogenesis (*genere* to produce) fibrinolysis {fibrinolytic} (*lyein* to loosen) fibrinopurulent (*puris* pus) fibrinorrhea (*rhein* to flow) fibrinoscopy (also called *inoscopy*) (*skopein* to examine) *fibro*: fibroadenoma (*aden* gland + *oma* tumor) fibroadipose (*adeps* fat + *ose* condition) fibroangioma (*angeion* blood vessel + *oma* tumor) fibroareolar (*areola* small space) fibroatrophy (atrophy: *a* negative + *trophein* to nourish) fibroblast {fibroblastic}, fibroblastoma (*blastos* bud + *oma* tumor) fibrobronchitis (also called *fibrinous bronchitis*) (*bronchos* windpipe + *itis* inflammation) fibrocalcific (calculus + *facere* to make) fibrocarcinoma (also called *scirrhous carcinoma*) (*karkinos* crab, cancer + *oma* tumor)

Element	From	Meaning	Examples
fibr (cont'd)		[fiber]	fibrocartilage {fibrocartilaginous}
			fibrocaseous (*caseus* cheese)
			fibrocellular
			fibrochondritis (*chondros* cartilage + *itis* inflammation)
			fibrochondroma (also called *chondrofibroma*) (*chondros* cartilage + *oma* tumor)
			fibrocollagenous (*kolla* glue + *genere* to produce)
			fibrocystic, fibrocystoma (*kystis* sac, bladder + *oma* tumor)
			fibrocyte, fibrocytogenesis (*kytos* cell + *genere* produce)
			fibrodysplasia (*dys* abnormal + *plassein* to form)
			fibroelastic, fibroelastoma (elastic + *oma* tumor)
			fibroenchondroma (*enchondroma* overgrowth of cartilage)
			fibroepithelioma (epithelium + *oma* tumor)
			fibrofolliculoma (follicle + *oma* tumor)
			fibrogenesis {fibrogenic} (*genere* to produce)
			fibroglia, fibrogliosis (*glia* glue + *osis* condition)
			fibrokeratoma (*keras* horn + *oma* tumor)
			fibrolamellar (*lamina* layer, plate)
			fibrolipoma {fibrolipomatous} (*lipos* fat + *oma* tumor)
			fibromembranous (*membrane* a thin skin)
			fibrometer (*metron* measure)
			fibromuscular (muscle)
			fibromyalgia (*myos* muscle + *algos* pain)
			fibromyxoma (also called *myxofibroma*) (*myxa* mucus + *oma* tumor)
			fibronectin (*nectere* to bind)
			fibroneuroma (also called *neurofibroma*) (*neuron* nerve + *oma* tumor)
			fibronuclear (made up of nucleated fibers)
			fibro-odontoma (*odontos* tooth + *oma* tumor)
			fibro-osseous (*osse* bone)
			fibro-osteoma (also called *ossifying fibroma*) (*osteon* bone + *oma* tumor)
			fibropapilloma (*papilla* nipple; from *papula* pimple + *oma* tumor)
			fibroplasia {fibroplastic} (*plassein* to form)
			fibropurulent (*puris* pus)
			fibroreticulate (*rete* network)
			fibrosarcoma (*sarkos* flesh + *oma* tumor)
			fibrosclerosis (*sklerosis* hardening)
			fibroserous (serum)
			fibrothorax (*thorax* chest)
			fibrovascular (*vas* vessel)
			fibroxanthoma (*xanthos* yellow + *oma* tumor)
			fibrom: fibromectomy (*oma* tumor + *ektome* excision)
			fibromat fibrous tumor:
			fibromatoid (*eidos* form)
			fibromatosis (*osis* condition)
			fibromato: fibromatogenic (*oma* tumor + *genere* to produce)
			TRAILING ROOT COMPOUND:
			fibril:
			myofibril (*myos* muscle)
			neurofibril (*neuron* nerve)
			tonofibril (*tonos* tone)
			fibro:
			myofibroblastoma (*myos* muscle + blastoma)

Element	From	Meaning	Examples
fibr (cont'd)		[fiber]	myofibroblastosis (*myos* muscle + blastosis)
			fibroma fibrous tumor:
			adenofibroma (*adenos* gland)
			angiofibroma (*angeion* blood vessel)
			chondrofibroma (*chondros* cartilage)
			cystofibroma (*kystis* sac, bladder)
			dermatofibroma (*dermatos* skin)
			elastofibroma (*elastos* ductile)
			epulofibroma (*epulis* gumboil)
			ganglioneurofibroma (ganglion + *neuron* nerve)
			lipofibroma (*lipos* fat)
			metrofibroma (*metra* uterus)
			myofibroma (*myos* muscle)
			myxofibroma (*myxa* mucus)
			neurofibroma (*neuron* nerve)
			osteofibroma (*osteon* bone)
			fibrosis fiber condition:
			adenofibrosis (*adenos* gland)
			angiofibrosis (*angeion* blood vessel)
			coniofibrosis (*konis* dust)
			myelofibrosis (*myelos* marrow)
			myofibrosis (*myos* muscle)
			osteofibrosis (*osteon* bone)
			phlebofibrosis (*phlebos* vein)
			siderofibrosis (*sideros* iron)
			venofibrosis (*vena* vein)
			fibrositis: myofibrositis (*myos* muscle + *itis* inflammation)
			fibrous:
			cellulofibrous (cellular)
			mucofibrous (mucus)
			osseofibrous (*os* bone)
			CROSS REFERENCE: in
fil	Latin *filum*	thread, filament	SIMPLE ROOT:
			filaceous (composed of filaments or threadlike structures)
			filament (a delicate fiber or thread) {filaceous}
			filamentous (composed of long, threadlike structures: said of bacterial colonies; also called *filar*)
			filamentum (pl., filamenta)
			filar (also called *filaceous, filamentous*), filaria (pl., filariae)
			filum (a threadlike structure or part; pl., fila)
			PREFIXED ROOT:
			filament:
			interfilamentous (*inter* between)
			microfilament (*mikros* small)
			monofilament (*monos* single)
			protofilament (*protos* first)
			filar:
			interfilar (*inter* between)
			intrafilar (*intra* within)
			LEADING ROOT COMPOUND:
			fili: filiform (threadlike; resembling filariae) (*forma* shape)
			filo:
			filopodium (pl., filopodia) (*pous* foot)
			filopressure (*premere* to press)

Element	From	Meaning	Examples
fil (cont'd)		[thread]	filovaricosis (*varix* dilated vein + *osis* condition) TRAILING ROOT COMPOUND: cytofilaments (*kytos* cell) myofilaments (*myos* muscle) neurofilament (*neuron* nerve) nucleofilaments (filamentary forms of chromosome) tonofilament (*tonos* tone, tension) CROSS REFERENCE: mit, nema
fistul	Latin *fistula* pipe, tube	tubelike passage	SIMPLE ROOT: fistula (an abnormal tubelike passage from a normal cavity or tube to a free surface or to another cavity; pl., fistulae, fistulas) {fistulous}, fistulation (or, fistulization) PREFIXED ROOT: intrafistular {intrafistularal; situated within a fissure, as of the brain) (*intra* within) perifistular (*peri* around) LEADING ROOT COMPOUND: *fistul*: fistulectomy (or, fistulotomy) (*ektome* excision) *fistula*: fistulatome (*tome* a cutting instrument) *fistulo*: fistuloenterostomy (*enteron* intestine + *stoma* mouth, opening) fistulography (*graphein* to write) TRAILING ROOT COMPOUND: tracheofistulization (creation of an opening in the trachea communicating with the cervical skin) (*trachea* windpipe) CROSS REFERENCE: salping, syring, tub[1]
fix	Latin *figere*	to fasten, attach	SIMPLE ROOT: fixation (the act of holding or fastening in a fixed position; immobilizing; making rigid), fixative (a substance used to make firm or rigid) PREFIXED ROOT: transfix (to pierce through with a sharp instrument), transfixion (an amputation maneuver) (*trans* through) TRAILING ROOT COMPOUND: colofixation (colon) pelvifixation (pelvis) uterofixation (also called *hysteropexy*) (uterus) vaginofixation (vagina) ventrofixation (also called *ventrosuspension*) (*venter* belly) vesicofixation (*vesica* bladder) CROSS REFERENCE: pact, pex
foll	Latin *follis* bellows	excretory or secretory sac or gland	SIMPLE ROOT: follicle {follicular}, folliculus (pl., folliculi) PREFIXED ROOT: interfollicular (*inter* between) intrafollicular (*intra* within) macrofollicular (*makros* large) parafollicular (*para* alongside) perifollicular (*peri* around) LEADING ROOT COMPOUND: folliculitis (*itis* inflammation) folliculoma (*oma* tumor) folliculosis (*osis* condition) TRAILING ROOT COMPOUND: angiofollicular (*angeion* blood vessel) fibrofolliculoma (fiber + *oma* tumor) trichofolliculoma (*trichos* hair + *oma* tumor) CROSS REFERENCE: None

Element	From	Meaning	Examples
for	Latin *forare* to bore	natural opening; passage	SIMPLE ROOT: foramen (a natural opening or passage, especially one into or through a bone; pl., foramina) foraminulum (a minute foramen) PREFIXED ROOT: biforate (having two foramina or openings) (*bi* two) biperforate (having two perforations) (*bi* two) imperforate (*im* negative + perforate) perforans (penetrating; perforating; a term applied to various muscles, nerves, arteries, and veins that perforate other structures) perforated (pierced with holes), perforation (the act of boring or piercing through a part; a hole made through a part or substance), perforator (*per* through) uniforate (having only one opening) (*uni* one) LEADING ROOT COMPOUND: foraminiferous (having foramina) (*ferre* to bear) foraminotomy (the operation of removing the roof of intervertebral foramina, done for the relief of nerve root oppression) (*tomy* incision) CROSS REFERENCE: or, pyl, stoma, tres
form	Latin *forma*	form, shape	SIMPLE ROOT: formatio (pl., formationes), formation, formative, formula (pl., formulas, or formulae), formulary TRAILING ROOT COMPOUND: (Examples of) aciniform (*acinus* grape; saclike dilatation) acneform (or, acneiform; resembling acne) adeniform (*adenos* gland) amebiform (ameba) bacilliform (shaped like bacteria; rodlike) baculiform (*baculum* a rod) cancriform (cancer) cartilaginiform (also called *chondroid*) (cartilage) cerebriform (cerebrum) chancriform (chancre) coliform (*colum* sieve) cordiform (*cordis* heart) cribriform (also called *cribrate, polyporous*) (*cribrum* sieve) cystiform (*kystis* sac, bladder) dentiform (*dens* tooth) gangliform (ganglion) lentiform (*lentis* pea) ossiform (*os* bone) pisiform (*pisum* pea) somatoform (*somatos* body) vermiform (*vermis* worm) CROSS REFERENCE: eid, ide, morph, oid, plas
fron	Latin *frons, frontis*	forehead, front	SIMPLE ROOT: frons (the region of the face above the eyes) frontad (toward a frontal aspect) frontal (pertaining to the forehead) frontalis (designates a relationship to the frontal or coronal plane) PREFIXED ROOT: confrontation (*com* with) hypofrontality (*hypo* under) interfrontal (*inter* between)

Element	From	Meaning	Examples
fron (cont'd)		[forehead, front]	medifrontal (*medius* middle)
			prefrontal (situated in the anterior part of the frontal lobe or region; the central part of the ethmoid bone) (*pre* before)
			subfrontal (*sub* under)
			transfrontal (*trans* across)
			LEADING ROOT COMPOUND:
			fronti: frontipetal (directed to the front) (*petere* to seek)
			fronto:
			frontomaxillary (*maxilla* upper jaw)
			frontonasal (*nasus* nose)
			frontooccipital (*occiput* back of head)
			frontoparietal (pertaining to the frontal and parietal bones)
			frontotemporal (pertaining to the frontal and temporal bones)
			frontozygomatic (also called *zygomaticofrontal*) (*zygon* yoke)
			TRAILING ROOT COMPOUND:
			ethmofrontal (*ethmos* sieve)
			nasofrontal (*nasus* nose)
			occipitofrontal (*occiput* back of head: *ob* against + *caput* head)
			parietofrontal (*paries* wall)
			sphenofrontal (*sphenos* wedge)
			squamofrontal (*squama* scale, plate)
			temporofrontal (temple)
			zygomaticofrontal (also called *frontozygomatic*) (*zygon* yoke: zygomatic process)
			CROSS REFERENCE: None
fund, **fus**	Latin *fundere*	to pour	SIMPLE ROOT: fusion (meeting and joining together through liquefaction by heat)
			PREFIXED ROOT:
			fund: infundibulum (any of various funnel-shaped organs or passages, as the extension of the third ventricle of the brain to the pituitary gland; the calyx of a kidney; or the ovarian end of a fallopian tube; also called *choana*) (*in* in)
			fus: diffusate (to pour in different directions; also called *dialysate*) (*dis* away)
			fusate: perfusate (the fluid used for perfusion) (*per* through)
			fuse:
			diffuse {diffusible}, diffusion (*dis* apart, away)
			effuse (spread out; profuse), effusion (*ex* out)
			superfuse (to flush a liquid over the top of a tissue) (*super* above)
			fusible: infusible (incapable of being melted) (*in* negative)
			fusion:
			autoreinfusion (*autos* self + reinfusion)
			autotransfusion (*autos* self + transfusion)
			infusion (the steeping of a substance in water for obtaining its proximate principles; the therapeutic introduction of a fluid other than blood, as a saline solution, into a vein; not to be confused with *injection, instillation,* or *insufflation*) (*in* in)
			microtransfusion (*mikros* small + transfusion)
			perfusion (the act of pouring over or through, especially the passage of a fluid through the vessels of a specific organ or body part), perfusionist (*per* through)
			transfusion (the introduction of whole blood, plasma substitutes, or other solution directly into the blood stream) (*trans* through)
			CROSS REFERENCE: chem, chys

Element	From	Meaning	Examples
funi	Latin *funis*	cord, rope (umbilical cord)	SIMPLE ROOT: funicle, funiculus (pl., funiculi) {funicular} funis (any cordlike structure; also called *umbilical cord*) {funic} LEADING ROOT COMPOUND: *funi:* funiform (*forma* shape) funipuncture (also called *cordocentesis*) (*pungere* to pierce) *funicul:* funiculitis (*itis* inflammation) *funis:* funisitis (*itis* inflammation) *funiculo:* funiculoepididymitis (inflammation of the spermatic cord and the epididymis) (*itis* inflammation) funiculopexy (*pexis* fixation) CROSS REFERENCE: chord
fus			See fund for *infusible*.

G

Element	From	Meaning	Examples
galact, **gala**, **galo**	Greek *gala, galaktos*	milk	SIMPLE ROOT: galactic (also called *lactic*), galactose PREFIXED ROOT: *galactia*: agalactia (absence of milk secretion after childbirth; also called *agalactosis*) {agalactous} (*a* privative) dysgalactia (*dys* abnormal) hypergalactia (also called *polygalactia*) {hypergalactous} (*hyper* above) hypogalactia {hypogalactous} (*hypo* under) polygalactia (also called *hypergalactia*) (*polys* much) *galactic*: antigalactic (also called *lactifuge*), antigalactagogue (*anti* against + *agein* to lead) *galactorrhea*: agalactorrhea (*a* privative + *rhein* to flow) *galactosis*: hypergalactosis (*hyper* above + *osis* condition) LEADING ROOT COMPOUND: *galact*: galactacrasia (or, galactocrasia; abnormal composition of breast milk) (*a* negative + *krasis* a mixing) galactagogue (or, galactogogue) (*agein* to lead) galactemia (*emia* blood condition) galactidrosis (*hidros* sweat + *osis* condition) [h of hidros elided] galactischia (also called *galactoschesis*) (*ischein* to suppress) galactoma (also called *galactocele*) (*oma* tumor) galactosis (*osis* condition) *galacto*: galactoblast (also called *colostrum corpuscle*) (*blastos* germ) galactocele (also called *lactocele*) (*kele* tumor) galactocrasia (or, galactacrasia) (*krasis* a mixing) galactogen {galactogenous} (*genere* to produce) galactogogue (or, galactagogue) (*agein* to lead) galactography (*graphein* to write) galactometer (*metron* measure) galactopexy {galactopexic} (*pexis* fixation) galactophagous (subsisting or feeding on milk; also called *lactivorous*) (*phagein* to consume) galactophlebitis (*phlebos* vein + *itis* inflammation) galactophlysis (*phlysis* eruption) galactophore {galactophorous; also called *lactiferous*}, galactophoritis (*pherein* to carry + *itis* inflammation) galactophygous (arresting the milk secretion) (*phyge* flight) galactoplania (*planan* to wander) galactopoiesis (also called *lactogenic*) (*poiesis* production) galactopyra (also called *milk fever*) (*pyr* fire, fever) galactorrhea (*rhein* to flow) galactoschesis (also called *galactischia*) (*schesis* suppression) galactoscope (also called *lactoscope*) (*skopein* to examine) galactostasia (or, galactostasis) (*stasis* stoppage) galactotoxin, galactotoxism (*toxin* poison) galactotrophy (*trophein* to nourish)

Element	From	Meaning	Examples
galact (cont'd)		[milk]	*galactos*: galactosemia (*emia* blood condition) galactosuria (*uria* urine condition) TRAILING ROOT COMPOUND: androgalactozemia (*andros* man + *zemia* loss) neogala (the first milk developed after childbirth) (*neos* new) oligogalactia (*oligos* little, scant) phygogalactic (also called *lactifuge*) (*phyge* flight) CROSS REFERENCE: lact
gam	Greek *gamos,* *gametes*	marriage; joined, united; sexual reproduction	SIMPLE ROOT: gamete (a mature male or female reproductive cell; the spermatozoon or ovum respectively) {gametic}, gamic, ga-mone (a hypothetical substance uniting the ovum and sperm) PREFIXED ROOT: *gamete*: agamete (any asexual unicellular organism) (*a* privative) anisogamete {anisogametic} (*aniso* unequal) heterogamete {heterogametic} (*heteros* other) homogamete {homogametic} (*homos* same) isogamete {isogametic} (*isos* equal) macrogamete (also called *megagamete*) (*makros* large) megagamete (also called *macrogamete*) (*megas* large) microgamete (*mikros* small) *gametic*: digametic (also called *heterogametic*) (*di* two) monogametic (*monos* single) *gametocyte* reproduction cell: macrogametocyte (*makros* large) microgametocyte (*mikros* small) *gamia*: apogamia (or, apogamy; unisexual reproduction; also called *parthenogenesis*) (*apo* from) *gamic*: agamic (reproducing asexually; asexual) (*a* negative) *gamo*: agamogenesis (also called *agamogony, schizogony*) {agamogenetic} (*a* negative + *genere* to produce) agamogony (also called *schizogony*) (*a* negative + *gonos* offspring) *gamont*: macrogamont (also called *macrogametocyte*) (*makros* large) microgamont (also called *microgametocyte*) (*mikros* small) *gamous*: agamous (also called *asexual*) (*a* privative) allogamous (*allos* other) anisogamous (*aniso* unequal; *an* negative + *isos* equal) autogamous (*autos* self) endogamous (*endon* within) heterogamous (*heteros* other) isogamous (*isos* equal) polygamous (*polys* many) progamous (previous to fertilization of the ovum) (*pro* before) *gamy*: allogamy (cross-fertilization) (*allos* other) aneugamy (lit., not well married; resulting in an abnormal number of chromosomes in the gamete) (*an* negative + *eugamy*) anisogamy (*aniso* unequal; *an* negative + *isos* equal) apogamy {apogamic} (*apo* away)

Element	From	Meaning	Examples
gam (cont'd)		[reproduction]	autogamy (self-fertilization) (*autos* self)
			endogamy (*endon* within)
			eugamy (the union of gametes, each of which contains the proper complement of chromosomes) (*eu* well)
			exogamy (*exo* outside)
			heterogamy (*heteros* other)
			hologamy (*holos* entire, whole)
			homogamy (*homos* same)
			isogamy (*isos* equal)
			macrogamy (*makros* large)
			microgamy (also called *merogamy*) (*mikros* small)
			monogamy (*monos* single)
			polygamy (*polys* many)
			syngamy (sexual reproduction; cell union as of gametes in fertilization) {syngamous} (*syn* with)
			LEADING ROOT COMPOUND:
			gam: gamont (also called *gametocyte*) (*on* being)
			gamet:
			gametangium (*angeion* blood vessel)
			gametoid (*eidos* form)
			gameto:
			gametocide {gametocidal} (*caedere* to cut, kill)
			gametocyte, gametocytemia (*kytos* cell + *emia* blood condition)
			gametogenesis (*genere* to produce)
			gametogony (*gone* seed)
			gametokinetic (*kinein* to move)
			gametophagia (or, gamophagia) (*phagein* to devour)
			gametophyte (*phyton* plant: growth)
			gamo:
			gamogenesis {gamogenetic} (*genere* to produce)
			gamogony (*gone* seed)
			gamophagia (the disappearance of the male or female element in the conjugation of unicellular organisms) (*phagein* to devour)
			TRAILING ROOT COMPOUND:
			apolegamy (selection, especially sexual selection in breeding) {apolegamic} (*apolegein* to pick out)
			karyogamy (*karyon* nut: nucleus)
			merogamy (also called *microgamy*) (*meros* part)
			misogamy (*misein* to hate)
			oogamy (the conjugation of two dissimilar gametes; also called *heterogamy*) {oogamous} (*oon* egg, ovum)
			plasmogamy (*plassein* to form)
			CROSS REFERENCE: None
gangli	Greek *ganglion* knot	knot, tumor, swelling	SIMPLE ROOT: ganglion (pl., ganglia, ganglions) {ganglial, ganglionic}, ganglionated (or, gangliated)
			PREFIXED ROOT:
			gangli:
			paraganglioma (*para* alongside + *oma* tumor)
			perigangliitis (*peri* around + *itis* inflammation)
			ganglion: paraganglion (pl., paraganglia) (*para* alongside)
			ganglionate: deganglionate (*de* negative)
			ganglionic:
			heteroganglionic (also called *interganglionic*) (*heteros* other)
			interganglionic (also called *heteroganglionic*) (*inter* between)

Element	From	Meaning	Examples
gangli (cont'd)		[knot]	multiganglionic (*multus* many)
			periganglionic (*peri* around)
			polyganglionic (*polys* many)
			postganglionic (*post* posterior)
			preganglionic (*pre* before)
			ganglionosis ganglion condition:
			hyperganglionosis (*hyper* above)
			hypoganglionosis (*hypo* under)
			LEADING ROOT COMPOUND:
			gangli:
			gangliectomy (*ektome* excision)
			gangliform (or, ganglioform) (*forma* shape)
			gangliitis (or, ganglionitis) (*itis* inflammation)
			ganglioma (*oma* tumor)
			ganglio:
			ganglioblast (*blastos* bud, shoot, germ)
			gangliocyte, gangliocytoma (*kytos* cell + *oma* tumor)
			ganglioform (or, gangliform) (*forma* shape)
			ganglioglioma (*glia* glue + *oma* tumor)
			ganglioglioneuroma (*glia* glue + *neuron* nerve + *oma* tumor)
			gangliolytic (*lyein* to dissolve)
			ganglioneuroblastoma (*neuron* nerve + *blastos* bud, shoot, germ + *oma* tumor)
			ganglioneurofibroma (*neuron* nerve + *fibra* fiber + *oma* tumor)
			ganglioneuroma (*neuron* nerve + *oma* tumor)
			ganglioplegic (*plessein* to strike)
			gangliospore (*sporos* seed)
			gangliosympathectomy (excision of a sympathetic ganglion)
			ganglion:
			ganglionectomy (*ektome* excision)
			ganglionitis (*itis* inflammation)
			gangliono:
			ganglionoplegic (*plessein* to strike)
			ganglionostomy (*stoma* mouth, opening)
			TRAILING ROOT COMPOUND:
			neurogangliitis, neuroganglion (*neuron* nerve + *itis* inflammation)
			pseudoganglion (a slight thickening of a nerve, resembling a ganglion) (*pseudes* false)
			vasoganglion (*vas* vessel)
			CROSS REFERENCE: cel^2, nod, onc
gast(r)	Greek *gaster*	stomach, belly	SIMPLE ROOT: gastric, gastricism, gastrin, gastrula, gastrulate
			PREFIXED ROOT:
			gaster:
			epigaster {epigastric} (*epi* upon)
			mesogaster (*mesos* middle)
			metagaster (*meta* after)
			progaster (the archenteron) (*pro* before)
			prosogaster (the foregut) (*proso* forward)
			protogaster (also called *archenteron*) (*protos* first)
			gastr:
			epigastralgia (*epi* upon + *algos* pain)
			hemigastrectomy (*hemi* half + *ektome* excision)
			gastria:
			agastria (absence of a stomach) (*a* privative)

Element	From	Meaning	Examples
gast(r) (cont'd)		[stomach]	megalogastria (also called *macrogastria*) (*megalos* large)
			macrogastria (also called *megalogastria*) (*makros* large)
			microgastria (*mikros* small)
			polygastria (excessive secretion of gastric juice) (*polys* much)
			gastric:
			digastric (*di* two)
			endogastric (*endon* within)
			epigastric (*epi* upon)
			exogastric (*exo* outside)
			intragastric (*intra* within)
			introgastric (*intro* into)
			monogastric (*monos* single)
			perigastric (*peri* around)
			trigastric (having three bellies; said of a muscle) (*tri* three)
			gastrin:
			pentagastrin (*penta* five)
			progastrin (*pro* before)
			gastrinemia: hypergastrinemia (*hyper* above + *emia* blood condition)
			gastritis inflammation of the stomach:
			endogastritis (*endon* within)
			esogastritis (*eso* inside)
			exogastritis (*exo* outside)
			perigastritis (inflammation of the peritoneal coat of the stomach) (*peri* around)
			gastrium:
			epigastrium {epigastric} (*epi* upon)
			mesogastrium {mesogastric} (*mesos* middle)
			hypogastrium {hypogastric} (*hypo* under)
			gastrius: engastrius (*en* in)
			gastroschisis fissure of the stomach:
			hologastroschisis (*holos* entire)
			hypogastroschisis (*hypo* under)
			gastrula: exogastrula (an abnormal embryo in which the primitive gut has been everted) (*exo* outside)
			LEADING ROOT COMPOUND:
			gastr:
			gastralgia, gastralgokenosis (*algos* pain + *kenosis* emptiness)
			gastratrophia (atrophic gastritis) (*a* negative + *trophein* to nourish)
			gastrectomy (*ektome* excision)
			gastritis {gastritic} (*itis* inflammation)
			gastrodynia (also called *gastralgia*) (*odyne* pain)
			gastrosis (also called *gastropathy*) (*osis* condition)
			gastro:
			gastroadenitis (*adenos* gland + *itis* inflammation)
			gastroadynamic (*a* privative + *dynamis* power)
			gastroblennorrhea (*blennos* mucus + *rhein* to flow)
			gastrocardiac (*kardia* heart)
			gastrocele (*kele* hernia)
			gastrochronorrhea (*chronos* time + *rhein* to flow)
			gastrocnemius (*kneme* leg)
			gastrocolic, gastrocolitis (*kolon* colon + *itis* inflammation)
			gastrocolostomy (colon + *stoma* mouth, opening)
			gastrocolotomy (colon + *tomy* incision)

Element	From	Meaning	Examples
gast(r) (cont'd)		[stomach]	gastrocutaneous (*cutis* skin)
			gastrocystoplasty (*kystis* bladder + *plassein* to form)
			gastrodermis (*derma* skin)
			gastroduodenectomy (duodenum + *ektome* excision)
			gastroduodenitis (duodenum + *itis* inflammation)
			gastroenteric (*enteron* intestine) [see separate entry: gastroenter-]
			gastroepiploic (*epiploon* omentum)
			gastroesophageal, gastroesophagitis (esophagus + *itis* inflammation)
			gastrogastrostomy (*stoma* mouth, artificial opening)
			gastrogenic (*genere* to produce)
			gastrohepatic, gastrohepatitis (*hepar* liver + *itis* inflammation)
			gastrohydrorrhea (*hydor* water + *rhein* to flow)
			gastroileac, gastroileitis (ileum + *itis* inflammation)
			gastroileostomy (ileum + *stoma* mouth, opening)
			gastrointestinal (also called *enterogastric, gastroenteric*)
			gastrojejunocolic (jejunum + colon)
			gastrokinesograph (*kinein* to move + *graphein* to write)
			gastrolienal (also called *gastrosplenic*) (*lien* spleen)
			gastrolith, gastrolithiasis (*lithos* stone + *iasis* condition)
			gastrology {gastrologist} (*logos* study)
			gastrolysis (*lyein* to dissolve)
			gastromalacia (*malakos* soft)
			gastromegaly (*megas* large)
			gastromelus (*melos* limb)
			gastromycosis (*mykes* fungus + *osis* condition)
			gastromyotomy (*myos* muscle + *tomy* incision)
			gastromyxorrhea (*myxa* mucus + *rhein* to flow)
			gastroparalysis (also called *gastroparesis*)
			gastroparesis (also called *gastroparalysis*) (*paresis* paralysis)
			gastroparietal (*paries* wall)
			gastropathy (also called *gastrosis*) {gastropathic} (*pathos* disease)
			gastroperiodynia (periodic attacks of pain in the stomach) (*periodos* period + *odyne* pain)
			gastropexy (*pexis* fixation)
			gastrophrenic (*phren* diaphragm)
			gastrophthisis (*phthisis* a wasting away)
			gastroplasty (*plassein* to form)
			gastroplegia (also called *gastroparesis*) (*plegia* paralysis)
			gastroplication (*plicare* to fold)
			gastropneumonic (*pneumon* lung)
			gastroptosis (or, gastroptosia) (*ptosis* prolapse: a falling)
			gastropulmonary (*pulmon* lung)
			gastropyloric (pylorus)
			gastrorenal (also called *renogastric*) (*ren* kidney)
			gastrorrhagia (*rhagia* bursting forth)
			gastrorrhaphy (*rhaphe* suture)
			gastrorrhea (*rhein* to flow)
			gastrorrhexis (*rhexis* rupture)
			gastroschisis (*schisis* fissure)
			gastroscope {gastroscopic}, gastroscopy (*skopein* to examine)
			gastrospasm (*spasmos* contraction)
			gastrosplenic (also called *gastrolienal*) (*splen* spleen)
			gastrostaxis (*staxis* a dripping)
			gastrostenosis (*stenosis* a narrowing; shrinkage)

Element	From	Meaning	Examples
gast(r) (cont'd)		[stomach]	gastrostoma, gastrostomy (*stoma* mouth, opening)
			gastrothoracopagus (conjoined twins united at the thorax and abdomen) (*thorax* chest + *pagos* fixed)
			gastrotome, gastrotomy (*tomy* incision)
			gastrotonometer, gastrotonometry (*tonos* tone + *metron* measure)
			gastrotoxin (*toxin* poison)
			gastrotropic (affecting the stomach) (*tropos* a turning)
			TRAILING ROOT COMPOUND:
			gastria:
			atretogastria (*atretos* not perforated: *a* negative + *tretos* perforated)
			tachygastria (*tachys* fast, swift)
			gastric:
			aortogastric (*aorta*)
			enterogastric (also called *gastrointestinal*) (*enteron* intestine)
			esophagogastric (also called *gastroesophageal*) (esophagus)
			hepatogastric (*hepatos* liver)
			nasogastric (*nasus* nose)
			nephrogastric (also called *gastrorenal*) (*nephros* kidney)
			neurogastric (*neuron* nerve)
			phrenogastric (*phrenos* diaphragm)
			pneumogastric (*pneumon* lung)
			renogastric (also called *gastrorenal*) (*ren* kidney)
			gastritis stomach inflammation:
			enterogastritis (*enteron* intestine)
			mycogastritis (*mykes* fungus)
			gastroschisis: thoracogastroschisis (thorax + *schisis* fissure)
			gastrula: merogastrula (*meros* part)
			gastry: bathygastry (also called *gastroptosis*) (*bathos* deep, low)
			CROSS REFERENCE: stomach, ventr
gastroenter	Greek *gaster* belly + *enteron* intestine	See Examples	SIMPLE ROOT: gastroenteric (also called *gastrointestinal*)
			LEADING ROOT COMPOUND:
			gastroenter:
			gastroenteralgia (*algos* pain)
			gastroenteritis (*itis* inflammation)
			gastroentero:
			gastroenterocolitis (colon + *itis* inflammation)
			gastroenterocolostomy (colon + *stoma* mouth, opening)
			gastroenterology (*logos* study)
			gastroenteropathy (*pathos* suffering)
			gastroenteroplasty (*plassein* to form)
			gastroenteroptosis (*ptosis* a falling)
			gastroenterostomy (*stoma* mouth, opening)
			gastroenterotomy (*tomy* incision)
			CROSS REFERENCE: None
gen	Latin *gignere* to beget; Greek *gignesthai* to be born	to originate, produce; race	SIMPLE ROOT:
			gender, gene {genic}
			generate (to produce; to procreate), generation {generative}
			generic (that which is not a trademark, as a generic medicine)
			genital (pertaining to reproduction, or to the organs of generation), genitals (the reproductive organs; organa genitalia), genitalia (also called *genitals*)
			PREFIXED ROOT:
			gen:
			antigen (antibody + gen) {antigenic} (*anti* against)

A Thesaurus of Medical Word Roots

Element	From	Meaning	Examples
gen (cont'd)		[to originate]	isoantigen (*isos* equal + antigen)
			polygene (*polys* many)
			superantigen (*super* above + antigen)
			transgene, transgenesis {transgenic} (*trans* across)
			genal:
			intergenal (between different genes) (*inter* between)
			intragenal (*intra* within)
			geneic:
			allogeneic (or, allogenic) (*allos* other)
			isogeneic (or, isogenic; also called *syngeneic*) (*isos* equal)
			syngeneic (also called *isogeneic, isogenic, isologous, isoplastic, syn-genic*) (*syn* with)
			geneity:
			heterogeneity (*heteros* other)
			homogeneity (*homos* same)
			gener:
			congener {congeneric}, congenerous (*con* with)
			degeneracy, degenerate (*de* negative)
			isogeneric (*isos* equal)
			generation:
			degeneration {degenerative} (*de* negative)
			regeneration (*re* again)
			super-regeneration (*super* over + regeneration)
			genesis:
			agenesis (absence or failure to form of any part) (*a* privative)
			anagenesis (regeneration of lost parts; repair of tissue) {anagenetic} (*ana* again, up)
			autogenesis {autogenetic} (*autos* self)
			cacogenesis (also called *dysgenesis*) (*kakos* bad)
			catagenesis {catagenetic} (*kata* down)
			digenesis {digenetic} (*di* two)
			diplogenesis (*diploos* double)
			dysgenesis (*dys* abnormal)
			epigenesis {epigenetic} (*epi* upon)
			heterogenesis {heterogenetic} (*heteros* other)
			hologenesis (*holos* entire, whole)
			homogenesis {homogenetic} (*homos* same)
			hypergenesis {hypergenetic} (*hyper* above)
			hypogenesis {hypogenetic} (*hypo* under)
			isogenesis (*isos* equal)
			metagenesis (*meta* change)
			microgenesis (*mikros* small)
			monogenesis {monogenic} (*monos* single)
			palingenesis (*palin* again, backward)
			pangenesis (*pan* all)
			syngenesis {syngenetic} (*syn* with, together)
			genetic:
			amphigenetic (*amphi* both)
			exogenetic (or, exogenous) (*exo* outside)
			heterogenetic (*heteros* other)
			monogenetic (*monos* single)
			genic:
			amphogenic (producing offspring of both sexes) (*ampho* both)
			antigenic (*anti* against)

Element	From	Meaning	Examples
gen (cont'd)		[to originate]	dysgenic, dysgenics (also called *cacogenics*) (*dys* abnormal) ectogenic (or, ectogenous) (*ektos* outside) endogenic (or, endogenous) (*endon* within) eugenics (*eu* well) heterogenic (*heteros* other) intragenic (within a gene) (*intra* within) isogenic (also called *syngeneic*) (*isos* equal) mesogenic (*mesos* middle) polygenic (*polys* many) transgenic (*trans* across) *genital*: congenital (occurring from birth, as a congenital disease) (*com* with) extragenital (outside of or unrelated to the genitals) (*extra* outside) paragenital (*para* alongside) pregenital (that period when erotic interest in the reproductive organs and functions is not yet organized) (*pre* before) progenital (on the external surface of the genitals) (*pro* before) *genitalism*: agenitalism (a condition due to lack of the internal secretion of the testicles or ovaries) (*a* privative) dysgenitalism (*dys* abnormal) hypergenitalism (also called *hypergonadism*) (*hyper* above) hypogenitalism (also called *hypogonadism*) (*hypo* under) microgenitalism (*mikros* small) paragenitalism (*para* alongside) *genito*: macrogenitosomia (excessive somatic growth, with unusual enlargement of the genital organs) (*makros* large + *soma* body) *genitor*: progenitor (*pro* before) *genous*: autogenous (also called *autologous*) (*autos* self) ectogenous (also called *exogenous*) (*ektos* outside) exogenous (or, exogenetic; also called *ectogenous*) (*exo* outside) heterogenous (*heteros* other) homogenous (*homos* same) indigenous (native) (*indu* within) isogenous (*isos* equal) monogenous (*monos* single) *genus*: subgenus (a taxonomic category between a genus and a species) (*sub* below) *geny*: endodyogeny (*endon* within + *dys* two) endopolygeny (*endon* within + *polys* many) progeny (offspring, or descendants) (*pro* before) LEADING ROOT COMPOUND: *genital*: genitaloid (*eidos* form) *genito*: genitocrural (also called *genitofemoral*) (*crus* leg) genitofemoral (also called *genitocrural*) (femur, thigh) genitoplasty (*plassein* to form) genitourinary (also called *urogenital, urinosexual*) (*ouron* urine) *geno*: genoblast (*blastos* germ) genodermatology (*dermatos* skin + *logos* study) genotoxic (*toxic* poisonous)

A Thesaurus of Medical Word Roots

Element	From	Meaning	Examples
gen (cont'd)		[to originate]	genotype {genotypic} (*typos* type)

TRAILING ROOT COMPOUND:

gen:

aerogen (*aer* air)

androgen (*andros* man)

hydrogen (*hydor* water)

opsinogen (opsonin)

oxygen (*oxys* sharp)

plasmagen (also called *protoplasm*) (plasma)

saprogen (*sapros* rotten)

trichogen (*trichos* hair)

genation:

miscegenation (marriage or interbreeding of individuals of different races) (*miscere* to mix)

oxygenation (*oxys* sharp)

genesis:

actinogenesis (*aktis* ray)

adipogenesis (*adeps* fat)

aerogenesis (*aer* air)

algogenesis (*algos* pain)

allantogenesis (*allantos* sausage)

amelogenesis (Middle English *amel* enamel)

amniogenesis (*amnion* fetal membrane)

amylogenesis (*amylon* starch)

androgenesis (*andros* man)

angiogenesis (also called *vasculogenesis*) (*angeion* blood vessel)

atherogenesis (*athere* gruel)

biligenesis (bile)

biogenesis (*bios* life)

blastogenesis (*blastos* germ, sprout)

bradygenesis (*bradys* slow)

cardiogenesis (*kardia* heart)

choriogenesis (*chorion* membrane)

chromogenesis (*chroma* color)

ciliogenesis (*cilium* eyelid, eyelash)

cystogenesis (*kystis* bladder, sac)

esthesiogenesis (the production of sensation, especially of nervous erethism, or irritability) (*esthesia* feeling)

fibrogenesis (*fibra* fiber)

gamogenesis (sexual reproduction) (*gamos* marriage)

glycogenesis (*glykys* sweet)

gonadogenesis (*gone* seed: procreation)

gynogenesis (*gyne* woman)

hematogensis (*hematos* blood)

histogenesis (*histos* web, tissue)

hormonogenesis (*hormaein* to excite; hormone)

hypnogenesis (*hypnos* sleep)

idiogenesis (of self-origin or origin without known cause, especially with reference to disease) (*idios* one's own)

inogenesis (*inos* fiber)

keratogenesis (*keratos* horn)

lipogenesis (*lipos* fat)

lithogenesis (*lithos* stone)

melanogenesis (*melas* black, dark)

Element	From	Meaning	Examples
gen (cont'd)		[to originate]	merogenesis {merogenetic} (*meros* part)
			myelinogenesis (myelin)
			myelogenesis (*myelos* marrow)
			neogenesis (*neos* new)
			odontogenesis (*odontos* tooth)
			omphalogenesis (*omphalos* umbilicus, navel)
			oncogenesis (*onkos* mass, bulk, tumor)
			ontogenesis (*ontos* existence)
			oogenesis (also called *ovigenesis*) (*oon* egg, ovum)
			orthogenesis (*orthos* straight)
			osteogenesis (*osteon* bone)
			ovigenesis (also called *oogenesis*) (*ovum* egg)
			parthenogenesis (*parthenos* virgin)
			physiogenesis (embryology) (*phyein* to grow)
			placentogenesis (placenta)
			psychogenesis (*psyche* mind)
			pyogenesis (also called *pyopoiesis*) (*pyon* pus)
			pythogenesis (origination from decaying matter) (*pythein* to rot)
			schizogenesis (*schizein* to split)
			somatogenesis (*somatos* body)
			spermatogenesis (*sperma* seed, sperm)
			sporogenesis (*sporos* seed)
			thermogenesis (*therme* heat)
			tumorigenesis (*tumor* swelling)
			vasculogenesis (also called *angiogenesis*) (*vasculum* small vessel)
			vitellogenesis (*vitellus* egg yolk)
			xenogenesis (*xenos* foreign, strange)
			genic(s):
			aerogenic (*aer* air)
			angiogenic (*angeion* blood vessel)
			cancerogenic (cancer)
			cardiogenic (*kardia* heart)
			cytogenic (*kytos* cell)
			deutogenic (*deuteros* second)
			meningogenic (*meningos* membrane)
			myogenic (*myos* muscle)
			nephritogenic (*nephros* kidney)
			oligogenic (*oligos* little, scant)
			orthogenics (also called *eugenics*) (*orthos* straight)
			otogenic (*otos* ear)
			ovariogenic (ovary)
			pathogenic (*pathos* disease)
			peptogenic (*peptein* to digest)
			phlogogenic (*phlogos* inflammation)
			phosgenic (*phos* light)
			pleurogenic (*pleura* side, rib)
			proctogenic (*proktos* anus, rectum)
			ptyalogenic (*ptyalon* saliva)
			pyrogenic (*pyr* fire, fever)
			sarcogenic (*sarkos* flesh)
			somatogenic (*somatos* body)
			spermatogenic (*sperma* seed, sperm)
			sporogenic (*sporos* seed)
			thymogenic (*thymos* mind, spirit)

Element	From	Meaning	Examples
gen (cont'd)		[to originate]	toxigenic (*toxikon* poison)
			tracheogenic (*trachea* windpipe)
			traumatogenic (*trauma* wound)
			tympanogenic (*tympanon* eardrum)
			ulcerogenic (ulcer)
			uterogenic (uterus)
			vertebrogenic (vertebra)
			vestibulogenic (vestibule)
			viscerogenic (*viscera* internal organs)
			zymogenic (*zyme* yeast)
			genous:
			acrogenous (*akros* extremity)
			adenogenous (*adenos* gland)
			adipogenous (also called *lipogenous*) (*adipos* fat)
			adrenogenous (adrenal gland; fr. *ad* to + *rene* kidney)
			aerogenous (producing gas, as certain bacteria) (*aer* air)
			androgenous (*andros* man)
			arthrogenous (*arthron* joint)
			ascogenous (*askos* bag, sac)
			blennogenous (also called *muciparous*) (*blenna* mucus)
			branchiogenous (*branchia* gills: pharyngeal arches)
			chondrogenous (*chondros* cartilage)
			chromatogenous (*chroma* color)
			cirrhogenous (*kirrhos* orange-yellow)
			cytogenous (*kytos* cell)
			desmogenous (*dein* to bind: ligament)
			diabetogenous (diabetes)
			enterogenous (*enteron* intestine)
			entomogenous (*entomon* insect)
			fibrinogenous (fibrin)
			galactogenous (*galaktos* milk)
			glycogenous (*glykys* sweet)
			goitrogenous (goiter)
			hematogenous (*hematos* blood)
			hepatogenous (*hepatos* liver)
			histogenous (*histos* web, tissue)
			hypnogenous (*hypnos* sleep)
			inogenous (*inos* fiber)
			keratogenous (*keratos* horn)
			lactigenous (*lac* milk)
			lipogenous (also called *adipogenous*) (*lipos* fat)
			lithogenous (*lithos* stone, calculus)
			lymphogenous (*lympha* water, lymph)
			metrogenous (*metra* uterus)
			morbigenous (*morbus* sickness)
			myelogenous (*myelos* marrow)
			myogenous (*myos* muscle)
			necrogenous (or, necrogenic) (*nekros* dead, death)
			nephrogenous (*nephros* kidney)
			neurogenous (*neuron* nerve)
			nitrogenous (nitrogen)
			obesogenous (obesity)
			odontogenous (*odontos* tooth)
			oncogenous (*onkos* mass, tumor)

Element	From	Meaning	Examples
gen (cont'd)		[to originate]	oophorogenous (*oophoros* bearing eggs)
			osteogenous (*osteon* bone)
			otogenous (*otos* ear)
			ovigenous (also called *oogenetic*) (*ovum* egg)
			ovulogenous (*ovule* small egg)
			pathogenous (*pathos* disease)
			phlebogenous (*phlebos* vein)
			phytogenous (*phyton* plant: growth)
			pleurogenous (*pleura* rib, side)
			proteinogenous (protein)
			pyogenous (also called *purulent*) (*pyon* pus)
			pythogenous (*pythein* to rot)
			rhinogenous (*rhinos* nose)
			schizogenous (*schizein* to split: fission)
			sclerogenous (*skleros* hard)
			sensigenous (sense, impulse)
			sialogenous (*sialon* saliva)
			siderogenous (*sideros* iron)
			skeletogenous (skeleton)
			spirochetogenous (spirochete)
			splenogenous (spleen)
			spodogenous (*spodos* ashes: waste materials)
			steatogenous (also called *lipogenic*) (*steatos* fat)
			stromatogenous (*stroma* supporting tissue)
			teratogenous (*teratos* fetal monster)
			tetanigenous (tetanus)
			thermogenous (*therme* heat)
			thyrogenous (thyroid gland)
			urogenous (*ouron* urine)
			xenogenous (caused by a foreign body) (*xenos* foreign)
			geny:
			dichogeny (*dicha* two)
			ectrogeny (congenital absence or defect of any body part) {ectrogenic} (*ektros* absence)
			PREFIXED TRAILING ROOT COMPOUND:
			adermogenesis (failure of or imperfection in the regeneration of skin, especially in the repair of a cutaneous effect) (*a* privative + *derma* skin)
			dysontogenesis (*dys* abnormal + *ontos* being)
			CROSS REFERENCE: gon[1], nat[1], par
geni[1]	Greek *geneion* chin	chin, jaw	SIMPLE ROOT: genial (or, genian; pertaining to the chin), genion
			PREFIXED ROOT:
			macrogenia (enlargement of the jaw, especially the chin, which may involve only the osseous or soft-tissue components of the bony and soft tissues) (*makros* large)
			microgenia (abnormal smallness of the chin) (*mikros* small)
			progenia (also called *prognathism*; a condition marked by abnormal protrusion of the mandible) (*pro* before)
			LEADING ROOT COMPOUND:
			genioglossus (either of a pair of lingual muscles with origin in the mandible, with insertion to the lingual fascia below the mucous membrane and epiglottis, with nerve supply from the hypoglossal nerve) (*glossa* tongue)
			geniohyoid (pertaining to the chin and hyoid bone)

Element	From	Meaning	Examples
geni[1] (cont'd)		[chin, jaw]	geniocheiloplasty (*cheilos* lip + *plassein* to form) genioplasty (*plassein* to form) TRAILING ROOT COMPOUND: opisthogenia (defective development of the jaws following ankylosis of the jaw; compare *retrognathism*) (*opisthen* behind) CROSS REFERENCE: gnath, maxill, ment
geni[2]	Latin *genu*	knee, kneelike bend	SIMPLE ROOT: genicular, geniculate (bent, like a knee), geniculum (pl., genicula), genu (pl., genua) {genual} PREFIXED ROOT: supergenual (*super* above) LEADING ROOT COMPOUND: genuclast (an instrument for breaking knee-joint adhesions) (*klaein* to break) genucubital (*cubitus* elbow) genupectoral (*pectus* chest) CROSS REFERENCE: gon[3], patell
ger[1], **gest**	Latin *gerere*	to carry, bear	SIMPLE ROOT: gestation (the period of development of the young in viviparous animals from time of fertilization of the ovum) PREFIXED ROOT: *gest*: congested, congestion {congestive} (*com* with) contragestation (capable of preventing gestation, either by preventing implantation or by causing the uterine lining to shed after implantation) (*contra* against) decongestant, decongestive (*de* negative + congestive) digest, digestant, digestible, digestion, digestive (*dis* apart) egesta, egestion (the casting out, or excretion from the body, of material which is indigestible) (*ex* out) exterogestate (*exterus* outside) hyperingestion (*hyper* over, beyond + ingestion) indigestion (*in* negative + digestion) ingest, ingestion {ingestive} (*in* in) maldigestion (*mal* ill, bad, abnormal + digestion) multigesta (also called *multigravida*) (*multus* many) predigestion (*pre* before + digestion) progestational, progestogen (*pro* before + *genesis* origin) suggestibility, suggestible, suggestion {suggestive} (*sub* under) LEADING ROOT COMPOUND: *gest*: gestosis (any disorder of pregnancy; pl., gestoses) (*osis* condition) *gesta*: gestagen (progestational agent) (*genere* to produce) TRAILING ROOT COMPOUND: *gerous*: calcigerous (*calx* limestone, calcium) cystigerous (also called *cystiferous*) (*kystis* sac, bladder) dentigerous (*dens* tooth) lactigerous (also called *lactiferous*) (*lactis* milk) ovigerous (*ovum* egg) pedigerous (*pes* foot) proligerous (*proles* offspring) setigerous (*seta* bristle) *gestation*: pseudogestation (*pseudes* false) uterogestation (normal pregnancy) (*uterus*) CROSS REFERENCE: fer, gen, phor

A Thesaurus of Medical Word Roots

Element	From	Meaning	Examples
ger[2]	Greek *geras, gerontos*	old age	SIMPLE ROOT: geratic (pertaining to old age), gerontal (pertaining to an old person or old age; senile) PREFIXED ROOT: agerasia (an unusually youthful appearance in a person of advanced years) (*a* privative) progeria (senility occurring in childhood) (*pro* before) LEADING ROOT COMPOUND: *ger*: geriatric, geriatrics (*iatrein* to heal) gerodontia (or, gerodontics), gerodontist (*odontos* tooth) *gerato*: geratology (or, gerontology) (*logos* study) *gero*: gerocomia (or, gerocomy; the care of old people (*komein* to care for) geroderma (or, gerodermia; dystrophy of the skin and genitals, producing the appearance of old age) (*dermia* skin condition) geromarasmus (*marasmos* a wasting away) geromorphism (premature senility) (*morphe* form) *geront*: gerontopia (also called *senopia*) (*opia* vision condition) *geronto*: gerontologist, gerontology (*logos* study) gerontophilia (sexual attraction to old people) (*philein* to love) gerontotherapeutics, gerontotherapy (*therapy* treatment) gerontotoxon (or, gerontoxon; degenerative circle about corneal exterior surface seen in the aged) (*toxon* poison) TRAILING ROOT COMPOUND: acrogeria (a condition in which the skin of the hands and feet shows signs of premature aging) (*akron* extremity) CROSS REFERENCE: presby
gest			See ger[1] for *gestation, congestion*.
geus	Greek *geusis, geuma*	taste	PREFIXED ROOT: *geusia*: ageusia (lack or impairment of the sense of taste) (*a* privative) ambageusia (*ambo* both + ageusia) cacogeusia (a bad taste) (*kakos* bad, abnormal) dysgeusia (a condition characterized by alterations of the sense of taste which may range from mild to severe, including gross distortions of taste quality; also called *parageusia*) (*dys* abnormal) hemiageusia (also called *hemigeusia*) (*hemi* half + ageusia) heterogeusia (*heteros* other) hemigeusia (or, hemiageustia) (*hemi* half) hypergeusia (also called *oxygeusia*) (*hyper* above, beyond) hypogeusia (also called *amblygeustia*) (*hypo* below) parageusia (also called *dysgeusia*) {parageusic} (*para* abnormal) TRAILING ROOT COMPOUND: *geusia*: glycogeusia (a sweet taste in the mouth) (*glykys* sweet) oxygeusia (also called *hypergeusia*) (*oxys* sharp) phantogeusia (a continuous abnormal taste in the mouth) (*phantom*) picrogeusia (a pathologic bitter taste) (*pikros* bitter) *geustia*: allotriogeustia (*allotrios* strange) amblygeustia (also called *hypogeusia*) (*amblys* dull) CROSS REFERENCE: None

Element	From	Meaning	Examples
gingiv	Latin *gingiva*	gums (of the mouth)	SIMPLE ROOT: gingiva (pl., gingivae) {gingival} gingivally (toward the gingivae) PREFIXED ROOT: macrogingivae (fibromatosis gingivae) (*makros* large) mesogingival (*mesos* middle) subgingival (*sub* beneath) LEADING ROOT COMPOUND: *gingiv*: gingivalgia (*algos* pain) gingivectomy (excision of diseased gum tissue in periodontal pa- thologies; also called *ulectomy*) (*ektome* excision) gingivitis (*itis* inflammation) gingivosis (*osis* condition) *gingivo*: gingivoaxial (*axis* axle) gingivobuccoaxial (*bucca* cheek + *axis* axle) gingivoglossitis (*glossa* tongue + *itis* inflammation) gingivolabial (*labium* lip) gingivoplasty (*plassein* to form) gingivostomatitis (*stoma* mouth + *itis* inflammation) TRAILING ROOT COMPOUND: buccogingival (relating to the cheek and the gums) (*bucca* cheek) dentogingival (*dens* tooth) distogingival (*distans* distant) linguogingival (*lingua* tongue) mucogingivitis (mucus + *itis* inflammation) CROSS REFERENCE: oulo

gland,
glans
	Latin
	glans
	acorn
		gland	NOTE: Root is so called from the gland being an aggregation of
			   cells, having the texture and shape of an acorn.
			SIMPLE ROOT:
			gland (pl., glandulae) {glandular; also called *adenic, adenous*},
			   glandule (pl., glandulae), glandulous
			glans (glans penis, the head or tip of the penis; glans clitoris, the
			   small mass of erectile tissue at the tip of the clitoris; pl., glandes)
			PREFIXED ROOT:
			glandular:
			homoglandular (*homos* same)
			hyperglandular (*hyper* above)
			hypoglandular (*hypo* under)
			intraglandular (*intra* within)
			multiglandular (also called *pluriglandular*) (*multus* many)
			periglandular, periglandulitis (*peri* around + *itis* inflammation)
			pluriglandular (also called *polyglandular*) (*pluris* more)
			polyglandular (also called *pluriglandular*) (*polys* many)
			uniglandular (*unus* one)
			glandulous: eglandulous (having no glands) (*ex* without)
			LEADING ROOT COMPOUND:
			glandi: glandilemma (*lemma* membrane, envelope)
			glanduli: glanduliform (*forma* shape)
			glandulo: glanuloplasty (*plassein* to form)
			TRAILING ROOT COMPOUND:
			epithelioglandular (epithelium)
			excitoglandular (causing glands to secrete)

Element	From	Meaning	Examples
gland (cont'd)		[gland]	lymphoglandular (*lympha* water, fluid) neuroglandular (*neuron* nerve) oculoglandular (*oculus* eye) pseudoglandular (a stage in the growth of the embryonic lung before ciliated cells are differentiated) (*pseudes* false) sensoriglandular (pertaining to the reflexive secretion by glands triggered by sensory stimulation of a nerve) ulceroglandular (*ulcer* sore) CROSS REFERENCE: acin, aden, thym[1]
gli	Greek *glia*	glue	NOTE: This root is extended to mean the "neuroglia"; as a word termination form, *-glia* means "a gluelike structure." SIMPLE ROOT: glia (the neuroglia), gliadin, glial (also called *neuroglial*) PREFIXED ROOT: ectoglia (*ektos* outside) macroglia (*makros* large, long) mesoglia (*mesos* middle) microglia (*mikros* small) LEADING ROOT COMPOUND: *gli*: glioma (a tumor composed of tissue which represents neuroglia in any one of its stages of development) {gliomatous}, gliomatosis (*oma* tumor + *osis* condition) gliosis (an excess of astroglia in damaged areas of the central nervous system) (*osis* condition) *glia*: gliacyte (a cell of the neuroglia) (*kytos* cell) *glio*: gliobacteria (*bakterion* rod-shaped bacterium) glioblast, glioblastoma (*blastos* germ, cell + *oma* tumor) gliococcus (*kokkos* berry-shaped bacterium) gliocyte, gliocytoma (*kytos* cell + *oma* tumor) gliofibrillary (*fibra* fiber) gliomyxoma (a tumor containing gliomatous and myxomatous elements) (*myxa* mucus + *oma* tumor) glioneuroma (also called *ganglioglioma*) (*neuron* nerve + *oma* tumor) gliophagia (*phagein* to devour, consume) gliopil (a dense feltwork of glial processes) (*pilos* felt) gliosarcoma (*sarkos* flesh + *oma* tumor) gliosome (*soma* body) gliotoxin (*toxin* poison) *gliomat*: gliomatosis (also called *neurogliomatosis*) (*oma* tumor + *osis* condition) TRAILING ROOT COMPOUND: *glia*: astroglia (the astrocytes) (*aster* star) inoglia (*inos* fiber) neuroglia (*neuron* nerve) oligodendroglia (*oligos* scarcity + *dendron* tree: growth) sarcoglia (*sarkos* flesh) teloglia (*telos* end) *glioma* glutinous tumor: angioglioma (a tumor that is a mixed glioma and angioma) (*angeion* blood vessel)

Element	From	Meaning	Examples
gli (cont'd)		[glue]	cryptoglioma (a stage of retinal glioma in which the eyeball shrinks, masking the presence of the growth) (*kryptos* hidden) fibroglioma (a glioma containing excessive fibrous tissue) ganglioglioma (*ganglion* swelling, knot) myxoglioma (*myxa* mucus) neuroglioma (*neuron* nerve) pseudoglioma (*pseudes* false) TERM: brainstem glioma (the primary brain tumor occurring in the pons or the medulla) CROSS REFERENCE: colla, glut²
glob, **glom**	Latin *globus* ball; *glomus* ball	ball, sphere	NOTE: Because of their similar meanings, the two roots are listed together here, although they are derived ultimately from different sources. SIMPLE ROOT: *glob*: globin (the protein constituent of hemoglobin) globose (globe-shaped; spherical) globular (like a globe or globule; composed of globules) globule, globulin, globulose, globulus (or, globule; pl., globuli) globus (encapsulated globular masses containing bacilli, seen in smears of lepromatous leprosy lesions; pl., globi) *globulin*: globulinuria (*uria* urine condition) *glom*: glomerate, glomerular, glomerule (or, glomerulus; pl., glomeruli), glomerulose glomus (pl., glomera) {glomal, glomic} PREFIXED ROOT: *globate*: conglobate (forming into a rounded mass or clump: used of certain glands), conglobation (*com* with) *globular*: interglobular (*inter* between) intraglobular (also called *intracorpuscular*) (*intra* within) *globulin*: antiglobulin (*anti* against) euglobulin (*eu* well) macroglobulin (*makros* large) metaglobulin (*meta* change) microglobulin (*mikros* small) paraglobulin (*para* alongside) *globulinemia* globulins in the blood: dysglobulinemia (*dys* abnormal) hyperglobulinemia (*hyper* above) macroglobulinemia (*makros* large) *globulose*: heteroglobulose (*heteros* other) protoglobulose (*protos* first, primary) *glom*: agglomerate {agglomerated}, agglomeration (aggregation) (*ad* to) conglomerate (heaped together) (*con* with) juxtaglomerular (*juxta* near) postglomerular (*post* after) LEADING ROOT COMPOUND: *glob*: globoid (globe-shaped; spheroid) (*eidos* form) *globino*: globinometer (*metron* measure)

Element	From	Meaning	Examples
glob (cont'd)		[ball, sphere]	*globuli*: globuliferous (*ferre* to bear, carry)
			globulin: globulinuria (*uria* urine condition)
			glom:
			glomangioma (*angeion* blood vessel + *oma* tumor)
			glomectomy (*ektome* excision)
			glomoid (*eidos* shape)
			glomerul: glomerulitis (*itis* inflammation)
			glomerulo:
			glomerulonephritis (*nephros* kidney + *itis* inflammation)
			glomerulopathy (*pathos* disease)
			glomerulosclerosis (*skleros* hard + *osis* condition)
			TRAILING ROOT COMPOUND:
			globulin:
			cryoglobulin (*kryos* cold)
			hemoglobin (*haima* blood)
			immunoglobulin (immunity)
			lactoglobulin (*lactis* milk)
			myoglobulin (*myos* muscle)
			ovoglobulin (*ovum* egg)
			pyroglobulin (*pyr* heat)
			pseudoglobulin (*pseudes* false)
			seroglobulin (*serum* whey)
			toxoglobulin (*toxikon* poison)
			globinuria: myoglobinuria (*myos* muscle + *uria* urine condition)
			globus:
			keratoglobus (also called *megalocornea*) (*keratos* horn: cornea)
			lentiglobus (exaggerated curvature of the lens of the eye) (*lentis* lens)
			glomerulus: pseudoglomerulus (*pseudes* false)
			CROSS REFERENCE: spher
gloss, **glott**	Greek *glossa*	tongue	SIMPLE ROOT:
			gloss:
			glossa (the tongue; lingua) {glossal}
			glossocoma (retraction of the tongue)
			glott:
			glottic (or, glottal; pertaining to the glottis; pertaining to the tongue)
			glottis (the vocal apparatus of the larynx, consisting of the true vocal cords and the opening between them; pl., glottides)
			PREFIXED ROOT:
			glossal:
			entoglossal (within the tongue) (*entos* inside)
			hemiglossal (relating to one lateral half of the tongue; also called *hemilingual*) (*hemi* half)
			hypoglossal (also called *sublingual*) (*hypo* under)
			subglossal (also called *sublingual*) (*sub* below)
			glossectomy: hemiglossectomy (*hemi* half + *ektome* excision)
			glossia:
			aglossia (congenital absence of the tongue) (*a* privative)
			diglossia (double tongue, or bifid tongue) (*di* two)
			macroglossia (also called *megaloglossia*) (*makros* large)
			megaloglossia (also called *macroglossia*) (*megalos* large)
			microglossia (*mikros* small)
			panglossia (abnormal or pathologic garrulity, or talkativeness) (*pan* all)
			glossis: proglossis (or, proglottid; the tip of the tongue) (*pro* before)

Element	From	Meaning	Examples
gloss (cont'd)		[tongue]	*glossitis* inflammation of the tongue:
			hemiglossitis (*hemi* half)
			periglossitis (*peri* around)
			subglossitis (*sub* under)
			glottic pertaining to the tongue, or the glottis:
			epiglottic (*epi* upon)
			infraglottic (also called *subglottic*) (*infra* below, beneath)
			periglottic (*peri* around, near)
			preepiglottic (*pre* before + epiglottic)
			subepiglottic (*sub* under + epiglottic)
			subglottic (also called *infraglottic*) (*sub* under)
			supraglottic (*supra* above)
			transglottic (*trans* across)
			glottis:
			epiglottis (a thin leaflike structure located immediately posterior to the root of the tongue) {epiglottic, epiglottidean} (*epi* upon)
			hypoglottis (or, hypoglossis) (*hypo* under)
			periglottis (*peri around*)
			proglottis (pl., proglottides) (*pro* before)
			supraglottis (*supra* above)
			glottitis inflammation of the tongue:
			epiglottitis (*epi* upon)
			supraglottitis (*supra* above)
			LEADING ROOT COMPOUND:
			gloss:
			glossagra (gouty pain of the tongue) (*agra* seizure)
			glossalgia (also called *glossodynia*) (*algos* pain)
			glossectomy (also called *glossosteresis*) (*ektome* excision)
			glossitis (*itis* inflammation)
			glossodontotropism (*odontos* tooth + *trope* a turning)
			glossodynia (also called *glossalgia*) (*odyne* pain)
			glossoncus (a swelling of the tongue) (*onkos* mass, tumor)
			glosso:
			glossocele (swelling and protrusion of the tongue) (*kele* tumor)
			glossodynamometer (*dynamis* power + *metron* measure)
			glossoepiglottic (or, glossoepiglottidean; pertaining to tongue and epiglottis, as glossoepiglottic folds)
			glossokinesthetic (*kinesis* movement + *esthesia* feeling)
			glossolalia (speech in an unknown or imaginary language; gibberish) (*lalein* to speak)
			glossology (the study of the tongue and its diseases) (*logos* study)
			glossolysis (also called *glossoplegia*) (*lyein* to loosen)
			glossopalatine (also called *palatoglossal*) (*palatum* roof of mouth)
			glossopathy (any disease of the tongue) (*pathos* disease)
			glossopexy (lip-tongue adhesion) (*pexis* fixation)
			glossopharyngeal (*pharynx* throat)
			glossophobia (also called *lalophobia*) (*phobia* fear)
			glossophytia (black tongue) (*phyton* plant: growth)
			glossoplasty (plastic surgery of the tongue) (*plassein* to form)
			glossoplegia (paralysis of the tongue) (*plessein* to strike)
			glossoptosis (downward placement or retraction of the tongue) (*ptein* to fall)
			glossopyrosis (burning tongue; also called *glossodynia*) (*pyr* fire, heat + *osis* condition)

A Thesaurus of Medical Word Roots

Element	From	Meaning	Examples
gloss (cont'd)		[tongue]	glossorrhaphy (*rhaphe* suture)
			glossoscopy (*skopein* to examine)
			glossospasm (*spasmos* contraction)
			glossosteresis (also called *glossectomy*) (*steresis* loss)
			glossotomy (*tomy* incision)
			glossotrichia (hairy tongue; also called *trichoglossia*) (*thrix* hair)
			glott: glottitis (*itis* inflammation)
			glotti: glottiscope (*skopein* to examine)
			glottido: glottidospasm (the sudden acute spasm of the vocal cords that can result in occlusion of the airway and death; also called *laryngospasm*) (*spasmos* contraction)
			glotto: glottology (also called *glossology*) (*logos* study)
			TRAILING ROOT COMPOUND:
			glossal:
			hyoglossal (*hyoid* U-shaped)
			palatoglossal (palate)
			pharyngoglossal (pharynx)
			platyglossal (*platys* flat)
			sternoglossal (*sternon* chest)
			thyroglossal (thyroid)
			glossia:
			ankyloglossia (restricted movement of the tongue, resulting in speech difficulty; also called *adherent tongue, lingua frenata, tongue-tie*) (*ankylos* bent, fused, crooked)
			baryglossia (in pathology, difficulty of speech; also called *baryphonia*) (*barys* heavy)
			bradyglossia (abnormal slowness of speech) (*bradys* slow)
			idioglossia (imperfect articulation, with the utterance of meaningless vocal sounds) {idioglottic} (*idios* one's own, peculiar)
			melanoglossia (also called *black tongue*) (*melas* dark, black)
			pachyglossia (abnormal thickness of the tongue) (*pachys* thick)
			schistoglossia (*schistos* split)
			trichoglossia (also called *glossotrichia, hairy tongue*) (*trichos* hair)
			glossitis inflammation of tongue:
			gingivoglossitis (*gingivae* gums)
			stomatoglossitis (*stomatos* mouth)
			uloglossitis (inflammation of the gums and the tongue) (*oulon* gums)
			glossus:
			genioglossus (also called *genioglossus muscle*) (*geneion* chin)
			hyobasioglossus (*ypsilon* U-shaped + *basis* base)
			styloglossus (styloid process)
			glottic: phrenoglottic (*phren* diaphragm)
			glottis:
			neoglottis (*neos* new)
			pseudoglottis {pseudoglottic} (*pseudes* false)
			PREFIXED TRAILING ROOT COMPOUND: hemimacroglossia (enlargement of half of the tongue) (*hemi* half + macroglossia)
			CROSS REFERENCE: lingu
gluc			See glyc- for *glucose*.
glut[1]	Greek *gloutos*	buttocks, rump	SIMPLE ROOT: gluteal (pertaining to the buttocks)
			PREFIXED ROOT:
			intergluteal (also called *internatal*) (*inter* between)
			intragluteal (*intra* within)
			mesogluteal (*mesos* middle)

Element	From	Meaning	Examples
glut[1] (cont'd)		[buttocks, rump]	LEADING ROOT COMPOUND: *glut*: glutitis (*itis* inflammation) *gluteo*: gluteofemoral (*femur* thigh) gluteoinguinal (*inguen* groin) TRAILING ROOT COMPOUND: ischiogluteal (*ischium*) CROSS REFERENCE: pyg
glut[2]	Latin *gluten*	glue	SIMPLE ROOT: gluten, glutinous (sticky; adhesive; gluey) PREFIXED ROOT: agglutinin, agglutinant, agglutination {agglutinable} (*ad* to) coagglutination (*com* with + agglutination) conglutinant, conglutination (*com* with) hetereoagglutinin (*heteros* other + agglutinin) isoagglutinin (antibody in a serum which agglutinates the blood cells of those of the same species from which it is derived) (*isos* equal + agglutinin) CROSS REFERENCE: colla, gli
glyc, **gluc**	Greek *glykys* sweet; *gleukos* sweetness	sweet, sugar; glucose	SIMPLE ROOT: *gluc*: glucal (a glycal of glucose), glucan gluconate, glucose, glucoside *glyc*: glycal, glycan, glycation, glycase glycerate, glyceride, glycerin, glycoside PREFIXED ROOT: *glucagon*: glucagonoma (a glucagon-producing tumor) (*oma* tumor) *glucagonemia* condition of glucagon in the blood: hyperglucagonemia (*hyper* above) hypoglucagonemia (*hypo* under) *glucoside*: polyglucoside (*polys* many) *glyc*: hyperglycistia (*hyper* above + *histia* tissue condition) [h of histia elided] *glyco*: hyperglycogenolysis (*hyper* above + *genere* to produce + *lysis* loosening) hyperglycorrhachia (*hyper* above + *rhachis* spine) hyperglycosemia (*hyper* above + *emia* blood condition) *glycemia* sugar condition of the blood: aglycemia (absence of sugar in the blood) (*a* privative) dysglycemia (any disorder of blood sugar metabolism) (*dys* abnormal) euglycemia (also called *normoglycemia*) {euglycemic} (*eu* well) hyperglycemia (opposite of *hypoglycemia*) (*hyper* above) hypoglycemia (opposite of *hyperglycemia*) {hypoglycemic} (*hypo* under) normoglycemia (also called *euglycemia*) (*norma* normal) *glycemic*: orthoglycemic (*orthos* straight + *emia* blood condition) *glycerid*: hyperglyceridemia (*hyper* above + *emia* blood condition) monoglyceride (*monos* single) *glyco*: hypoglycogenolysis (*hypo* under + *genere* to produce + *lysis* dissolution) hypoglycorrhachia (*hypo* under + *rhachis* spine)

A Thesaurus of Medical Word Roots

Element	From	Meaning	Examples
glyc (cont'd)		[sweet, sugar]	LEADING ROOT COMPOUND:
			gluc:
			glucagon (a pancreatic hormone that raises blood sugar), glucago-noma (*agein* to lead + *oma* tumor)
			glucemia (also called *glycemia*) (*emia* blood condition)
			gluco:
			glucofuranose (*furan* a heterocyclic compound)
			glucogenesis {glucogenic} (*genere* to produce)
			glucohemia (also called *glycemia*) (*hemia* blood condition)
			glucokinetic, glucokinin (*kinein* to move)
			glucolysis (*lyein* to loosen)
			gluconeogenesis (*neos* new + *genere* to produce)
			glucopenia (*penia* deficiency)
			glucophore (*pherein* to bear)
			glucoplastic (also called *glucogenic*) (*plassein* to form)
			glucos: glucosuria (also called *glycuresis*) (*uria* urine condition)
			glyc:
			glycemia (also called *glucemia*) (*emia* blood condition)
			glycuresis (also called *glucosuria*) (*uresis* urine excretion)
			glyco:
			glycogen, glycogenesis {glycogenous} (*genere* to produce)
			glycogeusia (*geusia* taste condition)
			glycohemia (also called *glucohemia*) (*hemia* blood condition)
			glycolysis (*lyein* to loosen)
			glycopenia (*penia* deficiency)
			glycopexis {glycopexic} (*pexis* fixation)
			glycophilia (*philein* to love)
			glycoprival (*privus* deprived of)
			glycoptyalism (also called *glycosialia*) (*ptyalon* saliva)
			glycorrhea (any sugary discharge from the body, as of urine) (*rhein* to flow)
			glycosialia (also called *glycoptyalism*), glycosialorrhea (excessive flow of saliva containing sugar) (*sialon* saliva + *rhein* to flow)
			glycotaxis (*tassein* to arrange)
			glycotrophic (also called *glycotropic*) (*trophe* nourishment)
			glycotropic (also called *glycotrophic*) (*trepein* to turn)
			glycos: glycosuria (also called *dextrosuria, glucosuria*) (*uria* urine condition)
			TRAILING ROOT COMPOUND:
			neuroglycopenia (*neuron* nerve + glycopenia)
			normoglycemia (also called *euglycemia*) (*norma* rule, normal + *emia* blood condition)
			CROSS REFERENCE: sacchar
gnath	Greek *gnathos*	jaw, mandible	SIMPLE ROOT:
			gnathic (pertaining to the jaw or cheek)
			gnathion (the lowest point on the median line of the mandible)
			PREFIXED ROOT:
			gnathia:
			agnathia {agnathous} (*a* privative)
			atelognathia (*ateles* incomplete: *a* privative + *telos* complete)
			dysgnathia {dysgnathic} (*dys* abnormal)
			eugnathia {eugnathic; pertaining to a normal state of the maxilla (upper jaw) and mandible (lower jaw)} (*eu* well)
			exognathia (also called *prognathism*) (*exo* outside)

A Thesaurus of Medical Word Roots

Element	From	Meaning	Examples
gnath (cont'd)		[jaw, mandible]	hemignathia (*hemi* half)
			macrognathia (also called *megagnathia*) (*makros* large)
			megagnathia (also called *macrognathia*) (*mega* large)
			micrognathia (also called *brachygnathia*) (*mikros* small)
			prognathia (or, prognathism; also called *progenia*) {prognathic, prognathous} (*pro* forward)
			retrognathia (or, retrognathism) {retrognathic} (*retro* backward)
			syngnathia (*syn* together)
			gnathic:
			eurygnathic (*eurys* wide)
			mesiognathic (*mesos* middle)
			gnathion:
			endognathion (*endon* within)
			exognathion (the alveolar process of the upper jaw) (*exo* outside)
			mesognathion (*mesos* middle)
			gnathism:
			eurygnathism {eurygnathous} (*eurys* wide)
			retrognathism (also called *opisthognathism*) (*retro* backward)
			gnathous:
			anisognathous (*aniso* unequal: *an* negative + *isos* equal)
			hypognathous (*hypo* under)
			isognathous (*isos* equal)
			mesognathous (*mesos* middle)
			prognathous (*pro* forward)
			gnathus:
			augnathus (also called *dignathus*) (*au* again)
			dignathus (a fetus with two lower jaws; also called *augnathus*) (*di* two)
			epignathus {epignathous} (*epi* upon)
			hypognathus {hypognathous} (*hypo* under)
			polygnathus (*poly* many)
			paragnathus (*para* abnormal)
			LEADING ROOT COMPOUND:
			gnath:
			gnathalgia (also called *gnathodynia*) (*algos* pain)
			gnathitis (*itis* inflammation)
			gnathodynia (also called *gnathalgia*) (*odyne* pain)
			gnatho:
			gnathocephalus (a malformed fetus in which the head consists primarily of the jaws) (*kephale* head)
			gnathodynamometer (*dynamis* power + *metron* measure)
			gnathography (*graphein* to write)
			gnathology {gnathologic} (*logos* study)
			gnathoplasty (*plassein* to form)
			gnathoschisis (congenital jaw cleft) (*schisis* fissure)
			gnathostatics (*static* pertaining to standing)
			TRAILING ROOT COMPOUND:
			gnathia:
			apertognathia (also called *open bite*) (*aperture* opening)
			brachygnathia (also called *micrognathia*) (*brachys* short)
			orthognathia {orthognathic} (*orthos* straight, normal)
			gnathic: stomatognathic (denoting the mouth and jaws collectively) (*stomatos* mouth)
			gnathism: opisthognathism (also called *retrognathism*) (*opisthein* behind)

Element	From	Meaning	Examples
gnath (cont'd)		[jaw, mandible]	*gnathous*: orthognathous (*orthos* straight, normal) pachygnathous (*pachys* thick) palatognathous (having a congenital cleft palate) *gnathus*: desmiognathus (*dein* to bind: ligament) myognathus (*myos* muscle) CROSS REFERENCE: geny, maxill
gnos, **gnot,** **gnom**	Greek *gignoskein* to know; *gnosis* knowledge	to know, discern	PREFIXED ROOT: *gnom*: paragnomen (an unexpected reaction) (*para* abnormal) *gnos*: agnosia (loss of comprehension of auditory, visual, or other sensations) (*a* privative) [see separate entry: agnos-] diagnose (lit., to know thoroughly) (*dia* across, through) dysgnosia (*dys* abnormal) eugnosia {eugnostic} (*eu* well, normal) hypergnosis (an exaggerated perception) (*hyper* above) prognose, prognosis {prognostic}, prognosticate (*pro* before) LEADING ROOT COMPOUND: gnotobiota (the specifically and entirely known microfauna and microflora of a specially reared laboratory animal) gnotobiote {gnotobiotic}, gnotobiotics (*bios* life) gnotophoresis (*phorein* to carry) TRAILING ROOT COMPOUND: *gnomic*: thanatognomonic (*thanatos* death) toxignomic (*toxic* poison) *gnomy*: pathognomy (the science of the signs and symptoms of disease) (*pathos* disease) physiognomy (also called *physiognosis*) (physical) *gnosis*: acroagnosis (*akron* extremity + *a* privative) barognosis (or, baragnosis) (*baros* weight) chronognosis (*chronos* time) hemodiagnosis (*haima* blood + diagnosis) immunodiagnosis (immune + diagnosis) lalognosis (*lalein* to speak) physiognosis (also called *physiognomy*) (*physis* nature) somatognosis (also called *cenesthesia*) (*somatos* body) stereognosis {stereognostic} (*stereos* solid) topognosis (also called *topesthesia*) (*topos* place) visuognosis (*videre* to see) *gnosy*: pharmacognosy (*pharmakon* medicine, drug) PREFIXED TRAILING ROOT COMPOUND: abarognosis (loss of sense of weight) (*a* privative + *baros* weight) astereognosis (*a* privative + *stereos* solid) CROSS REFERENCE: None
gon[1]	Greek *gonos* seed	seed, semen	NOTE: This root is extended to include "begetting" or "producing," and denoting "mother cell or structure." SIMPLE ROOT: gonad (the primary sex gland of either sex: ovary, testis) {gonadal} gonidium (the motile reproductive unit of certain nitrogen-fixing bacteria) (pl., gonidia)

Element	From	Meaning	Examples
gon[1] (cont'd)		[seed, semen]	PREFIXED ROOT:

gonad: agonad, agonadal (lacking gonads) (*a* privative)

gonadism:

agonadism (*a* privative)

amphigonadism (*amphi* both)

hypergonadism (*hyper* above)

hypogonadism (*hypo* below)

gonadotropic pertaining to gonad growth:

antigonadotropic (*anti* against)

hypergonadotropic (*hyper* above)

hypogonadotropic (*hypo* under)

gonal: epigonal (*epi* upon)

gonic:

dysgonic (*dys* abnormal)

eugonic (growing luxuriantly: said of bacterial cultures) (*eu* well)

syngonic (*syn* with, together)

gonocyte: protogonocyte (*protos* first + gonocyte)

gonoma: progonoma (*pro* before + *oma* tumor)

gonoplasm: protogonoplasm (*protos* first + *plassein* to form)

gonorrheal: paragonorrheal (*para* alongside + *rhein* to flow)

gonorrheic: antigonorrheic (curative of gonorrhea) (*anti* against + *rhein* to flow)

gony:

amphigony (sexual reproduction) (*amphi* both, around)

ectogony (the influence exerted on the mother by the developing embryo) (*ektos* outside)

heterogony (also called *heterogenesis*) (*heteros* other)

monogony (asexual reproduction) (*monos* single)

LEADING ROOT COMPOUND:

gon: gonacratia (spermatorrhea) (*acratia* incontinence)

gona: gonaduct (the duct of a gonad; an oviduct, or sperm duct) (a mesh of *gonad* + *duct*)

gonad:

gonadarche (the onset of gonadal functioning) (*archein* to begin)

gonadectomy (surgical removal of an ovary or a testis) (*ektome* excision)

gonado:

gonadoblastoma (*blastos* germ, bud, sprout + *oma* tumor)

gonadogenesis (*genesis* beginning)

gonadinhibitory (inhibiting or preventing gonadal activity)

gonadokinetic (stimulating gonadal activity) (*kinein* to move)

gonadopathy (any disease of the gonads) (*pathos* disease)

gonadotoxic {gonadotoxicity}, gonadotoxin (*toxic* poisonous)

gonadotrope (also called *gonadotroph*) {gonadotropic}, gonadotropin (*trepein* to turn)

gonadotroph (also called *gonadotrope*) (*trophein* to nourish)

gone:

gonecystitis (*kystis* bladder, sac + *itis* inflammation)

gonepoiesis {gonepoietic} (*poiein* to make, produce)

gono:

gonoblennorrhea (*blennos* mucus + *rhein* to flow)

gonocele (also called *spermatocele*) (*kele* tumor)

gonochorism (*chorizein* to separate)

gonococcemia (*kokkos* a bacterium + *emia* blood condition)

Element	From	Meaning	Examples
gon[1] (cont'd)		[seed, semen]	gonococcide (also called *gonocide*) (*caedere* to kill) gonococcus (a microorganism causing gonorrhea; pl., gonococci) {gonococcal, gonococcic} (*kokkos* berry: a spherical bacterium) gonocyte (*kytos* cell) gonomery (*meros* part) gononephrotome (*nephros* kidney + *tome* a section) gonophage (*phagein* to devour, consume) gonophore (*pherein* to bear) gonorrhea {gonorrheal} (*rhein* to flow) gonosome (also called *sex chromosome*) (*soma* body) gonotome (that part of the mesoderm which develops into the reproductive organs of the embryo) (*tome* a section) TRAILING ROOT COMPOUND: *gone*: androgone (a spermatogenic cell) (*andros* man) *gonium*: myelogonium (*myelos* marrow) oogonium (*oon* egg, ovum) spermatogonium (*sperma* seed, sperm) *gony*: archegony (spontaneous generation) (*archein* to be first) cytogony (cytogenic reproduction) (*kytos* cell) gametogony (*gamos* reproduction) merogony (*meros* part) schizogony (*schizein* to divide) sporogony (*sporos* seed) CROSS REFERENCE: blast, gen, oo, ov, semen, sperm, spor
gon[2]	Greek *gonia*	angle	SIMPLE ROOT: gonion (a cephalometric landmark, designating external angles of the mandible; pl., gonia) PREFIXED ROOT: *gonal*: trigonal (triangular) (*tri* three) *gonial*: bigonial (*bi* two) intergonial (*inter* between) *gonium*: pregonium (*pre* before) *gonum*: tetragonum (a platelike muscle) (*tetra* four) trigonum (pl., trigona) (*tri* three) LEADING ROOT COMPOUND: goniocraniometry (measurement of the cranial, or head, angles) (*kranion* skull + *metron* measure) goniodysgenesis (aberration of the anterior ocular segment) (*dys* abnormal + genesis) goniometer (an instrument for measuring angles; also called *pronometer*) (*metron* measure) goniophotography (photography of the angle of the anterior chamber of the eye) (*photos* light + *graphein* to write) goniopuncture (*pungere* to pierce) gonioscope {gonioscopy} (*skopein* to examine) goniosynechia (*synechia* adhesion of parts) goniotomy (*tomy* incision) TRAILING ROOT COMPOUND: stethogoniometer (an apparatus for measuring the curvature of the chest) (*stethos* chest + *metron* measure) CROSS REFERENCE: canth

Element	From	Meaning	Examples
gon[3]	Greek *gony*	knee	LEADING ROOT COMPOUND: *gon*: gonagra (gout in the knee) (*agra* seizure) gonalgia (*algos* pain) gonarthritis (*arthron* joint + *itis* inflammation) gonitis (or, goneitis) (*itis* inflammation) *gonato*: gonatocele (tumor of the knee) (*kele* tumor) *gono*: gonocampis (permanent flexion of the knee) (*kamptos* bent, curved) *gony*: gonycampis (abnormal curvature of the knee) (*kamptos* bent) gonycrotesis (also called *genu valgum*—knock-knee) (*krotesis* striking) gonyoncus (*onkos* bulk, tumor) *gonyo*: gonyocele (synovitis of the femorotibial joint) (*kele* tumor) TRAILING ROOT COMPOUND: hydropneumogony (the injection of air into a joint to determine the amount of effusion) CROSS REFERENCE: geni[2], patella
graft	Latin *graphium* fr. Greek *grapheion* stylus	bud, shoot	SIMPLE ROOT: graft (any tissue or organ for transplantation) PREFIXED ROOT: allograft (also called *homograft, allogeneic graft*) (*allos* other) autograft (tissue transplanted from one place to another on the same body) (*autos* self) endograft (*endon* within) heterograft (also called *xenograft*) (*heteros* other, different) homograft (*homos* same) isograft (also called *syngraft, isotransplant*) (*isos* equal) perigraft (*peri* around) syngraft (*syn* together) TRAILING ROOT COMPOUND: xenograft (also called *heterograft*) (*xenos* strange) CROSS REFERENCE: blast, germ, gon[1], sperm, spor
gram			See graph-.
gran	Latin *granum* a grain	grain, particle	SIMPLE ROOT: grana, granula (granule; pl., granulae) granular (made up of or marked by presence of granules or grains) granulatio (a granule, or granular mass; pl. granulationes) granulation (the division of hard or metallic substances into small particles) granule (or, granula) granulose (the main constituent of the starch grain or granule) PREFIXED ROOT: *granul*: paragranuloma (a type of Hodgkin's disease) (*para* alongside + *oma* tumor) *granular*: intergranular (between the granule cells of the brain) (*inter* between) subgranular (somewhat granular) (*sub* below) *granulo*: hypogranulocytosis (also called *granulocytopenia*) (*hypo* under + *kytos* cell + *osis* condition) progranulocyte (also called *promyelocyte*) (*pro* before + *kytos* cell) LEADING ROOT COMPOUND: *grano*: granoplasm (granular protoplasm) (*plassein* to form)

Element	From	Meaning	Examples
gran (cont'd)		[grain, particle]	*granul*: granuloma, granulomatosis (*oma* tumor + *osis* condition) granulosis {granulosity} (*osis* condition) *granuli*: granuliform (*forma* shape) *granulo*: granuloadipose (*adipose* fat) granuloblast (also called *myeloblast*) (*blastos* germ, sprout) granulocyte (*kytos* cell) granulomere (also called *chromomere*) (*meros* part) granulopenia (also called *granulocytopenia, agranulocytosis*) (*penia* deficiency) granuloplasm (the inner substance of an ameba, or other unicellular organism) {granuloplastic} (*plassein* to form) granulopoiesis {granulopoietic} (*poiein* to make, produce) granulopotent (*potis* ability, power) TRAILING ROOT COMPOUND: *granuloma* granulous tumor: angiogranuloma (an angioma containing granulation tissue) lipogranuloma (a nodule of lipoid material associated with granulomatous inflammation; also called *oleogranuloma*) (*lipos* fat) lymphogranuloma (Hodgkin's disease) (*lympha* water, liquid) oleogranuloma (also called *lipogranuloma*) (*oleum* oil) trichogranuloma (*trichos* hair) ulcerogranuloma (ulcer) xanthogranuloma (a tumor having histologic characteristics of both granuloma and xanthoma) (*xanthos* yellow) CROSS REFERENCE: chondr
graph, **gram**	Greek *graphein* to write *gramma* drawing	writing; record of writing	SIMPLE ROOT: graph (a diagram or curve representing clinical or experimental data), graphic, graphics, graphite PREFIXED ROOT: *gram*: agrammatism (inability to speak grammatical or intelligible sentences or to arrange words in grammatical sequence, due to a cerebral disease) (*a* privative) diagram {diagrammatic} (*dia* across) kilogram (*chilioi* thousand) polygram (*polys* many) program (a formal set of procedures for conducting an activity) *graph*: micrograph (*mikros* small) polygraph (*polys* many) pyelograph (*pyelos* pelvis) *graphia*: agraphia (loss of the ability to write) (*a* privative) dysgraphia (*dys* abnormal) palingraphia (writing backward) (*palin* backward) paragraphia (*para* abnormal) *graphy*: micrography (*mikros* small) retrography (mirror writing) (*retro* backward) LEADING ROOT COMPOUND: *graph*: graphanesthesia (*anesthesia* lack of perception) graphesthesia (*esthesia* perception)

A Thesaurus of Medical Word Roots

Element	From	Meaning	Examples
graph (cont'd)		[writing]	*grapho*: graphology (*logos* study) graphomotor (*movere* to move) graphophobia (*phobia* fear) graphorrhea (writing of many meaningless words and phrases) (*rhein* to flow) graphospasm (writer's cramp) (*span* to contract) TRAILING ROOT COMPOUND: (Examples) *gram*: actinogram (*aktis* ray) angiogram (*angeion* blood vessel) aortogram (aorta) arteriogram (artery) arthrogram (*arthron* joint) cardiogram (*kardia* heart) mammogram (*mamma* breast) nephrogram (*nephros* kidney) renogram (*renes* kidney) somatogram (*somatos* body) sonogram (*sonus* sound) thermogram (*therme* heat) tachogram (*tachys* swift, fast) *graphy*: adenography (*adenos* gland) amniography (*amnion* fetal membrane) angiography (*angeion* blood vessel) aortography (aorta) arteriography (artery) arthrography (*arthron* joint) anthropography (*anthropos* mankind; human beings) balneography (*balneum* bath) bronchography (*bronchos* windpipe) cardiography (*kardia* heart) craniography (*kranion* skull) desmography (*desmos* band: ligament) diskography (disk—of spine) echography (also called *ultrasonography*) enterography (*enteron* intestine) epidemiography (epidemic) fetography (fetus) hepatography (*hepatos* liver) histography (*histos* web, tissue) laryngography (larynx) lymphography (*lympha* water, fluid) mammography (*mamma* breast) myelography (*myelos* marrow) myography (*myos* muscle) nephrography (also called *renography*) (*nephros* kidney) nosography (*nosos* disease) odontography (*odontos* tooth) oncography (*onkos* mass, tumor) organography (organs) osteography (*osteon* bone) otography (*otos* ear)

A Thesaurus of Medical Word Roots

Element	From	Meaning	Examples
graph (cont'd)		[writing]	parietography (*paries* wall—of an organ)
			pathography (*pathos* disease)
			phlebography (also called *venography*) (*phlebos* vein)
			planigraphy (also called *tomography*) (*planus* plane)
			pleurography (*pleura* rib, side)
			pneumography (*pneuma* breath, gas)
			portography (portal vein)
			posturography (posture)
			proctography (*proktos* anus, rectum)
			ptyalography (also called *sialography*) (*ptyalon* saliva)
			pyelography (*pyelos* pelvis)
			rachigraphy (*rachis* spine)
			renography (*renes* kidney)
			salpingography (*salpingos* tube)
			saphenography (saphena—a type of vein)
			skeletography (skeleton)
			sphygmography (*sphygmos* pulse)
			splanchnography (*splanchnos* viscus)
			splenography (also called *lienography*, although this term is rarely used) (spleen)
			tachography (*tachys* swift, fast)
			tenontography (*tenontos* tendon)
			thermography (*therme* heat)
			tocography (*tokos* childbirth)
			tomography (*tomos* a cutting)
			tonography (*tonos* tension, pressure—of eye)
			ureterography (ureter)
			urethrography (urethra)
			urography (*ouron* urine: urinary tract)
			uterography (also called *hysterography*) (uterus)
			varicography (*varix* a varicose vein)
			vasography (also called *angiography*) (*vas* vessel)
			venography (also called *phlebography*) (*vena* vein)
			vesiculography (*vesicula* small bladder, sac)
			viscerography (*viscera* internal organs)
			CROSS REFERENCE: None
grav	Latin *gravis* heavy *gravida* pregnant	heavy; pregnant	SIMPLE ROOT:
			grave (serious, dangerous, severe)
			gravid (pregnant) {gravidic}, gravida (a pregnant woman)
			gravidism (pregnancy, or the sum of symptoms, signs, and conditions associated with it), graviditas (pregnancy)
			gravidity (pregnancy; the conditions of being pregnant, without regard to the outcome)
			gravitation, gravity
			PREFIXED ROOT:
			gravescent: ingravescent (increasing in severity) (*in* intensive)
			gravid: progravid (before or preceding pregnancy) (*pro* before)
			gravida:
			multigravida (*multus* many)
			nulligravida (*nullus* none)
			octigravida (*octo* eight)
			plurigravida (*plus* more, many)
			primigravida (*prima* first)
			secundigravida (written *gravida II*) (second)

Element	From	Meaning	Examples
grav (cont'd)		[heavy, pregnant]	septigravida (*septum* seven)
			sextigravida (written *Gravida VI*) (*sexti* six)
			tertigravida (written *Gravida III*) (*tertius* third)
			unigravida (also called *primigravida*) (*uni* one)
			LEADING ROOT COMPOUND:
			gravi:
			gravimeter {gravimetric; determined by weight) (*metron* measure)
			gravistatic (due to gravitation, as gravistatic pulmonary congestion) (*statikos* causing to stand)
			gravido:
			gravidocardiac (pertaining to cardiac disorders resulting from pregnancy) (*kardia* heart)
			gravidopuerperal (pertaining to pregnancy and puerperium, or the final stage of labor)
			gravito: gravitometer (*metron* measure)
			DISGUISED ROOT: grief (a normal response to an external loss)
			CROSS REFERENCE: bar, cyes
gyn	Greek *gyne* woman	woman; female sex [female reproductive organs]	SIMPLE ROOT: gynecic (pertaining to or associated with women)
			PREFIXED ROOT:
			digyny (or, digynia; fertilization of one ovum by more than one spermatazoon) (*di* two)
			polygyny (*polys* many)
			LEADING ROOT COMPOUND:
			gyn:
			gynander, gynandrism, gynandry (*andros* man)
			gynandroid (*andros* man + *eidos* form)
			gynandromorphism (an abnormal combination of male and female characteristics) (*andros* man + *morphe* shape)
			gynatresia (occlusion of some part of the female genital tract, especially of the vagina) (*atresis* imperforation)
			gyne:
			gyneduct (*ductere* to lead)
			gynephobia (*phobia* fear)
			gynec: gynecoid (*eidos* form)
			gyneco:
			gynecogen {gynecogenic} (*genere* to produce)
			gynecography (*graphein* to write)
			gynecology {gynecologic} (*logos* study)
			gynecomania (satyriasis) (*mania* craze)
			gynecomastia, gynecomastism (*mastos* breast)
			gynecopathy (*pathos* disease)
			gyno:
			gynogenesis (*genere* to produce)
			gynopathic, gynopathy (*pathos* disease)
			gynophobia (or, gynephobia) (*phobia* fear)
			gynoplasty (*plassein* to form)
			TRAILING ROOT COMPOUND:
			androgyny (sexual ambiguity, either physical or psychological) {androgynous} (*andros* man)
			hologynic (counterpart is *holandric*) (*holos* whole, entire)
			misogyny (an aversion or hatred of women) (*misein* to hate)
			pseudogynecomastia (enlargement of the male breast by an excess of adipose tissue) (*pseudes* false + *mastia* breast condition)
			CROSS REFERENCE: None

Element	From	Meaning	Examples
gyr	Greek *gyros* Latin *gyrare* to turn	ring, circle; convolution	SIMPLE ROOT: gyrate (twisted in a ring or spiral shape) gyration (a circular motion or revolution; arrangement of convolutions or gyri in the cerebral cortex) gyrose (or, gyrous; marked by curved lines or circles) gyrus (pl., gyri) PREFIXED ROOT: *gyral*: intergyral (*inter* between) intragyral (*intra* within) *gyria*: agyria {agyric} (*a* privative) macrogyria (also called *pachygyria*) (*makron* large) microgyria (also called *polymicrogyria*) (*mikros* small) pachygyria (also called *macrogyria*) (*pachys* thick) polygyria (also called *polymicrogyria*) (*polys* many) polymicrogyria (also called *polygyria*) (*polys* many + microgyria) *gyrus*: subgyrus (any gyrus that is partly concealed or covered by another or by others) (*sub* below) LEADING ROOT COMPOUND: *gyr*: gyrectomy (*ektome* excision) gyrencephalic (*enkephalon* brain) *gyro*: gyrochrome (*chroma* color) gyrometer (*metron* measure) gyrospasm (*span* to contract) TRAILING ROOT COMPOUND: *gyral*: dextrogyral (also called *dextrorotatory*) (*dexter* right) levogyral (*laevus* left) *gyration*: oculogyration (*oculus* eye) sinistrogyration (*sinister* left) *gyria*: ischogyria (a condition in which the cerebral convolutions have a jagged appearance, as in bulbar sclerosis) (*ischein* to suppress) oculogyria (the limits of rotation of the eyeballs) (*oculus* eye) pachygyria (also called *macrogyria*) (*pachys* thick) schizogyria (the presence of wedge-shaped cracks in the convolutions of the brain) (*schizein* to split) ulegyria (a cerebral cortex in which the gyri are narrow and distorted by scars) (*oule* scar, cicatrix) CROSS REFERENCE: an, cycl, orb

Element	From	Meaning	Examples
hal	Greek *hals*	salt	SIMPLE ROOT: halide (a compound of a halogen) PREFIXED ROOT: *alomenia* condition of salt in the blood: [h of halo elided] hyperalonemia (also called *hypersalemia*) (*hyper* above) hypoalonemia (also called *hyposalemia*) (*hypo* under) LEADING ROOT COMPOUND: *hal*: haloid (*eidos* form) *hali*: haliphagia (*phagein* to consume, devour) halisteresis (or, halosteresis) {halisteretic} (*steresis* loss, deprivation) *halo*: halobacterium (pl., halobacteria) halodermia (also called *halogenoderma*) (*derma* skin) haloduric (*durare* to last, endure) halogen, halogenoderma (*genere* to produce + *derma* skin) halophil, halophile, halophilic (*philein* to love—an affinity for) halosteresis (or, halisteresis; a loss or lack of the lime salts of bone; also called *osteomalacia*) (*steresis* loss) TRAILING ROOT COMPOUND: osteohalisteresis (a condition of soft bones caused by a loss or deficiency of mineral elements) (*osteon* bone + *steresis* deprivation) CROSS REFERENCE: sal
hapl-	Greek *haploos*	simple, single	See Appendix B for examples of words with this initial combining form. Others are listed with roots to which it is attached. CROSS REFERENCE: mono-
hapt, **haph,** **haps,** **hapte,** **aph,** **aps**	Greek *haptein* to touch Latin *apere* to reach	to touch, to seize upon, to hold fast; seizure	SIMPLE ROOT: hapten, haptene, heptenic, haptic, apsis PREFIXED ROOT: *aph*: diaphemetric (*dia* through + *metron* measure) [h is elided] *aphia*: [h is elided] amblyaphia (dull sense of touch) (*amblys* dull) anaphia (lack or loss of the sense of touch) {anaptic} (*an* privative) dysaphia (impairment of the sense of touch; also called *paraphia*, *pseudaphia*) {dysaphic} (*dys* abnormal) hyperaphia (also called *tactile hyperesthesia*) {hyperaphic} (*hyper* above) paraphia (also called *dysaphia, pseudaphia*) (*para* abnormal) pseudaphia (also called *dysaphia, paraphia*) (*pseudes* false) *apho*: synaphoceptors (*syn* together + receptor) [h is elided] *apsis*: [h is elided] metasynapsis (also called *metasyndesis*) (*meta* after + synapsis) parasynapsis (*para* alongside + synapsis) synapsis (*syn* with, together) *haph*: anhaphia (or, anaphia) (*an* privative) *haps*: ephapse {ephaptic} (*epi* upon) LEADING ROOT COMPOUND: *aph*: aphephobia (or, haphephobia) (*phobia* fear) *haph*: haphalgesia (*algos* pain) *haphe*: haphephobia (or, haptephobia; a morbid dislike or fear of being touched) (*phobia* fear)

Element	From	Meaning	Examples
hapt (cont'd)		[to touch]	*hapto*: haptodysphoria (an unpleasant sensation derived from touching certain objects) (*dys* abnormal + *phorein* to bear) haptoglobin (globin: the protein constituent of hemoglobin) haptometer (an instrument for measuring the sensitivity to touch) (*metron* measure) CROSS REFERENCE: palp
helc **(elc)**	Greek *helkos*	sore, ulcer	LEADING ROOT COMPOUND: *helc*: helcoid (resembling an ulcer) (*eidos* form) helcoma (corneal ulcer) (*oma* tumor, ulcer) helcosis (ulceration; the formation of an ulcer) (*osis* condition) *helco*: helcology (the scientific study of ulcers) (*logy* study) helcomenia (occurrence of ulcers at the time of a menstruation) (*menia* menstruation condition) helcoplasty (the act or process of repairing lesions made by ulcers, especially by plastic operation) (*plassein* to form) TRAILING ROOT COMPOUND: *elcosis* ulcerous condition: [h is elided] cystelcosis (*kystis* bladder) enterelcosis (*enteron* intestine) nephrelcosis (*nephros* kidney) omphalelcosis (*omphalos* navel, umbilicus) prostatelcosis (prostate) psorelcosis (ulceration of the skin resulting from scabies) (*psora* itch) splenelcosis (spleen) *helcosis* ulcerous condition: dacryohelcosis (*dacryon* tear) keratohelcosis (ulceration of the cornea) (*keratos* cornea) masthelcosis (*mastos* breast) othelcosis (ulceration of the auricle or external meatus of the ear; suppuration of the middle ear) (*otos* ear) CROSS REFERENCE: noma, ulc
helix, **helic**	Greek *helix*	coil, spiral	SIMPLE ROOT: *helic*: helical (or, helicine; of a spiral form; of or pertaining to the helix) *helix*: helix (a coiled structure, such as the coil of wire in an electromagnet; also, margin of the external ear; pl., helices) PREFIXED ROOT: *helic*: prehelicine (in front of the helix of the pinna) (*pre* before) superhelicity (*super* above) *helix*: anthelix (or, antihelix; curved prominence of the external ear parallel to and in front of the helix) (*anti* against) superhelix (*super* above) LEADING ROOT COMPOUND: *helic*: helicoid (*eidos* form) *helico*: helicopodia (a gait seen in some conversion reactions or hysteric disorders, in which feet imitate half circles) (*podos* foot) helicotrema (an opening at the apex of the cochlea) (*trema* hole) CROSS REFERENCE: cochl, spir

A Thesaurus of Medical Word Roots

Element	From	Meaning	Examples
helminth	Greek *helmins,* *helminthos*	worm	SIMPLE ROOT: helminth {helminthic}, helminthism PREFIXED ROOT: anthelminthic (or, anthelmintic; destructive to worms; an agent that is destructive to worms) (*anti* against) LEADING ROOT COMPOUND: *helminth*: helminthagogue (also called *anthelmintic, vermifuge*) (*agein* to lead) helminthemesis (*emesis* vomiting) helminthiasis (*iasis* condition) helminthoid (*eidos* form) helminthoma (*oma* tumor) *helmintho*: helminthology (*logos* study) helminthophobia (*phobia* fear of) TRAILING ROOT COMPOUND: nemathelminth (*nema* thread) platyhelminth (also called *flatworm*) (*platys* flat, broad) pseudohelminth (*pseudes* false) CROSS REFERENCE: scol
hem, **hemo,** **em,** **-emia** (see Appendix C)	Greek *haima,* *hematos*	blood	NOTE: The elided form of *haima* and *hematos* is *em;* a blood condition is indicated by the suffix *-emia.* SIMPLE ROOT: hemal, hematal, hematic (or, hemic), hematin PREFIXED ROOT: *emia* blood condition: anemia (a reduction in the number of circulating erythrocytes or in the quantity of hemoglobin) {anemic} (*an* privative) dysemia (*dys* abnormal) exemia (*ex* out) hyperemia {hyperemic}, hyperemization (*hyper* above) panhyperemia (*pan* all + *hyper* above, beyond) *emo*: anemotrophy (*an* privative + *trophe* nourishment) *hematocrit*: microhematocrit (*mikros* small + *krinein* to discern) *hematopenia*: panhematopenia (*pan* all + *penia* deficiency) *hematopoiesis* production of blood: anhematopoiesis (*an* privative) dyshematopoiesis (or, dyshemopoiesis) (*dys* abnormal) *hemo*: anhemolytic (*an* privative + *lyein* to loosen) antihemolysin (*anti* against + *lyein* to loosen) antihemorrhagic (*anti* against + *rhagic* bursting forth) autohemolysin, autohemolysis (*autos* self + *lyein* to loosen) autohemotherapy (also called *autotransfusion*) (*autos* self + *therapy* treatment) hyperhemoglobinemia (*hyper* above + hemoglobin + *emia* blood condition) isohemagglutination (*isos* equal + agglutination) isohemolysis {isohemolytic} (*isos* equal + *lysein* to loosen) parahemophilia (*para* abnormal + *philein* to love) posthemorrhagic (*post* following) LEADING ROOT COMPOUND: *hem*: hemadsorption (*ad* to + *sorbere* to suck) hemagogue {hemagogic} (*agein* to lead) hemamebiasis (any infection with ameboid forms of parasites in red blood cells, as in malaria)

Element	From	Meaning	Examples
hem (cont'd)		[blood]	hemanalysis (analysis)
			hemapheresis (*apheresis* removal)
			hemarthrosis (*arthron* joint + *osis* condition)
			hemerythrin (the coloring matter of the blood of earthworms which is contained in the plasma) (*erythros* red)
			hemisotonic (*isos* equal + *tonus* tone)
			hemophthalmia (*ophthalmia* eye condition)
			hema:
			hemachrome (*chroma* color)
			hemacytometer (or, hemocytometer) (*kytos* cell + *metron* measure)
			hemafacient (also called *hematopoietic*) (*facere* to make)
			hemaphein, hemapheism (*phaios* dusky)
			hemathermal, hemathermous (*therme* heat)
			hemado: hemadostenosis (the narrowing or obliteration of a blood vessel) (*stenos* narrow + *osis* condition)
			hemangi blood vessel:
			hemangiectasis (or, hemangiectasia) (*ektasis* a stretching)
			hemangioma, hemangiomatosis (*oma* tumor + *osis* condition)
			hemangio blood vessel:
			hemangioblast, hemangioblastoma (*blastos* germ + *oma* tumor)
			hemangioendothelioblastoma (endothelium + blastoma)
			hemangioendothelioma (endothelium + *oma* tumor)
			hemangiofibroma (fiber + *oma* tumor)
			hemangiolymphoangioma (lyphoma + angioma)
			hemangiopericytoma (pericyte + *oma* tumor)
			hemangiosarcoma (*sarkos* flesh + *oma* tumor)
			hemat:
			hematapostema (*apostema* abscess)
			hematemesis (*emesis* vomiting)
			hematencephalon (also called *cerebral hemorrhage*) (*enkephalos* brain)
			hematidrosis (*hidros* sweat) [h of hidros elided]
			hematoid (resembling blood) (*eidos* form)
			hematoma (*oma* tumor)
			hematomphalocele (*omphalos* umbilicus + *kele* hernia)
			hematopsia (also called *hemophthalmia*) (*opsia* vision condition)
			hematosis (*osis* condition)
			hematosteon (*osteon* bone)
			hematuria (*uria* urine condition)
			hemato:
			hematoblast (*blastos* bud, shoot, germ)
			hematocele (*kele* tumor)
			hematocephaly (*kephale* head)
			hematochezia (*chezein* to defecate)
			hematochlorin (*chloros* light green)
			hematochromatosis (*chroma* color + *osis* condition)
			hematochyluria (*chylos* chyle + *uria* urine condition)
			hematocoelia (also called *hemoperitoneum*) (*koilia* cavity)
			hematocolpometra (*kolpos* vagina + *metra* uterus)
			hematocolpos (*kolpos* vagina)
			hematocrit (*krinein* to separate)
			hematocryal (also called *poikilothermic*) (*kryos* cold)
			hematocyst (or, hematocystis) (*kystis* sac, bladder)
			hematocyte, hematocytoblast (*kytos* cell + *blastos* germ, cell)

Element	From	Meaning	Examples
hem (cont'd)		[blood]	hematodyscrasia (or, hemodyscrasia) (*dyscrasia* bad mixture)
			hematodystrophy (or, hemodystrophy) (*dystrophy* bad nourishment)
			hematoencephalic (*enkephalon* brain)
			hematogenesis (also called *hemopoiesis*) {hematogenic, hematogenous} (*genere* to produce)
			hematogone (*gone* seed)
			hematohidrosis (the excretion of blood or blood pigment in the sweat; also called *hemidrosis*) (*hidrosis* sweat condition)
			hematohistioblast (*histion* web, tissue + *blastos* germ, cell)
			hematology (*logy* study)
			hematolymphangioma (*lympha* water, liquid + *angeion* vessel + *oma* tumor)
			hematolysis {hematolytic} (*lyein* to dissolve)
			hematometra (*metra* uterus)
			hematometry (*metron* measure)
			hematomyelia, hematomyelitis (*myelos* marrow + *itis* inflammation)
			hematomyelopore (*myelos* marrow + *poros* pore)
			hematopathology, hematopathy (*pathos* disease + *logos* study)
			hematopenia (*penia* deficiency)
			hematoperitoneum (or, hemoperitoneum) (peritoneum)
			hematophagia (also called *hemoposia*; the drinking of blood, as by parasites) {hematophagous} (*phagein* to consume)
			hematoplastic (or, hemoplastic) (*plassein* to form)
			hematopoiesis (also called *hematogenesis, hemogenesis*) {hematopoietic} (*poiein* to make, produce)
			hematorrhachis (also called *hematomyelia*) (*rhachis* spine)
			hematorrhea (copious hemorrhage) (*rhein* to flow)
			hematosalpinx (*salpinx* tube)
			hematosepsis (also called *septicemia*) (*sepsis* decay)
			hematospectroscope (*specere* to see + *skopein* to examine)
			hematospermatocele (*spermatos* seed + *kele* tumor)
			hematothermal (or, homeothermic) (*therme* heat)
			hematotoxic, hematotoxicosis (*toxikosis* poisonous condition)
			hematotrachelos (*trachelos* neck—of uterus)
			hematotropic (*tropos* a turning)
			hematozemia (*zemia* loss)
			hematozoan (any living organism in the blood) (*zoon* animal)
			hemo:
			hemochromatosis (*chroma* color + *osis* condition)
			hemocyanin (*kyanos* the color blue)
			hemocyte (*kytos* cell)
			hematorrhachis (*rhachis* spine)
			hemodialysis (dialysis: *dia* across + *lyein* to loosen)
			hemodynamics (*dynamis* power)
			hemofiltration (filter)
			hemoflagellates (*flagellum* whip)
			hemoglobin (*globus* ball, sphere)
			hemohistioblast (*histion* web, tissue + *blastos* germ, cell)
			hemolymph (*lympha* water, fluid)
			hemolysin, hemolysis {hemolytic} (*lyein* to loosen)
			hemonephrosis (*nephrosis* kidney condition)
			hemopathology, hemopathy (*pathos* disease + *logy* study)
			hemopericardium (*peri* around + *kardia* heart)
			hemoperitoneum (peritoneum)

Element	From	Meaning	Examples
hem (cont'd)		[blood]	hemophile, hemophilia (*philein* to love—have an affinity for)
			hemophobia (*phobia* fear)
			hemorrhage (*rhage* bursting forth)
			hemorrhoid {hemorrhoidal}, hemorrhoidectomy (*rhein* to flow + *ektome* excision)
			hemosialemesis (*sialon* saliva + *emesis* vomiting)
			hemosiderosis (*sideros* iron + *osis* condition)
			hemospermia (blood in the semen) (*spermia* semen condition)
			hemosporidium (*sporidium* small seed)
			hemostasis {hemostatic} (*stasis* standing still)
			hemostaxis (*staxis* a dripping)
			hemostyptic (*styptikos* astringent)
			hemotachometer (or, hematachometer) (*tachos* swiftness + *metron* measure)
			hemotherapy (*therapy* treatment)
			hemothorax (or, hemathorax) (*thorax* chest)
			hemotoxic (or, hematotoxic, hematoxic) (*toxikon* poison)
			hemotroph (or, hemotrophe) {hemotrophic} (*trophe* nourishment)
			hemotropic (*trope* a turning)
			hemotympanum (or, hematotypanum) (*tympanon* eardrum)
			hemozoic (*zoion* animal)
			TRAILING ROOT COMPOUND:
			emia blood condition: (Examples)
			acidemia (acid)
			alkalemia (alkali)
			bacillemia (bacilli)
			bacteremia (bacteria)
			calcemia (also called *hypercalcemia*) (calcium)
			canceremia (cancer cells)
			chloremia (also called *chlorosis, hyperchloremia*) (*chloros* green)
			cholemia (*chole* bile)
			chylemia (*chylus* juice)
			fructosemia (fructose)
			fungemia (fungus)
			glycemia (*glykys* sweet, sugar)
			hydremia (*hydor* water)
			icteroanemia (*ikteros* jaundice + anemia)
			inosemia (*inos* fiber)
			ischemia (an insufficient supply of blood to an organ) (*ischein* to hold, suppress)
			ketonemia (ketone)
			leukemia (*leukos* white—blood cells)
			myelemia (*myelos* marrow, spinal cord)
			oligemia (*oligos* scant, little)
			parasitemia (parasites)
			pseudoanemia (*pseudes* false + anemia)
			pyemia (or, pyohemia) (*pyon* pus)
			septicemia (*sepsis* putrefaction)
			toxemia (also called *toxicohemia*) (*toxikon* poison)
			uremia (*ouron* urine)
			hemal: neurohemal (*neuron* nerve)
			hematoma blood tumor:
			cephalhematoma (or, cephalohematoma) (*kephale* head)
			meninghematoma (*meningos* membrane)

Element	From	Meaning	Examples
hem (cont'd)		[blood]	*hematuria*: icterohematuria (*ikteros* jaundice + *uria* urine condition) *hemoglobin*: myohemoglobin (*myos* muscle + hemoglobin) *hemophilia*: deuterohemophilia (*deuteros* second + *philein* to love) *hemorrhea*: dacryohemorrhea (*dakryon* tear + *rhein* to flow) PREFIXED TRAILING ROOT COMPOUND: *emia* blood condition: aglycemia (*a* privative + *glykys* sugar, sweet) aleukemia (also called *leukopenia*) (*a* privative + *leukos* white) anhydremia (*an* privative + *hydor* water, fluid) anoxemia (*an* privative + *oxys* sharp) dysglycemia (*dys* abnormal + *glykys* sweet: sugar) endotoxemia (*endon* within + *toxikos* poison) hypercalcemia (*hyper* above + calcium) hyperglycemia (*hyper* above + *glykys* sugar) hyperlipidemia (*hyper* above + *lipos* fat) hypervolemia (*hypo* under + volume) hypocalcemia (*hypo* under + calcium) hypoglycemia (*hypo* under + *glykys* sugar) hypovolemia (*hypo* under + volume) polycythemia (*polys* many + *kytos* cell) CROSS REFERENCE: sangui
hemi-	Greek prefix	half	See Appendix B for examples of words with this prefix. Others are listed with the root to which it is attached. CROSS REFERENCE: medi-
hepa	Greek *hepar,* *hepatos*	liver	SIMPLE ROOT: hepar, heparin, heparinate hepatic, hepatism (ill health due to liver disease), hepatization PREFIXED ROOT: *heparin*: hyperheparinemia (*hyper* above + *emia* blood condition) *hepatectomy*: hemihepatectomy (*hemi* half + *ektome* excision) *hepatia*: dyshepatia (disordered liver function) (*dys* abnormal) hyperhepatia (*hyper* over, beyond) hypohepatia (*hypo* under) megalohepatia (*megalos* large) microhepatia (*mikros* small) *hepatic*: extrahepatic (*extra* outside) infrahepatic (also called *subhepatic*) (*infra* below) intrahepatic (*intra* within) parahepatic (*para* alongside) perihepatic (*peri* around) posthepatic (*post* behind) subhepatic (also called *infrahepatic*) (*sub* below) suprahepatic (*supra* over) transhepatic (*trans* across) *hepatitis* inflammation of the liver: parahepatitis (*para* alongside) perihepatitis (inflammation of the peritoneal capsule of the liver and other nearby tissues) (*peri* around) *hepatized*: dehepatized (having the liver removed) (*de* negative) LEADING ROOT COMPOUND: *hepat*: hepatalgia (also called *hepatodynia*) (*algos* pain)

Element	From	Meaning	Examples
hepa (cont'd)		[liver]	hepatatrophia (or, hepatatrophy) (atrophy; *a* privative + *trophein* to nourish)
			hepatectomy (*ektome* excision)
			hepatitis {hepatitic} (*itis* inflammation)
			hepatodynia (also called *hepatalgia*) (*odyne* pain)
			hepatoid (*eidos* form; similar to)
			hepatoma (*oma* tumor)
			hepatomphalos, hepatomphalocele (*omphalos* navel + *kele* hernia)
			hepatosis (*osis* condition)
			hepatico:
			hepaticodochotomy (combined hepaticotomy and choledochotomy) (*tomy* incision)
			hepaticoduodenostomy (duodenum + *stoma* mouth, opening)
			hepaticoenterostomy (*enteron* intestine + *stoma* mouth, opening)
			hepaticogastrostomy (*gaster* stomach + *stoma* mouth, opening)
			hepaticolithotomy (*lithos* stone + *tomy* incision)
			hepaticolithotripsy (*lithos* stone + *tripsis* rubbing: friction)
			hepaticopulmonary (also called *hepatopneumonic*) (*pulmon* lung)
			hepaticostomy (*stoma* mouth, opening)
			hepaticotomy (*tomy* incision)
			hepato:
			hepatobiliary (bile)
			hepatoblastoma (*blastos* germ, cell + *oma* tumor)
			hepatobronchial (*bronchos* windpipe)
			hepatocarcinogenesis (*karkinos* cancer + *genere* to produce)
			hepatocele (*kele* hernia)
			hepatocholangitis (*chole* bile + *angeion* blood vessel + *itis* inflammation)
			hepatocirrhosis (*kirrhos* orange-yellow + *osis* condition)
			hepatocolic (*kolon* colon)
			hepatocystic (*kystis* bladder)
			hepatocyte (*kytos* cell)
			hepatoduodenal (duodenum)
			hepatoenterostomy (*enteron* intestine + *stoma* mouth, opening)
			hepatofugal (*fugere* to flee)
			hepatogastric (*gaster* stomach)
			hepatogenic (or, hepatogenous) (*genere* to produce)
			hepatogram, hepatography (*graphein* to write)
			hepatojugular (jugular vein)
			hepatolienal, hepatolienomegaly (*lien* spleen + *megalos* large)
			hepatolith, hepatolithectomy (*lithos* stone + *ektome* excision)
			hepatolithiasis (*lithos* stone + *iasis* condition)
			hepatology (*logy* study)
			hepatolysis {hepatolytic} (*lyein* to loosen)
			hepatomalacia (*malakos* soft)
			hepatomegaly (or, hepatomegalia) (*megalos* large)
			hepatomelanosis (*melanos* dark, black + *osis* condition)
			hepatometry (*metron* measure)
			hepatonecrosis (*nekrosis* death)
			hepatonephritis (*nephros* kidney + *itis* inflammation)
			hepatonephromegaly (*nephros* kidney + *megalos* large)
			hepatopathy {hepatopathic} (*pathos* disease)
			hepatoperitonitis (peritoneum + *itis* inflammation)
			hepatopetal (*petere* to seek)

A Thesaurus of Medical Word Roots

Element	From	Meaning	Examples
hepa (cont'd)		[liver]	hepatopexy (*pexis* fixation)
			hepatophlebitis (*phlebos* vein + *itis* inflammation)
			hepatophrenic (*phren* diaphragm)
			hepatophyma (*phyma* tumor, growth)
			hepatopleural (*pleura* rib, side)
			hepatopneumonic (*pneumon* lung)
			hepatoportal (*portal* entrance, gateway)
			hepatoptosis (*ptosis* a falling, prolapse)
			hepatopulmonary (also called *hepatopneumonic*) (*pulmon* lung)
			hepatorenal (*ren* kidney)
			hepatorrhagia (*rhagia* bursting forth)
			hepatorrhaphy (*rhaphe* suture)
			hepatorrhea (*rhein* to flow)
			hepatorrhexis (*rhexis* rupture)
			hepatoscopy (*skopein* to examine)
			hepatosplenitis (spleen + *itis* inflammation)
			hepatosplenomegaly (spleen + *megalos* large)
			hepatosplenopathy (spleen + *pathos* disease)
			hepatostomy (*stoma* mouth, opening)
			hepatotherapy (*therapy* treatment)
			hepatotomy (*tomy* incision)
			hepatotoxic (*toxic* poison)
			hepatotropic (*tropein* to turn)
			TRAILING ROOT COMPOUND:
			hepatic pertaining to the liver:
			adipohepatic (*adeps* fat)
			cardiohepatic (*kardia* heart)
			duodenohepatic (*duodenum*)
			enterohepatic (*enteron* intestine)
			gastrohepatic (*gaster* belly)
			phrenohepatic (*phren* diaphragm)
			pulmonohepatic (*pulmon* lung)
			hepatitis inflammation of the liver:
			gastrohepatitis (*gaster* stomach)
			icterohepatitis (*ikteros* jaundice)
			pleurohepatitis (*pleura* side, rib)
			purohepatitis (*puris* pus)
			steatohepatitis (*steatos* fat)
			hepato: splenohepatomegalia (spleen + *megalos* large)
			CROSS REFERENCE: None
heres, **eres**	Greek *hairein*	to take	PREFIXED ROOT:
			apheresis (withdrawal of blood from a donor) (*apo* away)
			dieresis (the division or separation of parts normally united; in surgery, the operative separation of parts by incision, electrosurgery, or cautery) (*dia* apart) [h is elided]
			exeresis (also called *excision*) (*ex* out) [h is elided]
			syneresis (a drawing together of the particles of the dispersed phase of a gel) (*syn* together) [h is elided]
			TRAILING ROOT COMPOUND:
			apheresis: [h is elided]
			erythrocytapheresis (*erythros* red + *kytos* cell)
			hemapheresis (also called *apheresis*) (*haima* blood)
			leukapheresis (*leukos* white)
			lymphapheresis (*lympha* fluid)

Element	From	Meaning	Examples
heres (cont'd)		[to take]	plasmapheresis (plasma) thrombocytapheresis (*thrombos* clot + *kytos* cell) *eresis*: [h is elided] cholaneresis (cholane) choleresis (*chole* bile) cytodieresis (*kytos* cell + dieresis) CROSS REFERENCE: apheres, lep[2]
hern	Latin *hernia*	protrusion, rupture	SIMPLE ROOT: hernia (the protrusion of a loop or knuckle of an organ or tissue through an abnormal opening; pl., herniae) {hernial}, herniated, herniation PREFIXED ROOT: endoherniotomy (*endon* within + *tomy* incision) perihernial (*peri* around) LEADING ROOT COMPOUND: *herni*: hernioid (*eidos* form) *hernio*: hernioappendectomy (appendix + *ektome* excision) hernioenterotomy (*enteron* intestine + *tomy* incision) herniography (*graphein* to write) herniolaparotomy (laparotomy for the treatment of hernia) (*lapara* flank, loins + *tomy* incision) hernioplasty (*plassein* to form) herniorrhaphy (surgical procedure for hernia) (*rhaphe* suture) herniotomy (also called *celotomy, kelotomy*) (*tomy* incision) TRAILING ROOT COMPOUND: pseudohernia (an inflamed sac or gland simulating strangulated hernia) (*pseudes* false) CROSS REFERENCE: rhex
heter-	Greek *heteros*	other, another, different	See Appendix B for examples of words with this prefix. Others are listed with the root to which it is attached. CROSS REFERENCE: all, alter, aniso
hidr	Greek *hidros*	sweat, perspiration	PREFIXED ROOT: *hidrosis* sweat condition: anhidrosis (an abnormal deficiency of sweat) {anhidrotic; or, *anidrotic*} (*an* privative) dyshidrosis (*dys* abnormal) hemihidrosis (*hemi* half) hemihyperhidrosis (excessive sweating on one side of the body only; also called *hemidiaphoresis*) (*hemi* half + hyperhidrosis) hyperhidrosis (also called *hyperidrosis, polyhidrosis, polyidrosis*) {hyperhidrotic} (*hyper* above) hypohidrosis (or, hyphidrosis) {hypohidrotic} (*hypo* under) panhidrosis (or, panidrosis; sweating of the entire surface of the body) (*pan* all) parahidrosis (or, paridrosis) (*para* abnormal) polyhidrosis (also called *hyperhidrosis*) (*polys* much) synhidrosis (sweating, especially excessive sweating associated with another condition) (*syn* with) LEADING ROOT COMPOUND: *hidr*: hidradenitis (or, hidrosadenitis, hydradenitis) (*adenos* gland + *itis* inflammation) hidrosis {hidrotic} (*osis* condition) *hidro*: hidroacanthoma (acanthoma) (*akantha* thorn + *oma* tumor)

Element	From	Meaning	Examples
hidr (cont'd)		[sweat]	hidrocystoma (also called *syringocystoma*) (*kystis* sac + *oma* tumor)
			hidromeiosis (*meiosis* a lessening)
			hidropoiesis {hidropoietic} (*poiein* to make, produce)
			hidrorrhea (profuse perspiration) (*rhein* to flow)
			hidroschesis (suppression of the perspiration) (*schesis* holding back)
			TRAILING ROOT COMPOUND:
			hidrosis sweat condition:
			acrohyperhidrosis (*akron* extremity + *hyper* above)
			bromhidrosis (also called *osmidrosis*) (*bromos* stench)
			chromhidrosis (*chroma* color)
			hematohidrosis (or, hematidrosis) (*hematos* blood)
			menhidrosis (*men* month: menstruation)
			urhidrosis (or, uridrosis) (*ouron* urine)
			idrosis sweat condition [h is elided]
			chylidrosis (sweating of a fluid resembling chyle)
			galactidrosis (sweating a milky fluid) (*gala* milk)
			osmidrosis (also called *bromhidrosis*) (*osme* smell)
			podobromidrosis (*podos* foot + *bromos* stench)
			CROSS REFERENCE: sud
hist	Greek *histos* loom, web	web, tissue (body tissue)	SIMPLE ROOT: histamine, histic, histidine, histidyl, histone
			PREFIXED ROOT:
			anhistic, anhistous (*an* privative)
			antihistamine (*anti* against)
			microhistology (*mikros* small + *logos* study)
			polyhistiocytoma (*polys* many + *kytos* cell + *oma* tumor)
			LEADING ROOT COMPOUND:
			hist:
			histanoxia (*an* privative + *oxia* oxygen condition)
			histoid (or, histioid) (*eidos* form)
			histoma (*oma* tumor)
			histamin: histaminemia (*emia* blood condition)
			histidin:
			histidinemia (*emia* blood condition)
			histidinuria (*uria* urine condition)
			histio:
			histioblast (or, histoblast) (*blastos* germ, cell)
			histiocyte {histiocytic}, histiocytoma (*kytos* cell + *oma* tumor)
			histiocytosis (*kytos* cell + *osis* condition)
			histo:
			histoblast (or, histioblast) (*blastos* germ)
			histoclastic (*klaein* to break)
			histocyte (*kytos* cell)
			histodiagnosis
			histodialysis (*dialysis* loosening)
			histogenesis {histogenetic}, histogenous, histogeny (*genere* to produce)
			histogram, histography (*graphein* to write)
			histohematogenous (*hematos* blood + *genere* to produce)
			histohydria (*hydria* water or liquid condition)
			histohypoxia (*hypo* under + *oxia* oxygen condition)
			histokinesis (*kinesis* motion)
			histology {histologic} (*logy* study)
			histolysis {histolytic} (*lyein* to loosen)
			histomorphology (*morphe* form + *logos* study)

Element	From	Meaning	Examples
hist (cont'd)		[tissue]	histonomy (a law of the development and structure of the tissues of the body) (*nomos* law) histopathogenesis (*pathos* disease + *genesis* origin) histopathology (*pathos* disease + *logos* study) histophagous (*phagein* to consume, devour) histophyly (the tribal history of cells; a division of morphophyly) (*phylon* race, tribe) histophysiology (*physis* nature + *logos* study) histoplasmoma (*plassein* to form + *oma* tumor) histoplasmosis (*plassein* to form + *osis* condition) historadiography (radium + *graphein* to write) historrhexis (*rhexis* rupture) histoteliosis (*telos* end + *osis* condition) histotherapy (*therapy* treatment) histotomy (also called *microtomy*) (*tomy* incision) histotoxic (*toxic* poisonous) histotroph {histotrophic} (*trophe* nourishment) histotropic (*tropos* a turning) histozoic (*zoion* animal) *histon*: histonuria (*uria* urine condition) PREFIXED TRAILING ROOT COMPOUND: hyperglycistia (excess of sugar in the bodily tissues) (*hyper* above + *glykys* sugar) [h is elided] CROSS REFERENCE: None
hol	Greek *holos*	whole, entire	See Appendix B for examples of words with this element. Others are placed with the roots to which it is attached. CROSS REFERENCE: pan
hom, **homeo**	Greek *homos* same	same, shared, similar, resembling	PREFIXED ROOT: anomaly (marked deviation from the normal standard) {anomalous} [h is elided] See Appendix B for examples of words with these initial combining forms. Others are listed with the roots to which they are attached. CROSS REFERENCE: cen, iso
humer	Latin *humerus* from Greek *omos* shoulder	upper arm	SIMPLE ROOT: humerus (the bone that extends from the shoulder to the elbow; pl., humeri) PREFIXED ROOT: subhumeral (*sub* below) transhumeral (*trans* across) LEADING ROOT COMPOUND: humeroradial (radius) humeroscapular (*scapula* shoulder blade) TRAILING ROOT COMPOUND: acromiohumeral (*acromion* high point of the shoulder) coracohumeral (of or relating to the coracoid process and the humerus) facioscapulohumeral (relating to or affecting the muscles of the face, scapula, and arm) glenohumeral (*glene* socket) radiohumeral (radius) scapulohumeral (*scapula* shoulder blade) thoracicohumeral (*thorax* chest) PREFIXED TRAILING ROOT COMPOUND: intercostohumeral (relating to an intercostal space and the arm) (*inter* between + *costa* rib, side) CROSS REFERENCE: None

Element	From	Meaning	Examples
hydr	Greek *hydor*	water	SIMPLE ROOT: hydrase, hydrate, hydrated, hydration hydride (any compound of hydrogen with an element or radical) hydrops (edema; also called *dropsy*) PREFIXED ROOT: *hydr:* anhydration (dehydration) {anhydrous}, anhydride (*an* privative) anhydrochloria (also called *anchlorohydria*) (*an* privative + *chloros* green) antihydropic (effective against dropsy) (*anti* against) dehydrant, dehydrate, dehydration (*de* negative) dihydrate {dihydric} (*di* two) euhydration (*eu* well) hyperhydration (also called *overhydration*) (*hyper* above) isohydric (*isos* equal) monohydrated, monohydric (*monos* single) polyhydric, polyhydruria (*polys* many + *uria* urine condition) trihydric (containing three hydrogen atoms) (*tri* three) *hydremia* condition of fluid in the blood: anhydremia (*an* privative) hypohydremia (*hypo* under) *hydro:* hyperhydropexy (*hyper* above + *pexis* fixation) *hydruria:* isohydruria (*isos* equal + *uria* urine condition) LEADING ROOT COMPOUND: *hydr:* hydraeroperitoneum (*aer* air + peritoneum) hydragogue (*agein* to lead) hydranencephaly (*an* privative + *enkephalon* brain) hydrarthrosis (*arthrosis* joint condition) hydraulics (*aulos* pipe) hydremia (*emia* blood condition) hydromphalus (*omphalos* navel) hydrophthalmos (*ophthalmos* eye) hydrovarium (ovary) hydruria {hydruric} (*uria* urine condition) *hydro:* hydroadipsia (*a* privative + *dipsia* thirst condition) hydrocele, hydrocelectomy (*kele* hernia + *ektome* excision) hydrocephalus, hydrocephaly {hydrocephalic} (*kephale* head) hydrochloric (*chloros* green) hydrocholecystis (*chole* bile + *kystis* bladder) hydrocholeresis {hydrocholeretic} (*chole* bile + *hairein* to take) [h is elided] hydrocholesterol (a reduced form of cholesterol) hydrocolpos (*kolpos* vagina) hydrocyst, hydrocystoma (*kystis*, sac, bladder + *oma* tumor) hydrocytosis (*kytos* cell + *osis* condition) hydrodipsia, hydrodipsomania (*dipsa* thirst + *mania* frenzy) hydrodiuresis (*diuresis* urination) hydrodynamics (*dynamis* power) hydroencephalocele (*enkephalon* brain + *kele* tumor) hydrogen, hydrogenate (*genere* to produce) hydrography (*graphein* to write) hydrohymenitis (*hymen* membrane + *itis* inflammation)

Element	From	Meaning	Examples
hydr (cont'd)		[water]	hydrokinetic(s) (*kinein* to move)
			hydrolabile {hydrolability} (*labilis* unstable)
			hydrology (*logy* study)
			hydrolymph (*lympha* water, liquid)
			hydrolysis {hydrolytic} (*lyein* to loosen)
			hydromeningitis (*meningos* membrane + *itis* inflammation)
			hydrometer {hydrometric} (*metron* measure)
			hydrometra (*metra* uterus)
			hydrometrocolpos (*metra* uterus + *kolpos* vagina)
			hydromyelia (*myelia* marrow condition)
			hydronephrosis (*nephrosis* kidney condition)
			hydropenia {hydropenic} (*penia* deficiency)
			hydropericarditis (pericardium + *itis* inflammation)
			hydroperitoneum (peritoneum)
			hydropexis {hydropexic} (*pexis* fixation)
			hydrophilic, hydrophilous (*philein* to love)
			hydrophobia (a former term for *rabies*, from the symptomatic in- ability to swallow liquids), hydrophobic (not capable of uniting with or absorbing water) (*phobia* fear)
			hydropneumatosis (*pneumatosis* the presence of air or gas)
			hydrorrhea (*rhein* to flow)
			hydrostabile (*stabilis* stable)
			hydrostat, hydrostatic, hydrostatics (*statikos* standing)
			hydrotaxis (*taxis* arrangement)
			hydrotherapy (*therapy* treatment)
			hydrothermal (*therme* heat)
			hydrotomy (*tomy* incision)
			hydrotropism (*trepein* to turn)
			PREFIXED TRAILING ROOT COMPOUND:
			achlorhydria (*a* privative + *chloros* green)
			hyperchlorhydria (*hyper* excessive + *chloros* green)
			CROSS REFERENCE: lymph
hymen	Greek *hymen,* *hymenos*	membrane, caul	SIMPLE ROOT:
			hymen (the membranous fold which partially or wholly occludes the external orifice of the vagina) {hymenal}
			hymenium (the fertile, or spore-producing, surface of a fungus, which is composed of hyphae living on the fruiting body)
			LEADING ROOT COMPOUND:
			hymen:
			hymenectomy (*ektome* excision)
			hymenitis (*itis* inflammation)
			hymeno:
			hymenology (*logy* study)
			hymenopterism (poisoning from a winged insect) (*pteron* wing)
			hymenorrhaphy (the closure of the vagina by sutures at the hymen; also called *hymen reconstruction surgery*) (*rhaphe* suture)
			hymenotome, hymenotomy (*tomy* incision)
			TRAILING ROOT COMPOUND:
			nymphohymeneal (*nymphe* labia minora)
			pachymenia (an abnormal thickness of the skin or other membrane) (*pachys* thick)
			phacohymenitis (also called *phacocystitis*: inflammation about the capsule of the crystalline lens) (*phakos* lens + *itis* inflammation)
			CROSS REFERENCE: chori, ependym, mening, pia

Element	From	Meaning	Examples
hyper-	Greek prefix	over, above	See Appendix B for examples of words with this prefix. Others are listed with the root to which it is attached. CROSS REFERENCE: super-
hypo-	Greek prefix	under, below	See Appendix B for examples of words with this prefix. Others are listed with the roots to which it is attached. CROSS REFERENCE: sub-
hypophys	Greek *hypo* under + *phyein* to grow	pituitary gland	SIMPLE ROOT: hypophysis (the pituitary gland, which is attached by a stalk to the hypothalamus) {hypophysial} PREFIXED ROOT: parahypophysis (*para* resembling) LEADING ROOT COMPOUND: *hypophys*: hypophysectomy (*ektome* excision) hypophysitis (*itis* inflammation) *hypophyseo*: hypophyseoportal (*porta* gate, opening) hypophyseoprivic (or, hypophysioprivic) (*privare* to deprive) *hypophysio*: hypophysiotropic (*tropein* to turn) TRAILING ROOT COMPOUND: adenohypophysis (the anterior lobe of the hypophysis, consisting of the distal part, intermediate part, and infundibular part) (*adenos* gland) neurohypophysis (also called *lobus nervosus*) (*neuron* nerve) CROSS REFERENCE: None
hyster	Greek *hystera*	womb, uterus	SIMPLE ROOT: hysteria (so called because the Ancients believed that women were more excitable than men; therefore, their excitability was due to the uterus overacting) {hysteric, hysterical}, hystericism, hysterics PREFIXED ROOT: anthysteric (or, antihysteric) (*anti* against) dihysteria (*di* two) panhysterectomy (*pan* all + *ektome* excision) LEADING ROOT COMPOUND: *hyster*: hysteralgia (also called *hysterodynia*) (*algos* pain) hysteratresia (*atresia* imperforate) hysterectomy (*ektome* excision) hystereurysis (*eurysis* dilation) hysterodynia (also called *hysteralgia*) (*odyne* pain) hysteroid (*eidos* form) *hysteri*: hysteriform (*forma* form, shape) *hystero*: hysterocatalepsy (hysteria with cataleptic manifestations) hysterocele (*kele* hernia) hysterocleisis (surgical occlusion of the uterus) (*kleisis* closure) hysterocolpectomy (*kolpos* vagina + *ektome* excision) hysterocolposcope (*kolpos* vagina + *skopein* to examine) hysterocystopexy (*kystis* bladder + *pexis* fixation) hysterogenic (or, hysterogeny) (*genere* to produce) hysterogram, hysterograph, hysterography (*graphein* to write) hysterolith (uterine calculus) (*lithos* stone) hysterolysis (*lyein* to loosen) hysterometer, hysterometry (*metron* measure) hysteromyomectomy (also called *myomectomy*) (*myoma* muscle tumor + *ektome* excision)

Element	From	Meaning	Examples
hyster (cont'd)		[womb, uterus]	hysteromyotomy (*myos* muscle + *tomy* incision)
			hystero-oophorectomy (*oophor* egg-bearing + *ektome* excision)
			hysteropathy (*pathos* disease)
			hysteropexy (*pexis* fixation)
			heteroplasty (also called *uteroplasty*) (*plassein* to form)
			hysteroptosia (or, hysteroptosis) (*ptein* to fall: prolapse)
			hysterorrhaphy (*rhaphe* suture)
			hysterorrhexis (also called *metrorrhexis*) (*rhexis* rupture)
			hysterosalpingectomy (*salpingos* tube + *ektome* excision)
			hysterosalpingography (also called *hysterotubography*) (*salpingos* tube + *graphein* to write)
			hysterosalpingo-oophorectomy (*salpingos* tube + *oophor* egg-bearing + *ektome* excision)
			hysterosalpingostomy (*salpingos* tube + *stoma* mouth, opening)
			hysteroscope {hysteroscopy} (*skopein* to examine)
			hysterospasm (*spasmos* contraction)
			heterosystole (*systole* contracting)
			hysterothermometry (measurement of uterine temperature) (*therme* heat + *metron* measure)
			hysterotomy (*tomy* incision)
			hysterotrachelectasia (*trachelos* cervix + *ektasia* dilatation)
			hysterotracheloplasty (*trachelos* cervix + *plassein* to form)
			hysterotrachelorrhaphy (*trachelos* cervix + *rhaphe* suture)
			hysterotrachelectomy (*trachelos* cervix + *ektome* excision)
			hysterotubography (also called *hysterosalpingography*) (tube + *graphein* to write)
			TRAILING ROOT COMPOUND:
			colpohysteropexy (the fixation of a displaced vagina and uterus) (*kolpos* vagina + *pexy* fixation)
			sonohysterography (*sonus* sound + *graphein* to write)
			CROSS REFERENCE: colp, metr, uter

A Thesaurus of Medical Word Roots

Element	From	Meaning	Examples
iat(r)	Greek *iatrein* to heal *iatreia* cure	healing, care, treatment, remedy	SIMPLE ROOT: iatric (pertaining to medicine or to a physician) {iatrical} LEADING ROOT COMPOUND: *iath*: iathergy (the state of immunity existing in an immunized organism in which the tuberculin skin sensitivity has been abolished by specific desensitization) (*ergon* work) *iatr*: iatraliptics (treatment by inunction and friction) {iatraliptic} (*aleiphein* to anoint) *iatro*: iatrogenesis {iatrogenic} (*genere* to produce) iatrology (*logos* study) iatrophysics (*physic* natural) TRAILING ROOT COMPOUND: *iater*: philiater (a person interested in medical science; particularly, a medical student) (*philein* to love) *iatria*: odontoiatria (dental therapeutics) (*odontos* tooth) *iatrics*: andriatrics (the study of diseases of men, especially of the genital organs) (*andros* man) bariatrics (the study of obesity) (*baros* weight) ephebiatrics (also called *hebiatrics*) (*ephebos* early manhood) geriatrics (*geras* old age) gyniatrics (*gyne* woman, female) hebiatrics (also called *ephebiatrics*) (*hebe* youth) kinesiatrics (also called *kinesitherapy*) (*kinein* to move) ophthalmiatrics (*ophthalmos* eye) pediatrics (*pais* child) phoniatrics (also called *logopedics*) (*phone* sound) physiatrics (or, physiatry) (*physikos* nature) podiatric (*podos* foot) ponesiatrics (*ponesis* toil, exertion) presbyatrics (also called *geriatrics*) (*presbys* old) psychiatrics (*psyche* mind) *iatry*: laliatry (the study of speech disorders) (*lalein* to babble) pediatry (also called *pediatrics*) (*pais* child) podiatry (*pous* foot) psychiatry (*psyche* soul, mind) CROSS REFERENCE: therap
ict	Latin *ictus*	stroke, seizure	SIMPLE ROOT: ictus {ictal} PREFIXED ROOT: interictal (*inter* between) intraictal (occurring during an attack or seizure) (*intra* within) postictal (*post* after) preictal (occurring before a stroke or an attack, as before an acute epileptic attack) (*pre* before) LEADING ROOT COMPOUND: ictometer (an apparatus for determining the force of the apex beat of the heart) (*metron* measure) CROSS REFERENCE: agra, crot, epilep, palp, pleg, sphygmo

Element	From	Meaning	Examples
ide	Greek *idein* to see	appearance, form	SIMPLE ROOT: idea, ideal, idealist, idealization, ideation PREFIXED ROOT: anideus {anidean}, anidous (without form due to arrested development) (*an* privative) monoideism (a marked preoccupation with one idea or subject; a slight degree of monomania) (*monos* single) LEADING ROOT COMPOUND: ideogenetic (or, ideogenous) (*genere* to produce) ideokinetic (also called *ideomotor*) (*kinein* to move) ideology (*logy* study) ideomotion (also called *ideokinetic*) {ideomotor} (*movere* to move) ideophobia (*phobia* fear) CROSS REFERENCE: eid, form, morph, phan, plas
idio	Greek *idios*	one's own; peculiar, separate	SIMPLE ROOT: idiocy, idiot (lit., a private person; orig., one incapable of holding public office) See Appendix B for examples of words with this combining form. Others are placed with the roots to which it is attached. CROSS REFERENCE: auto, noe
idrosis			See hidr-.
il-[1]	Latin prefix	in, on	See Appendix B (in-[1]) for examples of words with this prefix. Others are listed with the roots to which it is attached. CROSS REFERENCE: in[1]
il-[2]	Latin prefix	negative	See Appendix B (in-[2]) for examples of words with this prefix. Others are listed with the roots to which it is attached. CROSS REFERENCE: in[2]
ile	Greek *eilein* to roll up, to twist	ileum, lower abdomen; lower intestines	SIMPLE ROOT: ileum (the lower portion of the intestines, opening into the large intestine) {ileac, ileal} ileus (obstruction of the intestines) {ileac} LEADING ROOT COMPOUND: *ile*: ileectomy (*ektome* excision) ileitis (*itis* inflammation) *ileo*: ileocecum {ileocecal} (*caecum* blind: blind gut) ileocolic, ileocolitis (colon + *itis* inflammation) ileocolonic (or, ileocolic) (colon) ileocolostomy (colon + *stoma* mouth, opening) ileocystoplasty (*kystis* bladder + *plassein* to form) ileoileostomy (ileum + *stoma* mouth, opening) ileojejunitis (jejunum + *itis* inflammation) ileopexy (*pexis* fixation) ileoproctostomy (*proktos* anus, rectum + *stoma* mouth, opening) ileorectostomy (also called *ileoproctostomy*) (rectum + *stoma* mouth, opening) ileorrhaphy (*rhaphein* to suture) ileosigmoidostomy (sigmoid + *stoma* mouth, opening) ileostomy (*stoma* mouth, opening) ileotomy (*tomy* incision) ileovesical (also called *vesicoileal*) (*vesica* bladder) TRAILING ROOT COMPOUND: pseudoileus (*pseudes* false) ureteroileostomy (ureter + *stoma* mouth, opening) CROSS REFERENCE: abdom, cel[1], ventr

Element	From	Meaning	Examples
ilio	Latin *ilium*	ilium, iliac region, groin, flank	SIMPE ROOT: ilium [os ilii; the upper and largest part of the hip bone (os coxae); pl., ilia] {iliac} PREFIXED ROOT: bisiliac (*bis* two) subilium {subiliac} (*sub* under) transiliac (across or between the ilia) (*trans* across) LEADING ROOT COMPOUND: iliococcygeal (coccyx) iliocolotomy (*kolon* colon + *tomy* incision) iliocostal (*costa* rib) iliofemoral, iliofemoroplasty (femur + *plassein* to form) iliohypogastric (pertaining to the ilium and hypogastrium) ilioinguinal (*inguen* groin) iliolumbar (*lumbar* loin) iliometer (*metron* measure) iliopagus (*pagus* fixed) iliopectineal (*pectineal* combed, ridged) iliopelvic (pelvis) iliosacral (sacrum) iliosciatic (ischium) iliospinal (spine) iliothoracopagus (*thorax* chest + *pagos* fixed) iliotibial (tibia) iliotrochanteric (*trochanter* a runner) ilioxiphopagus (*xiphos* sword: xiphoid process + *pagos* fixed) TRAILING ROOT COMPOUND: femoroiliac (femur) lumboiliac (*lumbus* loin) sacroiliac, sacroiliitis (sacrum + *itis* inflammation) vertebroiliac (vertebra) CROSS REFERENCE: inguen
im-¹	Latin prefix	in, into, on	See Appendix B (in-¹) for examples of words with this prefix. Others are listed with the roots to which it is attached. CROSS REFERENCE: en-
im-²	Latin prefix	negative	See Appendix B (in-²) for examples of words with this prefix. Others are listed with the roots to which it is attached. CROSS REFERENCE: ab-, dis-
immun	Latin *im* negative + *munia* duties, functions	free, exempt	SIMPLE ROOT: immune, immunity, immunization, immunize PREFIXED ROOT: heteroimmune, heteroimmunity (*heteros* other) hyperimmune {hyperimmunity}, hyperimmunization (*hyper* above) isoimmunization (*isos* equal) nonimmune, nonimmunity (also called *aphylaxis*) (*non* negative) panimmunity (an immunity to many infectious diseases) (*pan* all) LEADING ROOT COMPOUND: immunoadjuvant (*adjuvant* helper) immunobiology {immunobiological} (*bios* life + *logy* study) immunoblast (also called *lymphoblast*) (*blastos* germ, cell) immunogen {immunogenic} (*genere* to produce) immunopathogenesis (*pathos* disease + *genere* to produce) immunostimulant (*stimulus* goad, incentive) immunotherapy (*therapy* treatment) immunotoxin (*toxin* poison) CROSS REFERENCE: lys

A Thesaurus of Medical Word Roots

Element	From	Meaning	Examples
in-[1]	Latin prefix	in	See Appendix B for examples of words with this prefix, together with assimilations and elisions. Others are attached to the roots to which it is attached. CROSS REFERENCE: en-
in-[2]	Latin prefix	negative	See Appendix B for examples of words with this prefix, together with assimilations and elisions. Others are attached to the roots to which it is attached. CROSS REFERENCE: a-, ab-, de-
in	Greek *inos*	fiber	See Appendix B for examples of words with this element. Others are placed with the roots to which it is attached. CROSS REFERENCE: fibr
infra-	Latin prefix	below, beneath	See Appendix B for examples of words with this prefix. Others are listed with the roots to which it is attached. CROSS REFERENCE: sub-
inguen, inguin	Greek *inguen*	the groin	SIMPLE ROOT *inguen*: inguen (the lowest part of the abdominal wall, near the junction of the trunk and thigh; also called *groin*; pl., inguina) *inguin*: inguinal (pertaining to the inguen, or groin) PREFIXED ROOT: infrainguinal (*infra* below, beneath) suprainguinal (*supra* superior to, over) LEADING ROOT COMPOUND: *inguin*: inguinodynia (*odyne* pain) *inguino*: inguinoabdominal (abdomen) inguinocrural (*crus* thigh) inguinolabial (*labium* lip—fleshy border) inguinoperitoneal (peritoneum) inguinoscrotal (*scrotum* bag: testicle pouch) TRAILING ROOT COMPOUND: gluteoinguinal (pertaining to the buttock and groin) (*gloutos* buttock) ilioinguinal (iliac) lumboinguinal (pertaining to the loins and the groin) (*lumbus* loin) ventroinguinal (pertaining both to the abdomen and groin, or to the abdomen and inguinal canal, as ventroinguinal hernia) (*venter* abdomen) CROSS REFERENCE: ili
ini	Greek *inion*	occiput: back of head	SIMPLE ROOT: iniad (toward the inion), inion {iniac, inial} See Appendix B for examples of words with this initial combining form. Others are listed with the roots to which it is attached. CROSS REFERENCE: occip
insul, isol	Latin *insula*	island	SIMPLE ROOT: *isol*: isolate, isolation, isolator *insul*: insula (pl., insulae) {insular}, insulate, insulation, insulator insulin, insulinase (an enzyme in body tissue which destroys or inactivates insulin), insulism (also called *hyperinsulinism*) PREFIXED ROOT: *insular*: circuminsular (*circum* around) contrainsular (*contra* against) hyperinsulinar (*hyper* above)

Element	From	Meaning	Examples
insul (cont'd)		[island]	peri-insular (*peri* around)
			retroinsular (*retro* behind)
			transinsular (*trans* across)
			insulin:
			anti-insulin (*anti* against)
			proinsulin (*pro* before)
			insulinism:
			hyperinsulinism (also called *hyperinsulinemia*) (*hyper* above)
			hypoinsulinism (deficient secretion of insulin by the pancreas, resulting in hyperglycemia) (*hypo* under)
			LEADING ROOT COMPOUND:
			insul:
			insulitis (*itis* inflammation)
			insuloma (or, insulinoma; an adenoma of the islands of Langerhans of the pancreas) (*oma* tumor)
			insulin:
			insulinemia (*emia* blood condition)
			insulinoid (resembling insulin; any substance with hypoglycemic properties like those in insulin) (*eidos* form)
			insulinoma (or, insuloma) (*oma* tumor)
			insulino:
			insulinogenesis {insulinogenic} (*genere* to produce)
			insulinopenic (*penia* deficiency)
			insulo: insulogenic (or, insulinogenic) (*genere* to produce)
			CROSS REFERENCE nesi
inter- **intero-**	Latin prefix	among, between	EXTENDED PREFIX: intern, internal, internalization, internist
			See Appendix B for examples of words with these prefixes. Others are attached to the roots to which they are attached.
			CROSS REFERENCE: None
intestin	Latin *intestinus* inward, internal	intestine	SIMPLE ROOT: intestine {intestinal}, intestinum (pl., intestina)
			PREFIXED ROOT:
			circumintestinal (also called *circumenteric*) (*circum* around)
			extraintestinal (*extra* outside)
			intraintestinal (*intra* within)
			juxtaintestinal (*juxta* near)
			supraintestinal (*supra* superior)
			LEADING ROOT COMPOUND:
			intestinocystoplasty (also called *enterocystoplasty*) (*kystis* bladder + *plassein* to form)
			intestino-intestinal (pertaining to two different portions of the intestine, as the intestino-intestinal reflex)
			TRAILING ROOT COMPOUND:
			cholecystointestinal (*chole* bile + *kystis* bladder)
			enterointestinal (also called *intestino-intestinal*) (*enteron* intestine)
			gastrointestinal (also called *gastroenteric*) (*gaster* belly, stomach)
			musculointestinal (muscle)
			renointestinal (also called *enterorenal*) (*ren* kidney)
			ureterointestinal (of, relating to, or connecting the intestine and a ureter, as in *ureterointestinal anastomosis*)
			vesicointestinal (also called *enterovesical*) (*vesica* bladder)
			CROSS REFERENCE: enter, visc
intra- **intro-**	Latin prefix	within	See Appendix B for examples of words with these prefixes. Others are attached to the roots to which they are attached.
			CROSS REFERENCE: endo-, ento-

Element	From	Meaning	Examples
iod	Greek *ioeides* violet-colored	violet, iodine	SIMPLE ROOT: iodide, iodinate {iodination}, iodine, iodism, iodize PREFIXED ROOT: deiodination (*de* opposite) hyperiodemia (*hyper* beyond + *emia* blood condition) hypoiodidism (*hypo* under) subiodide (*sub* under) triiodide (*tri* three) LEADING ROOT COMPOUND: *iod*: iodemia (*emia* blood condition) iodopsin (also called *visual violet*) (*ops* eye) ioduria (*uria* urine condition) *iodi*: iodimetry (*metron* measure) *iodino*: iodinophil {iodinophilous} (*philein* to love—an affinity for) *iodo*: iododerma (*derma* skin) iodoform, iodoformism (poisoning by iodoform) (*formyl*) iodogenic (*genere* to produce) iodoglobulin (an iodine containing globulin) iodometry {iodometric} (*metron* measure) iodophilia, iodophilous (*philein* to love—have an affinity for) iodophor (*pherein* to bear) iodotherapy (*therapy* treatment) CROSS REFERENCE: None
ir-[1]	Latin prefix	in, into, on	See Appendix B (in-[1]) for examples of words with this prefix. Others are listed with the roots to which it is attached. CROSS REFERENCE: en-
ir-[2]	Latin prefix	negative	See Appendix B (in-[2]) for examples of words with this prefix. Others are listed with the roots to which it is attached. CROSS REFERENCE: a-, ab-, de-, dis-
irid, iris	Greek *iris* rainbow	colored circle; iris (of the eye)	SIMPLE ROOT: iridescence, iridescent, iridization, iris (pl., irides) {iridal, iridial, iridian, iridic} PREFIXED ROOT: *iridia*: aniridia (absence of the iris) (*an* privative) retroiridian (*retro* posterior) *iris*: ectiris (*ektos* outside) entiris (*entos* inside) LEADING ROOT COMPOUND: *ir*: iritis {iritic} (*itis* inflammation) *iri*: iridesis (or, iridodesis) (*desis* binding: fixation) *irid*: iridalgia (*algos* pain) iridauxesis (thickening of the iris) (*auxein* to increase) iridectome, iridectomy (*ektome* excision) iridemia (*emia* blood condition) irideremia (congenital absence of the iris) (*eremia* absence) iridoncus (*onkos* mass, tumor) *irido*: iridoavulsion (complete tearing away of the iris from its periphery) (*re* back + *vellere* to pull) iridocapsulitis (capsule + *itis* inflammation)

Element	From	Meaning	Examples
irid (cont'd)		[iris]	iridocele (*kele* tumor) iridociliary (*cilium* eyelash) iridochoroiditis (*choroid* membranous + *itis* inflammation) iridocoloboma (*coloboma* defect) iridocorneal (cornea) iridocyclectomy (*kyklos* circle + *ektome* excision) iridocystectomy (*kystis* bladder, capsule + *ektome* excision) iridocyte (*kytos* cell) iridodialysis (*dialysis* loosening) iridodilator (*dilate* to widen) iridodonesis (*donesis* tremor) iridokeratitis (*keratos* cornea + *itis* inflammation) iridokinesia (or, iridokinesis) {iridokinetic} (*kinein* to move) iridoleptynsis (*leptynsis* attenuation) iridology (*logy* study) iridomalacia (*malakos* soft) iridomotor (*motor* movement) iridopathy (*pathos* disease) iridoperiphakitis (*peri* around + *phakos* lens + *itis* inflammation) iridoplegia (*plegia* paralysis) iridoptosis (*ptosis* a falling) iridopupillary (pertaining to the iris and the pupil) iridorhexis (rupture of the iris; the tearing away of the iris) (*rhexis* rupture) iridoschisis (*schisis* fissure) iridosclerotomy (sclera + *tomy* incision) iridosteresis (*steresis* loss) iridotasis (*tasis* stretching) iridotomy (*tomy* incision) TRAILING ROOT COMPOUND: keratoiridocyclitis (*keras* cornea + *kyklos* circle + *itis* inflammation) scleroiritis (*skleros* hard + *itis* inflammation) scleriritomy (*skleros* hard + *tomy* incision) CROSS REFERENCE: None
isch	Greek *ischein*	to suppress, check	SIMPLE ROOT: ischesis (retention or suppression of a discharge) LEADING ROOT COMPOUND: *isch*: ischemia (local loss of blood supply) {ischemic} (*emia* blood condition) ischuria {ischuretic} (*uria* urine condition) *ischo*: ischochymia (*chymos* chyme: gastric juice) ischogyria (*gyros* circle) TRAILING ROOT COMPOUND: galactischia (suppression of the secretion of milk) (*gala* milk) myoischemia (*myos* muscle + *emia* blood condition) CROSS REFERENCE: schesis
ischi	Greek *ischion* hip joint	hip, haunch	SIMPLE ROOT: ischial, ischiatic (sciatic; ischial), ischiaticus (sciatic) ischium (the inferior dorsal part of the hip bone; pl., ischia) PREFIXED ROOT: interischiadic (also called *intersciatic*) (*inter* between) postischial (*post* posterior) transischiac (between the two ischia) (*trans* across)

Element	From	Meaning	Examples
ischi (cont'd)		[hip, haunch]	LEADING ROOT COMPOUND: *ischi*: ischiadelphus (also called *ischiodidymus*) (*adelphos* brother) ischialgia (pain in the hip; also called *ischiodynia*) (*algos* pain) ischiectomy (*ektome* excision) ischiodynia (also called *ischialgia*) (*odyne* pain) *ischio*: ischioanal (anus) ischiobulbar (bulb—of the penis) ischiocapsular (pertaining to the ischium and the capsular ligament of the hip joint) ischiocavernous (relating to the ischium and the corpus cavernosum, or the columns of erectile tissue of the clitoris or penis) ischiocele (hernia through the sciatic notch) (*kele* hernia) ischiococcygeus {ischiococcygeal} (coccyx) ischiodidymus (also called *ischiadelphus*) {ischiodymia} (*didymos* twin) ischiofemoral (*femur* thigh) ischiofibular (*fibula* clasp, pin—fibula) ischiohebotomy (*hebes* pubes + *tomy* incision) ischiomelus (*melos* limb) ischioneuralgia (*neuron* nerve + *algos* pain) ischiopagia (or, ischiopagy), ischiopagus (*pagos* fixed) ischioperineal (perineum) ischiopubic (*pubes* groin) ischiorectal (also called *rectischiac*) (rectum) ischiosacral (sacrum) ischiothoracopagus (also called *iliothoracopagus*) (*thorax* chest + *pagus* fixed) ischiotibial (tibia) ischiovaginal (vagina) ischiovertebral (vertebra) *ischion*: ischionitis (*itis* inflammation) TRAILING ROOT COMPOUND: rectischiac (rectum) DISGUISED ROOT: sciatic (pertaining to the hip or ischium) sciatica (severe pain in the leg along the course of the sciatic nerve) intersciatic (between the two ischia) (*inter* between) CROSS REFERENCE: cox
-ism (see Appendix C)	Greek *-izo* + *-mos*	state, condition, fact of being; process or result of an action	SUFFIXED ROOT: achromatism (*a* privative + *chroma* color) acrotism (*a* privative + *krotos* beat, pulse) albinism (congenital absence of pigmentation) (*albus* white) anorchism (*a* privative + *orchis* testis) arachnidism (*arachne* spider) autism (*autos* self) blepharism (*blepharizein* to wink) erythrism (*erythros* red) flavism (*flavus* yellow) gravidism (*gravida* pregnant) gustatism (also called *pseudogeusia*) (*gustare* to taste) gynandrism (*gyne* woman + *andros* man) herpetism (herpes) holism (*holos* whole)

Element	From	Meaning	Examples
-ism (cont'd)		[condition]	hypnotism (*hypnos* sleep)
			labialism (*labium* lip)
			melanism (*melas* black)
			nanism (*nanos* dwarf)
			oneirism (*oneiros* dream)
			ophidism (*ophidian* serpent, snake)
			paludism (*palus* marsh; thus, malaria)
			priapism (*priapus* penis)
			puerilism (*puer* child)
			syndactylism (*syn* with + *daktylos* finger, toe)
			teratism (*teratos* fetal monster)
			thyroidism (thyroid)
			CROSS REFERENCE: oid
iso-	Greek *isos*	same, equal	See Appendix B for examples of words with this prefix. Others are placed with the roots to which it is attached.
			NOTE: See separate entry: aniso-.
			CROSS REFERENCE: hom
-itis	Greek suffix	inflammation	TRAILING ROOT COMPOUND:
			Examples
			achillobursitis (Achilles tendon + *bursa* bag)
			acinitis (*acinus* berry: gland)
			acrodermatitis (*akros* extremity + *derma* skin)
			acroposthitis (*posthe* the prepuce—foreskin)
			adenitis (*adenos* gland)
			adiposities (also called *panniculitis*) (*adipos* fat)
			alveolitis (*alveolus* hollow sac, especially a tooth socket)
			amygdalitis (or, amigdalitis; also called *tonsillitis*) (*amygdal* tonsil)
			angiitis (*angeion* vessel)
			antritis (*antrum* cavity, especially within a bone)
			aortitis (*aorta*)
			appendicitis (appendix)
			arachnoiditis (arachnoid)
			arthritis (*arthron* joint)
			balanitis (*balanos* acorn: glans penis)
			bronchitis (*bronchus* windpipe)
			bulbitis (bulb of the urethra)
			bursitis (*bursa* bag, pouch)
			canthitis (canthus—angle of the eye)
			celitis (*koilia* belly—stomach, abdomen)
			cheilitis (also called *chilitis*) (*cheilos* lip)
			chondritis (*chondros* cartilage)
			chorditis (vocal or spermatic cord)
			clitoritis (clitoris)
			cloacitis (cloaca—drain)
			colonitis (or, colitis) (colon)
			colpitis (also called *vaginitis*) (*kolpos* vagina)
			conchitis (concha—of the nose)
			corditis (spermatic cord)
			coxitis (*coxa* hip)
			cryptitis (crypt)
			cyclitis (ciliary body)
			cystitis (cyst)
			dactylitis (*daktylos* finger, toe)
			dermatitis (*dermatos* skin)

Element	From	Meaning	Examples
itis (cont'd)		[inflammation]	desmitis (*desmos* band: ligament)
			didymitis (*didymos* twin: testis, testicle)
			duodenitis (duodenum)
			encephalitis (*enkephalon* brain)
			enteritis (*enteron* intestine)
			epididymitis (epididymis)
			fibrositis (fibrous tissue; also called *muscular rheumatism*)
			gastritis (*gaster* stomach, belly)
			gingivitis (*gingivae* gums—of the mouth)
			glossitis (*glossa* tongue)
			hepatitis (*hepatos* liver)
			initis (*inos* fiber)
			laryngitis (larynx)
			mastitis (*mastos* breast)
			melitis (*melon* cheek)
			meningitis (*meningos* membrane)
			myelitis (*myelos* marrow)
			myositis (*myos* muscle)
			myringitis (also called *tympanitis*) (*myringa* eardrum)
			nephritis (*nephros* kidney)
			neuritis (also called *neuropathy*) (*neuron* nerve)
			odontitis (also called *pulpitis*) (*odontos* tooth)
			orchitis (or, orchiditis; also called *testitis*) (*orchis* testicle)
			otitis (*otos* ear)
			panniculitis (also called *adipositis*) (*pannus* cloth—layer of fat)
			pharyngitis (also called *sore throat*) (*pharynx* throat)
			phlebitis (*phlebos* vein)
			pimelitis (also called *panniculitis*) (*pimele* fat tissue)
			prostatitis (prostate)
			pyelitis (*pyelos* pelvis)
			pyloritis (pylorus—the aboral outlet of the stomach)
			rhinitis (also called *nasal catarrh*) (*rhinos* nose)
			sinusitis (sinus)
			tonsillitis (also called *amygdalitis,* or *amigdalitis*) (tonsil)
			uteritis (also called *metritis*) (uterus)
			vaginitis (vagina)
			CROSS REFERENCE: caum, febr, phleg, pyr

A Thesaurus of Medical Word Roots

J

Element	From	Meaning	Examples
jejun	Latin *jejunus* lacking food	empty, hungry	SIMPLE ROOT: jejunum [the middle part of the small intestine (originally thought to be empty after death) between the duodenum and the ileum] {jejunal} PREFIXED ROOT: mesojejunum (the mesentery of the jejunum) (*mesos* middle) perijejunitis (*peri* around + *itis* inflammation) LEADING ROOT COMPOUND: *jejun*: jejunectomy (*ektome* excision) jejunitis (*itis* inflammation) *jejuno*: jejunocecostomy (*cecum* blind gut + *stoma* mouth, opening) jejunocolostomy (*colon* + *stoma* mouth, opening) jejunoileal, jejunoileitis (*ileum* + *itis* inflammation) jejunoileostomy (*ileum* + *stoma* mouth, opening) jejunojejunostomy (an anastomosis between two portions of the jejunum) (*stoma* mouth, opening) jejunoplasty (*plassein* to form) jejunorrhaphy (operative repair of the jejunum) (*rhaphe* suture) jejunostomy (operative establishment of a fistula from the jejunum to the abdominal wall) (*stoma* mouth, opening) jejunotomy (incision into the jejunum) (*tomy* incision) TRAILING ROOT COMPOUND: gastrojejunostomy (*gaster* stomach + *stoma* mouth, opening) CROSS REFERENCE: None
jug, junct, joint	Latin *jungere*	to join	SIMPLE ROOT: *joint*: joint (the point of juncture between two bones) *jug*: jugal (connecting like a yoke; pertaining to the cheek) jugale (the jugal joint), jugate (locked together; marked by ridges) jugular (pertaining to the neck) jugulation (from *jugulare*, lit., to cut the throat of; the sudden and rapid arrest of disease by therapeutical measures) jugum (a depression or ridge connecting two structures; pl., juga) *junct*: junction {junctional} junctura (also called *joint, junction*; pl., juncturae), juncture PREFIXED ROOT: *join*: conjoined (joined together; as conjoined twins) (*con* with) *joint*: disjoint (*dis* apart) *jugal*: conjugal (*com* with) subjugal (situated below the zygomatic bone) (*sub* below) *jugular*: intrajugular (*intra* within) *jugant*: conjugant (*con* with, together) *jugate*: conjugate (opposite of *disjugate*), conjugated (*com* with) disconjugate (*dis* apart + conjugate) disjugate (not joined together in position or action; not acting in common; the opposite of *conjugate*) (*dis* apart)

A Thesaurus of Medical Word Roots

Element	From	Meaning	Examples
jug (cont'd)		[to join]	*junct*: adjunct (in addition to the principal procedure or course of therapy) {adjunctive} (*ad* to) disjunct, disjunction (or, dysjunction) {disjunctive} (*dis* apart) *junctiv*: conjunctiva (the delicate membrane that lines the eyelids and covers the exposed surface of the eyeball; also called *tunica conjunctiva*; pl., conjunctivae) {conjunctival} conjunctivitis (inflammation of the conjunctiva, the mucous membrane lining the inner surface of the eyelids and covering the front part of the eyeball) (*com* with + *itis* inflammation) LEADING ROOT COMPOUND: jugomaxillary (*maxilla* jaw) TRAILING ROOT COMPOUND: maxillojugal (*maxilla* jaw) CROSS REFERENCE: zyg
juxta-	Latin *juxta*	near	See Appendix B for examples of words with this prefix. Others are attached to the roots to which it is attached. CROSS REFERENCE: None

A Thesaurus of Medical Word Roots

$\mathcal{K}$

Element	From	Meaning	Examples
karyo, **caryo**	Greek *karyon* nut, kernel	nucleus, kernel	SIMPLE ROOT: karyon (the nucleus of a cell), karyonide PREFIXED ROOT: *caryote*: acaryote (or, akaryocyte) (*a* privative) eucaryote (or, eukaryote) (*eu* well) procaryote (or, prokaryote) (*pro* before) *karyoblast*: megakaryoblast (or, megacaryoblast) (*megas* large + *blastos* germ) *karyocyte* cell nucleus: akaryocyte (*a* privative) megakaryocyte (or, megacaryocyte) (*megas* large) pleokaryocyte (*pleion* more) polykaryocyte (*polys* many) promegakaryocyte (*pro* before + *megas* large) *karyon*: amphikaryon (a diploid nucleus) (*amphi* around) dikaryon {dikaryotic} (*di* two) diplokaryon (*diploos* double) eukaryon (*eu* well) hemikaryon (a cell nucleus which contains the haploid number of chromosomes) (*hemi* half) heterokaryon (*heteros* other) homokaryon (*homos* same) monokaryon (a mononuclear spore or cell of a fungus that produces a dikaryon in its life cycle) (*monos* single) perikaryon (also called *neurosome*; pl., perikarya) (*peri* around) prokaryon (*pro* before) synkaryon (or, syncaryon; a nucleus resulting from fusion of two pronuclei) (*syn* with) *karyosis* cell condition: anisokaryosis (*aniso* unequal: *an* negative + *isos* equal) dyskaryosis {dyskaryotic} (*dys* abnormal) eukaryosis (the state of having a true nucleus) {eukaryotic} (*eu* well) heterokaryosis (*heteros* other) megakaryocytosis (*megas* large + *kytos* cell) prokaryosis (*pro* before) LEADING ROOT COMPOUND: *kary*: karyapsis (union of nuclei in a conjugating cell) (*haptein* to touch) [h of haptein elided] *karyo*: karyochrome (a nerve cell the nucleus of which is deeply stainable, while the body is not) (*chroma* color) karyochylema (nuclear sap) (*chylus* juice) karyoclasis (or, karyoklasis; the fragmentation of a cell nucleus; also called *karyorrhexis*) (*klaein* to break) karyocyte (a nucleated cell; an early normoblast) (*kytos* cell) karyogamy (union of nuclei in cell conjugation) {karyogamic} (*gamos* marriage: reproduction) karyogenesis {karyogenic} (*genere* to produce)

Element	From	Meaning	Examples
karyo (cont'd)		[nucleus]	karyogonad (also called *micronucleus*) (*gone* seed)
			karyokinesis (the phenomena involved in division of the nucleus, usually an early stage in the process of cell division, or mitosis) {karyokinetic} (*kinein* to move)
			karyology (*logy* study)
			karyolymph (the liquid part of a cell nucleus, as contrasted with the chromatin and linin) (*lymph* liquid, water)
			karyolysis (a form of necrobiosis in which the nucleus of a cell swells and loses its chromatin) {karyolytic} (*lyein* to loose)
			karyomegaly (abnormal enlargement of the nucleus of a call, not caused by polyploidy) (*megalos* large)
			karyomere (a vesicle containing only a small portion of the typical nucleus, usually following abnormal mitosis) (*meros* part)
			karyometry (*metron* measure)
			karyomicrosome (*mikros* small + *soma* body)
			karyomitosis (division of the nucleus of a cell preceding mitosis) {karyomitotic} (*mitos* thread + *osis* condition)
			karyomorphism (the shape of a cell nucleus) (*morphe* form)
			karyophage (a protozoan that exercises phagocytic action on the nucleus of the cell it infects) (*phagein* to devour, consume)
			karyoplasm (the nucleoplasm, or protoplasm of the nucleus of a cell) {karyoplasmic} (*plassein* to form)
			karyoplast (the nucleus of a cell), karyoplastin (the substance of a miotic spindle; the parachromatin) (*plassein* to form)
			karyopyknosis {karyopyknotic} (*pyknosis* density)
			karyoreticulum (also called *karyomitome*) (*reticulum* network)
			karyorrhexis (rupture of the cell nucleus in which the chromatin disintegrates into formless granules which are extruded from the cell; also called *karyoclasis*) (*rhexis* rupture)
			karyosome (*soma* body)
			karyostasis (the so-called resting stage of the nucleus between mitotic divisions) (*stasis* stoppage)
			karyotheca (also called *nuclear envelope*) (*theke* sheath)
			karyotype {karyotypic} (*typos* type, model)
			karyozoic (existing in or inhabiting the nuclei of cells, as do certain protozoa) (*zoon* animal)
			TRAILING ROOT COMPOUND:
			archikaryon (the nucleus of a zygote) (*archein* to begin)
			pleokaryocyte (*pleon* more + *kytos* cell)
			CROSS REFERENCE: nuc(le), pyren
kerat, **cerat,** **ceros**	Greek *keras* horn	horn, cornea	SIMPLE ROOT:
			keratic (pertaining to horn; pertaining to the cornea)
			keratin (a scleroprotein which is the principal constituent of epidermis, hair, nails, horny tissues, and the organic matrix of the enamel of the teeth) {keratinous}, keratinization, keratinize
			PREFIXED ROOT:
			ceros: megaloceros (a fetus having projections from the forehead resembling horns) (*megalos* large)
			keratic: perikeratic (also called *pericorneal*) (*peri* around)
			keratin:
			eukeratin (a true keratin found in hair, nails, feathers, and bones) (*eu* well)
			prekeratin (a fibrous protein synthesized by basal cells of the epidermis) (*pre* before)

Element	From	Meaning	Examples
kerat (cont'd)		[horn, cornea]	*kerato*:
			epikeratophakia (*epi* upon + *phakos* lens)
			epikeratoprosthesis (*epi* upon + *prosthesis* an addition)
			heterokeratoplasty (*heteros* other + *plassein* to form)
			homokeratoplasty (*homos* same + *plassein* to form)
			keratoma: dyskeratoma (*dys* abnormal + *oma* tumor)
			keratosis horny or corneal condition:
			akeratosis (deficiency of the horny tissue) (*a* privative)
			dyskeratosis {dyskeratotic} (*dys* abnormal)
			hyperkeratosis (*hyper* above)
			hypokeratosis (*hypo* under)
			parakeratosis (*para* alongside)
			LEADING ROOT COMPOUND:
			cerato:
			ceratocricoid (or, keratocricoid; pertaining to the posterior horn of the thyroid cartilage and the cricoid cartilage)
			ceratohyal (pertaining to a cornu minus of the hyoid bone)
			kera:
			keratome, keratomy (*tomy* incision)
			keratorus (*torus* swelling, knot, bulge)
			keratosis (pl., keratoses) (*osis* condition)
			kerat:
			keratalgia (pain in the cornea) (*algos* pain)
			keratectasia (or, keratoectasia; protrusion of the cornea; also called *corneal ectasia*) (*ektasis* dilatation)
			keratectomy (*ektome* excision)
			keratitis (*itis* inflammation)
			keratoid (*eidos* form)
			keratoma (*oma* tumor)
			keratose, keratosis {keratotic} (*osis* condition)
			keratin: keratinoid (*eidos* form)
			keratino:
			keratinocyte (*kytos* cell)
			keratinophilic (*philein* to love: attraction for)
			keratinosome (*soma* body)
			kerato:
			keratoacanthoma (*akantha* thorn + *oma* tumor)
			keratoangioma (also called *angiokeratoma*) (*angeion* vessel + *oma* tumor)
			keratocele (*kele* hernia)
			keratocentesis (*kentein* to puncture)
			keratoconjunctivitis (inflammation of the cornea and the conjunctiva) (*itis* inflammation)
			keratoconus (*konos* cone)
			keratocyst (*kystis* sac)
			keratocyte (*kytos* cell)
			keratoderma (*derma* skin)
			keratodermatocele (*dermatos* skin + *kele* hernia)
			keratodermitis (*derma* skin + *itis* inflammation)
			keratoectasia (*ektasis* dilatation)
			keratoelastoidosis (elastic + *eidos* form + *osis* condition)
			keratoepithelioplasty (epithelium + *plassein* to form)
			keratogenesis {keratogenetic, keratogenous} (*genere* to produce)
			keratoglobus (*globus* ball)

Element	From	Meaning	Examples
kerat (cont'd)		[horn, cornea]	keratohelcosis (*helcosis* ulceration)
			keratohemia (*hemia* blood condition)
			keratoleptynsis (*leptynsis* attenuation—making thin)
			keratoleukoma (*leukoma* whiteness)
			keratolysis {keratolytic} (*lyein* to loosen)
			keratomalacia (*malakos* soft)
			keratometer {keratometric} (*metron* measure)
			keratomileusis (*smileusis* carving) [s is elided]
			keratomycosis (a fungal disease of the cornea) (*mykes* fungus + *osis* condition)
			keratonosus (*nosos* disease)
			keratonyxis (also called *aqueous paracentesis*) (*nyxis* puncture)
			keratopathy (or, keratopathia) (*pathos* disease)
			keratophakia (*phakos* lens)
			keratoplasty (also called *corneal transplantation*) (*plassein* to form)
			keratoprosthesis (*prosthesis* addition)
			keratorrhexis (*rhexis* rupture)
			keratoscleritis (sclera + *itis* inflammation)
			keratoscope, keratoscopy (*skopein* to examine)
			keratotome, keratotomy (*tomy* incision)
			keratotorus (or, keratorus) (*torus* protuberance)
			TRAILING ROOT COMPOUND:
			keratin:
			cytokeratin (*kytos* cell)
			neurokeratin (*neuron* nerve)
			pseudokeratin (*pseudes* false)
			keratitis: sclerokeratitis (*skleros* hard + *itis* inflammation)
			kerato:
			acanthokeratoderma (*akanthos* thorn + *derma* skin)
			orthokeratology (*orthos* straight + *logy* study)
			prosthokeratoplasty (prosthesis + *plassein* to form)
			keratoma corneal tumor:
			angiokeratoma (*angeion* blood vessel)
			fibrokeratoma (fiber)
			keratosis corneal or horny condition:
			acrokeratosis (*akros* extremity, tip)
			leukokeratosis (also called *leukoplakia*) (*leukos* white)
			melanokeratosis (*melanos* dark)
			orthokeratosis (*orthos* correct, straight)
			pharyngokeratosis (pharynx)
			porokeratosis (*poros* pore)
			splenokeratosis (or, splenoceratosis) (spleen)
			sudorikeratosis (*sudor* sweat)
			CROSS REFERENCE: cerebr, corn
keto	Greek *keto*	ketone (a substance containing the carbonyl group, CO)	NOTE: The root *keto* is a back-formation of *ketone*, an arbitrary variation of *acetone*, the base of which is *aceto* acid, sour.
			SIMPLE ROOT:
			ketene, ketol, ketone
			ketonization (conversion into ketone)
			ketose, ketoside
			PREFIXED ROOT:
			antiketogenic (*anti* against + ketogenic)
			hyperketonemia (*hyper* above + ketonemia)
			hyperketonuria (*hyper* above + ketonuria)

Element	From	Meaning	Examples
keto (cont'd)		[ketone]	hyperketosis (also called *ketosis*) (*hyper* beyond + ketosis) LEADING ROOT COMPOUND: *ket*: ketosis (also called *hyperketosis*) {ketotic} (*osis* condition) *keto*: ketoacid (*acid* sour) ketogenesis (also called *ketoplasia*) {ketogenetic, ketogenic} (*genere* to produce) ketoheptose (any ketose containing seven carbon atoms) (*hepta* seven) ketohexose (*hex* six) ketolysis {ketolytic} (*lyein* to dissolve) ketopentose (*penta* five) ketoplasia (also called *ketogenesis*) (*plassein* to form) ketosteroid (*stereos* solid + *eidos* form) *keton*: ketonemia (an excess of ketone bodies in the blood, as in starvation and diabetes mellitus) (*emia* blood condition) ketonuria (ketone bodies in the urine, as in diabetes mellitus; also called *acetonuria, hyperketonuria*) (*uria* urine condition) *ketos*: ketosuria (*uria* urine condition) CROSS REFERENCE: None
kine			See cine- for *kinesis*.
klept, **clep**	Greek *kleptein*	to steal	LEADING ROOT COMPOUND: kleptomania, kleptomaniac (*mania* madness) kleptophobia (or, cleptophobia) (*phobia* fear) TRAILING ROOT COMPOUND: amnioclepsis (*amnion* membrane) uroclepsis (the unconscious escape of urine) (*ouron* urine) CROSS REFERENCE: None
klon			See clon- for *logoklony*.
koilo			See cel¹ for *koilocyte*.
koni			See coni- for *koniocortex*.
kyph, **cyph**	Greek *kyphos*	humped	SIMPLE ROOT: kyphos (the convex prominence of the spine in kyphosis), kyphosis {kyphotic} LEADING ROOT COMPOUND: kyphoplasty (*plassein* to form) kyphoscoliosis (*skoliosis* curving) kyphotone (a brace for use in tuberculosis of the spine) (*tonos* tension) TRAILING ROOT COMPOUND: ithyokyphosis (or, ithycyphos; backward projection of the spinal column) (*ithys* straight, erect + *osis* condition) rachiocyphosis (also called *kyphosis*) (*rhachis* spine) rhinokyphosis (*rhinos* nose + *osis* condition) scoliokyphosis (combined lateral and posterior curvature of the spine) (*skolios* twisted + *osis* condition) CROSS REFERENCE: None

A Thesaurus of Medical Word Roots

$\mathcal{L}$

Element	From	Meaning	Examples
labi[1]	Latin *labium* lip	lip, edge; lip-shaped structure; fleshy border; vulva	SIMPLE ROOT: *labi*: labial {labially}, labialism, labialize, labium (pl., labia) *labr*: labrum (a lip; a lip-shaped structure; pl., labra) PREFIXED ROOT: *labe*: bilabe (an instrument for taking small calculi from the bladder through the urethra) (*bi* two) *labia*: macrolabia (also called *macrocheilia*) (*makros* large) *labial*: interlabial (*inter* between) mesiolabial (*mesos* middle) prolabial (*pro* before) proximolabial (*proximo* next to, close) LEADING ROOT COMPOUND: labiocervical (also called *cervicolabial*) (*cervix* neck—of a tooth) labiochorea (a chronic spasm of the lips) (*chorea* dance, twitch) labioclination (*clinere* to lean) labiodental (*dens* tooth) labiogingival (also called *gingivolabial*) (*gingivae* gums) labioglossolaryngeal (*glossa* tongue + larynx) labioglossopharyngeal (*glossa* tongue + pharynx) labiograph (*graphein* to write) labiolingual (*lingua* tongue) labiology {labiologic} (*logy* study) labiomental (also called *mentolabial*) (*mentum* chin) labiomycosis (*mykes* fungus + *osis* condition) labionasal (also called *nasolabial*) (*nasus* nose) labiopalatine (*palatum* roof of mouth) labioplacement (positioning more forward toward the lips than normal) labioplasty (also called *cheiloplasty*) (*plassein* to form) labiotenaculum (*tenere* to hold) labioversion (*vertere* to turn) TRAILING ROOT COMPOUND: alveololabial (*alveolus* little hollow—of the upper or lower jaw) axiolabial (*axis*—of tooth) buccolabial (*bucca* cheek) cervicolabial (also called *labiocervical*) (*cervix* neck—of tooth) dentilabial (*dens* tooth) distolabial (*distans* distant, remote) gingivolabial (*gingivae* gums) incisolabial (*incisor*—tooth) inguinolabial (*inguen* groin) maxillolabial (*maxilla* upper jaw) mentolabial (*mentum* chin) nasolabial (*nasus* nose) nympholabial (*nymph* a developmental stage) proximolabial (*proximus* nearest, next to) rectolabial (rectum) vaginolabial (vagina) CROSS REFERENCE: cheil, episio

Element	From	Meaning	Examples
labi[2]	Latin *labilis*	unstable	SIMPLE ROOT: labile, lability TRAILING ROOT COMPOUND: hydrolabile (compare *hydrostabile*) (*hydor* water) thermolabile (easily altered or decomposed by heat; also called *heat labile*) (*therme* heat) siccolabile (altered or destroyed by drying) (*siccus* dry) thixolabile (*thixis* a touch) vasolabile (*vas* vessel) CROSS REFERENCE: None
labyrinth	Greek *labyrinthos*	maze	SIMPLE ROOT: labyrinth (intricate communicating passages; the internal ear consisting of osseous and membranous labyrinths) labyrinthine (pertaining to a labyrinth; intricate or involved) labyrinthus (also called *convoluted part of kidney lobule*; pl., labyrinthi) PREFIXED ROOT: perilabyrinth, perilabyrinthitis (also called *circumscribed labyrinthitis*) (*peri* around + *itis* inflammation) retrolabyrinthine (*retro* backward) LEADING ROOT COMPOUND: *labyrinth*: labyrinthectomy (*ektome* excision) labyrinthitis (*itis* inflammation) *labyrintho*: labyrinthotomy (*tomy* incision) TRAILING ROOT COMPOUND: neurolabyrinthitis (idiopathic inflammation of the vestibular nerve) (*neuron* nerve + *itis* inflammation) CROSS REFERENCE: None
lacri, lachry	Latin *lacrima*	teardrop	SIMPLE ROOT: *lacri*: lacrima (pl., lacrimae), lacrimal (or, lachrymal), lacrimation, lacrimator, lacrimatory *lachry*: lachrymal (or, lacrimal) PREFIXED ROOT: delacrimation (excessive and abnormal flow of tears) (*de* intensive) prelacrimal (in front of the lacrimal sac) (*pre* before) LEADING ROOT COMPOUND: lacrimotomy (*tomy* incision) TRAILING ROOT COMPOUND: ethmolacrimal (pertaining to the ethmoid and the lacrimal bones) (*ethmos* sieve) nasolacrimal (*nasus* nose) CROSS REFERENCE: dacry
lact	Latin *lac*	milk	SIMPLE ROOT: lac (pl., lacta), lactase, lactate, lactation {lactational} lacteal, lactescence, lactescent lactic, lactim, lactin (lactose, sugar of milk) lactinated (containing or prepared with milk sugar) lactone, lactose (also called *milk sugar*) PREFIXED ROOT: delactation (weaning; the cessation of lactation) (*de* opposite) hyperlactation (also called *superlactation*) (*hyper* over) hypolactasia (*hypo* under) prolactin, prolactinoma (also called *prolactin-producing adenoma*) (*pro* before + *oma* tumor) superlactation (also called *hyperlactation*) (*super* over, above)

Element	From	Meaning	Examples
lact (cont'd)		[milk]	LEADING ROOT COMPOUND: *lact*: lactacidemia (also called *lactic acidemia*) (acid + *emia* blood condition) lactacidosis (acidosis due to increased lactic acid) lactaciduria (acid + *uria* urine condition) lactagogue (*agein* to lead) lactalbumin (a simple, highly nutritious protein found in milk) *lacti*: lactiferous (*ferre* to bear) lactifuge {lactifugal} (*fugere* to flee) lactimorbus (also called *milk disease*) (*morbus* disease) lactigenous (*genere* to produce) lactivorous (also called *galactophagous*) (*vorare* to eat, consume) *lacto*: lactobacillus (*bacillus* rod-shaped organism) lactochrome (also called *lactoflavin*) (*chroma* color) lactocrit (*krinein* to separate) lactoferrin (*ferrum* iron) lactoflavin (also called *lactochrome, riboflavin*) (*flavus* yellow) lactogen, lactogenesis {lactogenic} (*genere* to produce) lactoglobulin (*globus* globe) lactometer (*metron* measure) lactoprotein (a protein derived from milk) lactorrhea (also called *galactorrhea*) (*rhein* to flow) lactoscope (also called *galactoscope*) (*skopein* to examine) lactotherapy (*therapy* treatment) lactotoxin (*toxon* poison) *lactos*: lactosuria (*uria* urine condition) CROSS REFERENCE: galact
lal	Greek *lalein*	to speak, prattle	SIMPLE ROOT: lallation (a babbling form of speech), lalling (a form of stammering in which the speech is almost unintelligible) PREFIXED ROOT: alalia (loss of ability to speak) (*a* privative) allolalia (*allos* other) dyslalia (also called *paralalia*) (*dys* abnormal) heterolalia (also called *heterophasia*) (*heteros* other) palilalia (also called *palinphrasia*) (*palin* backward, again) paralalia (also called *dyslalia, mogilalia*) (*para* abnormal) LEADING ROOT COMPOUND: *lal*: laliatry (*iatrein* to heal, cure) *lalio*: laliophobia (or, lalophobia; extreme dislike of speaking) (*phobia* fear) *lalo*: lalochezia (emotional relief by using indecent or vulgar language) (*chezein* to defecate) lalognosis (the understanding of speech) (*gnosis* knowledge) lalopathy (any disorder of speech) (*pathos* disease) laloplegia (also called *logoplegia*) (*plessein* to strike) TRAILING ROOT COMPOUND: barylalia (*barys* heavy) bradylalia (also called *bradyarthria*) (*bradys* slow) coprolalia (excessive use of obscene language) (*kopros* dung: filthy) echolalia (also called *embolalia*) (echo)

Element	From	Meaning	Examples
lal (cont'd)		[to speak, prattle]	embolalia (or, embololalia; the interpolation of meaningless words into the speech) (*emballein* to insert)
			glossolalia (*glossa* tongue)
			idiolalia (a condition marked by the use of invented language) (*idios* one's own: peculiar)
			mogilalia (also called *paralalia*) (*mogis* with difficulty)
			neolalia (*neos* new)
			rhinolalia (also called *rhinism, rhinophonia*) (*rhinos* nose)
			stomatolalia (also called *hyponasality, rhinophonia*) (*stoma* mouth)
			CROSS REFERENCE: phas, phem, phen[1], phon[2], phras
lam	Greek *lamina* thin sheet	layer, plate	SIMPLE ROOT:
			lamella (pl., lamellae) {lamellar}, lamellate (or, lamellated)
			lamin, lamina (pl., laminae), laminar, laminin, lamination
			PREFIXED ROOT:
			lamellar:
			bilamellar (*bi* two)
			epilamellar (*epi* upon)
			interlamellar (*inter* between)
			intralamellar (*intra* within)
			lamin:
			delamination (separation of the blastoderm into the epiblast and hypoblast) (*de* apart)
			eulaminate (*eu* well)
			unilaminate (or, unilaminar) (*uni* one)
			laminar:
			bilaminar (having or pertaining to two layers) (*bi* two)
			trilaminar (*tri* three)
			unilaminar (having only one layer) (*uni* one)
			laminectomy: hemilaminectomy (*hemi* half + *ektome* excision)
			LEADING ROOT COMPOUND:
			lamelli: lamelliform (resembling lamellae) (*forma* shape)
			lamin:
			laminectomy (*ektome* excision)
			laminitis (*itis* inflammation)
			lamina: laminaplasty (or, laminoplasty) (*plassein* to form)
			lamino:
			laminogram, laminograph (*graphein* to write)
			laminoplasty (or, laminaplasty) (*plassein* to form)
			laminotomy (*tomy* incision)
			TRAILING ROOT COMPOUND: fibrolamellar (fiber)
			CROSS REFERENCE: cort, plat
lapar	Greek *lapara*	loin, flank; abdomen	PREFIXED ROOT: minilaparotomy (*mini* small + laparotomy)
			LEADING ROOT COMPOUND:
			lapar: laparectomy (*ektome* excision)
			laparo:
			laparocele (ventral hernia) (*kele* hernia)
			laparocystectomy (*kystis* bladder + *ektome* excision)
			laparocystotomy (*kysis* bladder + *tomy* incision)
			laparoendoscopic (*endon* within + *skopein* to examine)
			laparoenterostomy (or, enterostomy) (*enteron* intestine + *stoma* mouth, opening)
			laparogastroscopy (*gaster* stomach + *skopein* to examine)
			laparohysterectomy (*hystera* womb + *ektome* excision)
			laparomonodidymus (*monos* single + *didymos* twin, double)

A Thesaurus of Medical Word Roots

Element	From	Meaning	Examples
lapar (cont'd)		[loin, flank]	laparomyositis (or, laparomyitis) (*myos* muscle + *itis* inflammation)
			laparonephrectomy (*nephros* kidney + *ektome* excision)
			laparorrhaphy (*rhaphe* suture)
			laparosalpingo-oophororectomy (removal of the uterine tube and ovary through an abdominal incision) (*ektome* excision)
			laparoscope, laparoscopy (*skopein* to examine)
			laparotome, laparotomy (also called *celiotomy*) (*tomy* incision)
			TRAILING ROOT COMPOUND:
			laparotomy loin incision:
			herniolaparotomy (hernia)
			splenolaparotomy (spleen)
			thoracolaparotomy (thorax)
			CROSS REFERENCE: cel[1], lumb, stoma, ventr
laryn	Greek *larynx*	larynx, windpipe	SIMPLE ROOT: larynx (pl., larynges) {laryngeal}
			PREFIXED ROOT:
			laryng: hemilaryngectomy (*hemi* half + *ektome* excision)
			laryngeal:
			endolaryngeal (*endon* within)
			intralaryngeal (*intra* within)
			perilaryngeal, perilaryngitis (*peri* around + *itis* inflammation)
			prelaryngeal (*pre* anterior)
			larynx: hypolarynx (also called *cavitas infraglottica*) (*hypo* under)
			LEADING ROOT COMPOUND:
			laryng:
			laryngalgia (*algos* pain)
			laryngectomy (*ektome* excision)
			laryngemphraxis (*emphraxis* stoppage, obstruction)
			laryngendoscope (*endon* within + *skopein* to examine)
			laryngitis (*itis* inflammation)
			laryngo:
			laryngocele (*kele* hernia)
			laryngocentesis (*kentesis* puncture)
			laryngofissure (*fissure* a splitting)
			laryngogram, laryngograph (*graphein* to write)
			laryngomalacia (*malakos* soft)
			laryngometry (*metron* measure)
			laryngoparalysis (also called *laryngoplegia*)
			laryngopathy (*pathos* disease, disorder)
			laryngopharyngitis (pharynx + *itis* inflammation)
			laryngophthisis (tuberculosis of the larynx) (*phthisis* a wasting)
			laryngophony (*phone* sound)
			laryngoplasty (*plassein* to form)
			laryngoplegia (also called *laryngoparalysis*) (*plege* stroke)
			laryngoptosis (an abnormally low position of the larynx) (*ptosis* a falling)
			laryngorhinology (*rhinos* nose + *logos* study)
			laryngorrhagia (*rhagia* bursting forth)
			laryngorrhaphy (*rhaphe* suture)
			laryngorrhea (*rhein* to flow)
			laryngoscleroma (*skleroma* an induration)
			laryngoscope, laryngoscopy {laryngoscopic} (*skopein* to examine)
			laryngospasm (*spasmos* contraction)
			laryngostasis (*stasis* stoppage)
			laryngostenosis (*stenosis* contracture)

Element	From	Meaning	Examples
laryn (cont'd)		[larynx]	laryngostomy (*stoma* mouth, opening)
			laryngotomy (*tomy* incision)
			laryngotracheal (also called *tracheolaryngeal*), laryngotracheitis (*trachea* windpipe + *itis* inflammation)
			laryngoxerosis (*xerosis* dryness)
			TRAILING ROOT COMPOUND:
			labioglossolaryngeal (*labium* lip + *glossa* tongue)
			otolaryngology (*otos* ear + *logy* study)
			pharyngolaryngeal, pharyngolaryngitis (pharynx + *itis* inflammation)
			presbylaryngitis (*presbys* old age + *itis* inflammation)
			rhinolaryngitis (*rhinos* nose + *itis* inflammation)
			stylolaryngeus (*stylos* pillar)
			thyrolaryngeal (thyroid)
			tracheolaryngeal (also called *laryngotracheal*) (*trachea* windpipe)
			CROSS REFERENCE: bronch, trache
later, **late**	Latin *latus*	side, wide	SIMPLE ROOT:
			laterad (toward the side)
			lateral (denoting a position farther from the median plane or midline of the body or of a structure; pertaining to a side)
			laterality (a relationship to one side, such as a tendency, in voluntary motor acts, to use preferentially the organs of the same side)
			lateralization (the tendency for certain processes to be more highly developed on one side of the brain than the other)
			latus (broad, wide)
			PREFIXED ROOT:
			lat: dilatancy (an increasing viscosity with increasing rate of shear accompanied by volumetric expansion) (*dis* apart, away)
			late: dilate (to make wider or larger), dilated, dilatation, dilation, dilator (*dis* apart, away)
			lateral:
			ambilateral (relating to or affecting both sides) (*ambi* both)
			anterolateral (in front and to the side) (*antero* front)
			bilateral (having two sides, or pertaining to both sides; also called *ambilateral*), bilateralism (bilateral symmetry) (*bi* two)
			collateral (not direct or immediate; a small side branch, as of a blood vessel or nerve) (*com* with)
			contralateral (also called *heterolateral*; opposed to *homolateral* and *ipsilateral*) (*contra* against)
			hemilateral (*hemi* half)
			heterolateral (also called *contralateral*) (*heteros* different)
			homolateral (also called *ipsilateral*) (*homos* same)
			inferolateral (*inferior* lower)
			ipsilateral (also called *homolateral*) (*ipsi* same)
			mediolateral (*medius* middle)
			quadrilateral (*quattuor* four)
			superolateral (*superior* above)
			translateral (*trans* across)
			trilateral (*tri* three)
			unilateral (*uni* one)
			LEADING ROOT COMPOUND:
			lateroabdominal (abdomen)
			laterodeviation (*deviation* a turning aside)
			lateroduction (movement of an eye to either side) (*ducere* to lead)

Element	From	Meaning	Examples
later (cont'd)		[side, wide]	lateroflexion (or, lateriflexion) (*flectere* to bend)
			lateroposition (displacement to one side) (*ponere* to place)
			lateropulsion (involuntary tendency in cerebellar and labyrinthine disease to fall to one side; an involuntary tendency to go to one side while walking) (*pellere* to beat)
			laterotorsion (twisting of the vertical meridian of the eye to the right or to the left) (*torquere* to twist)
			laterotrusion (*trudere* to thrust)
			lateroversion (a turning to one side) (*vertere* to turn)
			TRAILING ROOT COMPOUND:
			basilateral, basolateral (basis)
			ventrolateral (both ventral and lateral) (*venter* belly)
			CROSS REFERENCE: canth, cost, eury, pleur
lecith	Greek *lekithos*	egg yolk, ovum	SIMPLE ROOT: lecithal, lecithinase (also called *phospholipase*)
			PREFIXED ROOT:
			alecithal (without yolk; also called *oligolecithal*) (*a* privative)
			centrolecithal (Greek *kentron* point; Latin *centrum* center)
			ectolecithal (*ektos* outside)
			isolecithal (*isos* equal)
			macrolecithal (also called *megalecithal, polylecithal*) (*makros* large)
			medialecithal (*medius* middle)
			megalecithal (also called *macrolecithal*) (*megalos* large)
			mesolecithal (*mesos* middle)
			microlecithal (also called *miolecithal*) (*mikros* small)
			miolecithal (also called *microlecithal*) (*meion* smaller)
			polylecithal (also called *macrolecithal*) (*polys* many)
			LEADING ROOT COMPOUND:
			lecithin: lecithinemia (*emia* blood condition)
			lecitho:
			lecithoblast (*blastos* bud, shoot, germ)
			lecithoprotein
			lecithovitellin (a saline extract of egg yolks used in egg-yolk agar to test for bacterial lecithinase) (*vitellus* egg yolk)
			TRAILING ROOT COMPOUND:
			oligolecithal (also called *alecithal*) (*oligos* scarce)
			telolecithal (*telos* end)
			tropholecithus {tropholecithal} (*trophe* nutrition)
			CROSS REFERENCE: ov, vitell
leio	Greek *leios*	smooth	LEADING ROOT COMPOUND:
			leiodermia (abnormal glossiness and smoothness of the skin) (*dermia* skin condition)
			leiodystonia (dystonia of a smooth muscle) (*dys* abnormal + *tonia* tone condition)
			leiomyoblastoma (*myos* muscle + *blastos* germ + *oma* tumor)
			leiomyofibroma (*myos* muscle + *fibra* fiber + *oma* tumor)
			leiomyomatosis (*myos* muscle + *oma* tumor + *osis* condition)
			leiomyomectomy (*myos* muscle + *oma* tumor + *ektome* excision)
			leiomyosarcoma (*myos* muscle + *sarkos* flesh + *oma* tumor)
			leiotrichous (*trichos* hair)
			CROSS REFERENCE: None
lemma	Greek *lemma*	husk, sheath	SIMPLE ROOT: lemma (the three egg membranes)
			PREFIXED ROOT:
			alemmal (*a* privative)
			epilemma (also called *endoneurium*) {epilemmal} (*epi* upon)

Element	From	Meaning	Examples
lemma (cont'd)		[husk, sheath]	hypolemmal (located beneath a sheath) (*hypo* under)
			LEADING ROOT COMPOUND:
			lemmoblast (*blastos* bud, shoot, germ)
			lemmocyte (*kytos* cell)
			TRAILING ROOT COMPOUND:
			axilemma (or, axolemma; the plasma membrane of an axon; also called *Mauthner's sheath*) (*axon* axle, axis)
			cytolemma (cell membrane) (*kytos* cell)
			glandilemma (gland)
			myolemma (plasma membrane of a striated muscle fiber; also called *sarcolemma*) (*myos* muscle)
			neurilemma (or, neurolemma) (*neuron* nerve)
			nucleolemma (*nux* nut: central core; nucleus)
			oolemma (*oon* egg, ovum)
			plasmalemma (*plassein* to form—plasma)
			sarcolemma (*sarkos* flesh)
			trichilemmoma (*trichos* hair + *oma* tumor)
			NB: *Dilemma*, from *di*, two + *lemma*, proposition, is not related to this family, and is not otherwise listed.
			CROSS REFERENCE: theca, vagina
lens, lent	Latin *lens, lentis* pea	lens, pea-shaped	SIMPLE ROOT:
			lens: lens
			lent:
			lenticel (a lens-shaped gland)
			lenticula (the lenticular nucleus) {lenticular}, lenticulus (pl., lenticuli)
			lentigo (a tan or brown macule on the skin; pl., lentigines)
			PREFIXED ROOT:
			lental:
			circumlental (also called *perilenticular*) (*circum* around)
			retrolental (behind the crystalline lens) (*retro* behind)
			lenticular:
			perilenticular (also called *circumlental*) (*peri* around)
			retrolenticular (also called *retrolental, behind the lentiform nucleus of the brain*) (*retro* behind)
			LEADING ROOT COMPOUND:
			lens: lensectomy (*ektome* excision)
			lenso:
			lensometer (*metron* measure)
			lensopathy (*pathos* disease)
			lenti:
			lenticonus (*conus* cone)
			lentiform (*forma* shape)
			lentiglobus (*globus* globe: eyeball)
			lenticulo:
			lenticulooptic (*optikos* eye)
			lenticulopapular (*papula* pimple)
			lenticulostriate (*striatus* furrow)
			lenticulothalamic (thalamus)
			TRAILING ROOT COMPOUND:
			capsulolenticular (capsule)
			hepatolenticular (*hepatos* liver)
			thalamolenticular (thalamus)
			CROSS REFERENCE: phac

Element	From	Meaning	Examples
lep¹	Greek *lepos* husk, rind, scale	scale	SIMPLE ROOT: leper, lepidic (relating to scales or a scaly covering layer) leprid (early cutaneous lesion of leprosy), leprosy {leprotic, leprous} PREFIXED ROOT: *lepid*: epilepidoma (*epi* upon + *oma* tumor) *leprosis*: paraleprosis (*para* alongside + *osis* condition) *leprotic*: antileprotic (*anti* against + *osis* condition) LEADING ROOT COMPOUND: *lepo*: lepothrix (also called *trichomycosis axillaris, Paxton's disease*) (*thrix* hair) *lepr*: leproma {lepromatous} (*oma* tumor) *lepro*: leprostatic (*statikos* standing, inhibiting) *lepros*: leprosarium (a hospital especially designed for the care of or those suffering from leprosy), leprosery (*arium* a place for) CROSS REFERENCE: lam, squam
lep²	Greek *lambanein* to seize	to seize, hold, take, grasp; seizure	PREFIXED ROOT: *lepsis*: analepsis (flashback) {analeptic} (*ana* again) prolepsis {proleptic} (*pro* before) *lepsy*: catalepsy {cataleptic}, cataleptiform (or, cataleptoid) (*kata* down + *forma* shape) epilepsy {epileptic} (*epi* upon) [see separate entry: epilep-] paralepsy (also called *psycholepsy*) (*para* alongside, abnormal) *leptic*: analeptic (counteracting drowsiness or the effects of sedatives; re-storative) (*ana* again) polyleptic (*polys* many) proleptic (*pro* before) TRAILING ROOT COMPOUND: *lepsy*: narcolepsy {narcoleptic} (*narkoun* to benumb) nympholepsy (*nymph* nymphae, or labia minora) psycholepsy (also called *paralepsy*) (*psyche* mind) *leptic*: neuroleptic (*neuron* nerve) organoleptic (*organon* organ) thymoleptic (*thymos* mind) CROSS REFERENCE: agra, epilep, heres
lept	Greek *leptos* slender	delicate, fine, small, slender, thin, weak	SIMPLE ROOT: leptin (a helical protein secreted by adipose tissue) See Appendix B for examples of words with this element. Others are placed with the roots to which it is attached. CROSS REFERENCE: mano, micro, nan
les	Latin *laedere* to hurt	lesion, wound	SIMPLE ROOT: lesion (a wound or injury; a pathologic change in the tissues) PREFIXED ROOT: *lesion*: hemilesion (a lesion on one side of the spinal cord) (*hemi* half) microlesion (*mikros* small) *lesional*: intralesional (*intra* within) perilesional (*peri* around) sublesional (*sub* beneath) CROSS REFERENCE: trauma

A Thesaurus of Medical Word Roots

Element	From	Meaning	Examples
leuk, **leuc**	Greek *leukos* light	white	SIMPLE ROOT: leucine, leukoma (pl., leukomata) leukon (the total mass of circulating leukocytes) PREFIXED ROOT: *leukia*: aleukia (*a* privative) *leukoblast* white germ cell: macroleukoblast (*makros* large) microleukoblast (*mikros* small) *leukocyte* white blood cell: proleukocyte (also called *leukoblast*) (*pro* before) protoleukocyte (*protos* first) *leukocytic*: intraleukocytic (*intra* within + *kytos* cell) *leukocytosis* white cell condition: aleukocytosis (*a* privative) hyperleukocytosis (*hyper* over) LEADING ROOT COMPOUND: *leuc*: leucitis (also called *scleritis, sclerotitis*) (*itis* inflammation) *leucin*: leucinuria (*uria* urine condition) *leuco*: leucocyte (or, leukocyte) (*kytos* cell) leucoplakia (or, leukoplakia) (*plax* plate; flat area) leucoplast (*plassein* to form) leucotomy (or, leukotomy) (*tomy* incision) *leuk*: leukapheresis (*apheresis* removal) leukemia (*emia* blood condition) [see separate entry: leukem-] leukencephalitis (*enkephalon* brain + *itis* inflammation) leukodontia (*odontos* tooth) leukonychia (*onyx* nail) *leuko*: leukobilbin (also called *white bile*) leukoblast, leukoblastosis (*blastos* germ + *osis* condition) leukochloroma (*chloros* green + *oma* tumor) leukocidin (*caedere* to cut, kill) leukocoria (or, leukokoria) (*kore* pupil—of eye) leukocyte {leukocytic} (*kytos* cell) leukoderma (also called *hypomelanosis*) {leukodermatous} (*derma* skin) leukodystrophy (*dys* abnormal + *trophein* to nourish) leukoencephalitis (*enkephalon* brain + *itis* inflammation) leukoencephalopathy (*enkephalon* brain + *pathos* disease) leukoerythroblastosis (*erythrys* red + blastosis) leukokeratosis (oral leukoplakia) (*keratosis* horny growth) leukokinesis {leukokinetic} (*kinein* to move) leukokoria (or, leukocoria) (*kore* pupil—of eye) leukomalacia (softening of the brain's white matter) (*malakos* soft) leukomyelitis (inflammation of white matter of the spinal cord) (*myelos* marrow + *itis* inflammation) leukomyelopathy (*myelos* marrow + *pathos* disease) leukonecrosis (*nekrosis* death) leukopathia (or, leukopathy) (*pathos* disease) leukopedesis (*pedan* to leap) leukopenia {leukopenic} (*penia* deficiency) leukoplakia (also called *leukoplasia*) (*plax* plate)

Element	From	Meaning	Examples
leuk (cont'd)		[white]	leukopoiesis (also called *leukocytogenesis, leukocytopoiesis*) {leukopoietic} (*poiein* to make, produce) leukorrhagia (*rhagia* bursting forth) leukorrhea {leukorrheal} (*rhein* to flow) leukosarcoma (*sarkos* flesh + *oma* tumor) leukoscope (*skopein* to examine) leukostasis (*stasis* stoppage) leukotaxis {leukotactic} (*taxis* arrangement) leukotome, leukotomy (prefrontal lobotomy) (*tomy* incision) leukotoxic (*toxic* poison) leukotrichia (*trichos* hair) TRAILING ROOT COMPOUND: melanoleukoderma (a mottled appearance of the skin, as in chronic arsenic poisoning) (*melanos* dark + *derma* skin) CROSS REFERENCE: album
leukem	Greek *leukos* white + *emia* blood condition	leukemia	SIMPLE ROOT: leukemia PREFIXED ROOT: aleukemia (also called *leukopenia*) {aleukemic} (*a* privative) amphileukemia (*amphi* around) hypoleukemia (also called *subleukemia*) (*hypo* under) subleukemia (also called *hypoleukemia*) (*sub* under) LEADING ROOT COMPOUND: *leukem*: leukemoid (leukemia + *eidos* form, resemblance) *leukemo*: leukemogenesis (leukemia + *genere* to produce) TRAILING ROOT COMPOUND: chloroleukemia (*chloros* green) erythroleukemia (*erythros* red) myeloleukemia (*myelos* marrow) CROSS REFERENCE: None
lev	Latin *laevus* left-handed	left; left hand	PREFIXED ROOT: ambilevosity (the inability to perform acts requiring manual skill with either hand) (*ambi* both) LEADING ROOT COMPOUND: levocardia, levocardiogram (*kardia* heart + *graphein* to write) levoclination (rotating of the upper poles of the vertical meridians of the eyes to the left; also called *levotorsion*) (*clinare* to lean) levocycloduction (*kyklos* circle + *ducere* to lead) levoduction (*ducere* to lead) levogyration (also called *levorotation*) (*gyrare* to turn) levorotation (also called *levogyration*), levorotatory (*rotare* to turn) levotorsion (also called *levoclination*) (*torquere* to twist) levoversion (*vertere* to turn) CROSS REFERENCE: sinist
lex	Greek *legein* to speak	reading, word	SIMPLE ROOT: lexical PREFIXED ROOT: alexia (inability to read; word-blindness) {alexic} (*a* privative) dyslexia (also called *paralexia*) {dyslexic} (*dys* abnormal) hyperlexia (in retarded children, the presence of relatively advanced reading ability) (*hyper* over, above) paralexia (also called *dyslexia*) (*para* abnormal) CROSS REFERENCE: logo
lien	Latin *lien*	spleen	SIMPLE ROOT: lien {lienal; also called *splenic*}, lienunculus (an accessory spleen) PREFIXED ROOT: alienia (absence of the spleen; also called *asplenia*) (*a* privative) [do not confuse with *alienism*, mental disorder]

A Thesaurus of Medical Word Roots

Element	From	Meaning	Examples
lien (cont'd)		[spleen]	LEADING ROOT COMPOUND: *lien*: lienitis (also called *splenitis*) (*itis* inflammation) *lieno*: lienocele (also called *splenocele*) (*kele* hernia) lienomalacia (abnormal softness of the spleen; also called *sple-nomalacia*) (*malakos* soft) lienomedullary (also called *splenomyelogenous*) (*medulla* marrow) lienomyelogenous (also called *lienomedullary*) (*myelos* marrow + *genere* to produce) lienopancreatic (pancreas) lienopathy (also called *splenopathy*) (*pathos* disease) lienorenal (also called *splenorenal*) (*ren* kidney) lienotoxin (*toxin* poison) CROSS REFERENCE: splen
lig	Latin *ligare* to bind, tie	ligament	SIMPLE ROOT: ligament, ligamentum (or, ligament; pl. ligamenta), ligand, ligate, ligation, ligator, ligature PREFIXED ROOT: *ligamen*: superligamen (a retentive dressing; a bandage retaining a surgical dressing already in place) (*super* over) *ligation*: alligation (the act of tying together or attaching by some bond, or the state of being attached) (*ad* to, toward) colligation {colligative} (*com* with) deligation (the application of a ligature or bandage) (*de* down) obligation (*ob* against) ultraligation (*ultra* beyond) *ligamentous*: extraligamentous (*extra* outside) interligamentous (or, interligamentary) (*inter* between) intraligamentous (*intra* within) periligamentous (*peri* around) LEADING ROOT COMPOUND: ligamentopexy (or, ligamentopexis) (*pexis* fixation) TRAILING ROOT COMPOUND: *ligamentous*: osseoligamentous (made of bone and ligament) (*osseo* bond) tuboligamentous (*tubus* tube) *ligation*: vasoligation (ligation of the ductus vas deferens, as a means of sterilization) (*vas* vessel) CROSS REFERENCE: desm
lingu, **linct**	Latin *lingua* tongue Greek *leikhein* to lick	tongue, speech; language; to lick	SIMPLE ROOT: *linct*: lincture (or, linctus; an electuary; a medicinal substance mixed with honey or sugar to form a paste suitable for oral consumption) *lingu*: lingua (a tongue, or an organ resembling a tongue; pl., lin-guae) {lingual}, lingualis, lingually (toward the tongue), lingula (pl. lingulae) PREFIXED ROOT: hemilingual (also called *hemiglossal*) (*hemi* half) intralingual (*intra* within) mesiolingual (*mesos* middle) perlingual (*per* through) postlingual (*post* after) prelingual (*pre* before) proximolingual (*proximus* nearest)

Element	From	Meaning	Examples
lingu (cont'd)		[tongue]	retrolingual (behind the tongue) (*retro* behind)
			sublingual, sublinguitis (*sub* under + *itis* inflammation)
			LEADING ROOT COMPOUND:
			lingui: linguiform (*forma* shape)
			linguo:
			linguoaxial (axis—of a tooth)
			linguoaxiogingival (axis + *gingivae* gums—of the mouth)
			linguocervical (*cervix* neck—of a tooth)
			linguoclination (*clinare* to lean)
			linguodental (*dens* tooth)
			linguodistal (*distal* distant)
			linguogingival (*gingivae* gums—of the mouth)
			linguo-occlusal (occlusion—of teeth)
			linguopapillitis (*papilla* pimple)
			linguoplate (also called *lingual plate*)
			linguopulpal (*pulpus* pulp)
			linguoversion (*vertere* to turn)
			TRAILING ROOT COMPOUND:
			lingual:
			alveololingual (*alveolo* cavity, socket—of tooth)
			axiolingual (*axon* axis—of a tooth)
			brachiofaciolingual (*brachium* arm + face)
			buccolingual (*bucca* cheek)
			cervicolingual (also called *linguocervical*) (*cervix* neck—of a tooth)
			dentilingual (*dens* tooth)
			distolingual (*distans* distant, remote)
			faciolingual (*facies* face)
			incisolingual (incisor—biting tooth)
			labiolingual (*labium* lip)
			orolingual (*oris* mouth)
			thyrolingual (also called *thyroglossal*) (thyroid)
			linguistics: psycholinguistics (the study of the influence of psychological factors of development of language) (*psyche* mind)
			CROSS REFERENCE: gloss, lal, phas, phem, phon, phras
lip	Greek	fat, fatty; oily	SIMPLE ROOT: lipase, lipid {lipidic}, lipin (a complex lipid)
	lipos fat		PREFIXED ROOT:
	liparos		*lipase*: colipase (*co* with)
	fatty, oily		*lipemia* condition of fat in the blood:
			antilipemic (preventing or counteracting the accumulation of fatty substances in the blood) (*anti* against)
			hyperlipemia {hyperlipemic} (*hyper* above)
			hypolipemia {hypolipemic} (*hypo* under)
			lipidemia condition of lipids in the blood:
			dyslipidemia (*dys* abnormal)
			hyperlipidemia (*hyper* above)
			lipo: alipotropic (*a* privative + *tropos* a turning)
			lipoid: alipoid (*a* privative + *eidos* form)
			lipoma: polymicrolipomatosis (*polys* many + *mikros* small + lipoma + *osis* condition)
			liposis fat condition:
			dyslipidosis (*dys* abnormal)
			hyperliposis (an excess of fat in the blood serum or tissues) (*hyper* beyond)
			hypoliposis (*hypo* under)

A Thesaurus of Medical Word Roots

Element	From	Meaning	Examples
lip (cont'd)		[fat]	LEADING ROOT COMPOUND:

lip:

lipacidemia (*acidus* sharp: acid + *emia* blood condition)

lipaciduria (*acidus* sharp: acid + *uria* urine condition)

lipectomy (*ektome* excision)

lipedema (*edema* swelling)

lipemia (also called *lipidemia*) {lipemic} (*emia* blood condition)

lipoid, lipoidosis (*eidos* form + *osis* condition)

lipoma (*oma* tumor)

liposis (*osis* condition)

lipuria (*uria* urine condition)

liparo:

liparocele (scrotal hernia containing fat) (*kele* tumor, hernia)

liparodyspnea (*dys* abnormal + *pnein* to breathe)

lipas: lipasuria (presence of lipase in the urine) (*uria* urine condition)

lipid:

lipidemia (also called *lipemia*) (*emia* blood condition)

lipidosis (any disorder of fat metabolism) (*osis* condition)

lipiduria (*uria* urine condition)

lipido: lipidolysis (*lyein* to loosen)

lipo:

lipoadenoma (*aden* gland + *oma* tumor)

lipoarthritis (inflammation of the fatty tissues of the joints) (*arthron* joint + *itis* inflammation)

lipoatrophy (or, lipotrophia) (*atrophy* wasting away)

lipoblast {lipoblastic}, lipoblastoma, lipoblastomatosis (*blastos* germ + *oma* tumor + *osis* condition)

lipocardiac (*kardia* heart)

lipocele (also called *adipocele*) (*kele* hernia)

lipocere (also called *adipocere*) {lipoceratous} (*cera* wax)

lipochondrodystrophy (*chondros* cartilage + *dys* abnormal + *trophein* to nourish)

lipochondroma (*chondros* cartilage + *oma* tumor)

lipochrome (also called *chromolipid*), lipochromemia (*chroma* color + *emia* blood condition)

lipoclasis {lipclastic; also called *lipolytic*} (*klaein* to break)

lipocyte (*kytos* cell)

lipodermoid (congenital, yellowish-white, fatty, benign tumor located subconjunctivally) (*derma* skin + *eidos* form)

lipodieresis (also called *lipolysis*) (*dieresis* division)

lipodystrophy (or, lipodystrophia) (*dys* abnormal + *trophein* to nourish)

lipoferous (*ferre* to bear, carry)

lipofibroma (fiber + *oma* tumor)

lipofuscin (*fuscus* brown)

lipogenesis {lipogenetic, lipogenous} (*genere* to produce)

lipogranuloma (*granule* small grain + *oma* tumor)

lipohemarthrosis (*haima* blood + *arthron* joint + *osis* condition)

lipohypertrophy (*hyper* above, over + *trophein* to nourish)

lipolysis (also called *lipodieresis*) {lipolytic} (*lyein* to loosen)

lipomyxoma (also called *myxolipoma*) (*myxa* mucus + *oma* tumor)

lipopathy (*pathos* disease)

lipopenia {lipopenic} (*penia* deficiency)

lipopexia (the accumulation of fat in the tissues) (*pexia* fixation)

Element	From	Meaning	Examples
lip (cont'd)		[fat]	lipophagy (also called *lipolysis*) (*phagein* to devour, consume) lipophil, lipophilia {lipophilic} (*philein* to love—have an affinity for) lipoplasty (liposuction) (*plassein* to form) lipoprotein (protein) liposarcoma (*sarkos* flesh + *oma* tumor) liposoluble (soluble in fats) liposome (*soma* body) lipotrophy {lipotrophic} (*trophein* to nourish) lipotropic (*tropikos* turning) TRAILING ROOT COMPOUND: *lipidosis* fatty condition: cardiomyoliposis (*kardia* heart + *myos* muscle) mucolipidosis (mucus) sphingolipidosis (*sphingein* to bind fast) *lipids*: proteolipids (protein) *lipoma* fatty tumor: adenolipoma (*adenos* gland) angiolipoma (*angeion* blood vessel) chondrolipoma (*chondros* cartilage) dermolipoma (*derma* skin) fibrolipoma (*fibra* fiber) myelolipoma (*myelos* marrow) myolipoma (*myos* muscle) myxolipoma (*myxa* mucus) nevolipoma (*nevus* mole) osteolipoma (*osteon* bone) pseudolipoma (*pseudes* false) topholipoma (*tophus* porous stone) CROSS REFERENCE: adip, ather, piar, pimel, stear
list			See olist- for *anterolisthesis*.
lith, **lite**	Greek *lithos*	stone, calculus	SIMPLE ROOT: lithiasis (the formation or presence of abnormal calculi or other concretions) {lithiasic}, lithium (Li) {lithic} PREFIXED ROOT: antilithic (preventing the formation or development of calculi, as of the urinary tract) (*anti* against) endolith (*endon* within) heterolith (an intestinal concretion not formed of mineral matter) (*heteros* other) hyperlithuria (*hyper* above + *uria* urine condition) microlith, microlithiasis (*mikros* small + *iasis* condition) LEADING ROOT COMPOUND: *lith*: lithagogue (a remedy that expels calculi) (*agein* to lead) lithangiuria (calculous disease of the urinary tract) (*angeion* vessel + *uria* urine condition) litharge (fused lead protoxide, PbO; also called *lead monoxide*) (*argyros* silver) lithectomy (*ektome* excision) lithiasis (*iasis* condition) lithoid (*eidos* form) lithuresis (*uresis* urine excretion) lithuria (*uria* urine condition) *litho*: lithocenosis (*kenosis* evacuation)

Element	From	Meaning	Examples
lith (cont'd)		[stone]	lithoclast (also called *lithotrite*) (*klaein* to break)
			lithocystotomy (*kystis* bladder + *tomy* incision)
			lithogenesis (or, lithogeny; also called *calculogenesis*) {lithogenic, lithogenous} (*genere* to produce)
			litholapaxy (the crushing of a calculus in the bladder, followed by the washing out of the fragments) (*lapaxis* evacuation)
			litholysis {litholytic}, litholyte (*lyein* to dissolve)
			lithomyl (an instrument for pulverizing a stone in the bladder) (*myle* mill)
			lithonephritis (*nephron* kidney + *itis* inflammation)
			lithopedion (or, lithopedium; a dead fetus that has become stony or petrified) (*pais* child)
			lithotome, lithotomy (*tomy* incision)
			lithotresis (*tresis* a boring)
			lithotripsy {lithotriptic}, lithotriptor, lithotriptoscopy (*tribein* to rub + *skopein* to examine)
			lithotrite (also called *lithoclast*) (*tribein* to rub)
			lithotroph (also called *autotroph*) (*trophein* to nourish)
			TRAILING ROOT COMPOUND:
			lith:
			allotriolith (*allotrios* strange)
			angiolith (*angeion* blood vessel)
			appendicolith (appendix)
			arteriolith (artery)
			arthrolith (*arthron* joint)
			broncholith (*bronchos* windpipe)
			bursolith (*bursa* sac)
			canalith (canal)
			cholelith (a gallstone) {cholelithic} (*chole* bile)
			coprolith (also called *fecalith*) (*kopros* dung)
			cryptolith (*kryptos* hidden)
			cystolith {cystolithic} (*kystis* bladder)
			dacryolith (also called *ophthalmolith*) (*dakryon* teardrop)
			encephalolith (*enkephale* brain)
			enterolith (*enteron* intestine)
			fecalith (also called *coprolith, stercolith*) (*faex* refuse, dung)
			gastrolith (*gaster* stomach)
			hemolith (*haima* blood)
			hepatolith (*hepatos* liver)
			hysterolith (*hystera* uterus)
			inolith (a fibrous concretion) (*inos* fiber)
			nephrolith (*nephros* kidney)
			odontolith (dental calculus) (*odontos* tooth)
			ophthalmolith (also called *dacryolith*) (*ophthalmos* eye)
			oscheolith (*osche* scrotum—testicle pouch)
			otolith (or, otolite: also called *statolith*) (*otos* ear)
			pharyngolith (pharynx)
			phlebolith (*phlebos* vein)
			pleurolith (*pleura* rib, side)
			pneumolith (also called *pulmolith*) (*pneumon* lung)
			postholith (also called *preputial calculus*) (*posthe* prepuce)
			prostatolith (also called *prostatic calculus*) (prostate)
			ptyalolith (also called *sialolith*) (*ptyalon* saliva)
			pulmolith (also called *pneumolith*) (*pulmon* lung)

Element	From	Meaning	Examples
lith (cont'd)		[stone]	rhinolith (also called *nasal calculus*) (*rhinos* nose)
			sebolith (*sebum* suet, fat)
			sialolith (also called *ptyalolith, salivary calculus*) (*sialon* saliva)
			spermolith (also called *seminal vesicle calculus*) (*sperma* seed)
			spherolith (*sphaira* ball, globe, sphere)
			splanchnolith (*splanchnos* viscus)
			statolith (also called *otolith*) (*statos* standing)
			stercolith (also called *coprolith, fecalith*) (*stercus* feces, excrement)
			tonsillolith (also called *tonsillar calculus*) (tonsil)
			tricholith (a hairy concretion) (*trichos* hair)
			ureterolith (ureter)
			urolith (*ouron* urine)
			uterolith (also called *hysterolith*) (uterus)
			lithiasis calculus condition:
			arthrolithiasis (*arthron* joint)
			broncholithiasis (*bronchos* windpipe)
			cholelithiasis (*chole* bile)
			dacryolithiasis (*dakryon* teardrop)
			enterolithiasis (*enteron* intestine)
			gastrolithiasis (*gaster* stomach, belly)
			hepatolithiasis (*hepatos* liver)
			nephrolithiasis (*nephros* kidney)
			odontolithiasis (*odontos* tooth)
			phlebolithiasis (*phlebos* vein)
			pneumolithiasis (*pneumon* lung)
			pseudolithiasis (*pseudes* false)
			rhinolithiasis (*rhinos* nose)
			salpingolithiasis (*salpingos* tube)
			typhlolithiasis (*typhlon* blind gut)
			ureterolithiasis (ureter)
			urolithiasis (*ouron* urine)
			vesicolithiasis (also called *cystolithiasis*) (*vesica* bladder)
			lithectomy excision of calculus:
			cystolithectomy (*kystis* bladder)
			hepatolithectomy (*hepatos* liver)
			pancreatolithectomy (pancreas)
			lithotomy incision of calculus:
			cystolithotomy (also called *cystolithectomy*) (*kystis* bladder)
			nephrolithotomy (*nephros* kidney)
			pelvilithotomy (or, pelviolithotomy) (pelvis)
			pyelolithotomy (or, pelvilithotomy) (*pyelos* pelvis)
			ureterolithotomy (ureter)
			lithotripsy: cholelithotripsy (*chole* bile + *tripsis* crushing)
			CROSS REFERENCE: calc, petr
lob	Greek *lobos*; Latin *lobus*	lobe	SIMPLE ROOT:
			lobe {lobar, lobate, lobose}, lobite (limited to a definite lobe)
			lobulate (or, lobulated), lobule (a small lobe) {lobular}
			lobulose, lobulous, lobulus (pl., lobuli), lobus (pl., lobi)
			PREFIXED ROOT:
			lobar:
			interlobar (*inter* between)
			intralobar (*intra* within)
			multilobar (or, multilobate, multilobed) (*multi* many)
			perilobar (*peri* around)

A Thesaurus of Medical Word Roots

Element	From	Meaning	Examples
lob (cont'd)		[lobe]	unilobar (consisting of only one lobe) (*uni* one)
			lobate:
			bilobate (or, bilobed) (having two lobes) (*bi* two)
			multilobate (or, multilobar) (*multus* many)
			trilobate (or, trilobed) (*tri* three)
			lobe: sublobe (a division of a lobe) (*sub* below, part of)
			lobectomy: bilobectomy (*bi* two + lobectomy)
			lobitis: interlobitis (*inter* between + lobitis)
			lobul: perilobulitis (*peri* around + *itis* inflammation)
			lobular:
			bilobular (having two lobules) (*bi* two)
			centrilobular (or, centrolobular) (*kentron* center)
			interlobular (*inter* between)
			intralobular (*intra* within)
			multilobular (*multi* many)
			sublobular (*sub* under)
			lobus: mesolobus (*mesos* middle)
			LEADING ROOT COMPOUND:
			lob:
			lobectomy (*ektome* excision)
			lobitis (*itis* inflammation)
			lobo:
			lobomycosis (*mykes* fungus + *osis* condition)
			lobopodium (pl., lobopodia) (*podos* foot)
			lobotomy (*tomy* incision)
			CROSS REFERENCE: None
loc	Latin *locos*	place	SIMPLE ROOT:
			local (pertaining to one place or part; not general)
			localization (the determination of the site or place of any process or lesion), localized, localizer, locator
			loculate, loculus (cell, compartment; pl., loculi) {locular}
			locum, locus (pl., loci)
			PREFIXED ROOT:
			local:
			multilocal (*multus* many)
			unilocal (*uni* one)
			location:
			antelocation (the forward displacement of an organ) (*ante* before)
			dislocation (*dis* apart)
			translocation (*trans* across)
			locular:
			bilocular (or, biloculate; having two compartments) (*bi* two)
			intralocular (*intra* within)
			monolocular (also called *unilocular*) (*monos* single)
			multilocular (*multus* many)
			plurilocular (*plus* more)
			quadrilocular (*quattuor* four)
			trilocular (*tri* three)
			unilocular (also called *monolocular*) (*uni* one)
			LEADING ROOT COMPOUND: locomotorium (*movere* to move)
			FRENCH:
			accouchement (confinement for giving birth to a child)
			milieu (lit., middle of the place; surroundings; environment)
			CROSS REFERENCE: top

Element	From	Meaning	Examples
lochi	Greek *lochios* of child-birth	vaginal discharge	SIMPLE ROOT: lochia (the vaginal discharge that occurs during the first week or two after childbirth) {lochial} PREFIXED ROOT: alochia (absence of the lochia) (*a* privative) dyslochia (disordered lochial discharge) (*dys* abnormal) LEADING ROOT COMPOUND: lochiocolpos (distention of the vagina by retained lochia) (*kolpos* vagina) lochiometra, lochiometritis (*metra* uterus + *itis* inflammation) lochiopyra (puerperal fever) (*pyr* fire, fever) lochiorrhagia (*rhagia* bursting forth) lochiorrhea (an abnormally profuse discharge of the lochia) (*rhein* to flow) lochioschesis (also called *lochiostasis*) (*schesis* retention) lochiostasis (also called *lochioschesis*) (*stasis* halting) TERM: lochia alba (the final vaginal discharge after parturition, when the amount of blood decreases) CROSS REFERENCE: None
logo, **-logy** (see Appendix C)	Greek *logos* word	speech; reasoning give an account of; proportion; study of	PREFIXED ROOT: *logia*: alogia (inability to express oneself through speech; aphasia) (*a* privative) catalogia (verbigeration) (*kata* completely) dyslogia (impairment of the reasoning power; also, impairment of the speech, due to mental disorders) (*dys* abnormal) hyperlogia (morbid verbosity or loquacity) (*hyper* above) hypologia (*hypo* under) paralogia (or, paralogism, paralogy; false reasoning; self-deception) (*para* false, abnormal) polylogia (continuous and often incoherent speech) (*polys* many, much) *logous*: analogous (*ana* again, back, up) autologous (related to self) (*autos* self) heterologous (made up of tissue not normal to the part) (*heteros* other) isologous (*isos* equal) LEADING ROOT COMPOUND: *log*: logagraphia (*a* privative + *graphein* to write) logamnesia (amnesia: *a* privative + *mneme* memory) logaphasia (motor aphasia) (*a* privative + *phanai* to speak) logasthenia (*asthenia* weakness: *a* privative + *sthenos* strength) *logo*: logoclonia (or, logoklony) (*klonein* to agitate) logopedia (or, logopedics) (*pais* child) logoplegia (also called *laloplegia*; paralysis of the speech organs) (*plessein* to strike) logorrhea (unusual loquacity seen in insanity) (*rhein* to flow) logospasm (*spasmos* contraction) logotherapy (*therapy* treatment) TRAILING ROOT COMPOUND: *logia*: pseudologia (pathologic lying in speech or writing) (*pseudes* false)

Element	From	Meaning	Examples
logo (cont'd)		[word, speech]	*logism*: neologism (a meaningless word uttered by a psychotic or delirious person) (*neos* new) *logy*: (examples) adenology (*adenos* gland) allergology (allergies) angiology (*angeion* vessel—blood vessel) arthrology (*arthron* joint) audiology (*audire* to hear) cancerology (cancer) cardiology (*kardia* heart) dermatology (*dermatos* skin) gastrology (*gaster* stomach, belly) histology (*histos* tissue) myology (*myos* muscle) nephrology (*nephros* kidney) neurology (*neuron* nerve) oncology (*onkos* mass, tumor) otology (*otos* ear) pathology (*pathos* feeling, disease) psychology (*psyche* mind) proctology (*proktos* anus, rectum) rhinology (*rhinos* nose) CROSS REFERENCE: lal, lingu, loqui, or, phan, phras
loqui	Latin *loqui*	to speak	TRAILING ROOT COMPOUND: *loquism*: capriloquism (also called *egophony*) (*caper* goat) maniloquism (also called *dactylology, signing*) (*manus* hand) somniloquism (*somnus* sleep) *loquy*: bronchiloquy (*bronchos* windpipe) pectoriloquy (*pectus* chest) CROSS REFERENCE: fab, lal, lingu, logo, phas
lum	Latin *lumen*	light	SIMPLE ROOT: lumen (the space within an artery, vein, intestine, or tube; also, unit of light; pl., lumina) {luminal, luminalis} luminance, luminescence, luminous PREFIXED ROOT: illumination (the lighting up of a part, cavity, organ, or object for inspection) illuminism (a state marked by delusions of communication with supernatural beings) (*in* in) intraluminal (also called *intratubal, endoluminal*) (*intra* within) subluminal (*sub* below, beneath) transillumination (*trans* across + illumination) LEADING ROOT COMPOUND: *lumi*: lumichrome (*chroma* color) lumiflavin (*flavus* yellow) lumirhodopsin (*rhodon* rose + *opsis* vision) *lumini*: luminiferous (conveying light or propagating those vibrations which constitute light) (*ferre* to bear) *lumino*: luminophore (a chemical group that gives the property of luminescence to organic compounds) (*pherein* to bear) CROSS REFERENCE: phos

Element	From	Meaning	Examples
lumb	Latin *lumbus*	loin	SIMPLE ROOT: lumbago (pain in mid and lower back; a descriptive term not specifying cause; also called *lumbodynia*) lumbarization (a congenital anomaly of the lumbosacral junction) lumbus (the part of the back between the thorax and the pelvis; also called *loin*; pl., lumbi) {lumbar} PREFIXED ROOT: paralumbar (next to the lumbar side) (*para* alongside) prelumbar (situated immediately in front of the loins; applied to the dorsal part of the abdomen) (*pre* before) sublumbar (*sub* below) supralumbar (*supra* above) translumbar (*trans* across, through) LEADING ROOT COMPOUND: *lumb*: lumbodynia (also called *lumbago*) (*odyne* pain) lumbovarian (ovary) *lumbo*: lumboabdominal (relating to the sides and front of the abdomen) lumbocolostomy (the operation of forming a permanent opening into the colon by an incision through the lumbar region) (colon + *stoma* mouth, opening) lumbocolotomy (colon + *tomy* incision) lumbocostal (*costa* rib, side) lumbocrural (*crus* leg; *crura* legs) lumbodorsal [pertaining to the lumbar and thoracic (formerly called *dorsal*) regions] (*dorsum* back) lumboiliac (also called *lumboinguinal, iliolumbar*) (ilium) lumboinguinal (pertaining to the loins and the groin) (*inguen* groin) lumbosacral (sacrum) TRAILING ROOT COMPOUND: dorsolumbar (*dorsum* back) iliolumbar (also called *lumboiliac*) (ilium) sacrolumbar (pertaining to the sacrum and the lumbar) thoracolumbar (*thorakos* chest) CROSS REFERENCE: lapar
lut	Latin *luteus*	yellow [See Root Note]	ROOT NOTE: Also refers to the corpus luteum, a yellow glandular mass in the ovary. SIMPLE ROOT: luteal, lutein (a yellow pigment {luteal, luteinic} luteinization, luteinize; luteolin LEADING ROOT COMPOUND: *lute*: luteectomy (*ektome* excision) luteoma (or, luteinoma) (*oma* tumor) *luteo*: luteolysin (a substance that causes degeneration of the corpus luteum) {luteolytic} (*lyein* to dissolve) luteotropic (*tropein* to turn) CROSS REFERENCE: cirrh, xanth
lymph	Latin *lympha* water	fluid (of the body)	SIMPLE ROOT: lymph (or, lympha; a transparent, slightly yellow liquid of alkaline reaction, found in the lymphatic vessels) {lymphatic, lymphous}, lymphatism, lymphization

A Thesaurus of Medical Word Roots

Element	From	Meaning	Examples
lymph (cont'd)		[body fluid]	PREFIXED ROOT:

lympha:

endolympha (or, endolymph) {endolymphic} (*endon* within)

perilympha {perilymphatic} (*peri* around)

lymphemia lymphatic blood condition:

hypolymphemia (also called *sublymphemia*) (*hypo* under)

sublymphemia (also called *hypolymphemia*) (*sub* below)

lymphia: alymphia (absence or deficiency of lymph) (*a* privative)

lymphocyte white blood cell:

mesolymphocyte (*mesos* medium)

prolymphocyte (*pro* before)

LEADING ROOT COMPOUND:

lymph:

lymphadenoma (*aden* gland + *oma* tumor)

lymphagogue (an agent that promotes the production of lymph) (*agein* to lead)

lymphangial (*angeion* vessel—blood vessel)

lymphapheresis (*apheresis* removal)

lymphectasia (*ectasia* distention, a stretching)

lymphedema (*edema* swelling)

lymphemia (*emia* blood condition)

lymphenteritis (*enteron* intestine + *itis* inflammation)

lymphnoditis (also called *lymphadenitis*) (*nodus* knot + *itis* inflammation)

lymphoid, lymphoidectomy (*eidos* form + *ektome* excision)

lymphoma {lymphomatous}, lymphomatosis (*oma* tumor + *osis* condition)

lymphosis (*osis* condition)

lymphuria (*uria* urine condition)

lymphat: lymphatitis (*itis* inflammation)

lymphatico: lymphaticostomy (*stoma* mouth, opening)

lymphato:

lymphatogenous (*genere* to produce)

lymphatology (*logos* study)

lymphatolysis {lymphatolytic} (*lyein* to dissolve)

lympho:

lymphoblastoma (*blastos* germ + *oma* tumor)

lymphoblastosis (*blastos* germ + *osis* condition)

lymphocele (also called *lymphocyst*) (*kele* tumor)

lymphocerastism (*kerastos* mixed)

lymphocinesia (also called *lymphokinesis*) (*kinein* to move)

lymphocyst (also called *lymphocele*) (*kystis* bladder, sac)

lymphocyte (*kytos* cell)

lymphoduct (a lymphatic vessel) (*ducere* to lead)

lymphogenesis {lymphgenic, lymphogenous} (*genesis* beginning)

lymphoglandula (a lymph node) (*glans* acorn: gland)

lymphogranuloma, lymphogranulomatosis (*granulum* little grain + *oma* tumor + *osis* condition)

lymphography (*graphein* to write)

lymphohistiocytosis (proliferation or infiltration of lymphocytes and histiocytes) (*histos* web + *kytos* cell + *osis* condition)

lymphokinesis (*kinein* to move)

lympholeukocyte (also called *lymphocyte*) (*leukos* white + *kytos* cell)

lymphology (*logos* study)

A Thesaurus of Medical Word Roots

Element	From	Meaning	Examples
lymph (cont'd)		[body fluid]	lympholysis {lympholytic} (*lyein* to loosen)
			lymphomyxoma (*myxa* mucus + *oma* tumor)
			lymphonodus (also called *lymph node*; pl., lymphonodi) (*nodus* knot)
			lymphopathy (or, lymphopathia) (*pathos* disease)
			lymphopenia (*penia* deficiency)
			lymphoplasia, lymphoplasm (*plassein* to form)
			lymphopoiesis {lymphopoietic} (*poiein* to produce)
			lymphoreticular, lymphoreticulosis (*ret* net + *osis* condition)
			lymphorrhagia (also called *lymphorrhea*) (*rhagia* bursting forth)
			lymphorrhea (also called *lymphorrhagia*) (*rhein* to flow)
			lymphosarcoma (*sarkos* flesh + *oma* tumor)
			lymphostasis (*stasis* standing)
			lymphotaxis (*taxis* arrangement)
			lymphotoxicity, lymphotoxin (*toxin* poison)
			lymphotrophy (*trophein* to nourish)
			lymphotropic (*tropein* to turn)
			TRAILING ROOT COMPOUND:
			lymph:
			cortilymph (similar to *perilymph*) (organ of Corti)
			cytolymph (*kytos* cell)
			hemolymph (*haima* blood)
			karyolymph (also called *nucleolymph*) (*karyon* nucleus of a cell)
			nucleolymph (also called *karyolymph*) (*nucleus* nut, kernel)
			lymphatic:
			pyelolymphatic (*pyelos* pelvis)
			splenolymphatic (spleen)
			vasculolymphatic (*vascule* small vessel)
			lymphitis inflammation of lymph gland:
			adenolymphitis (also called *lymphadenitis*) (*adenos* gland)
			angiolymphitis (also called *lymphangitis*) (*angeion* vessel)
			lymphocyte: pseudolymphocyte (*pseudes* false + lymphocyte)
			lymphoma lymph tumor:
			adenolymphoma (*aden* gland)
			neurolymphomatosis (*neuron* nerve + *osis* condition)
			pseudolymphoma (*pseudes* false)
			CROSS REFERENCE: hydr, ser
lys, **lyt,** **lyz**	Greek *lyein* to loosen	to loosen, dissolve, free; also, to weaken, esp. at the side	SIMPLE ROOT:
			lysate (material produced by the destructive process of lysis)
			lysin, lysis (the process of cell destruction through the action of specific lysins; the gradual ending of disease symptoms)
			lytic (pertaining to lysis or to a lysin; producing lysis)
			PREFIXED ROOT:
			lysin:
			heterolysin (*heteros* other)
			isolysin (*isos* equal)
			lysis:
			analysis (as opposed to *synthesis*) {analytic} (*ana* again)
			antilysis {antilytic} (*anti* against)
			autolysis {autolytic} (*autos* self)
			catalysis {catalytic} (*kata* down)
			dialysis {dialytic} (*dia* across) [see separate entry: dialys-]
			ectolysis (lysis of the ectoplasm) (*ektos* outside)
			endolysis (*endon* inside)

Element	From	Meaning	Examples
lys (cont'd)		[to loosen]	heterolysis {heterolytic} (*heteros* different) homolysis (*homos* same) isolysis {isolytic} (*isos* equal) paralysis (pl., paralyses) {paralytic} (*para* beside) *lyst*: analyst (*ana* again) catalyst (*kata* down) *lytic*: intradialytic (taking place during hemodialysis) (*intra* within + *dia* through) *lyto*: paralytogenic (*para* alongside + *genere* to produce) *lyze*: analyze, analyzer (*ana* again) autolyze (*autos* self) catalyze (*kata* down) dialyze (*dia* across) paralyze {paralyzant} (*para* beside) LEADING ROOT COMPOUND: *lyo*: lyoenzyme (enzyme) lyolysis (also called *solvolysis*) lyophil {lyophilic} (*philein* to love—have an affinity for) lyophobic (not having an affinity for solution) (*phobia* fear) lyosorption (*sorbere* to suck in) lyotropic (also called *lyophilic*) (*tropic* turning) *lys*: lysemia (*emia* blood condition) lysinosis (lung disease due to inhaling cotton fibers, as in cotton mills) (*inos* fiber + *osis* condition) *lysin*: lysinuria (*uria* urine condition) *lysino*: lysinogenic (*genere* to produce) *lyso*: lysogenesis {lysogenic} (*genere* to produce) lysosome (*soma* body) lysotype lysozyme (*zyme* ferment, leaven) TRAILING ROOT COMPOUND: acantholysis (atrophy of the prickle cell layer of the epidermis) (*akanthos* thorny) adipolysis {adipolytic} (*adeps* fat) aminolysis (amine) angiolysis (*angeion* blood vessel) arthrolysis (*arthron* joint) biolysis {biolytic} (*bios* life) blastolysis {blastolytic} (*blastos* bud, shoot, germ) cancerolytic (also called *carcinolytic*) (cancer) cantholysis (*kanthos* eye angle) carcinolysis (also called *cancerolytic*) (*karkinos* crab, cancer) cardiolysis (*kardia* heart) catholysis (cathode) ceruminolysis (*cerumen* waxlike secretion) chemolysis (chemical) chondrolysis (*chondros* cartilage) chromatolysis (*chromatos* color) cololysis (colon)

A Thesaurus of Medical Word Roots

Element	From	Meaning	Examples
lys (cont'd)		[to loosen]	corelysis (*kore* pupil of eye)
			cryolysis (*kryos* cold)
			cytolysis (*kytos* cell, vessel)
			dermatolysis (*dermatos* skin)
			duodenolysis (duodenum)
			elastolysis (*elastos* ductile)
			electrolysis (electricity)
			enzymolysis (enzyme; *en* in + *zyme* leaven)
			fibrinolysis (fibrin)
			gangliolysis (*ganglion* knot)
			gastrolysis (*gaster* stomach, belly)
			glycolysis (or, glucolysis) (*glykys* sweet)
			hemolysis (or, hematolysis) (*haima* blood)
			hepatolysis (*hepatos* liver)
			histolysis (*histos* web, tissue)
			hydrolysis (*hydor* water)
			hysterolysis (*hystera* uterus)
			karyolysis (*karyon* nut: nucleus)
			leukolysis (also called *leukocytolysis*) (*leukos* white)
			lipolysis (*lipos* fat)
			lymphatolysis (*lympha* water: body fluid)
			morpholysis (*morphe* form)
			mucolysis (mucus)
			myelinolysis (also called *myelinosis*) (myelin)
			myolysis (*myos* muscle)
			necrolysis (*nekros* dead)
			nephrolysis (*nephros* kidney)
			neurolysis (*neuron* nerve)
			odontolysis (*odontos* tooth)
			oncolysis (*onkos* mass, bulk: tumor)
			onycholysis (*onychos* nail)
			osteolysis (*osteon* bone)
			peptolysis {peptolytic} (peptone)
			phacolysis (or, phakolysis) {phacolytic} (*phakos* lens)
			phagolysis (also called *phagocytolysis*) (*phagein* to consume)
			pharyngolysis (pharynx)
			photolysis (*photos* light)
			physiolysis (*phyein* to grow)
			plasmolysis (*plassein* to form)
			pleurolysis (*pleura* side, rib)
			pneumolysis (*pneumon* lung)
			proteolysis (protein)
			pyrolysis (*pyr* fire, heat, fever)
			rachilysis (*rhachis* spine, backbone)
			rhizolysis (*rhiza* root)
			salpingolysis (*salpingos* tube)
			spermatolysis (*spermatos* seed, sperm)
			sphincterolysis (*sphingein* to draw tight)
			splenolysis (*splen* spleen)
			spondylolysis (*spondylos* vertebra)
			steatolysis (*steatos* fat)
			tenolysis (or, tendolysis) (*tenon* tendon)
			thermolysis (*therme* heat)
			thrombolysis (*thrombos* clot)

269

Element	From	Meaning	Examples
lys (cont'd)		[to loosen]	thymolysis (thymus)
			trypanolysis (*trypanon* a borer)
			ureterolysis (ureter)
			lyte:
			actinolyte (*aktis* ray)
			photolyte (a substance decomposed by light) (*photos* light)
			lytic:
			adipolytic (*adipos* fat)
			adrenolytic (adrenal glands)
			amylolytic (*amylon* starch)
			cytolytic (*kytos* cell)
			elastolytic (elastic)
			enzymolytic (enzyme)
			epitheliolytic (epithelium)
			hemolytic (*haima* blood)
			hepatolytic (*hepatos* liver)
			mucinolytic (mucin)
			nephrolytic (*nephros* kidney)
			neurolytic (*neuron* nerve)
			ovolytic (*ovum* egg)
			peptidolytic (peptide)
			spasmolytic (spasm)
			thermolytic (*therme* heat)
			thrombolytic (*thrombos* clot)
			thyrolytic (thyroid gland)
			lyze:
			electrolyze (to decompose by the direct action of electricity)
			hemolyze (*haima* blood)
			hydrolyze (*hydor* water)
			thermolyze (*therme* heat)
			CROSS REFERENCE: clas, lept, pares

Element	From	Meaning	Examples
macr-	Greek prefix *makros*	long, large; abnormal length or size	TRAILING ROOT COMPOUND: acromacria (abnormal length and slenderness of the fingers and toes; also called *arachnodactyly*) (*akros* extremity) See Appendix B for examples of words with this element used as a prefix. Others are listed with the root to which it is attached. CROSS REFERENCE: dolicho, mega
macul	Latin *macula* spot	spot, blemish, stain	SIMPLE ROOT: macula (or, macule; a stain or spot; used in anatomical nomenclature to designate an area distinguishable from its surroundings; pl., maculae) {macular, maculate} PREFIXED ROOT: emaculation (*ex* out) LEADING ROOT COMPOUND: maculocerebral (pertaining to the macula retinae and the brain) (*cerebrum* brain) maculoerythematous (*erythrys* red) maculopapule {maculopapular} (*papula* pimple) maculopathy (*pathos* disease) maculovesicular (both macular and vesicular) (*vesica* blister) TERMS: macula lutea (a part of the retina) macula retinae (a yellowish depression on the retina) CROSS REFERENCE: punct
mal-	Latin prefix	bad, abnormal	EXTENDED PREFIX: mal (a disease or disorder), maladie (or, malady; a disease) malaria (lit., bad air; a disease caused by certain mosquitoes) {malarial, malarious} malignant, malum (a disease) FRENCH: malaise (a vague feeling of bodily discomfort and fatigue) See Appendix B for examples of words with this element used as a prefix. Others are listed with the root to which it is attached. CROSS REFERENCE: cac-, dys-
malac, malag, malax	Greek *malakos*	abnormal softness	SIMPLE ROOT: *malac*: malacia (also called *malacosis*) {malacic}, malacotic (said of teeth), malactic (softening; emollient; an emollient medicine) *malag*: malagma (an emollient or cataplasm) *malax*: malaxation (formation of ingredients into a mass for pills and plasters) LEADING ROOT COMPOUND: *malac*: malacoma (*oma* tumor) malacosis (also called *malacia*) {malacotic} (*osis* condition) malacosteon (also called *osteomalacia*) (*osteon* bone) *malaco*: malacoplakia (*plax* plaque) TRAILING ROOT COMPOUND: adenomalacia (*adenos* gland) arteriomalacia (*arteria* artery) bronchomalacia (*bronchos* windpipe) cardiomalacia (*kardia* heart) cerebromalacia (*cerebrum* skull)

Element	From	Meaning	Examples
malac (cont'd)		[abnormal softness]	chondromalacia (*chondros* cartilage)
			craniomalacia (*kranion* skull)
			encephalomalacia (*enkephale* brain)
			esophagomalacia (esophagus)
			gastromalacia (*gaster* stomach, belly)
			hepatomalacia (*hepatos* liver)
			iridomalacia (*iridos* rainbow: iris)
			keratomalacia (also called *xerotic keratitis*) (*keras* horn: cornea)
			laryngomalacia (also called *chondromalacia of larynx*)
			leukomalacia (softening of the white matter of the brain)
			lienomalacia (also called *splenomalacia*) (*lien* spleen)
			lunatomalacia (osteochondrosis of the semilunar bone) (*luna* moon)
			meningomalacia (*meningos* membrane)
			metromalacia (*metra* uterus)
			myelomalacia (*myelos* marrow)
			myomalacia (*myos* muscle)
			nephromalacia (*nephros* kidney)
			neuromalacia (*neuron* nerve)
			onychomalacia (*onychos* nail)
			ophthalmomalacia (*ophthalmos* eye)
			osteomalacia (also called *malacosteon*) (*osteon* bone)
			phacomalacia (softening of the lens) (*phakos* lens)
			pneumomalacia (*pneumon* lung)
			retinomalacia (retina)
			scleromalacia (degenerative thinning of the sclera) (sclera)
			splenomalacia (also called *lienomalacia*) (spleen)
			spondylomalacia (*spondylos* vertebra)
			stomatomalacia (*stomatos* mouth)
			tarsomalacia (*tarsos* eyelid)
			tephromalacia (*tephros* gray—gray matter of brain or spinal cord)
			tracheomalacia (*trachea* windpipe)
			CROSS REFERENCE: pia
mamm	Latin *mamma* breast	breast, nipple	SIMPLE ROOT:
			mamma (gland for secreting milk; pl. mammae)
			mammal, mammary
			mamilla (pl., mamillae), mamillary (also spelled *mammillary*)
			mamillate (or, mammillate, mamillated; also, mammillated; having nipple-like projections), mamillation
			PREFIXED ROOT:
			mammae: multimammae (also called *polymastia*) (*multus* many)
			mammary:
			inframammary (below the mammary gland) (*infra* below)
			intermammary (between the breasts) (*inter* between)
			intramammary (*intra* within)
			retromammary (*retro* behind)
			submammary (*sub* under)
			supramammary (*supra* above, superior to)
			mamillary:
			inframamillary (inferior to the nipple) (*infra* below)
			intermamillary (between the nipples) (*inter* between)
			LEADING ROOT COMPOUND:
			mamill: mamillitis (or, mammillitis) (*itis* inflammation)
			mamm:
			mammalgia (also called *mastalgia, mastodynia*) (*algos* pain)

Element	From	Meaning	Examples
mamm (cont'd)		[breast, nipple]	mammectomy (also called *mastectomy*) (*ektome* excision)
			mammose (*osis* condition)
			mamma:
			mammaplasty (*plassein* to form)
			mammatroph (also called *lactotroph*) (*trophein* to nourish)
			mammi:
			mammiform (*forma* shape)
			mammiplasia (or, mammoplasia) (*plassein* to form)
			mammill: mammillitis (*itis* inflammation)
			mammilla: mammillaplasty (*plassein* to form)
			mammilli:
			mammilliform (*forma* shape)
			mammilliplasty (also called *theleplasty*) (*plassein* to form)
			mammo:
			mammogen, mammogenesis (*genere* to produce)
			mammogram, mammography (*graphein* to write)
			mammoplasia, mammoplasty (*plassein* to form)
			mammotomy (also called *mastotomy*) (*tomy* incision)
			mammotroph (also called *lactotroph*) (*trophe* nourishment)
			mammotropic (also called *mammotrophic*) (*trepein* to turn)
			TRAILING ROOT COMPOUND:
			thalamomamillary (*thalamus* inner chamber)
			vertebromammary (*vertebra*)
			CROSS REFERENCE: mast, papill, pector, stern, steth, thel
mandib	Latin *mandere* to chew	lower jawbone	SIMPLE ROOT: mandibula (pl., mandibulae), mandible (or, mandibulum) {mandibular}
			PREFIXED ROOT:
			mandible: micromandible (*mikros* small)
			mandibular:
			circummandibular (*circum* around)
			epimandibular (situated upon the lower jaw) (*epi* upon)
			inframandibular (also called *submandibular*) (*infra* below)
			perimandibular (*peri* around)
			retromandibular (*retro* behind)
			submandibular (also called *inframandibular*) (*sub* below)
			supramandibular (*supra* above)
			LEADING ROOT COMPOUND:
			mandibul: mandibulectomy (*ektome* excision)
			mandibulo:
			mandibulofacial (face)
			mandibulooculofacial (*oculus* eye + face)
			mandibulopharyngeal (pharynx)
			TRAILING ROOT COMPOUND:
			maxillomandibular (*maxilla* upper jaw)
			oromandibular (*oris* mouth)
			stylomandibular (styloid process)
			temporomandibular (temporal bone)
			tympanomandibular (*tympanom* drum: eardrum)
			CROSS REFERENCE: geny, gnath, maxill
mania	Greek *mania*	madness for; insanity; mental aberration	SIMPLE ROOT: mania, maniac {maniacal}, manicky
			PREFIXED ROOT:
			hypomania {hypomanic} (*hypo* under)
			monomania {monomaniacal} (*monos* one, single)
			premaniacal (preceding a manic attack) (*pre* before)

Element	From	Meaning	Examples
mania (cont'd)		[madness]	LEADING ROOT COMPOUND: maniaphobia (*phobia* fear) TRAILING ROOT COMPOUND: ablutomania (*ablutio* washing, especially of the hands) dipsomania (*dipsa* thirst) doromania (*doron* gift) erotomania (*eros* sexual desire) kleptomania (*kleptein* to steal) megalomania (delusion of grandeur) {megalomaniac} (*megalos* large) phagomania (*phagein* to eat) pyromania (obsessive preoccupation with fires) (*pyr* fire) toxicomania (addiction to a drug) (*toxikon* poison) CROSS REFERENCE: None
mano	Greek *manos*	thin	LEADING ROOT COMPOUND: manometer (an instrument for measuring the pressure or tension of liquids or gases, as the blood, etc.; also called *manoscopy*) {manometric} (*metron* measure) manoscopy (the measurement of the density of gases; also called *manometer*) (*skopein* to examine) TRAILING ROOT COMPOUND: nasomanometer (a manometer for measuring intranasal pressure; also called *rhinomanometry*) (*nasus* nose) phlebomanometer (*phlebos* vein) rhinomanometry (also called *nasomanometer*) (*rhinos* nose) sphygmomanometer (*sphygmos* pulse) CROSS REFERENCE: lept
mast, maz	Greek *mastos; mazos* breast	breast; mammary gland	PREFIXED ROOT: *mast:* postmastectomy (*post* after + *ektome* excision) *mastia:* amastia (or, amazia; lack of breast development) (*a* privative) anisomastia (*aniso* unequal: *an* negative + *isos* equal) gigantomastia (extreme macromastia) (*gigantos* giant) hypermastia (also called *gigantomastia, macromastia, polymastia*) (*hyper* above, over) hypomastia (abnormal smallness of the mammary glands; also called *micromastia*) (*hypo* under) macromastia (also called *polymastia*) (*makros* large) micromastia (also called *hypomastia*) (*mikros* small) pleomastia (also called *polymastia*) (*pleion* excessive) polymastia (also called *hypermastia, macromastia*) (*polys* many) tetramastia (also called *tetramazia*) (*tetra* four) *mastitis* inflammation of the breast: paramastitis (*para* alongside) perimastitis (*peri* around) *mastoid* similar to a breast: bimastoid (*bi* two) postmastoid (*post* posterior) retromastoid (*retro* posterior) supramastoid (*supra* above) *mazia:* amazia (lack of the development of the breasts) (*a* privative) macromazia (also called *macromastia*) (*makros* large) micromazia (also called *micromastia*) (*mikros* small) pleomazia (also called *polymastia*) (*pleion* excessive)

Element	From	Meaning	Examples
mast (cont'd)		[breast]	polymazia (also called *polymastia*) (*polys* many)

polymazia (also called *polymastia*) (*polys* many)
tetramazia (also called *tetramastia*) (*tetra* four)
LEADING ROOT COMPOUND:
mast:
mastadenitis (inflammation of the mammary gland; also called *mas-titis*) (*adenos* gland + *itis* inflammation)
mastadenoma (*adenos* gland + *oma* tumor)
mastalgia (pain in the mammary gland) (*algos* pain)
mastatrophia (or, mastatrophy; atrophy of the mammary gland) (*a* negative + *trephein* to nourish)
mastauxe (*auxein* to increase)
mastectomy (*ektome* excision)
mastitis (also called *mastadenitis*) (*itis* inflammation)
mastoccipital (*occiput* back of the head: *ob* against + *caput* head)
mastodynia (or, mazodynia) (*odyne* pain)
mastoid (*eidos* form)
mastoncus (*onkos* mass, tumor)
masto:
mastocytoma (a neoplasm containing mastocytes) (*kytos* cell + *oma* tumor)
mastocytosis (an overproduction of mast cells in body tissues) (*kytos* cell + *osis* condition)
mastomenia (*mene* menses)
mastooccipital (or, mastoccipital) (*occiput* back of the head)
mastopathia (or, mastopathy) (*pathos* disease)
mastopexy (also called *mazopexy*) (*pexis* fixation)
mastoplasia (also called *mammoplasia*) (*plassein* to form)
mastoptosis (pendulous breasts) (*ptein* to fall)
mastorrhagia (*rhagia* bursting forth)
mastoscirrhus (*skirrhos* hardness)
mastosquamous (*squama* scale)
mastostomy (*stoma* mouth, opening)
mastosyrinx (*syrinx* tube)
mastotomy (*tomy* incision)
mastoid:
mastoidalgia (*algos* pain)
mastoidectomy (*ektome* excision)
mastoiditis (*itis* inflammation)
mastoido: mastoidotomy (*tomy* incision)
mazo:
mazopexy (also called *mastopexy*) (*pexis* fixation)
mazoplasia (*plassein* to form)
TRAILING ROOT COMPOUND:
mast: acromastitis (*akron* extremity + *itis* inflammation)
mastia: pseudogynecomastia (*pseudes* false + *gyneco* woman)
mastoid:
otomastoiditis (*otos* ear + *itis* inflammation)
petromastoid (also called *otocranium*) (*petra* stone)
squamomastoid (*squama* scale, plate)
sternomastoid (*sternon* chest, breast)
stylomastoid (styloid process)
tympanomastoiditis (*tympanon* eardrum + *itis* inflammation)
NB: *Mastication*, from *masticare*, to chew, is not in this family.
CROSS REFERENCE: mamm, pect, stern, steth, thora

Element	From	Meaning	Examples
mastig	Greek *mastix* lash, whip	flagellum	SIMPLE ROOT: mastigote (an individual flagellate) PREFIXED ROOT: amastigote (*a* privative) epimastigote (*epi* upon) heteromastigote (*heteros* other) holomastigote (*holos* entire) isomastigote (*isos* equal) monomastigote (*monos* single) paramastigote (*para* alongside) polymastigote (*polys* many) promastigote (*pro* before) tetramastigote (*tetra* four) trimastigote (*tri* three) TRAILING ROOT COMPOUND: choanomastigote (*choane* funnel) opisthomastigote (*opisthen* behind, at the back) trypomastigote (*trypanon* borer) CROSS REFERENCE: None
maxill	Latin *maxilla* jaw	jawbone; upper jaw	SIMPLE ROOT: maxilla (pl., maxillas, maxillae) {maxillary} PREFIXED ROOT: *maxill*: hemimaxillectomy (*hemi* half + maxillectomy) *maxillary*: admaxillary (toward the maxilla) (*ad* to) bimaxillary (*bi* two) inframaxillary (also called *submaxillary, mandibular*) (*infra* below) intermaxillary (*inter* between) monomaxillary (*monos* one) premaxillary (*pre* before) submaxillary (*sub* under) supramaxillary (*supra* above) LEADING ROOT COMPOUND: *maxill*: maxillectomy (*ektome* excision) maxillitis (*itis* inflammation) *maxillo*: maxilloethmoidectomy (ethmoid process + *ektome* excision) maxillojugal (*jugum* yoke) maxillolabial (*labium* lip) maxillomandibular (*mandible* the lower jaw) maxillopalatine (also called *palatomaxillary*) maxillopharyngeal (*pharynx* throat) maxillotomy (*tomy* incision) TRAILING ROOT COMPOUND: buccomaxillary (*bucca* cheek) ethmomaxillary (ethmoid process) frontomaxillary (*frons* front: frontal bone) jugomaxillary (also called *zygomaticomaxillary*) (*jugum* a yoke) oromaxillary (*oris* mouth) palatomaxillary (also called *maxillopalatine*) pharyngomaxillary (also called *maxillopharyngeal*) (*pharynx* throat) sphenomaxillary (*sphenos* wedge) stylomaxillary (styloid process) zygomaxillary (*zygon* yoke) CROSS REFERENCE: geny, gnath

Element	From	Meaning	Examples
mazo			See mast.
meat	Latin *meare* to go, pass	passage	SIMPLE ROOT: meatus (a passage or opening in the body; pl., meatus, or meatuses) {meatal}
			PREFIXED ROOT:
			meable:
			impermeable (*im* negative + permeable)
			permeable {permeability}, permeant, permeate, permeation (*per* through)
			semipermeable (*semi* half + permeable)
			meant: impermeant (*im* negative)
			meatal:
			parameatal (situated near or around a meatus) (*para* alongside)
			suprameatal (*supra* above)
			LEADING ROOT COMPOUND:
			meatometer (an instrument for measuring the urinary meatus) (*metron* measure)
			meatoplasty (*plassein* to form)
			meatorrhaphy (suture of the severed end of the urethra to the glans penis following surgical procedure to enlarge the meatus) (*rhaphe* suture)
			meatoscope, meatoscopy (*skopein* to examine)
			meatotome, meatotomy (incision of the urinary meatus in order to enlarge it; also called *porotomy*) (*tomy* incision)
			CROSS REFERENCE: for, por
medi	Latin *medius*	middle	SIMPLE ROOT:
			media (plural of *medium*; middle)
			mediad (toward a median line or plane)
			medial, medialization, median, medianus
			mediate, mediation, mediator, medium (pl., media)
			PREFIXED ROOT:
			medial:
			admedial (situated toward the median plane) (*ad* to)
			submedial (or, submedian) (*sub* below)
			superomedial (*super* above)
			median:
			anteromedian (*antero* front)
			inferomedian (*inferus* low)
			paramedian (*para* alongside)
			postmedian (*post* posterior)
			posteromedian {posteromedial} (*posterior* behind)
			submedian (or, submedial) (*sub* below)
			mediary: intermediary (*inter* between)
			mediate: intermediate (*inter* between)
			medius: intermedius (*inter* between)
			LEADING ROOT COMPOUND:
			medi:
			medicephalic (*kephale* head)
			medifrontal (pertaining to the middle of the forehead)
			medioccipital (*occiput* back of head: *ob* against + *caput* head)
			medisect (to divide or dissect medially) (*sectare* to cut)
			mediao: mediaometer (an instrument for detecting and measuring refractive errors of the dioptric media) (*metron* measure)
			medio:
			mediocarpal (midcarpal) (*karpos* wrist)

Element	From	Meaning	Examples
medi (cont'd)		[middle]	mediodens (also called *mesiodens*) (*dens* tooth)
			mediodorsal (*dorsum* back)
			mediolateral (*laterus* side)
			medionecrosis (necrosis of a tunica media) (*nekrosis* death)
			mediotarsal (*tarsus* ankle)
			mediotrusion (*trudere* to thrust)
			TRAILING ROOT COMPOUND:
			dorsomedian (*dorsum* back of body)
			ventromedian (*venter* belly)
			CROSS REFERENCE: meso
medull	Latin *medulla*; from *medius* middle	marrow	SIMPLE ROOT:
			medulla (the middle, inmost part of an organ or structure; pl., medullas, or medullae) {medullary}
			medullated (also called *myelinated*), medullation, medullization
			PREFIXED ROOT:
			medullary:
			extramedullary (*extra* outside)
			intramedullary (*intra* within)
			juxtamedullary (*juxta* near, close by)
			perimedullary (*peri* around)
			medullate:
			emedullate (to extract bone marrow) (*ex* out)
			nonmedullated (also called *unmyelinated*) (*non* negative)
			LEADING ROOT COMPOUND:
			medull:
			medullectomy (excision of the medulla of an organ, as of the adrenal gland) (*ektome* excision)
			medullitis (*itis* inflammation)
			medulloid (*eidos* form)
			medullosis (*osis* condition)
			medullo:
			medulloadrenal (also called *adrenomedullary*) (*adrenal* pertaining to the kidneys)
			medulloarthritis (*arthron* joint + *itis* inflammation)
			medulloblast, medulloblastoma (*blastos* germ + *oma* tumor)
			medulloepithelioma (epithelium + *oma* tumor)
			medullomyoblastoma (*myos* muscle + *blastos* germ + *oma* tumor)
			TRAILING ROOT COMPOUND:
			adrenomedullary (also called *medulloadrenal*)
			cerebellomedullary (cerebellum)
			corticomedullary (*cortex* rind; outer portion of an organ)
			lienomedullary (also called *splenomedullary*) (*lien* spleen)
			pontomedullary (*pontis* bridge)
			radiculomedullary (*radix* root)
			renomedullary (*ren* kidney)
			splenomedullary (also called *lienomedullary*) (*splen* spleen)
			TERM: medulla oblongata (lit., elongated marrow; the nervous tissue at the bottom of the brain that controls respiration, circulation, and certain other bodily functions)
			CROSS REFERENCE: myel
mega(ly)	Greek *megas*, *megalos* very large	great, large	See Appendix B for examples of words beginning with this element. Others are placed with the roots to which it is attached.
			See Appendix C for examples of words ending with –megaly.
			CROSS REFERENCE: macr

Element	From	Meaning	Examples
meio			See mio-.
mel[1]	Greek *melos*	limb, member	PREFIXED ROOT: *melia* limb condition: amelia (congenital absence of one or more limbs; also called *lipomeria*) (*a* privative) anisomelia (*aniso* unequal: *an* negative + *isos* equal) cacomelia (congenital deformity of a limb) (*kakos* bad) diamelia (absence of two limbs) (*di* two + amelia) dimelia (*di* two) dysmelia (*dys* abnormal) hemiectromelia (*hemi* half + *ektrosis* imperfect development) hemimelia (*hemi* half) hypomelia (*hypo* under) macromelia (also called *megalomelia*) (*makros* large) megalomelia (also called *macromelia*) (*megalos* large) mesomelia (*mesos* middle) micromelia (*mikros* small) polymelia (*polys* many) symmelia (or, symelia; also called *sirenomelia*) (*sym* with) tetraamelia (*tetra* four + amelia) triamelia (absence of three limbs) (*tri* three + amelia) *melic*: monomelic (affecting one limb) (*monos* single) *melus*: tetramelus (*tetra* four) LEADING ROOT COMPOUND: *mel*: melagra (muscular pain in the limbs) (*agra* seizure) melalgia (pain of neural origin in the limbs) (*algos* pain) *melo*: melodidymus (an individual with a supernumerary limb) (*didymos* twin) melomelus (a fetus with normal limbs and rudimentary supernumerary limbs) (*melos* limb) [root is doubly used] melorheostosis (*rhein* to flow + *osteon* bone + *osis* condition) *melos*: melosalgia (pain in the lower limbs) (*algos* pain) TRAILING ROOT COMPOUND: *melia* limb condition: brachymelia (*brachys* short) camptomelia (*kampsis* bent) dolichostenomelia (*dolichos* long + *stenos* narrow) ectromelia (*ektrosis* congenital absence) meromelia (*meros* part) peromelia (or, peromely) (*peros* maimed) rhizomelic (*rhiza* root) schistomelia (*schistos* split) *melic*: orthomelic (*orthos* straight) rhizomelic (*rhiza* root) *melus*: ectromelus (*ektrosis* congenital absence) notomelus (*noton* back of body) peromelus (*peros* maimed) pleuromelus (*pleura* rib, side) pygomelus (*pyge* rump, buttocks) CROSS REFERENCE: brachi, member, scel

279

Element	From	Meaning	Examples
mel[2]	Greek *melon*	cheek	LEADING ROOT COMPOUND: *mel*: melitis (*itis* inflammation) melotia (a developmental anomaly characterized by displacement of the ear onto the cheek) (*otos* ear) *melo*: meloplasty (or, melonoplasty) (*plassein* to form) meloschisis (also called *oblique facial cleft*) (*schisis* fissure) *melono*: melonoplasty (or, meloplasty; plastic surgery of the cheek) (*plassein* to form) CROSS REFERENCE: bucc
melan	Greek *melas, melanos*	black, dark	SIMPLE ROOT: melanin, melanism (abnormal black pigmentation of the organs and tissues) {melanistic} melanous (having black or dark skin and hair) melasma (a patchy pigmentation of sun-exposed skin) melena (the passage of dark and pitchy stools stained with blood pigments or with altered blood; black vomit) PREFIXED ROOT: *melanosis* dark condition: amelanosis (complete lack of melanin in the tissues) (*a* privative) hypermelanosis (*hyper* beyond) hypomelanosis (*hypo* below) *melanosome*: macromelanosome (*makros* large + *soma* body) LEADING ROOT COMPOUND: *melan*: melancholia (a depressed and unhappy emotional state with abnormal inhibition of mental and bodily activity) (*chole* bile) melanemesis (black vomit; also called *melenemesis*) (*emein* to vomit) melanemia (*emia* blood condition) melanoid (resembling melanin; of a dark color; a material resembling melanin) (*eidos* form) melanoma (a malignant, pigmented mole or tumor), melanomatosis (*oma* tumor + *osis* condition) melanonychia (*onychos* nail) melanosis {melanotic} (*osis* condition) melanuria (dark pigments in the urine) (*uria* urine condition) *melani*: melaniferous (*ferre* to bear) *melano*: melanoacanthoma (*akantha* thorn + *oma* tumor) melanoblast, melanoblastoma (*blastos* germ, cell + *oma* tumor) melanocarcinoma (*karkinos* cancer + *oma* tumor) melanocyte, melanocytosis (*kytos* cell + *osis* condition) melanodermatitis (*dermatos* skin + *itis* inflammation) melanogenesis {melanogenic}, melanogenemia (*genere* to produce + *emia* blood condition) melanoglossia (black hairy tongue) (*glossa* tongue) melanokeratosis (*keratos* cornea + *osis* condition) melanoleukoderma (a mottled appearance of the skin, as in chronic arsenic poisoning) (*leukos* white + *derma* skin) melanopathy (*pathos* disease) melanophage (*phagein* to eat, consume) melanophore (*pherein* to bear) melanoplakia (*plax* plate, plaque)

Element	From	Meaning	Examples
melan (cont'd)		[black, dark]	melanoprotein (a protein complex containing melanin)
			melanorrhagia (also called *melena*) (*rhagia* bursting forth)
			melanorrhea (also called *melena)* (*rhein* to flow)
			melanosarcoma (*sarkos* flesh + *oma* tumor)
			melanosome (*soma* body)
			melanotonin (a hormone secreted by the pineal gland)
			melanotroph (also called *melanotropin*) (*trophein* to nourish)
			melanotropic, melanotropin (*tropic* turning)
			melanotrichous (*trichos* hair)
			TRAILING ROOT COMPOUND:
			melanosis excessive pigmentation:
			cardiomelanosis (*kardia* heart)
			hepatomelanosis (*hepatos* liver)
			myomelanosis (*myos* muscle)
			ophthalmomelanosis (*ophthalmos* eye)
			pneumomelanosis (*pneumon* lung)
			pseudomelanosis (a staining of the tissue after death with pigments from the blood) (*pseudes* false)
			CROSS REFERENCE: scoto
membran	Latin *membrana*	a thin skin	SIMPLE ROOT:
			membrana (a thin layer of tissue covering a surface, lining a cavity, or dividing a space or organ; pl., membranae) {membranaceous}
			membrane, membranelle, membranous (or, membranaceous), membrum (pl., membra)
			PREFIXED ROOT:
			intermembranous (*inter* between)
			intramembranous (*intra* within)
			semimembranous (*semi* half, partly)
			submembranous (*sub* below)
			transmembrane (*trans* across)
			LEADING ROOT COMPOUND:
			membran:
			membranectomy (removal of the membranes of a subdural hematoma) (*ektome* excision)
			membranoid (also called *membraniform*) (*eidos* form)
			membrani: membraniform (also called *membranoid*) (*forma* shape)
			membrano: membranocartilaginous (cartilage)
			TRAILING ROOT COMPOUND:
			membrane:
			biomembrane (any membrane, e.g., the cell membrane, of an organism) {biomembranous} (*bios* life)
			cytomembrane (also called *plasma membrane, cell membrane*) (*kytos* cell)
			neomembrane (also called *false membrane*) (*neos* new)
			pseudomembrane (also called *false membrane*) (*pseudes* false)
			membranous:
			biomembranous (*bios* life)
			fibromembranous (*fibra* fiber)
			mucomembranous (mucus)
			musculomembranous (muscle)
			pseudomembranous (*pseudes* false)
			seromembranous (serum)
			ulceromembranous (ulcer)
			CROSS REFERENCE: mening, myring

Element	From	Meaning	Examples
men, **mens**	Greek *mene*, *mensis*	moon, crescent (menses, menstruation)	NOTE: See note under Latin mens-. SIMPLE ROOT: meniscus (a crescent or crescent-shaped thing) [see separate entry: menisc-] menses (the monthly flow of blood from the genital tract of women) [also listed under mens-] PREFIXED ROOT: *men*: emmenagogue (also called *menagogue*) {emmenagogic} (*em* in + *agein* to lead) *menarch*: premenarche {premenarchal} (*pre* before + menarche) *menia*: catamenia (monthly menstrual discharge) {catamenial} (*kata* down) emmenia (also called *menses*) {emmenic} (*em* in) paramenia (also called *dysmenorrhea*) (*para* abnormal) polymenia (also called *polymenorrhea*) (*polys* much) *meniopathy*: emmeniopathy (a menstrual disorder) (*em* in + *pathos* disease) *meno*: emmenology (*em* in + *logos* study) epimenorrhagia (menstruation that is unusually prolonged and profuse) (*epi* upon + *rhagia* excessive flow) *menopause*: perimenopause (*peri* around) postmenopause (*post* after) *menorrhea* menstrual flow: amenorrhea (absence or suppression of menstruation) (*a* privative) dysmenorrhea (the occurrence of painful cramps during menstruation; also called *paramenia*) (*dys* abnormal) epimenorrhea (also called *polymenorrhea*) (*epi* upon) eumenorrhea (normal menstruation) (*eu* well) hypermenorrhea (excessively prolonged or profuse menstrual flow; also called *menorrhagia, menostaxis*) (*hyper* over, beyond) hypomenorrhea (diminution of menstrual flow or duration) (*hypo* under) plurimenorrhea (also called *polymenorrhea*) (*pluris* more) polyhypermenorrhea (*polys* much + *hyper* over) polyhypomenorrhea (*polys* much + *hypo* below) polymenorrhea (also called *epimenorrhea*) (*polys* much) *menstrual*: intermenstrual (*inter* between) midmenstrual (Old English *midd* middle) postmenstrual (*post* after) premenstrual (*pre* before) *menstruum*: intermenstruum (*inter* between) premenstruum (*pre* before) LEADING ROOT COMPOUND: *men*: menacme (the height of menstrual activity) (*akme* top) menagogue (also called *emmenagogue*) (*agein* to lead) menalgia (*algos* pain) menarche (the beginning of menstruation; also, the first menstrual cycle of an individual) {menarchal} (*archein* to begin) menhidrosis (*hidros* sweat)

A Thesaurus of Medical Word Roots

Element	From	Meaning	Examples
men (cont'd)		[menstruation]	*meni*: menischesis (or, menoschesis) (*schesis* retention)
			meno:
			menolipsis (also called *menopause*) (*leipein* to fail)
			menopause (also called *menolipsis*) (*pauein* to cease)
			menophania (first appearance of the menses at puberty) (*phanein* to appear, show)
			menoplania (vicarious menstruation) (*planan* to wander)
			menorrhagia (excessive menstrual flow; also called *hypermenorrhea*) (*rhagia* bursting forth)
			menorrhalgia (also called *dysmenorrhea*) (*rhein* to flow + *algos* pain)
			menorrhea (normal menstrual flow; also, profuse menstruation) {menorrheal} (*rhein* to flow)
			menoschesis (or, menischesis; suppression of menstruation) (*schesis* retention)
			menostasia (or, menostasis) (*stasis* halting)
			menostaxis (excessively prolonged menstruation) (*staxis* dripping, dropping)
			TRAILING ROOT COMPOUND:
			menia menstrual condition:
			cephalomenia (*kephale* head)
			enteromenia (*enteron* intestine)
			helcomenia (*helkos* ulcer)
			myelomenia (*myelos* spinal cord)
			xenomenia (*xenos* strange)
			xeromenia (*xeros* dry)
			menorrhea flowing of menses:
			bromomenorrhea (*bromos* stench)
			cryptomenorrhea (*kryptos* hidden)
			oligomenorrhea (*oligos* little)
			stomatomenia (*stomatos* mouth)
			CROSS REFERENCE: mens
mening, **meninx**	Greek *meninx*	membrane	SIMPLE ROOT:
			meningism (the signs of meningitis associated with acute febrile illness but without actual inflammation of the meninges)
			meninx (any membrane, but especially one of the coverings of the brain or spinal cord; pl., meninges) {meningeal}
			PREFIXED ROOT:
			meningeal:
			intermeningeal (*inter* between)
			intrameningeal (*intra* within)
			submeningeal (*sub* below)
			meningitis inflammation of membrane:
			perimeningitis (also called *peripachymeningitis*) (*peri* around)
			peripachymeningitis (inflammation of the dura mater)
			LEADING ROOT COMPOUND:
			mening:
			meninghematoma (epidural hematoma) (*hematos* blood + *oma* tumor)
			meningitis (pl., meningitides) {meningitic} (*itis* inflammation)
			meningosis (*osis* condition)
			meninguria (*uria* urine condition)
			meninge: meningeoma (or, meningioma) (*oma* tumor)
			meningeo: meningeorrhaphy (*rhaphe* suture)
			meningi: meningioma (or, meningeoma), meningiomatosis (*oma* tumor + *osis* condition)

Element	From	Meaning	Examples
mening (cont'd)		[membrane]	*meningo*: meningoarteritis (*arteria* artery + *itis* inflammation) meningocele (*kele* hernia) meningocephalitis (also called *meningocerebritis*) (*kephale* head + *itis* inflammation) meningocerebritis (also called *meningoencephalitis*) (*cerebrum* brain + *itis* inflammation) meningococcemia (*kokkos* berry + *emia* blood condition) meningocortical (*cortex* rind—the outer portion of an organ) meningocyte (*kytos* cell) meningoencephalitis (*enkephalon* brain + *itis* inflammation) meningoencephalocele (*enkephalon* brain + *kele* hernia) meningoencephalomyelitis (*enkephalon* brain + *myelos* marrow + *itis* inflammation) meningoencephalopathy (*enkephalon* brain + *pathos* disease) meningogenic (*genere* to produce) meningohydroencephalocele (*hydor* water + *enkephalon* brain + *kele* hernia) meningomalacia (*malakos* soft) meningomyelitis (*myelos* marrow + itis inflammation) meningomyelocele (*myelos* marrow + *kele* tumor) meningopathy (*pathos* disease) meningorachidian (*rhachis* spine) meningoradicular (*radix* root) meningorecurrence (syphilitic meningitis induced in a syphilitic patient by antisyphilitic treatment) meningorrhagia (also called *meningorrhea*) (*rhagia* bursting forth) meningorrhea (also called *meningorrhagia*) (*rhein* to flow) meningothelioma (*thele* nipple + *oma* tumor) meningovascular (*vas* vessel: blood vessel) *menix*: pachymenix (also called *dura mater*) (*pachys* thick) TRAILING ROOT COMPOUND: *meningitis* inflammation of the meninges: arthromeningitis (also called *synovitis*) (*arthron* joint) cerebromeningitis (also called *meningocephalitis*) (*cerebrum* brain) choriomeningitis (*chorion* membrane) encephalomeningitis (*encephalon* brain) gonarthromeningitis (*gony* knee + *arthron* joint) hydromeningitis (*hydor* water) leptomeningitis (*leptos* thin) [leptomeninges: the pia mater and arachnoid considered together as one functional unit] orrhomeningitis (*orrhos* whey, serum + *itis* inflammation) pachymeningitis (inflammation of the dura mater) (*pachys* thick) pseudomeningitis (*pseudes* false) uveomeningitis (uvea) *meningocele* hernia of the meninges: craniomeningocele (*kranion* skull) encephalomeningocele (also called *encephalocele*, *meningoencephalocele* (*enkephalon* brain) hydromeningocele (*hydor* water) lipomeningocele (*lipos* fat) myelomeningocele (*myelos* spinal cord) syringomeningocele (*syringos* pipe) CROSS REFERENCE: hymen, membran, myring

Element	From	Meaning	Examples
menisc	Greek *meniskos*	crescent	SIMPLE ROOT: meniscus (a cartilage disk acting as a cushion between the ends of bone that meet in a joint; pl., menisci) PREFIXED ROOT: parameniscus (the structure or area around the menisci—semilunar firbrocartilages—of the knee) parameniscitis (*para* alongside + *itis* inflammation) LEADING ROOT COMPOUND: *menisc*: meniscectomy (excision of a meniscus, usually from the knee joint) (*ektome* excision) meniscitis (*itis* inflammation) *menisco*: meniscocyte (sickle cell) (*kytos* cell) meniscopexy (also called *meniscorrhaphy*) (*pexis* fixation) meniscorrhaphy (also called *meniscopexy*) (*rhaphe* suture) meniscotome (an instrument used in the removal of a meniscus) (*tome* a cutting instrument) meniscosynovial (synovial: *syn* with + *oon* egg) CROSS REFERENCE: men
mens, mest	Latin *mensis*	month, measure	NOTE: This root is originally from IE *men-*, month, and from which are derived Latin *mensis*, Greek *men*, both meaning "month"; Greek *mene*, moon (from its cycle of 28 days). The ovulation cycle in humans is called *menstruation*, a period of 28 days. SIMPLE ROOT: mensal (occurring monthly) menses [also listed under men-] menstrual, menstruate, menstruation, menstruous PREFIXED ROOT: bimester (a period of two months) (*bi* two) trimester (*tri* three) TRAILING ROOT COMPOUND: pseudomenstruation (*pseudes* false) CROSS REFERENCE: men
ment	Latin *mentum* chin	chin; projecting, as though jutting out with the chin	SIMPLE ROOT: mental (also called *genial*), mentalis, mentum PREFIXED ROOT: submental (*sub* below) supramental (*supra* above) LEADING ROOT COMPOUND: *ment*: mentagra (*agra* seizure) *mento*: mentoanterior (*anterior* before) mentolabial (*labium* lip) mentoplasty (*plassein* to form) mentoposterior (*posterior* after) TRAILING ROOT COMPOUND: labiomental (*labium* lip) verticomental (relating to the crown of the head and the chin) CROSS REFERENCE: geni[1]
mer	Greek *meros*	part, share	SIMPLE ROOT: mere (any one of the parts into which the substance of a zygote of a cell sometimes divides; meres in turn develop into blasts), merisis, merism, meristic PREFIXED ROOT: *mer*: anomer {anomeric} (*ano* up)

Element	From	Meaning	Examples
mer (cont'd)		[part, share]	dimer {dimeric, dimerous} (*di* two)
			epimer (*epi* upon)
			hexamer {hexameric} (*hex* six)
			isomer {isomeric, isomerous} (*isos* equal)
			monomer {monomeric} (*monos* single)
			polymer {polymeric} (*polys* many)
			protomer (*protos* first)
			mere:
			antimere (*anti* against)
			centromere (*kentron* point, center)
			ectomere (*ektos* outside)
			entomere (*enton* within, inner)
			epimere (*epi* upon)
			hypomere (*hypo* under)
			macromere (*makros* long, large)
			mesomere (*mesos* middle)
			metamere {metameric} (*meta* different)
			merism:
			amerism {ameristic} (*a* privative)
			alloisomerism (*allos* other + isomerism)
			allomerism (*allos* other)
			isomerism {isomeric} (*isos* equal)
			mesomerism (*mesos* middle)
			metamerism (*meta* after, beyond, over)
			meristic: ameristic (not divided into parts or segments) (*a* negative)
			merization:
			epimerization (*epi* upon)
			isomerization, isomerize (*isos* equal)
			polymerization, polymerize (*polys* many)
			merogony incomplete development of an ovum:
			endomerogony (*endon* within)
			ectomerogony (*ektos* outside)
			LEADING ROOT COMPOUND:
			mer:
			meront (*ontos* being)
			meropia (partial blindness) (*opia* vision condition)
			merosmia (a disorder of the sense of smell in which certain odors are not perceived) (*osmia* smell condition)
			merostotic (affecting only a part of a bone) (*osteon* bone)
			meri: merispore (*sporos* seed)
			mero:
			meroacrania (*a* privative + *kranion* skull)
			meroanencephaly (*an* privative + *enkephalon* brain)
			meroblastic (*blastos* bud, shoot, germ)
			merocrine (*krinein* to separate)
			merocyst (*kystis* sac, bladder)
			merocyte (*kytos* cell)
			merodiastolic (partially diastolic)
			merogamy (also called *microgamy*; *merogony*) (*gamos* reproduction)
			merogenesis {merogenetic, merogenic} (*genere* to produce)
			merogony (the incomplete development of an ovum that has been disorganized) {merogonic} (*gonos* procreation)
			meromelia (*melos* limb)
			meromicrosomia (*mikros* small + *soma* body)

A Thesaurus of Medical Word Roots

Element	From	Meaning	Examples
mer (cont'd)		[part]	meromorphosis (*morphe* form + *osis* condition)
			merorachischisis (or, merorhachischisis (*rhachis* spine + *schisis* fissure)
			merosystolic (partially systolic; relating to a portion of the systole of the heart)
			merotomy (*tomy* incision)
			merozygote (*zygotos* yoked)
			TRAILING ROOT COMPOUND:
			mer: oligomer (a molecule consisting of only a few monomeres) (*oligos* few, scant, little)
			mere:
			adenomere (*adenos* gland)
			blastomere (*blastos* bud, shoot, germ)
			branchiomere (*branchia* gills)
			chondromere (*chondros* cartilage)
			chromomere (also called *idiomere, granulomere*) (*chroma* color)
			cryptomere (*kryptein* to hide)
			dermatomere (*dermatos* skin)
			elastomer (a synthetic rubber used in dentistry as an impression material) (*elaunein* to set in motion)
			encephalomere (*enkephalos* brain)
			enteromere (*enteron* intestine)
			granulomere (also called *chromomere, idiomere*) (*granum* grain)
			hyalomere (*hyalos* glass)
			idiomere (also called *chromomere*) (*idios* one's own)
			karyomere (*karyon* nucleus)
			leptomere (*leptos* slender)
			myelomere (*myelos* marrow)
			myomere (also called *myotome*, a device for cutting muscle) (*myos* muscle)
			nephromere (*nephros* kidney)
			neuromere (*neuron* nerve)
			osteomere (*osteon* bone)
			rhombomere (also called *neuromere*) (*rhombos* rhomb)
			sarcomere (*sarkos* flesh)
			scleromere (*skleros* hard)
			telomere (*telos* end, complete)
			meria: lipomeria (congenital absence of a limb; also called *amelia*) (*leipein* to leave)
			merism: tautomerism {tautomeric} (*tautos* the same)
			mero: andromerogony (*andros* man + *gone* seed)
			CROSS REFERENCE: None
meso	Greek *mesos*	middle	SIMPLE ROOT: mesiad (or, mesad, mesially; toward the middle), mesial (situated in the middle), mesion {mesien}, meson
			PREFIXED ROOT:
			ectomesoblast (*ektos* outside + *blastos* bud, shoot, germ)
			paramesial (also called *paramedian*) (*para* alongside)
			LEADING ROOT COMPOUND:
			mes:
			mesectoblast (also called *ectomesoblast*) (*ektos* outer + *blastos* bud)
			mesectoderm (*ektos* outer + *derma* skin)
			mesencephalon {mesencephalic} (*enkephalon* brain)
			mesenchyme (*enchyma* cell tissue of a specified type)
			mesentery (*enteron* intestine)

Element	From	Meaning	Examples
meso (cont'd)		[middle]	mesodont {mesodontic} (*odontos* tooth)
			mesophryon (also called *glabella*) (*ophrys* eyebrow)
			mesopia {mesopic} (*opsis* sight)
			mesorchium {mesorchial} (*orchis* testicle)
			mesoropter (the normal eye position with muscles at rest) (*horos* boundary + *opter* observer) [h of horos elided]
			mesovarium (also called *mesoarium*) (ovary)
			mesio:
			mesiobuccal (pertaining to the mesial and buccal surfaces of a tooth) (*bucca* cheek)
			mesiocervical (*cervix* neck—of tooth)
			mesioclusion (*claudere* to close)
			mesiodens (pl., mesiodentes) (*dens* tooth)
			mesiodistal (distal—referring to a tooth)
			mesiogingival (*gingivae* gums)
			mesiognathic (*gnathos* jaw)
			mesioincisal (incisor—of teeth)
			mesiolabial (*labium* lip—of teeth)
			mesiolingual (pertaining to the mesial and lingual surfaces of a tooth) (*lingua* tongue)
			mesiopulpal (pulp—of tooth)
			mesioversion (*vertere* to turn)
			meso:
			mesoaortitis (aorta + *itis* inflammation)
			mesoappendix (appendix)
			mesoblast {mesoblastic}, mesoblastema {mesoblastemic} (*blastos* bud, shoot, germ)
			mesocardia (atypical location of the heart in the middle line of the thorax), mesocardium (pl., mesocardia) (*kardia* heart)
			mesocarpal (also called *midcarpal*) (*karpos* wrist)
			mesocaval (pertaining to or connecting the superior mesenteric vein and inferior vena cava)
			mesocecum {mesocecal} (*cecum* blind gut)
			mesocephalic (or, mesocephalous) (*kephale* head)
			mesochondrium (the matrix of cartilage) (*chondros* cartilage)
			mesocolon, mesocolopexy (colon + *pexis* fixation)
			mesocoloplication (colon + *plicare* to fold)
			mesocord (umbilical cord)
			mesocyst (*kytis* bladder)
			mesoderm {mesodermal, mesodermic} (*derma* skin)
			mesoduodenum {mesoduodenal}
			mesoepididymis
			mesoesophagus
			mesogaster (or, mesogastrium) {mesogastric} (*gaster* stomach)
			mesogenic (*genere* to produce)
			mesoglia (also called *microglia*) (*glia* glue)
			mesogluteus {mesogluteal} (*gloutos* buttock)
			mesognathion {mesognathic, mesognathous} (*gnathos* jaw)
			mesoileum
			mesojejunum
			mesolymphocyte (*lympha* fluid + *kytos* cell)
			mesomelia {mesomelic: pertaining to the midportion of the arm or leg} (*melos* limb)
			mesomere, mesomerism {mesomeric} (*meros* part)

Element	From	Meaning	Examples
meso (cont'd)		[middle]	mesometrium (*metra* uterus)
			mesomorph {mesomorphic} (*morphe* shape, form)
			mesonasal (*nasus* nose)
			mesonephroma (*nephros* kidney + *oma* tumor)
			mesoneuritis (*neuron* nerve + *itis* inflammation)
			mesophile {mesophilic: fond of moderate temperature: said of bacteria which develop best between 20° and 55° C.} (*philein* to love—have an affinity for)
			mesophlebitis (*phleps* vein + *itis* inflammation)
			mesopneumonium (*pneumon* lung)
			mesoprosopic (having a face of moderate width) (*prosopon* face)
			mesopulmonum (the mesentery of the embryonic lung) (*pulmon* lung)
			mesorectum (mesentery of the rectum)
			mesorrhaphy (also called *mesenteriorrhaphy*) (*rhaphe* suture)
			mesorrhine (*rhis* nose)
			mesosalpinx (*salpinx* tube)
			mesoscope (*skopein* to view)
			mesoseme (having a medium orbital index; having orbits neither broad nor narrow) (*sema* sign)
			mesosigmoid (sigmoid)
			mesosome (*soma* body)
			mesosternum (the corpus sterni) (*sternon* sternum)
			mesosystolic (systole)
			mesotendineum (or, mesotendon, mesotenon) (tendon)
			mesotropic (*tropein* to turn)
			mesotympanum (*tympanon* eardrum)
			TRAILING ROOT COMPOUND:
			axiomesial (axis—of tooth)
			buccomesial (*bucca* cheek)
			dorsomesial (*dorsum* back)
			linguomesial (*lingua* tongue)
			CROSS REFERENCE: medi
meta-	Greek prefix	after, beyond, over	See Appendix B for examples of words with this prefix. Others are listed with the root to which it is attached.
			CROSS REFERENCE: para-, ultra-
meter, **metrio,** **metro,** **-metry,** **-metric**	Greek *metron*	measure	NOTE: Because of the number of words ending with this root, see the root to which *meter* is suffixed, e.g., thermometer; see Appendix C for –metric.
			SIMPLE ROOT: meter (a linear standard of measurement in the international standards of weights and measures, equaling 39.37 inches) {metric}
			PREFIXED ROOT:
			meter:
			diameter (*dia* through)
			micrometer (*mikros* small)
			parameter {parametric} (*para* alongside)
			perimeter {perimetric}, perimetry (*peri* around)
			metric: isometric (*isos* equal)
			metropia vision measurement condition:
			ametropia (*a* privative)
			anisometropia (*aniso* unequal: *an* negative + *isos* equal)
			emmetropia (*em* in)
			heterometropia (*heteros* different)

Element	From	Meaning	Examples
meter (cont'd)		[measurement]	hypermetropia (*hyper* above)
			isometropia (*isos* equal)
			opsia: dysmetropsia (*dys* abnormal + *opsia* vision condition)
			metry:
			asymmetry {asymmetrical} (*a* negative + symmetry)
			endometry (*endon* within)
			symmetry (*sym* together)
			LEADING ROOT COMPOUND:
			metrio: metriocephalic (*metrios* moderate + *kephale* head)
			metro:
			metrology (*logos* study)
			metrostasis (a state in which the length of a muscle fiber is relatively fixed, and at which length it contracts and relaxes)
			TRAILING ROOT COMPOUND: (Examples)
			acoumeter (*akouein* to hear)
			algometer (or, algesimeter) (*algos* pain)
			arthrometer (*arthron* joint)
			cephalometer (*kephale* head)
			dosimeter (dose—of radiation)
			necrometer (*nekros* death)
			orthometer (*orthos* straight)
			pachymeter (or, pachometer) (*pachys* thick)
			phacometer (*phakos* lens)
			photometer (*photos* light)
			pyknometer (*pyknos* thick, compact)
			pyrometer (*pyr* fire, heat)
			rachiometer (*rhachis* spine)
			rhinometer (*rhinos* nose)
			metry:
			algometry (also called *algesimetry*) (*algos* pain)
			arthrometry (*arthron* joint)
			cardiometry (*kardia* heart)
			cephalometry (*kephale* head)
			craniometry (*kranion* skull)
			cytometry (*kytos* cell)
			hysterometry (*hystera* uterus, womb)
			psychometry (*psyche* mind)
			CROSS REFERENCE: mens
metr	Greek *metra*	uterus, womb	SIMPLE ROOT: metra (pl., metrae), metria
			PREFIXED ROOT:
			ametria (congenital absence of the uterus) (*a* privative)
			endometrium (*endon* within)
			mesometrium (*mesos* middle)
			parametrium {pl., parametria}, parametritis {parametritic} (*para* alongside + *itis* inflammation)
			perimetrium, perimetritis (*peri* around + *itis* inflammation)
			perimetrosalpingitis (*peri* around + *salpinx* tube + *itis* inflammation)
			protometrocyte (*protos* first + metrocyte)
			LEADING ROOT COMPOUND:
			metr:
			metratonia (*atonia* lack of tension: *a* privative + *tonos* tension)
			metratrophia (atrophy: *a* privative + *trephein* to nourish)
			metrectomy (also called *hysterectomy*) (*ektome* excision)
			metrectopia (*ektopia* displaced)

Element	From	Meaning	Examples
metr (cont'd)		[womb]	metreurynter (*eurynein* to stretch)
			metritis (*itis* inflammation)
			metrodynia (also called *hysteralgia*) (*odyne* pain)
			metro:
			metrocele (also called *hysterocele*) (*kele* hernia)
			metrocolpocele (*kolpos* vagina + *kele* hernia)
			metrocyte (also called *mother cell*) (*kytos* cell)
			metrodynamometer (instrument for measuring the force of uterine contractions) (*dynamis* power + *metron* measure)
			metroendometritis (combined inflammation of the uterus and its mucous membranes) (*endon* within + *itis* inflammation)
			metrofibroma (*fibra* fiber + *oma* tumor)
			metrogenous (*genere* to produce)
			metrography (also called *hysterography*) (*graphein* to write)
			metrolymphangitis (*lympha* fluid + *angeion* vessel + *itis* inflammation)
			metromalacia (softening of the uterus) (*malakos* soft)
			metromenorrhagia (also called *menometrorrhagia*) (*meno* menstrual + *rhagia* excessive flow)
			metroparalysis (paralysis of the uterus)
			metropathy (also called *hysteropathy*) (*pathos* disease)
			metroperitonitis (peritoneum + *itis* inflammation)
			metrophlebitis (*phleps* vein + *itis* inflammation)
			metroplasty (*plassein* to form)
			metropolis (the area in which a particular species of organisms commonly occurs) (*polis* lit., city; place)
			metroptosis (prolapse of the uterus) (*ptein* to fall)
			metrorrhagia (*rhagia* bursting forth)
			metrorrhea (abnormal uterine discharge) (*rhea* flow)
			metrorrhexis (*rhexis* rupture)
			metrosalpingitis (*salpingos* tube + *itis* inflammation)
			metroscope (*skopein* to examine)
			metrostaxis (*staxis* a dripping)
			metrostenosis (*stenosis* contraction)
			metrotomy (also called *hysterotomy*) (*tomy* incision)
			TRAILING ROOT COMPOUND:
			metra:
			hematometra (or, hemometra) (*hematos* blood)
			hydrophysometra (collection of fluid and gas in the uterus; also called *physohydrometra*) (*hydor* water + *physa* air)
			lochiometra (*lochia* vaginal discharge)
			physometra (*physa* air)
			pyometra (*pyon* pus)
			pyophysometra (*pyon* pus + *physa* air)
			metrium: myometrium {myometrial} (*myos* muscle)
			metritis inflammation of the uterus:
			adenomyometritis (*adenos* gland + *myos* muscle)
			myometritis (*myos* muscle)
			phlebometritis (*phlebos* vein)
			septimetritis (*sepsis* putrefaction)
			pyometritis (*pyon* pus)
			PREFIXED TRAILING ROOT COMPOUND: intramyometrial (*intra* within + *myometrial*)
			CROSS REFERENCE: colp, hyster[1], uter

Element	From	Meaning	Examples
micro-	Greek *mikros*	small	See Appendix B for examples of words with this prefix. Others are listed with the root to which it is attached. CROSS REFERENCE: lept, nan
migraine			See Disguised Root under cran-.
milieu			See French under loc-.
mim	Greek *mimos* imitator, actor	imitate, mimic	SIMPLE ROOT: mimesis (imitation, mimicry; a disease which exhibits symptoms of another disease) {mimetic}, mimic PREFIXED ROOT: amimia (*a* privative) hypermimia (*hyper* over, beyond) paramimia (the use of gestures unsuited to the words which they accompany) (*para* alongside) TRAILING ROOT COMPOUND: *mimesis*: necromimesis (*nekros* dead) pathomimesis (intentional imitation of a disease, particularly malingering) (*pathos* disease) *mimetic*: adrenomimetic (also called *sympathomimetic*) (adrenal gland) andromimetic (producing male characteristics) (*andros* man) neuromimetic (*neuron* nerve) sympathomimetic (mimicking the effects of impulses conveyed by adrenergic postganglionic fibers of the sympathetic nervous system; also called *adrenomimetic*) thyromimetic (thyroid gland) vagomimetic (*vagus* wandering) *mimia*: echomimia (also called *echopathia*, *echopraxia*) CROSS REFERENCE: None
mio, mei	Greek *meion* smaller, less	less, decreasing	SIMPLE ROOT: meiosis (or, miosis: a lessening) {miotic} PREFIXED ROOT: postmeiotic (*post* after) premeiotic (*pre* before) LEADING ROOT COMPOUND: *mi*: miopus (unequal conjoined twins with heads united in such a manner that one face is rudimentary) (*ops* face) miosis (or, meiosis; abnormal contraction of the pupils) {miotic} (*osis* condition) *mio*: miocardia (systolic lessening of heart's volume; not to be confused with *myocardia*) (*kardia* heart) miodidymus (*didymos* twin) miolecithal (containing little yolk) (*lekithos* yolk) miopragia (decreased functional activity) (*prassein* to perform) TRAILING ROOT COMPOUND: hidromeiosis (*hidros* sweat + *osis* condition) osteomiosis (*osteon* bone + *osis* condition) CROSS REFERENCE: None
misc, mix	Latin *miscere*	to mix	SIMPLE ROOT: *misc*: miscible (capable of being mixed) *mix*: mixture (a combination of different drugs or ingredients) PREFIXED ROOT: *misc*: immiscible (incapable of being mixed or blended) (*in* not) *mixia*: panmixia (or, panmixis; also called *random mating*) (*pan* all)

Element	From	Meaning	Examples
misc (cont'd)		[to mix]	*mixis*: amphimixis (*amphi* both) apomixis (also called *parthenogenesis*) (*apo* from) automixis (also called *autogamy*) (*autos* self) endomixis (*endon* within) panmixis (also called *random mating*) (*pan* all) LEADING ROOT COMPOUND: *misc*: miscegenation (the intermarriage or union of persons of different races, or the procreation of persons of mixed race) (*genere* to produce) *mixo*: mixoscopia (or, mixoscopy; sexual perversion in which gratification is obtained by the sight of one's love object engaged in sexual intercourse with another) (*skopein* to see) mixotroph {mixotrophic} (*trophein* to nourish) CROSS REFERENCE: cras
mit	Greek *mitos*	thread	SIMPLE ROOT: mitome (a thready network of the protoplasm of a cell) PREFIXED ROOT:: intramitochondrial (*intra* within + *chondros* granule) premitochondrial (*pre* before + *chondros* granule) *mitome*: paramitome (the fluid portion of the protoplasm of a cell) (*para* alongside) *mitosis* thread condition: amitosis (direct cell division; simple division of the nucleus and cell without the changes in the nucleus that characterize mitosis) (*a* privative) endomitosis {endomitotic} (*endon* within) *mitotic* pertaining to mitosis: amitotic (*a* privative) antimitotic (inhibiting or preventing mitosis) (*anti* against) intermitotic (*inter* between) postmitotic (*post* after, behind) premitotic (*pre* before) *mitus*: polymitus (also called *exflagellation*) (*polys* many) LEADING ROOT COMPOUND: *mit*: mitapsis (*hapsis* joining) [h of hapsis elided] mitosis (pl., mitoses) {mitotic} (*osis* condition) *mito*: mitochondrion (pl., mitochondria) (*chondrion* granule) mitogenesis (or, mitogenesia) {mitogenetic} (*genere* to produce) mitokinetic (*kinein* to move) mitoplasm (*plassein* to form) mitoschisis (*schisis* fissure) mitosome (a body formed from the spindle fibers of the preceding mitosis; a spindle remnant) (*soma* body) mitospore (an asexual spore, so called because it is produced by mitosis) TRAILING ROOT COMPOUND: karyomitosis {karyomitotic} (*karyon* kernel + *osis* condition) teleomitosis (a completed mitosis) (*telos* end + *osis* condition) CROSS REFERENCE: fil, nema
mix			See misc- for *mixotrophic*.

Element	From	Meaning	Examples
mne(m)	Greek *mneme*	memory, remember	PREFIXED ROOT: *mnesia*: amnesia (loss of memory) {amnesic, amnestic} (*a* privative) automnesia (spontaneous revival of memories of an earlier condition of life) (*autos* self) dysmnesia (a naturally poor or an impaired memory; disordered memory) {dysmnesic} (*dys* abnormal) ecmnesia (forgetfulness of recent events with normal memory for remote ones) (*ek* out) hypermnesia (unusual clarity of memory) {hypermnesic} (*hyper* above) hypomnesia (memory impairment) (*hypo* below) paramnesia (a disturbance of memory in which reality and fantasy are confused) (*para* beside) *mnesis*: anamnesis (a patient's recital of his or her medical history to a doctor) {anamnestic} (*ana* again) catamnesis (the follow-up history of a patient after being discharged from treatment) {catamnestic} (*kata* down) palinmnesis (memory for past events and experiences; also called *remote memory*) (*palin* again, backward) TRAILING ROOT COMPOUND: cryptomnesia (the recall of memories not recognized as such but thought to be original creations) (*kryptein* to hide) logamnesia (also called *receptive aphasia*) (*logos* word) pseudomnesia (a subjective impression of memory of events that have not occurred) (*pseudes* false) CROSS REFERENCE: None
mob			See mot- for *mobilize*.
mol	Latin *moles*	shapeless mass	SIMPLE ROOT: mole {molar; relating to a mass; not molecular}, molarity, molecule {molecular}, molecularity PREFIXED ROOT: bimolecular (*bi* two) equimolecular (*equi* equal) intermolecular (*inter* between) intramolecular (*intra* within) macromolecular (*makros* large) micromolecular (*mikros* small) monomolecular (*monos* single) orthomolecular (*orthos* straight) termolecular (*ter* three) TRAILING ROOT COMPOUND: biomolecular (a molecule produced by living cells) (*bios* life) pseudomonomolecular (*pseudes* false + monomolecular) CROSS REFERENCE: cel^2, gangli, onc, phyma
mono	Greek *monos*	one, alone; single, sole, unit	NOTE: In chemistry, this root is extended to mean containing one atom or one group (of a specified element). SIMPLE ROOT: monad (single-celled protozoon or a single-cell coccus; a univalent radical or element) PREFIXED ROOT: metamonad (a group of protozoa comprising most of the zooflagellates) (*meta* change) See Appendix B for examples of words beginning with this element. Others are listed with the root to which it is attached. CROSS REFERENCE: hapl, sol^2

Element	From	Meaning	Examples
morph	Greek *morphe*	form, shape	ROOT NOTE: This root derives from the Greek god Morpheus, one who shapes dreams.

SIMPLE ROOT:

morphea, morpheme (a meaningful unit of sound), morphia

morphine {morphinic}, morphinism, morphium

morphon (an individual organism or structural unit)

PREFIXED ROOT:

morph:

ectomorph {ectomorphic} (*ektos* outside)

endomorph {endomorphic} (*endon* within)

hypermorph (*hyper* over, above)

hypomorph (*hypo* under)

mesomorph {mesomorphic} (*mesos* middle)

polymorph (*polys* many)

morphia:

amorphia (state of being without definite form) (*a* negative)

dysmorphia (or, dysmorphism) (*dys* abnormal)

pantamorphia (complete or general deformity) (*panta* all + amorphia)

pantomorphia (the condition of an organism, such as an ameba, that is capable of assuming all shapes; perfect symmetry) (*pantos* all)

morphic:

dysmorphic (*dys* abnormal)

epimorphic (*epi* upon)

isomorphic (*isos* equal)

heteromorphic (or, heteromorphous) (*heteros* other)

homomorphic (*homos* same)

monomorphic (*monos* one)

trimorphic (or, trimorphous) (*tri* three)

morphism:

allomorphism (*allos* other)

eumorphism (retention of the normal form of a cell) (*eu* well)

heteromorphism (*heteros* different)

isomorphism (*isos* equal)

monomorphism (*monos* single)

morpho:

dysmorphogenesis (*dys* abnormal + *genesis* beginning)

dysmorphology (*dys* abnormal + *logos* study)

dysmorphopsia (*dys* abnormal + *opsia* vision condition)

metamorphopsia (*meta* beyond + *opsia* vision condition)

morphosis form condition:

anamorphosis (*ana* up, again)

dysmorphosis (malformation) (*dys* abnormal)

epimorphosis (*epi* upon)

heteromorphosis (*heteros* different)

holomorphosis (*holos* whole)

hypermorphosis (*hyper* above)

metamorphosis {metamorphotic} (*meta* after)

retromorphosis (also called *cataplasia*) (*retro* backward)

morphous:

amorphous (*a* privative)

dimorphous (*di* two)

heteromorphous (or, heteromorphic) (*heteros* other)

isomorphous (*isos* equal)

submorphous (*sub* under)

Element	From	Meaning	Examples
morph (cont'd)		[form, shape]	LEADING ROOT COMPOUND: *morph*: morphallaxis (*allaxis* exchange) morphosis {morphotic} (*osis* condition) *morpho*: morphogenesis {morphogenetic} (*genere* to produce) morphology (the science of the forms and structure of human be- ings) (*logy* study) morpholysis (destruction of form) (*lyein* to dissolve) morphometry {morphometric} (*metron* measure) morphophyly (*phylon* race, tribe) morphophysiology (also called *functional anatomy*) morphotype (*typos* type) TRAILING ROOT COMPOUND: *morph*: allelomorph (*allos* other) neomorph (*neos* new) pseudomorph (*pseudes* false) *morphic*: bathomorphic (having a deep or myopic eye) (*bathos* deep) brachymorphic (also called *brachytypical*) (*brachys* short) dolichomorphic (also called *longilineal*) (*dolichos* long) oligomorphic (*oligos* little, scant) platymorphic (*platys* flat) pleomorphic (*pleon* excessive) pyknomorphic (*pyknos* thick, dense, compact) *morphism*: geromorphism (premature senility) (*geras* old age) neomorphism (*neos* new) pathomorphism (*pathos* disease) pedomorphism (*paidos* child) *morphous*: adelomorphous (compare *delomorphous*) (*adelos* uncertain) delomorphous (of definite form and shape) (*delos* manifest) cystomorphous (*kystis* bladder) embryomorphous (embryo) homeomorphous (*homeo* similar, same) *morphus*: gastromorphus (*gaster* belly, abdomen, stomach) pygoamorphus (*pyge* buttocks + *a* negative) CROSS REFERENCE: eid, form, ide, phan, plas
mort, **mors**	Latin *mors,* *mortis*	death	SIMPLE ROOT: mors (death); mortal, mortality, mortician, mortu- ary (relating to death or to burial) PREFIXED ROOT: antemortem (occurring before death; see Term) (*ante* before) postmortal, postmortem (*post* after) premortal (occurring just before death) (*pre* before) LEADING ROOT COMPOUND: mortification (gangrene or sphace- lus; molar death) (*facere* to make) TRAILING ROOT COMPOUND: natimortality (the proportion of stillbirths to the general birth rate; also called *fetal death rate*) (*nasci* to be born) TERMS: ante mortem (before death); post mortem (after death) CROSS REFERENCE: necr

Element	From	Meaning	Examples
mot, mob, mov	Latin *movere*	to move	SIMPLE ROOT: mobilize (to make mobile or capable of movement) motile, motility, motion, motivation, motive, motor, motoricity movement, mover PREFIXED ROOT: *mob*: immobilization, immobilize (*im* negative) *mot*: promote, promoter, promotion (*pro* before) *motility*: dysmotility (*dys* abnormal) hypermotility (*hyper* over, above) hypomotility (also called *hypokinesis*) (*hypo* under) supermotility (*super* over, beyond) *motio*: emotiovascular (*e* out + vascular) *motion*: emotion {emotional} (*ex* out) *motivity*: ultromotivity (power of spontaneous movement—on one's own part) (*ultra* beyond) LEADING ROOT COMPOUND: motoceptor (*capere* to take, seize) motofacient (*facere* to make) motoneuron (*neuron* nerve) TRAILING ROOT COMPOUND: *motility*: cardiomotility (*kardia* heart) nervimotility (also called *neurimotility*) (*nervus* nerve) neurimotility (also called *nervimotility*) (*neuron* nerve) *motor*: algiomotor (producing painful movements or contractions, such as spasm or dysperistalsis) (*algos* pain) arteriomotor (artery) bronchomotor (*bronchus* windpipe) capillariomotor (capillary) cephalomotor (*kephale* head) iridomotor (*iridos* rainbow: iris) nervimotor (also called *neuromotor*) (nerve) neuromotor (also called *nervimotor*) (*neuron* nerve) oculomotor (*oculus* eye) pilomotor (*pilus* hair) pseudomotor (also called *dyskinetic*) (*pseudes* false) psychomotor (*psyche* mind) pupillomotor (pupil of eye) sensorimotor (*sentire* to feel, perceive) vasomotor (*vas* vessel) venomotor (*vena* vein) visceromotor (*viscus* internal organs) visuomotor (*videre* to see) CROSS REFERENCE: cin
muc	Latin *mucus*	moldy, sticky, mucous	SIMPLE ROOT: mucid (also called *muciferous*) mucilage {mucilaginous}, mucilago (or, mucilage) mucin (a glycoprotein found in mucus, and is present in saliva and bile and in salivary glands, in the skin, connective tissues, tendon and cartilage), mucinous mucosa (a mucous membrane, or tunica mucosa) {mucosal} mucus {mucous}

Element	From	Meaning	Examples
muc (cont'd)		[moldy, sticky, mucus]	PREFIXED ROOT: demucosation (*de* removal) paramucin (*para* alongside) submucous {submucosal} (*sub* below) LEADING ROOT COMPOUND: *muc*: mucitis (also called *mucositis*) (*itis* inflammation) mucoid (*eidos* form) *muci*: muciferous (also called *muciparous*) (*ferre* to bear) mucification (*facere* to make) mucigenous (also called *muciparous*) (*genere* to produce) muciparous (also called *blennogenic, muciferous*) (*parere* to bear) *mucin*: mucinemia (*emia* blood condition) mucinoid (*eidos* form) mucinosis (*osis* condition) mucinuria (*uria* urine condition) *mucino*: mucinoblast (*blastos* germ) mucinolytic (*lysis* dissolution) *muco*: mucocele (*kele* tumor) mucociliary (*cilium* eyelash) mucoclasis (*klaein* to break) mucocolitis (also called *mucous colitis*) (colon + *itis* inflammation) mucocolpos (*kolpos* vagina) mucocutaneous (*cutis* skin) mucocyst (*kystis* sac, cyst) mucoenteritis (*enteron* intestine + *itis* inflammation) mucofibrous (*fibre* fiber) mucoflocculent (*flocculus* tuft) mucogingivitis (*gingivae* gums + *itis* inflammation) mucolipidosis (*lipos* fat + *osis* condition) mucolysis {mucolytic} (*lyein* to loosen) mucomembranous (*membrane* a thin skin) mucopurulent (*puris* pus) mucosanguineous (*sanguis* blood) mucoserous (*serum* whey) mucostatic (*stasis* standing) *mucos*: mucosectomy (*ektome* excision) mucositis (also called *mucitis*) (*itis* inflammation) TRAILING ROOT COMPOUND: *mucin*: elastomucin (the mucoprotein of connective tissue) osseomucin (*osse* bone) pseudomucin {pseudomucinous} (*pseudes* false) tendomucin (tendon) *mucous*: puromucous (also called *mucopurulent*) (*puris* pus) pyromucous (*pyros* fire) *mucus*: seromucus {seromucous} (*serum* whey) CROSS REFERENCE: blenn, myx

Element	From	Meaning	Examples
multi-	Latin prefix	many, much	See Appendix B for examples of words with this prefix. Others are placed with the roots to which it is attached. CROSS REFERENCE: poly-
musc	Latin *musculus* little mouse	muscle	PREFIXED ROOT: intermuscular (*inter* between) intramuscular (*intra* within) LEADING ROOT COMPOUND: musculoaponeurotic (*aponeurosis* a sheetlike tendinous expansion, connecting a muscle with the parts it moves) musculocutaneous (also called *musculodermic*) (*cutis* skin) musculodermic (also called *musculocutaneous*) (*derma* skin) musculoelastic (elastic tissue) (*elauein* to stretch) musculomembranous (*membrane* a thin skin) musculophrenic (*phren* diaphragm) musculotendinous (tendon) musculotropic (*tropein* to turn) TRAILING ROOT COMPOUND: algiomuscular (*algos* pain) cardiomuscular (*kardia* heart) electro-muscular (pertaining to the contraction of the muscles under electricity) epitheliomuscular (epithelium) excitomuscular (causing muscular activity) fibromuscular (fiber) galvanomuscular (denoting the effect of the application of a galvanic, or direct, current to a muscle) idiomuscular (*idios* one's own, separate) nervimuscular (also called *neuromyological*) (nerve) neuromuscular (*neuron* nerve) peritoneomuscular (peritoneum) radiomuscular (going from the radial artery or nerve to the muscles) striomuscular (pertaining to or composed of striated muscle) CROSS REFERENCE: my
muta	Latin *mutare*	to change	SIMPLE ROOT: mutant, mutase, mutation, mutational mutualism (symbiosis in which both populations, or individuals, gain from the association and are unable to survive without it) mutualist (an organism associated with another in symbiosis; also called *symbion*) PREFIXED ROOT: *mutagen*: antimutagen (*anti* against + *genere* to produce) *mutation*: dismutation (*dis* apart) hypermutation (*hyper* above) permutation (complete change; transformation; act of altering objects in a group) (*per* intensive) transmutation (*trans* across) LEADING ROOT COMPOUND: mutagen, mutagenesis {mutagenic}, mutagenicity (*genere* to produce) CROSS REFERENCE: all
my	Greek *myos* mouse	muscle	NOTE: The Greek roots for *muscle*, *mussel*, and *mouse* (my-) and spinal cord (myelo-) are the same; all three originated from the root *myos*, mouse. Latin *muscle*, for instance, is "small mouse," from the rippling effect of flexing the biceps.

Element	From	Meaning	Examples
my (cont'd)		[muscle]	PREFIXED ROOT:

my: amyous (deficient in muscular tissue or strength) (*a* privative)

myasthen muscle strength:

amyasthenia (or, amyosthenia) {amyosthenic} (*a* privative)

antimyasthenic (*anti* against)

myocardial pertaining to heart muscle:

endomyocardial (*endon* within)

intramyocardial (*intra* within)

myocarditis inflammation of heart muscle:

endomyocarditis (*endon* within)

perimyocarditis (combined pericarditis and myocarditis)

myoesthesia: amyoesthesia (muscular anesthesia; inability to sense motion, weight, and balance) (*a* privative + *esthesia* feeling)

myometritis: endomyometritis (*endon* within + *metra* uterus + *itis* inflammation)

myoplasia: amyoplasia (*a* privative + *plassein* to form)

myoplegia: monomyoplegia (paralysis limited to a single muscle) (*monos* single + myoplegia)

myositis inflammation of muscle:

monomyositis (*monos* single)

perimyositis (*peri* around)

polymyositis (*polys* many)

myostasia: amyostasia {amyostatic} (*a* privative + *stasis* standing)

myosthenia: amyosthenia (or, amyasthenia) {amyosthenic} (*a* privative + *sthenos* strength)

myotaxy: amyotaxy (or, amyotaxia) (*a* negative + *taxis* order)

myotonia muscle tone condition:

amyotonia (*a* privative)

dysmyotonia (also called *dystonia*) (*dys* abnormal)

hypermyotonia (*hyper* over)

hypomyotonia (*hypo* below)

paramyotonia (*para* alongside)

myotrophy nutrition of muscle tissue:

amyotrophy {amyotrophic} (*a* privative)

hypermyotrophy (*hyper* above)

mysium:

endomysium (*endon* within)

epimysium (the fibrous sheath about an entire muscle) (*epi* upon)

exomysium (also called *perimysium*) (*exo* outside)

perimysium (connective tissue covering and binding together bundles of muscle fibers; pl., perimysia) {perimysial} (*peri* around)

LEADING ROOT COMPOUND:

my:

myalgia (also called *myodynia*) (*algos* pain)

myasthenia {myasthenic} (*asthenia* weakness)

myatonia (*a* privative + *tonos* tension)

myatrophy (*a* privative + *trephein* to nourish)

mycerosis (or, myokerosis) (*keros* wax)

myectomy (*ektome* excision)

myectopia (or, myectopy) (*ektopia* displaced)

myenteron {myenteric} (*enteron* intestine)

myesthesia (also called *kinesthetic sense*) (*esthesia* feeling)

myoculator (*oculus* eye)

myodynia (also called *myalgia*) (*odyne* pain)

Element	From	Meaning	Examples
my (cont'd)		[muscle]	myoid, myoidema (or, myoedema) (*eidos* form + *edema* swelling)
			myoma (a tumor consisting of muscle tissue) {myomatous} (*oma* tumor)
			myonymy (nomenclature of the muscles) (*onyma* name)
			myofunctional (*function* use)
			myogen {myogenic} (*genere* to produce)
			myoglobin, myoglobinuria (*globus* ball + *uria* urine condition)
			myognathus (*gnathos* jaw)
			myogram, myograph {myographic} (*graphein* to write)
			myohemoglobin (also called *myoglobin*) (*haima* blood + *globus* ball)
			myoischemia (*ischemia* blood deficiency)
			myokinesimeter (*kinesis* movement + *metron* measure)
			myokymia (*kyma* wave)
			myolemma (also called *sarcolemma*) (*lemma* husk)
			myolipoma (*lipos* fat + *oma* tumor)
			myology (or, myologia; the study of muscles, and the body of knowledge pertaining to muscles) (*logos* study)
			myolysis (*lysis* dissolution)
			myomalacia (*malakos* soft)
			myomelanosis (*melanosis* excessive pigmentation)
			myomere (also called *myotome*) (*meros* a part)
			myometer (*metron* measure)
			myometrium {myometrial}, myometritis (*metra* uterus + *itis* inflammation)
			myomitochondrion (mitochondrion: *mitos* thread + *chondros* cartilage)
			myonecrosis (*nekros* dead + *osis* condition)
			myoneme (*nema* thread)
			myoneural, myoneuroma (*neuron* nerve + *oma* tumor)
			myopachynsis (hypertrophy, or overgrowth, of muscle) (*pachys* thick)
			myopalmus (muscle twitching) (*palmos* pulsation, vibration)
			myoparesis (*paresis* slight paralysis)
			myopathy {myopathic} (*pathos* disease)
			myopericarditis (pericardium + *itis* inflammation)
			myoperitonitis (peritoneum + *itis* inflammation)
			myophage (*phagein* to devour, consume)
			myophone (*phone* sound)
			myoplasm, myoplasty {myoplastic} (*plassein* to form)
			myopolar (pole)
			myoprotein (protein)
			myorrhaphy (also called *myosuture*) (*rhaphe* suture)
			myorrhexis (*rhexis* rupture)
			myosalpingitis, myosalpinx (*salpingos, salpinx* uterine tube + *itis* inflammation)
			myosarcoma (*sarkos* flesh + *oma* tumor)
			myosclerosis (*sklerosis* hardening)
			myoseptum (also called *myocomma*; the connective tissue septum separating adjacent myotomes) (*septus* wall, partition)
			myospasm (or, myospasmus) (*spasmos* contraction)
			myospherulosis (*spherula* small sphere + *osis* condition)
			myosthenometer (*sthenos* strength + *metron* measure)
			myostroma (*stroma* mattress, foundation)
			myosuture (also called *myorrhaphy*) (*suere* to sew)

Element	From	Meaning	Examples
my (cont'd)		[muscle]	myotactic (*tactus* a touching)
			myotasis {myotatic} (*tasis* stretching)
			myotenositis (tendon + *itis* inflammation)
			myotenotomy (tendon + *tomy* incision)
			myothermic (*therme* heat)
			myotome, myotomy (*tomy* incision)
			myotone (or, myotony; muscular tone or tension), myotonia {myotonic}, myotonoid (*tonos* tone, tension + *eidos* resemblance)
			myotrophy {myotrophic} (*trophein* to nourish)
			myotropic (*tropic* turning to)
			myotube (a developing skeletal muscle cell or fiber with a tubular appearance)
			myovascular (*vas* vessel—blood vessel)
			myom: myomectomy (myoma + *ektome* excision)
			myomo: myomotomy (myoma + *tomy* incision)
			myos: myositis {myositic} (*itis* inflammation)
			TRAILING ROOT COMPOUND:
			myalgia: fibromyalgia (fiber + *algos* pain)
			myasthenia: neuromyasthenia (*neuron* nerve + myasthenia)
			myectomy: fibromyectomy (fiber + *ektome* excision)
			myitis muscle inflammation:
			fibromyitis (fiber)
			stethomyitis (*stethos* chest)
			laparomyitis (*lapara* abdominal, lumbar)
			myoblastoma: medullomyoblastoma (*medulla* marrow + blastoma)
			myocardiac: angiomyocardiac (*angeion* vessel + *kardia* heart)
			myoid muscle form:
			conomyoidin (*konos* cone)
			platymyoid (*platys* flat)
			myoma muscle tumor:
			adenomyoma (*adenos* gland)
			angiomyoma (*angeion* vessel—blood vessel)
			chondromyoma (*chondros* cartilage)
			cystomyoma (*kystis* bladder, cyst)
			dermatomyoma (*dermatos* skin)
			fibromyoma (fiber)
			hydromyoma (*hydor* water)
			hystermyoma (*hystera* uterus)
			leiomyoma (*leios* smooth)
			lipomyoma (also called *myolipoma*) (*lipos* fat)
			myxomyoma (*myxa* mucus)
			pyomyoma (*pyon* pus)
			rhabdomyoma (*rhabdos* rod)
			myomatosis: phlebomyomatosis (*phlebos* vein + myoma + *osis* condition)
			myopathy muscle disease:
			cardiomyopathy (*kardia* heart)
			neuromyopathy (*neuron* nerve)
			myoplasty plastic surgery of muscle tissue:
			cardiomyoplasty (*kardia* heart)
			tenomyoplasty (tendon)
			myosarcoma malignant muscle neoplasm:
			adenomyosarcoma (*adenos* gland)
			angiomyosarcoma (*angeion* blood vessel)

A Thesaurus of Medical Word Roots

Element	From	Meaning	Examples
my (cont'd)		[muscle]	leiomyosarcoma (*leios* smooth)
			rhabdomyosarcoma (*rhabdos* rod)
			myosis: adenomyosis (*adenos* gland + *osis* condition)
			myositis muscle inflammation:
			celiomyositis (*koila* belly)
			dermatomyositis (*dermatos* skin)
			inomyositis (also called *fibromyositis*) (*inos* fiber)
			laparomyositis (*lapara* flank, loins)
			neuromyositis (*neuron* nerve)
			ophthalmomyositis (*ophthalmos* eye)
			pyomyositis (*pyon* pus)
			stethomyositis (or, stethmyitis) (*stethos* chest)
			myotomy muscle incision:
			cardiomyotomy (also called *esophagomyotomy*) (*kardia* heart)
			esophagomyotomy (also called *cardiomyotomy*) (esophagus)
			ophthlmomyotomy (*ophthalmos* eye)
			pyloromyotomy (pylorus)
			seromyotomy (*serum* whey)
			tenomyotomy (tendon)
			myotonia muscle tone condition:
			acromyotonia (*akron* extremity)
			neuromyotonia (*neuron* nerve)
			CROSS REFERENCE: musc
myc	Greek *mykes* fungus	fungus, mushroom	SIMPLE ROOT: mycete, mycetism (or, mycetismus; poisoning from eating fungi, especially poisonous mushrooms)
			PREFIXED ROOT:
			antimycotic (counteracting the growth of fungi; also called *antifungal*) (*anti* against)
			deuteromycete (also called *imperfect fungus*) (*deuteros* second)
			eumycetes (the true fungi) (*eu* well)
			LEADING ROOT COMPOUND:
			myc:
			mycelium (the mass of threadlike processes constituting the fungal thallus; pl., mycelia) {mycelian} (*helos* nail) [h is elided]
			mycosis (pl., mycoses) {mycotic} (*osis* condition)
			mycet:
			mycethemia (also called *fungemia*) (*hemia* blood condition)
			mycetoma (a chronic infection of the feet; pl., mycetomas, mycetomata) (*oma* tumor)
			myceto: mycetogenic (or, mycetogenetic) (*genere* to produce)
			myco:
			mycobacterium (pl., mycobacteria), mycobacteriosis (*bakterion* rod-shaped organism + *osis* condition)
			mycocide (also called *fungicide*) (*caedere* to kill)
			mycoderma (*derma* skin)
			mycodermatitis (also called *dermatomycosis*) (*dermatos* skin + *itis* inflammation)
			mycogastritis (*gaster* stomach, belly + *itis* inflammation)
			mycology {mycologist} (*logos* study)
			mycopathology (*pathos* disease + *logos* study)
			mycophage (a virus that infects fungi), mycophagy (ingestion of mushrooms and other fungi) (*phagein* to devour, consume)
			mycopus (a nonpurulent discharge; a mixture of mucous material and pus; also called *mucopus*) (pus)

Element	From	Meaning	Examples
myc (cont'd)		[fungus, mushroom]	mycostasis (prevention of the growth or multiplication of fungi; also called *fungistasis*) {mycostatic; also called *fungistatic*} (*stasis* stoppage)
			mycotoxicosis, mycotoxin (*toxikon* poison + *osis* condition)
			TRAILING ROOT COMPOUND:
			mycete:
			actinomycete (*aktis* ray)
			ascomycete (*askos* bag)
			basidiomycete (*basidium* base)
			blastomycete (*blastos* germ)
			hyphomycete (*hyphe* web)
			myxomycete (a member of Myxomycetes, a class of fungi containing slime molds) (*myxa* mucus)
			phycomycete (*phykos* seaweed)
			mycoma fungal tumor:
			actinomycoma (a swelling caused by an actinomycete) (*aktis* ray)
			botryomycoma (*botrys* bunch of grapes)
			mycosis fungus condition:
			actinomycosis (*aktinos* ray)
			esophagomycosis (esophagus)
			hyphomycosis (*hyphe* web, tissue)
			labiomycosis (*labium* lip)
			myringomycosis (*maringa* membrane)
			oculomycosis (*oculus* eye)
			oomycosis (*oon* egg, ovum)
			onychomycosis (*onyx* nail)
			ophthalmomycosis (*ophthalmos* eye)
			otomycosis (*otos* ear)
			pharyngomycosis (pharynx)
			rhinomycosis (*rhinos* nose)
			stomatomycosis (*stomatos* mouth)
			tonsillomycosis (tonsil)
			trichomycosis (*trichos* hair)
			vaginomycosis (vagina)
			zygomycosis (*zygon* yoke)
			CROSS REFERENCE: fung
myel	Greek *myelos*	marrow (spinal cord)	SIMPLE ROOT:
			myelic (pertaining to the spinal cord, or bone marrow)
			myelin (a fatlike substance forming a sheath around the axons of certain nerves) {myelinic}, myelinated (also called *medullated*), myelination (or, myelization)
			myeloic, myelon (the spinal cord) {myelonic}
			PREFIXED ROOT:
			myel: perimyelis (also called *endosteum*), perimyelitis (also called *endosteitis*) (*peri* around + *itis* inflammation)
			myelia:
			amyelia (congenital absence of the spinal cord) (*a* privative)
			diplomyelia (*diploos* double)
			micromyelia (abnormal smallness or shortness of the spinal cord) (*mikros* small)
			myelination:
			demyelination (also called *myelinolysis*) (*de* opposite)
			dysmyelination (*dys* abnormal)
			hypomyelination (also called *hypomyelinogenesis*) (*hypo* under)

Element	From	Meaning	Examples
myel (cont'd)		[spinal cord]	nonmyelinated (also called *unmyelinated*) (*non* negative)
			myeloblast marrow germ:
			macromyeloblast (*makros* large)
			micromyeloblast (*mikros* small)
			premyeloblast (*pre* before)
			myelocyte marrow cell:
			metamyelocyte (*meta* after)
			premyelocyte (or, promyelocyte) (*pre* before)
			myelograph: perimyelography (*peri* around + *graphein* to write)
			myelopath: panmyelopathy (*pan* all + *pathos* disease)
			myelopoiesis: dysmyelopoiesis (also called *myelodysplasia*) (*dys* abnormal + *poiein* to make, produce)
			myelosis: panmyelosis (*pan* all + *osis* condition)
			LEADING ROOT COMPOUND:
			myel:
			myelalgia (pain in the spinal cord) (*algos* pain)
			myelapoplexy (also called *hematomyelia*) (*apoplexy* stroke)
			myelatelia (*atelos* incomplete: *a* negative + *telos* complete)
			myelauxe (*auxein* to increase)
			myelemia (*emia* blood condition)
			myelencephalon (also called *medulla oblongata*) (*enkephalos* brain)
			myelitis (inflammation of the spinal cord or the bone marrow) {myelitic} (*itis* inflammation)
			myeloid, myeloidosis (*eidos* form + *osis* condition)
			myeloma, myelomatoid (*oma* tumor + *eidos* form)
			myelosis (*osis* condition)
			myelin: myelinosis (*osis* condition)
			myelino:
			myelinoclasis (also called *demyelination*) (*klasis* a breaking)
			myelinogenesis (also called *myelization*) (*genere* to produce)
			myelinolysis (also called *demyelination*) (*lyein* to dissolve)
			myelinopathy (*pathos* disease)
			myelinotoxic (*toxikon* poison)
			myelo:
			myeloblastoma (*blastos* germ + *oma* tumor)
			myelocele[1] (*kele* hernia)
			myelocele[2] (*koilia* a hollow)
			myelocyst {myelocystic}, myelocystocele (*kystis* sac + *kele* tumor)
			myelocystomeningocele (*kystis* sac, bladder + *meningos* membrane + *kele* tumor)
			myelocyte (*kytos* cell)
			myelodiastasis (*diastasis* separation)
			myelodysplasia (also called *myelodyspoiesis*) (*dysplasia* abnormal molding)
			myelodyspoiesis (also called *myelodysplasia*) (*dyspoiesis* abnormal producing)
			myeloencephalic (also called *cerebrospinal*), myeloencephalitis (*encephalon* brain + *itis* inflammation)
			myelofibrosis (*fibra* fiber + *osis* condition)
			myelogenesis {myelogenetic, myelogenic} (*genere* to produce)
			myelogone (or, myelogonium) (*gone* seed)
			myelogram, myelography (*graphein* to write)
			myeloleukemia (*leukos* white + *emia* blood condition)
			myelolipoma (*lipos* fat + *oma* tumor)

A Thesaurus of Medical Word Roots

Element	From	Meaning	Examples
myel (cont'd)		[spinal cord]	myelolymphocyte (*lympha* fluid + *kytos* cell)
			myelolysis (also called *demyelination*) (*lyein* to dissolve)
			myelomalacia (morbid softening of the spinal cord) (*malakos* soft)
			myelomenia (vicarious menstrual hemorrhage into the spinal cord) (*menia* menstrual condition)
			myelomeningitis (*meningos* membrane + *itis* inflammation)
			myelomeningocele (also called *meningomyelocele*) (*meningos* membrane + *kele* hernia)
			myelomere (*meros* part)
			myelomonocyte (*monos* single + *kytos* cell)
			myeloneuritis (also called *neuromyelitis*) (*neuron* nerve + *itis* inflammation)
			myeloparalysis (also called *spinal paralysis*)
			myelopathy {myelopathic} (*pathos* disease)
			myelopetal (*petere* to seek)
			myelophage (*phagein* to devour)
			myelophthisis {myelophthistic} (*phthisis* a wasting)
			myeloplast (*plassein* to form)
			myeloplegia (also called *spinal paralysis*) (*plege* stroke, paralysis)
			myelopoiesis (the formation of bone marrow or the cells that arise from it; also called *myelogenesis*) {myelopoietic} (*poiein* to form)
			myelopore (*poros* opening)
			myeloradiculitis (*radix* root + *itis* inflammation)
			myelorrhagia (also called *hematomyelia*) (*rhagia* bursting forth)
			myelorrhaphy (*rhaphe* suture)
			myelosarcoma (also called *myeloma*) (*sarkos* flesh + *oma* tumor)
			myeloschisis (*schisis* fissure)
			myelosclerosis (*skleros* hard + *osis* condition)
			myeloscope, myeloscopy (*skopein* to examine)
			myelospongium (*spongos* sponge)
			myelotherapy (*therapy* treatment)
			myelotome, myelotomy (*tomy* incision)
			myelotoxic (*toxikon* poison)
			TRAILING ROOT COMPOUND:
			myelia:
			atelomyelia (*atelos* incomplete)
			diastematomyelia (*diastema* an interval)
			hematomyelia (also called *myelorrhagia*) (*hematos* blood)
			hydromyelia (*hydor* water, fluid)
			syringomyelia (*syringos* pipe, tube, fistula)
			myelitis inflammation of the spinal cord:
			encephalomyelitis (*enkephale* brain)
			hematomyelitis (*hematos* blood)
			leukomyelitis (*leukos* white—matter of the spinal cord)
			meningomyelitis (*meningos* membrane)
			neuromyelitis (*neuron* nerve)
			osteomyelitis (*osteon* bone)
			periosteomyelitis (*periosteum*)
			poliomyelitis (*polios* gray)
			rachiomyelitis (*rhachis* spine)
			tephromyelitis (*tephrys* gray)
			myelocele spinal cord hernia:
			encephalomyelocele (*enkephale* brain)
			meningomyelocele (*meningos* membrane)

A Thesaurus of Medical Word Roots

Element	From	Meaning	Examples
myel (cont'd)		[spinal cord]	*myelogenous* marrow producing: lienomyelogenous (also called *splenomyelogenous*) (*lien* spleen) splenomyelogenous (also called *lienomyelogenous*) (spleen) *myelomalacia*: splenomyelomalacia (spleen + *malakos* soft) *myelopathy* spinal cord disease: poliomyelopathy (*polios* gray) radiculomyelopathy (also called *myeloradiculopathy*) (*radicule* small root) CROSS REFERENCE: medull
myring	Latin *myringa*	drum membrane	See Appendix B for examples of words with this combining form. Others are listed with the roots to which it is attached. CROSS REFERENCE: hymen, membr, mening, tympan
myx	Greek *myxa*	mucus, slime	PREFIXED ROOT: amyxia (absence or deficiency of mucus) (*a* privative) amyxorrhea (absence of mucus secretion) (*a* privative + *rhein* to flow) hypomyxia (diminished secretion of mucus) (*hypo* under) LEADING ROOT COMPOUND: *myx*: myxadenitis (*adenos* gland + *itis* inflammation) myxadenoma (*adenos* gland + *oma* tumor) myxasthenia (*asthenia* weakness: *a* negative + *sthenos* strength) myxedematoid (*edema* swelling + *eidos* form) myxemia (also called *mucinemia*) (*emia* blood condition) myxoid (resembling mucus) (*eidos* form) myxoma, myxomatosis (*oma* tumor + *osis* condition) *myxo*: myxoblastoma (also called *myxoma*) (*blastos* germ + *oma* tumor) myxochondroma (a chondroma in which the stroma resembles primitive mesenchymal tissue) (*chondros* cartilage + *oma* tumor) myxocystitis (*kystis* sac, bladder + *itis* inflammation) myxocystoma (*kystis* sac, bladder + *oma* tumor) myxofibroma, myxofibrosarcoma (*fibra* fiber + *sarkos* flesh + *oma* tumor) myxolipoma (*lipos* fat + *oma* tumor) myxoneuroma (*neuron* nerve + *oma* tumor) myxopapilloma (*papilla* a nipple + *oma* tumor) myxopoiesis (*poiesis* producing) myxorrhea (also called *blennorrhea*) (*rhein* to flow) myxosarcoma (*sarkos* flesh + *oma* tumor) TRAILING ROOT COMPOUND: *myxoma* mucous tumor: angiomyxoma (*angeion* blood vessel) chondromyxoma (*chondros* cartilage) cystomyxoma (*kystis* sac, bladder) fibromyxoma (*fibra* fiber) gliomyxoma (*glia* glue) lipomyxoma (*lipos* fat) lymphomyxoma (*lympha* water, fluid) osteochondromyxoma (*osteon* bone + *chondros* cartilage) rhabdomyomyxoma (*rhabdos* rod + *myos* muscle) CROSS REFERENCE: blenn, muc

N

Element	From	Meaning	Examples
nan	Greek *nanos* Latin *nanus*	dwarf, small	SIMPLE ROOT: nanism (dwarfishness; marked undersize), nanous (dwarfish), nanus (dwarf) LEADING ROOT COMPOUND: *nan*: nanoid (*eidos* form) nanophthalmos (or, nanophthalmia) (*ophthalmos* eye) *nano*: nanocephalia (also called *microcephaly*) (*kephale* head) nanocormia (abnormally dwarfed trunk or body) (*kormus* trunk) nanomelia (also called *micromelia*), nanomelus (*melos* limb) nanosoma (dwarfism), nanosomia, nanosomus (*soma* body) CROSS REFERENCE: lept, micro, mio
nari	Latin *naris*	nostril	SIMPLE ROOT: naris (pl., nares) PREFIXED ROOT: *narial*: internarial (*inter* between) intranarial (*intra* within) postnarial (*post* behind) *naris*: postnaris (also called *choana*) (*post* after, behind) prenaris (pl., prenares) (*pre* before) CROSS REFERENCE: nas
nas	Latin *nasus*	nose	SIMPLE ROOT: nasal (also called *rhinal*) nasion (an anthropometric landmark) nasus (the nose, as well as the prolongation on the front of the head of a crane fly or of certain termites) PREFIXED ROOT: *nasal*: endonasal (also called *intranasal*) (*endon* within) internasal (*inter* between) intranasal (also called *endonasal*) (*intra* within) mesonasal (*mesos* middle) paranasal (*para* beside) pernasal (*per* through) postnasal (*post* posterior) prenasal (*pre* before) retronasal (*retro* behind) subnasal (*sub* under) supranasal (*supra* above) *nasality*: denasality (also called *hyponasality*) (*de* negative) hypernasality (*hyper* over, beyond) hyponasality (also called *denasality*) (*hypo* under) LEADING ROOT COMPOUND: *nas*: nasitis (also called *rhinitis*) (*itis* inflammation) *naso*: nasoantral, nasoantritis (*antron* cavity + *itis* inflammation) nasociliary (*cilium* eyebrow)

Element	From	Meaning	Examples
nas (cont'd)		[nose]	nasofrontal (pertaining to the nasal and frontal bones) (*frons* front)
			nasogastric (*gaster* stomach, belly)
			nasolabial (*labium* lip)
			nasolacrimal (*lacrima* teardrop)
			nasomanometer (a manometer for measuring intranasal pressure) (*manos* thin + *metron* measure)
			nasopalatine (palate: roof of mouth)
			nasopharyngeal (also called *pharyngonasal*) (pharynx)
			nasoscope (*skopein* to examine)
			nasoseptal, nasoseptitis (*septum* wall + *itis* inflammation)
			nasosinusitis (also called *rhinosinusitis*) (*sinus* a hollow + *itis* inflammation)
			nasotracheal (*trachea* windpipe)
			TRAILING ROOT COMPOUND:
			alinasal (pertaining to the sides or wings of the nose)
			alveolonasal (*alveus* hollow)
			antronasal (*antrum* cavity)
			aurinasal (*auris* ear)
			basinasal (basion)
			dorsonasal (*dorsum* back: the bridge of the nose)
			ethmonasal (*ethmos* sieve)
			frontonasal (*frontis* front)
			inferonasal (*inferus* low)
			labionasal (*labium* lip)
			lacrimonasal (*lacrima* teardrop)
			oculonasal (*oculus* eye)
			orbitonasal (orbit—eye socket)
			oronasal (*oris* mouth)
			palatonasal (palate: roof of mouth)
			pharyngonasal (also called *nasopharyngeal*) (*pharynx* throat)
			septonasal (*septum* partition)
			vomeronasal (pertaining to the vomer and nasal bone) (*vomer* plowshare: a flat bone)
			CROSS REFERENCE: nari, rhin
nat, **nas**	Latin *nasci* to be born	birth	SIMPLE ROOT:
			nas: nascent (just born; just coming into existence; also, just liberated from a chemical combination)
			nat: natal, natality, native
			PREFIXED ROOT:
			antenatal (also called *prenatal*) (*ante* before)
			intranatal (occurring during birth) (*intra* within)
			perinatal, perinatologist, perinatology (*peri* around + *logos* study)
			postnatal (*post* after)
			prenatal (also called *antenatal*) (*pre* before)
			LEADING ROOT COMPOUND:
			natimortality (the proportion of stillbirths to the general birth rate) (*mors* death)
			neonatal, neonatologist (*neos* new + *logos* study)
			CROSS REFERENCE: gen, par, toc
necr	Greek *nekros* dead	death; corpse	PREFIXED ROOT:
			medionecrosis (*medius* middle + necrosis)
			postnecrotic (after death of a tissue or part) (*post* after)
			synnecrosis (*syn* with + necrosis)

Element	From	Meaning	Examples
necr (cont'd)		[death]	LEADING ROOT COMPOUND: *necr*: necrectomy (*ektome* excision) necropsy (examination of a body after death) (*opsis* view) necrose, necrosis (pl., necroses) {necrotic} (*osis* condition) necrosteon (or, necrosteosis) (*osteon* bone) *necro*: necrobiosis {necrobiotic} (*bios* life + *osis* condition) necrocytosis (*kytos* cell + *osis* condition) necrogenic, necrogenous (*genere* to produce) necrolysis (*lysis* dissolution) necromania (*mania* craze) necromimesis (*mimesis* imitation) necroparasite (also called *saprophyte*) necropathy (*pathos* disease) necrophagous (*phagein* to devour, consume) necrophilia (or, necrophily) {necrophilic} (*philein* to love) necrophobia (*phobia* fear) necrosadism (mutilation of a corpse for sexual gratification) necroscopy (*skopein* to examine) necrosectomy (*secare* to cut) necrospermia (*sperma* seed, sperm) necrotomy (*tomy* incision) necrotoxin (*toxikon* poison) TRAILING ROOT COMPOUND: *necrosis* deadness: adiponecrosis (*adeps* fat) angionecrosis (*angeion* vessel: blood vessel) arterionecrosis (*arteria* artery) cardionecrosis (*kardia* heart) chondronecrosis (*chondros* cartilage) cytonecrosis (*kytos* cell) hepatonecrosis (*hepatos* liver) leukonecrosis (also called *white gangrene*) (*leukos* white) myonecrosis (*myos* muscle) osteonecrosis (*osteon* bone) rhinonecrosis (*rhinos* nose) steatonecrosis (also called *fat necrosis*) (*steatos* fat) stomatonecrosis (also called *noma*) (*stomatos* mouth) CROSS REFERENCE: mort
nema	Greek *nema*	thread, threadlike (nematode)	SIMPLE ROOT: nema (a nematode) {nemaline} nematization (infestation with nematodes or roundworms) PREFIXED ROOT: diplonema (*diploos* double) microneme (also called *sarconeme*) (*mikros* small) mononeme (*monos* single) LEADING ROOT COMPOUND: *nemat*: nemathelminthiasis (also called *nematodiasis*) (*helminth* worm + *iasis* condition) nematode (the phylum that includes true roundworms or threadworms, many species of which are parasitic) {nemic} (*eidos* form)

Element	From	Meaning	Examples
nema (cont'd)		[thread]	nematoid (resembling a thread; pertaining to a nematode parasite) (*eidos* form)
			nematosis (also called *nematodiasis*) (*osis* condition)
			nemati: nematicidal (or, nematocidal) (*caedere* to kill)
			nemato:
			nematoblast (also called *spermatid*) (*blastos* germ, sprout)
			nematocyst (*kystis* sac, bladder)
			nematodesma (also called *trichite*) (*desmos* band)
			nematology (*logos* study)
			nematospermia (spermatozoa having elongated tails) (*sperma* seed)
			nematod: nematodiasis (also called *nematosis*) (*iasis* condition)
			TRAILING ROOT COMPOUND:
			axoneme (axis)
			leptonema (*leptos* slender)
			myoneme (*myos* muscle)
			pachynema (also called *pachytene*) (*pachys* thick)
			sarconeme (also called *microneme*) (*sarkos* flesh)
			CROSS REFERENCE: fil, mit, trich
neo	Greek *neos*	new, recent, young	See Appendix B for examples of words beginning with this element. Others are placed with the roots to which it is attached.
			CROSS REFERENCE: None
nephr	Greek *nephros*	kidney	SIMPLE ROOT:
			nephric (also called *renal*)
			nephron (a long, convoluted, tubular structure in the kidney, consisting of the renal corpuscle, the proximal tubule, the nephronic loop, and the distal tubule)
			PREFIXED ROOT:
			nephrectomy excision of kidney:
			epinephrectomy (also called *adrenalectomy*) (*epi* upon)
			heminephrectomy (*hemi* half)
			uninephrectomy (excision of a single kidney) (*uni* one)
			nephric pertaining to the kidneys:
			anephric (*a* privative)
			paranephric (*para* alongside)
			perinephric (also called *circumrenal*) (*peri* around)
			uninephric (*uni* one)
			nephritic pertaining to kidney inflammation:
			antinephritic (*anti* against)
			perinephritic (*peri* around)
			nephritis inflammation of the kidney:
			epinephritis (*epi* upon)
			paranephritis (*para* alongside)
			perinephritis (*peri* around)
			nephrium: perinephrium (pl., perinephria) (*peri* around)
			nephrogen kidney formation:
			anephrogenesis (*a* privative)
			metanephrogenic (or, metanephrogenous) (*meta* after)
			nephroid: hypernephroid (*hyper* above + *eidos* form)
			nephroma kidney tumor:
			hypernephroma (*hyper* over, beyond)
			mesonephroma (also called *clear cell adenocarcinoma*) (*mesos* middle)
			paranephroma (tumor of the adrenal gland) (*para* alongside)

Element	From	Meaning	Examples
nephr (cont'd)		[kidney]	*nephron*: deutonephron (also called *mesonephros*) (*deuteros* second) mesonephron (or, mesonephros) (*mesos* middle) *nephros*: epinephros (also called *suprarenal gland*) (*epi* upon) mesonephros (pl., mesonephroi) {mesonephric} (*mesos* middle) metanephros (pl., metanephroi) {metanephric} (*meta* after) paranephros (an adrenal gland) {paranephric} (*para* alongside) pronephros (or, pronephron; also called *protonephros*; pl., pronephroi, protonephra) {pronephric} (*pro* before) LEADING ROOT COMPOUND: *nephr*: nephradenoma (*adenos* gland + *oma* tumor) nephralgia {nephralgic} (*algos* pain) nephrapostasis (*apostasis* suppuration) nephrauxe (also called *nephromegaly*) (*auxein* to increase) nephrectasia (or, nephrectasis) (*ektasis* dilatation) nephrectomy {nephrectomize} (*ektome* excision) nephredema (also called *nephremia*) (*edema* swelling) nephrelcosis (*helkosis* ulceration) [h of helkosis elided] nephremia (congestion of the kidney) (*emia* blood condition) nephritis {nephritic} (*itis* inflammation) nephroid (*eidos* form) nephroma (*oma* tumor) nephrosis (pl., nephroses) {nephrotic} (*osis* condition) *nephrito*: nephritogenic (causing nephritis) (*genere* to produce) *nephro*: nephroabdominal (abdomen) nephroangiosclerosis (*angeion* blood vessel + *sklerosis* hardening) nephroblastoma (*blastos* bud, shoot, germ + *oma* tumor) nephrocalcinosis (calcium + *osis* condition) nephrocardiac (*kardia* heart) nephrocele (*kele* hernia) nephrocolic (*kolon* colon) nephrocystitis (*kystis* bladder + *itis* inflammation) nephrocystosis (*kystis* bladder + *osis* condition) nephrogastric (*gaster* stomach, belly) nephrogenic, nephrogenous (*genere* to produce) nephrogram, nephrography (*graphein* to write) nephrolith, nephrolithiasis (*lithos* stone + *iasis* condition) nephrology (*logos* study) nephrolysis {nephrolytic} (*lyein* to loosen) nephromalacia (*malakos* soft) nephromegaly (also called *nephrauxe*) (*megalos* large) nephromere (*meros* part) nephropathy {nephropathic} (*pathos* disease) nephropexy (*pexis* fixation) nephrophthisis (*phthisis* wasting) nephropoietic (*poiein* to produce) nephroptosis (*ptosis* falling) nephropyosis (*pyosis* suppuration) nephrorrhagia (*rhagia* bursting forth) nephrorrhaphy (*rhaphe* suture) nephrosclerosis (*sklerosis* hardening)

Element	From	Meaning	Examples
nephr (cont'd)		[kidney]	nephroscope, nephroscopy (*skopein* to examine) nephrostoma (*stoma* mouth, opening) nephrotomy (*tomy* incision) nephrotoxic (*toxic* poison) nephrotropic (*trepein* to turn) *nephrono*: nephronophthisis (renal tuberculosis) (*phthisis* wasting) TRAILING ROOT COMPOUND: *nephric*: cardionephric (*kardia* heart) hepatonephric (*hepatos* liver) neuronephric (*neuron* nerve) splenonephric (spleen) *nephritis* inflammation of a kidney or the kidneys: glomerulonephritis (*glomerulus* a small ball) hepatonephritis (*hepatos* liver) lithonephritis (*lithos* stone) pyelonephritis (*pyelos* pelvis) pyonephritis (*pyon* pus) ureteropyelonephritis (ureter + *pyelos* pelvis) *nephroptosis*: splenonephroptosis (spleen + *ptosis* a falling) *nephrosis* kidney condition: cystonephrosis (*kystis* bladder) hematonephrosis (or, hemonephrosis) (*hematos* blood) hydronephrosis {hydronephrotic} (*hydor* water) pyelonephrosis (*pyelos* pelvis) pyonephrosis (*pyon* pus) CROSS REFERENCE: ren

nesi	Greek
	nesidion
		islet
		(isles of the
		Langerhans)
			PREFIXED ROOT: polynesic (multiple and insular; occurring in
			    many foci) (*polys* many)
			LEADING ROOT COMPOUND:
			nesidi: nesidiectomy (excision of the pancreatic islets) (*ektome* exci-
			    sion)
			nesidioblast islet shoot, bud, germ:
			nesidioblast (any one of the cells that build up the islet cells of the
			    pancreas)
			nesidioblastoma (islet cell adenoma) (*oma* tumor)
			nesidioblastosis (*osis* condition)
			CROSS REFERENCE: insul

neur	Greek *neuron*	nerve, nerves, nervous system	SIMPLE ROOT: neuridine (a base isolated from fresh human brain, identical with spermine) neurility (the sum of the attributes and functions of nerve tissue) neuron (or, neurone) {neural, neuronal} neurula, neurulation PREFIXED ROOT: *neural*: abneural (also called *abnerval*) (*ab* away) adneural (also called *adnerval*) (*ad* to) diploneural (*diploos* double) endoneural (also called *intraneural*) (*endon* within) epineural (*epi* upon) intraneural (also called *endoneural*) (*intra* within) mononeural (*monos* single)

Element	From	Meaning	Examples
neur (cont'd)		[nerve]	paraneural (*para* alongside)
			perineural (*peri* around)
			polyneural (or, polyneuric) (*polys* many)
			subneural (below the neural axis) (*sub* below)
			supraneural (*supra* above)
			neuralgia: antineuralgia {antineuralgic} (*anti* against + neuralgia)
			neurine: aneurine (also called *thiamine*) (*a* negative)
			neuritic pertaining to nerve inflammation:
			antineuritic (counteracting neuritis) (*anti* against)
			perineuritic (*peri* around)
			polyneuritic (*polys* many)
			postneuritic (*post* after)
			neuritis nerve inflammation:
			endoneuritis (*endon* within)
			mesoneuritis (*mesos* middle)
			mononeuritis (*monos* single)
			perineuritis (*peri* around)
			polyneuritis (*polys* many)
			pseudoneuritis (*pseudes* false)
			radiculoneuritis (*radix* root)
			neurium:
			endoneurium (*endon* within)
			epineurium {epineurial} (*epi* upon, over)
			perineurium (*peri* around)
			neuro:
			aneurogenic (*a* privative + *genere* to produce)
			interneuromeric (*inter* between + *meros* part)
			microneurography (*mikros* small + *graphein* to write)
			microneurosurgery (*mikros* small + surgery)
			neuron:
			paraneuron (*para* alongside)
			interneuron (*inter* between)
			protoneuron (*protos* first)
			neuropathy nerve disease:
			mononeuropathy (*monos* single)
			polyneuropathy (*polys* many)
			neurosis nerve condition:
			aponeurosis (*apo* from)
			dystrophoneurosis (*dys* abnormal + *trophein* to nourish)
			synneurosis (also called *syndesmosis*) (*syn* with, together)
			LEADING ROOT COMPOUND:
			neur:
			neuragmia (the tearing of a nerve trunk) (*agmos* break)
			neuralgia {neuralgic}, neuralgiform (resembling neuralgia) (*algos* pain + *forma* shape)
			neurapophysis (*apophysis* offshoot)
			neurapraxia (*apraxia* failure: *a* privative + *prassein* to do)
			neurarchy (*arche* rule, dominant)
			neurasthenia (*asthenia* weakness: *a* negative + *sthenos* strength)
			neuraxis {neuraxial} (*axis* axle)
			neurectasia (also called *neurotony*) (*ektasis* dilatation)
			neurectomy (*ektome* excision)
			neurectopia (*ektopia* displaced)
			neurenteric (*enteron* intestine)

Element	From	Meaning	Examples
neur (cont'd)		[nerve]	neurergic (*ergon* work)
			neurexeresis (nerve avulsion) (*exeresis* excision)
			neuriatry (*iatrein* to heal)
			neuritis (pl., neuritides) {neuritic} (*itis* inflammation)
			neurodynia (also called *neuralgia*) (*odyne* pain)
			neuroid (*eidos* form)
			neuroma {neuromatous} (*oma* tumor)
			neurosis (pl., neuroses) {neurotic} (*osis* condition)
			neuri:
			neurilemma {neurilemmal}, neurilemmitis (*lemma* sheath + *itis* inflammation)
			neurilemmoma (*lemma* sheath + *oma* tumor)
			neurimotility (also called *nervimotility*), neurimotor (also called *nervimotor*) (*movere* to move)
			neuro:
			neuroanatomy (anatomy)
			neuroarthropathy (*arthron* joint + *pathos* disease)
			neuroaugmentation {neuroaugmentative} (*augere* to increase)
			neurobiology (biology)
			neurobiotaxis (*bios* life + *taxis* arrangement)
			neuroblast, neuroblastoma (*blastos* germ, shoot + *oma* tumor)
			neurocardiac (*kardia* heart)
			neuroceptor (*capere* to hold)
			neurochondrite (*chondros* cartilage + *ite* mineral)
			neurocladism (*klados* branch)
			neurocranium (*kranion* the upper part of the head—the skull)
			neurocutaneous (*cutis* skin)
			neurocytology (*kytos* cell + *logos* study)
			neurocytolysis (*kytos* cell + *lysis* dissolution)
			neurodendrite (also called *dendrite*) (*dendron* tree: growth)
			neuroderm, neurodermatitis (*derma* skin + *itis* inflammation)
			neurodynamic (*dynamis* force)
			neuroectoderm {neuroectodermal} (*ektos* outside + *derma* skin)
			neuroencephalomyelopathy (*enkephale* brain + *myelos* spinal cord + *pathos* disease)
			neuroepithelium {neuroepithelial} (epithelium)
			neurofiber, neurofibril (a delicate thread) (fiber)
			neurofibroma (also called *fibroneuroma*), neurofibromatosis (fiber + *oma* tumor + *osis* condition)
			neurofilament (*filum* thread)
			neurogangliitis (*ganglion* knot + *itis* inflammation)
			neurogastric (*gaster* stomach)
			neurogenesis {neurogenetic, neurogenic} (*genere* to produce)
			neuroglia {neuroglial, neurogliar}, neurogliacyte (*glia* glue + *kytos* cell)
			neuroglycopenia (*glykys* sweet + *penia* deficiency)
			neurogram, neurography (*graphein* to write)
			neurohemal (*haima* blood)
			neurohistology (*histos* tissue + *logos* study)
			neurohormone {neurohormonal} (*hormaein* to set in motion)
			neurohypophysis (also called *lobus nervosus*)
			neurolabyrinthitis (labyrinth + *itis* inflammation)
			neurolemma (or, neurilemma) (*lemma* sheath)
			neuroleptic (*lepsis* a taking hold)

A Thesaurus of Medical Word Roots

Element	From	Meaning	Examples
neur (cont'd)		[nerve]	neurolipomatosis (*lipos* fat + *oma* tumor + *osis* condition)
			neurology {neurologic}, neurologist (*logos* study)
			neurolymphomatosis (lymphoma + *osis* condition)
			neurolysis {neurolytic} (*lyein* to loosen)
			neuromalacia (*malakos* soft)
			neuromere (*meros* part)
			neuromimetic (*mimetic* imitating)
			neuromuscular (also called *neuromyal*)
			neuromyal (also called *neuromuscular*) (*myos* muscle)
			neuromyasthenia (*myasthenia* muscle weakness)
			neuromyelitis (*myelos* marrow + *itis* inflammation)
			neuromyopathy (*myos* muscle + *pathos* disease)
			neuromyositis (*myos* muscle + *itis* inflammation)
			neuronephric (*nephros* kidney)
			neuronevus (*nevus* birthmark)
			neuronyxis (acupuncture of a nerve) (*nyxis* pricking)
			neurooncology (*onkos* mass + *logos* study)
			neuroophthalmology (*ophthalmos* eye + *logos* study)
			neurootology (*otos* ear + *logos* study)
			neuropathogenesis (*pathos* disease + *genesis* beginning)
			neuropathology, neuropathy (*pathos* disease + *logos* study)
			neurophilic (also called *neurotropic*) (*philein* to love—affinity for)
			neurophonia (*phone* sound)
			neurophysiology
			neuropil (or, neuropile) (*pilos* felt)
			neuroplasm {neuroplasmic}, neuroplasty (*plassein* to form)
			neuropore (*poros* pore)
			neuroprobasia (*pro* forward + *basis* walking, moving)
			neuropsychiatry (*psyche* mind + *iatria* healing)
			neuroretinitis (retina + *itis* inflammation)
			neuroretinopathy (retina + *pathos* disease)
			neurorrhaphy (also called *neurosuture*) (*rhaphe* suture)
			neurosarcocleisis (*sarkos* flesh + *kleisis* closure)
			neurosarcoma (*sarkos* flesh + *oma* tumor)
			neurosome (*soma* body)
			neurospasm (*spasmos* contraction)
			neurosplanchnic (also called *neurovisceral*) (*splanchnon* viscus)
			neurosuture (also called *neurorrhaphy*) (*suere* to sew)
			neurotaxis (*taxis* arrangement)
			neurotendinous (tendon)
			neurothele (also called *nerve papilla*) (*thele* nipple)
			neurotmesis (a type of axon loss lesion resulting from focal peripheral nerve injury)
			neurotome, neurotomy (*tomy* incision)
			neurotony (also called *neurestasia*) {neurotonic} (*teinein* to stretch)
			neurotoxin {neurotoxic} (*toxikon* poison)
			neurotrauma (also called *neurotrosis*) (*trauma* injury)
			neurotripsy (*tripsy* a crushing)
			neurotrophy {neurotrophic} (*trophein* to nourish)
			neurotropy {neurotropic} (*tropein* to turn)
			neurotrosis (also called *neurotrauma*) (*trosis* a wounding)
			neurovascular (*vas* vessel)
			neurovirulence, neurovirus (*virus* poison)
			neurovisceral (also called *neurosplanchnic*) (*viscera* internal organs)

Element	From	Meaning	Examples
neur (cont'd)		[nerve]	*neuron*: neuronitis (*itis* inflammation) *neurono*: neuronopathy (*pathos* disease) neuronophage, neuronophagia (*phagein* to consume) neuronotropic (*tropic* turning) TRAILING ROOT COMPOUND: *neural* pertaining to a nerve: adenoneural (*adenos* gland) cardioneural (*kardia* heart) myoneural (*myos* muscle) psychoneural (*psyche* mind) sensorineural (*sentire* to experience, to feel) *neuralgia* nerve pain: angioneuralgia (*angeion* vessel—blood vessel) ischioneuralgia (*ischion* hip joint) myoneuralgia (*myos* muscle) odontoneuralgia (facial neuralgia caused by a carious tooth) (*odontos* tooth) orchioneuralgia (also called *orchialgia*) (*orchis* testicle) osteoneuralgia (*osteon* bone) otoneuralgia (*otos* ear) *neure*: esthesioneure (a sensory neuron) (*esthesia* feeling) *neuritis* inflammation of a nerve: actinoneuritis (*aktis* ray) celluloneuritis (inflammation of neurons) (cell) enteroneuritis (*enteron* intestine) ganglioneuritis (*ganglion* a swelling, knot) myeloneuritis (also called *neuromyelitis*) (*myelos* marrow) pseudoneuritis (*pseudes* false) radioneuritis (X-ray) septineuritis (neuritis due to sepsis) (*septikos* putrefaction) *neuroma* nerve tumor: fibroneuroma (fiber) ganglioneuroma (*ganglion* knot, swelling) glioneuroma (also called *ganglioglioma*) (*glia* glue) myoneuroma (*myos* muscle) myxoneuroma (*myxa* mucus) pseudoneuroma (*pseudes* false) *neuromere*: hodoneuromere (*hodos* road, path + *meros* part) *neuron*: motoneuron (also called *motor neuron*) (*movere* to move) protoneuron (*protos* first) teleneuron (*telos* end) *neuropathy*: vasoneuropathy (*vas* vessel + *pathos* disease) *neurosis* nerve condition: acroneurosis (*akron* extremity) dermatoneurosis (*dermatos* skin) kinesioneurosis (*kinein* to move) pathoneurosis (*pathos* disease) psychoneurosis (*psyche* mind) thermoneurosis (*therme* heat) trophoneurosis (*trophein* to nourish) vasoneurosis (also called *angioneuropathy*) (*vas* vessel) CROSS REFERENCE: None

Element	From	Meaning	Examples
neutr	Latin *ne* not + *uter* either	neither, neutral	SIMPLE ROOT: neutral {neutrality}, neutralism, neutralization, neutralize neutrino (an elementary particle that has no electric charge and no mass), neutron (an electrically neutral subatomic particle) PREFIXED ROOT: antineutrino (*anti* against) metaneutrophil (or, metaneutrophile; not reacting normally with neutral dyes) (*meta* after + neutrophil) orthoneutrophil (also called *orthochromophil*) (*orthos* straight + neutrophil) LEADING ROOT COMPOUND: neutroclusion (*claudere* to close) neutrocyte (also called *neutrophil*) (*kytos* cell) neutropenia (*penia* deficiency) neutrophil (or, neutrophile) {neutrophilic} (*philein* to love) neutrotaxis (*tassein* to arrange) CROSS REFERENCE: None
noct	Latin *nox*	night	SIMPLE ROOT: nocturnal (pertaining to the night; opposed to *diurnal*) LEADING ROOT COMPOUND: noctalbuminuria (albuminuria in urine secreted at night) (*uria* urine condition) noctambulation (sleepwalking; also called *somnambulation*) (*ambulare* to walk) nocturia (excessive urination during the night; also called *nycturia*) (*uria* urine condition) TERMS: nocturnal emission (harmless involuntary discharge of semen during sleep and usually occurring during an erotic dream) nocturnal enuresis (urinary incontinence during sleep at night; also called *bedwetting*) CROSS REFERENCE: nyct
nod	Latin *nodus* knot	knot, protuberance	SIMPLE ROOT: node (pl., nodi) {nodal} nodose, nodosity nodular (marked with, or resembling, nodules) nodulation, nodule, nodulus (pl., noduli), nodus (pl., nodi) PREFIXED ROOT: internode {internodal}, internodular (*inter* between) macronodular (*makros* large) micronodular (*mikros* small) multinodular (or, multinodal, multinodulate) (*multus* many) TRAILING ROOT COMPOUND: trichonodosis (*trichos* hair) FRENCH: serrenoeud (device for tightening ligatures) (*serrer* to squeeze) CROSS REFERENCE: condyl, gangli
noe, noo, noema, noum	Greek *noema*	thoughts	SIMPLE ROOT: noematic, noesis (the operation of the intellect; cognition) {noetic} noumenal (pertaining to rational intuition independent of sensory perception) PREFIXED ROOT: *noetic*: anoetic (*a* privative)

Element	From	Meaning	Examples
noe (cont'd)		[thoughts]	dianoetic (of or proceeding from logical reasoning rather than intuition) (*dia* through) *noia*: hypernoia (*hyper* above) hyponoia (sluggish mental activity) (*hypo* below) paranoia {paranoiac}, paranoid (*para* abnormal + *eidos* form) LEADING ROOT COMPOUND: *noema*: noematachograph (device for recording time taken in mental activity) (*tachys* swift + *graphein* to write) noematachometer (a device for registering the time required in a mental operation) (*tachys* swift + *metron* measure) *noo*: nootropic (*tropikos* turning) CROSS REFERENCE: auto, idi
noma	Greek *nome*	spreading, wandering (ulcer)	SIMPLE ROOT: noma (gangrenous stomatitis) nomadic (wandering; unsettled; free) TRAILING ROOT COMPOUND: angionoma (ulceration of a blood vessel) (*angeion* vessel) stomatonoma (also called *noma*) (*stomatos* mouth) urinoma (*ouron* urine) CROSS REFERENCE: helc, plan², rad¹, ulc, vag
norm	Latin *norma* carpenter's square	rule, normal, usual	SIMPLE ROOT: norm, norma (a line established to define the aspects of the cranium), normal, normality, normalization, normative PREFIXED ROOT: *normal*: abnormal, abnormality (*ab* away) hypernormal (*hyper* beyond, above) paranormal (*para* alongside; beyond—in this word) seminormal (*semi* half) subnormal {subnormality} (*sub* below) supernormal (*super* over, above) supranormal (*supra* above) *normoblast* normal germ, bud: macronormoblast (*makros* large) micronormoblast (*mikros* small) pronormoblast (*pro* before) LEADING ROOT COMPOUND: normoblast {normoblastic}, normoblastosis (*blastos* bud, shoot, germ + *osis* condition) normocalcemia {normocalcemic} (*calx* calcium + *emia* blood condition) normocapnia (a normal tension of carbon dioxide in the blood) {normocapnic} (*kapnos* smoke) normocephalic (also called *mesocephalic*) (*kephale* head) normocholesterolemia {normocholesterolemic} (cholesterol + *emia* blood condition) normochromasia (a normal staining reaction in a cell or tissue; normal color of the red blood cells), normochromia (*chroma* color) normocyte, normocytosis (*kytos* cell + *osis* condition) normoglycemia (*glykos* sugar + *emia* blood condition) normosthenuria (*sthenos* strength + *uria* urine condition)

Element	From	Meaning	Examples
norm (cont'd)		[rule, normal]	normotension, normotensive (*tendere* to stretch)
			normothermia {normothermic} (*therme* heat)
			normotonia {normotonic} (*tonos* tension)
			normotrophic (*trephein* to nourish)
			CROSS REFERENCE: arch, orth
noso	Greek *nosos*	disease	SIMPLE ROOT: nosema, nosode (any product of disease used as a remedy)
			PREFIXED ROOT:
			anosodiaphoria (indifference to the existence of disease) (*a* negative + *diaphoria* difference)
			anosognosia {anosognosic} (*a* negative + *gnosis* knowledge)
			epinosis (an imaginary feeling of illness following an actual illness) {epinosic} (*epi* upon, after)
			LEADING ROOT COMPOUND:
			nos:
			nosencephalus (*enkephalon* brain)
			nosetiology (*aitia* cause + *logos* study)
			noso:
			nosochthonography (the geography of epidemic or other diseases; also called *geomedicine*) (*chthon* earth + *graphein* to write)
			nosocomial (originating or taking place in a hospital, as a nosocomial infection), nosocomium (*komeion* to take care of)
			nosogenesis {nosogenic} (*genere* to produce)
			nosogeography (*geos* earth + *graphein* to write)
			nosography {nosographic} (*graphein* to write)
			nosology (also called *nosonomy, nosotaxy*) (*logos* study)
			nosomania (an unfounded morbid belief that one is suffering from some special disease) (*mania* frenzy, madness)
			nosomycosis (also called *mycosis*) (*mykes* fungus + *osis* condition)
			nosonomy (also called *nosology*) (*nomos* law)
			nosophilia (a morbid desire to be sick or ill) (*philein* to love, desire)
			nosophobia (*phobia* fear)
			nosophyte (*phyton* plant: growth)
			nosopoietic (*poiein* to produce)
			nosotaxy (also called *nosology, nosonomy*) (*taxis* arrangement)
			nosotoxicosis, nosotoxin {nosotoxic, for both terms} (*toxikon* poison + *osis* condition)
			nosotrophy (care of the sick) (*trophein* to nourish) [term rarely used]
			nosotropic (*trepein* to turn)
			TRAILING ROOT COMPOUND:
			nosology study of disease:
			dermonosology (or, dermatonosology) (*derma* skin)
			odontonosology (also called *dentistry*) (*odontos* tooth)
			psychonosology (*psyche* mind)
			nosus, nosis:
			cirrhonosus (*kirrhos* yellow)
			hypsonosus (mountain sickness) (*hypsos* height)
			keratonosus (any disease of the cornea) (*keratos* cornea)
			myonosus (also called *myopathy*) (*myos* muscle)
			phytonosis (*phyton* plant: growth)
			sapronosis (*sapros* rotten)
			trichonosis (also called *trichopathy*) (*trichos* hair)
			xeronosus (also called *xerosis*) (*xeros* dry)
			CROSS REFERENCE: path

Element	From	Meaning	Examples
noto	Greek *noton*	the back (of the body)	SIMPLE ROOT: notum (the dorsal part of the body) {notal} PREFIXED ROOT: subnotochordal (*sub* under + notochord) LEADING ROOT COMPOUND: *not*: notalgia (pain in the back; also called *dorsalgia*) (*algos* pain) notancephalia (*an* privative + *kephale* head) notanencephalia (*an* privative + *enkephalon* brain) notencephalocele (*enkephalon* brain + *kele* hernia) *noto*: notochord, notochordoma (also called *chordoma*) (*chord* cord + *oma* tumor) notogenesis (*genere* to produce) notomelus (*melos* limb, member) CROSS REFERENCE: dors, rachi, spin, spondyl, vertebr
nour			See nur- for *nourishment*.
nuc(le)	Latin *nux* nut	nut, nucleus kernel [a spheroid body within a cell]	SIMPLE ROOT: nuclear, nucleated, nucleation, nucleide, nucleolus (pl., nucleoli) {nucleolar} nucleon, nucleotide nucleus (pl., nuclei) {nuclear: relating to a nucleus, either cellular or atomic} PREFIXED ROOT: *nuclear*: anuclear (*a* negative) antinuclear (*anti* against) binuclear (having two nuclei) (*bi* two) circumnuclear (also called *perinuclear*) (*circum* around) ectonuclear (*ektos* outside) endonuclear (*endon* within) extranuclear (*extra* outside, beyond) heteronuclear (*heteros* different) homonuclear (*homos* same) infranuclear (*infra* below, beneath) internuclear (*inter* between) intranuclear (*intra* within) mononuclear (*monos* single) multinuclear (also called *plurinuclear*) (*multi* many) paranuclear (or, paranucleate) (*para* beside) perinuclear (also called *circumnuclear*) (*peri* around) plurinuclear (also called *multinuclear*) (*pluris* more) polynuclear (also called *polynucleate*) (*polys* many) supranuclear (*supra* above) uninuclear (*uni* one) *nuclease*: endonuclease (*endon* within) *nucleate*: binucleate (or, binuclear), binucleation (*bi* two) mononucleate (*monos* single) multinucleate (*multus* many) paranucleate (also called *paranuclear*) (*para* beside) polynucleate (also called *polynuclear*) {polynucleated} (*polys* many) *nucleated*: anucleated (also called *denucleated*) (*a* privative) denucleated (also called *anucleated*) (*de* negative)

Element	From	Meaning	Examples
nuc(le) (cont'd)		[nucleus]	uninucleated (*uni* one)
			nucleation:
			binucleation (*bi* two)
			enucleation (*ex* out)
			nucleolar:
			intranucleolar (*intra* within)
			polynucleolar (having several nucleoli) (*polys* many)
			nucleolate: binucleolate (having two nucleoli) (*bi* two)
			nucleolus:
			endonucleolus (*endon* within)
			amphinucleolus (*amphi* both, around)
			paranucleolus (*para* alongside)
			nucleosis nucleus condition:
			mononucleosis (*monos* single)
			multinucleosis (also called *polynucleosis*) (*multus* many)
			polynucleosis (also called *multinucleosis*) (*polys* many)
			nucleus:
			amphinucleus (also called *centronucleus*) (*amphi* around)
			macronucleus (also called *meganucleus*) (*makros* large)
			meganucleus (also called *macronucleus*) (*megas* large)
			metanucleus (*meta* beyond)
			micronucleus (*mikros* small)
			paranucleus (*para* alongside)
			pronucleus (pl., pronuclei) (*pro* before)
			subnucleus (a secondary nucleus) (*sub* under)
			LEADING ROOT COMPOUND:
			nucle:
			nucleoid (resembling a nucleus; a nucleus-like body sometimes seen in the center of an erythrocyte) (*eidos* form)
			nucleosis (*osis* condition)
			nuclei: nucleiform (*forma* shape)
			nucleo:
			nucleocapsid (a unit of viral structure)
			nucleochylema (also called *karyolymph*) (*chylos* juice)
			nucleochyme (also called *karyolymph*) (*chymos* juice)
			nucleocytoplasmic (*kytos* cell + *plassein* to form)
			nucleofugal (moving away from a nucleus) (*fugere* to flee)
			nucleoglucoprotein (a combination of nucleoprotein with a carbohydrate) (*glykys* sweet + protein)
			nucleolymph (also called *karyolymph*) (*lympha* water, liquid)
			nucleomicrosome (also called *karyomicrosome*) (*mikros* small + *soma* body)
			nucleopetal (moving toward a nucleus) (*petere* to seek)
			nucleophagocytosis (*phagein* to consume + *kytos* cell + *osis* condition)
			nucleophil (or, nucleophile) {nucleophilic} (*philein* to love)
			nucleoplasm (also called *karyolymph*) (*plassein* to form)
			nucleoprotein (any of a class of conjugated proteins that consist of nucleic acids and simple proteins, such as the histones)
			nucleoreticulum (*reticulum* network)
			nucleorrhexis (*rhexis* rupture)
			nucleosome (*soma* body)
			nucleospindle (the spindle-shaped body in mitosis)
			nucleotoxin (*toxikon* poison)

Element	From	Meaning	Examples
nuc(le) (cont'd)		[nucleus]	*nucleol*: nucleoloid (also called *nucleoliform*) (*eidos* form)
			nucleoli: nucleoliform (also called *nucleoloid*) (*forma* shape)
			nucleolo: nucleolonema (or, nucleoloneme) (*nema* thread)
			TRAILING ROOT COMPOUND:
			centronucleus (also called *amphinucleus*) (*kentron* point)
			kinetonucleus (also called *kinetoplast*) (*kinein* to move)
			maritonucleus (the nucleus of the ovum after the sperm has entered it) (*maritus* married)
			trophonucleus (also called *macronucleus*) (*trophein* to nourish)
			PREFIXED TRAILING ROOT COMPOUND: polymorphonuclear (*poly* many + *morphe* form)
			CROSS REFERENCE: karyo, pyren
nur, **nutr,** **nour**	Latin *nutrire*	to nourish	SIMPLE ROOT:
			nour: nourishment (act of nourishing or of being nourished)
			nur: nurse (a person who takes care of the sick, wounded, or enfeebled, especially one who makes a profession of it)
			nutr:
			nutrient (nourishing; affording nutriment; as a noun, a substance which affects the nutritive or metabolic processes of the body)
			nutrilites, nutriment, nutrition {nutritional, nutritive, nutritious}
			nutriture (the status of the body in relation to nutrition, generally or in regard to a specific nutrient, such as protein)
			PREFIXED ROOT:
			nutrient:
			macronutrient (*makros* large)
			micronutrient (*mikros* small)
			nutrition:
			denutrition (*de* negative)
			hypernutrition (also called *hyperalimentation*) (*hyper* over)
			malnutrition (also called *subnutrition*) (*malus* ill, bad)
			subnutrition (also called *malnutrition*) (*sub* under)
			supernutrition (also called *hypernutrition*) (*super* above)
			LEADING ROOT COMPOUND: nutriology (*logos* study)
			CROSS REFERENCE: al, troph
nux			See nucl-.
nyct	Greek *nyx, nyktos* night	night, darkness	LEADING ROOT COMPOUND:
			nyct:
			nyctalgia (pain that occurs in sleep only, thus at night) (*algos* pain)
			nyctalopia (night blindness (*alaos* blind, obscure + *opia* vision condition)
			nyctanopia (also called *nyctalopia*) (*an* privative + *opia* vision condition) [in *nyctalopia,* the middle root is from *alaos,* obscure]
			nyctaphonia (*a* privative + *phonia* voice condition)
			nycturia (frequent urination during the night, especially more at night than during the day; also called *nocturia*) (*uria* urine condition)
			nyctero: nycterohemeral (or, nyctohemeral) (*hemera* day)
			nycto:
			nyctohemeral (or, nycterohemeral) (*hemera* day)
			nyctophilia (also called *scotophilia*) (*philein* to love)
			nyctophobia (morbid fear of darkness) (*phobia* fear)
			nyctophonia (compare *nyctaphonia,* above)
			CROSS REFERENCE: melan, noct, scoto

Element	From	Meaning	Examples
nymph	Greek *nymphe*; Latin *nympha*	bride; maiden labia minora	SIMPLE ROOT: nympha (labium minus pudendi; pl., nymphae) {nymphal} [labium minus pudendi: also called *small pudendal lip*] LEADING ROOT COMPOUND: *nymph*: nymphectomy (*ektome* excision) nymphitis (*itis* inflammation) nymphoncus (swelling of the nymphae) (*onkos* mass, tumor) *nympho*: nymphohymenal (pertaining to the labia minora and the hymen) nympholepsy (ecstatic frenzy) (*lepsis* a seizure) nymphomania {nymphomaniacal}, nymphomaniac (*mania* madness) nymphotomy (*tomy* incision) CROSS REFERENCE: None
nystagm, nyxtaxis	Greek *nystazein, nystagmos*	to doze, nod	SIMPLE ROOT: nystagmus {nystagmic}; nystaxis (or, nystagmus) PREFIXED ROOT: *nystagm*: micronystagmus (*mikros* small) *nyxtaxis*: dysnyxtaxis (a condition of half sleep; also called *light sleep*) (*dys* abnormal) LEADING ROOT COMPOUND: *nystagm*: nystagmoid (also called *nystagmiform*) (*eidos* form) *nystagmi*: nystagmiform (also called *nystagmoid*) (*forma* shape) *nystagmo*: nystagmogram. nystagmograph (*graphein* to write) TRAILING ROOT COMPOUND: pseudonystagmus (also called *end-position nystagmus*) (*pseudes* false) NB: Do not confuse this root with the coined *nystatin,* from *New York State* + *in*, an antibiotic developed in New York State. CROSS REFERENCE: None
nyx	Greek *nyttein*	to prick	SIMPLE ROOT: nyxis (puncture, or paracentesis) TRAILING ROOT COMPOUND: hyalonyxis (the surgical puncturing of the vitreous body) (*hyalos* glass) keratonyxis (also called *aqueous paracentesis*) (*keratos* cornea) neuronyxis (*neuron* nerve) scleronyxis (the surgical pricking of the sclera, the tough, white supporting tunic of the eyeball) (*skleros* hard) CROSS REFERENCE: cente, punct

A Thesaurus of Medical Word Roots

O

Element	From	Meaning	Examples
ob-	Latin prefix	against, opposite, intensive	See Appendix B for examples and assimilations of this prefix. Others are placed with the roots to which it is attached. CROSS REFERENCE: anti-, contra-, de-
occip	Latin *ob* against + *caput* head	back of the head	SIMPLE ROOT: occipitalis (the posterior portion of the occipitofrontalis muscle at the back of the head), occiput {occipital} PREFIXED ROOT: exoccipital (pertaining to a bone or region on each side of the great foramen of the skull) (*exo* out) midoccipital (also called *medioccipital*) (*Anglo-Saxon midd* middle) paroccipital (near the occipital bone) (*para* alongside) suboccipital (*sub* below) supraoccipital (or, superoccipital) (*supra* above) LEADING ROOT COMPOUND: occipitoanterior (*anterior* before) occipitoatloid (atlas + *eidos* form) occipitoaxial (or, occipitoaxoid) (axis) occipitobasilar (*basis* base) occipitobregmatic (*bregma* brow) occipitocervical (*cervix* neck) occipitofacial (the face) occipitofrontal (forehead) occipitomastoid (mastoid process) occipitomental (*mentum* chin) occipitoparietal (*paries* wall) occipitotemporal (temporal region) occipitothalamic (thalamus) TRAILING ROOT COMPOUND: atlanto-occipital (relating to the atlas and the occipital bone) basioccipital (base) cervico-occipital (*cervix* neck) fronto-occipital (*frons* front, forehead) masto-occipital (*mastos* breast) parieto-occipital (*parietas* wall) petro-occipital (or, petroccipital) (*petra* stone) spheno-occipital (*sphenos* wedge) squamo-occipital (*squama* a scale or platelike structure) temporo-occipital (temporal bone) CROSS REFERENCE: ini
ocul	Latin *oculus*	eye	SIMPLE ROOT: oculist (also called *ophthalmologist*) oculus (the organ of vision—the eye; pl., oculi) {ocular} PREFIXED ROOT: *ocular*: binocular (pertaining to both eyes) (*bin* two, both) circumocular (also called *periocular*) (*circum* around) extraocular (*extra* outside) intraocular (*intra* within) monocular (*monos* single) periocular (also called *circumocular*) (*peri* around)

Element	From	Meaning	Examples
ocul (cont'd)		[eye]	postocular (*post* posterior)
			retroocular (also called *retrobulbar*) (*retro* behind)
			subocular (*sub* below)
			supraocular (*supra* above)
			telebinocular (*tele* afar + binocular)
			transocular (*trans* across)
			uniocular (pertaining to or affecting but one eye) (*uni* one)
			oculate: inoculate (lit., to plant an eye into; to engraft an eye or bud from one organism to another) (*in* in)
			oculation:
			autoinoculation (*auto* self + inoculation)
			inoculation (*in* in)
			reinoculation (*re* again + inoculation)
			oculum: inoculum (the material that is inoculated) (*in* in)
			oculus: monoculus (also called *cyclops*) (*monos* single)
			LEADING ROOT COMPOUND:
			oculocardiac (*kardia* heart)
			oculocephalogyric (*kephale* head + *gyros* circle)
			oculocerebrorenal (*cerebrum* brain + *ren* kidney)
			oculocutaneous (*cutis* skin)
			oculofacial (face)
			oculogyration {oculogyric} (*gyros* circle)
			oculomotor (*movere* to move)
			oculomycosis (also called *ophthalmomycosis*) (*mykes* fungus + *osis* condition)
			oculonasal (*nasus* nose)
			oculopathy (also called *ophthalmopathy*) (*pathos* disease)
			oculoplethysmography (*plethymos* increase + *graphein* to write)
			oculopupillary (pupil of eye)
			oculospinal (spine)
			oculovertebral (vertebra)
			oculozygomatic (zygomatic process)
			TRAILING ROOT COMPOUND:
			dextrocular (right-eyed) (*dexter* right)
			sinistrocular (having the left eye dominant; left-eyed) (*sinister* left)
			vestibulo-ocular (vestibule)
			CROSS REFERENCE: optic, ophthalm
odont	Greek *odontos*	tooth	SIMPLE ROOT: odontic (also called *dental*)
			PREFIXED ROOT:
			odont:
			haplodont (*haplos* single)
			heterodont (having teeth of different types, such as incisors and molars) (*heteros* other)
			hypsodont (*hypso* high)
			macrodont (or, macrodontism) (*makros* long, large)
			megadont (also called *macrodont*), megadontism (also called *macrodontia*) (*mega* big)
			microdont (*mikros* small)
			odontalg: antodontalgic (or, antiodontalgic) (*anti* against + *algos* pain)
			odontia tooth condition:
			anodontia (or, anodontism) (*an* privative)
			endodontia (or, endodontics; the branch of dentistry concerned with the tooth pulp), endodontist (*endon* within)

Element	From	Meaning	Examples
odont (cont'd)		[tooth]	exodontia (or, exodontics) (*exo* out)
			hyperdontia (*hyper* above, over)
			hypodontia (*hypo* under)
			macrodontia (also called *megadontism*) (*makros* long, large)
			megadontia (or, megalodontia; also called *macrodontia*) (*megas, megalos* big, large)
			microdontia (or, microdontism) {microdontic} (*mikros* small)
			periodontia (or, periodontics) (*peri* around)
			polyodontia (also called *polydentia*) (*polys* many)
			odontiasis: dysodontiasis (*dys* abnormal + *iasis* condition)
			odontic:
			endodontic (*endon* within)
			isodontic (*isos* equal)
			periodontics, periodontist, periodontium (the tissues investing and supporting the teeth; pl., periodontia) (*peri* around)
			odontitis inflammation of the teeth:
			endodontitis (inflammation of the tooth pulp; also called *pulpitis*) (*endon* within)
			periodontitis (inflammation of the gums) (*peri* around)
			odontium:
			endodontium (the dental pulp), endodontologist (*endon* within + *logos* study)
			periodontium (pl., periodontia) (*peri* around)
			odontoclasia: periododontoclasia (*peri* around + *klasis* breaking)
			odontogenesis: dysodontogenesis {dysodontogenetic} (*dys* abnormal + *genesis* origin)
			odontology: periodontology (*peri* around + *logos* study)
			odontolysis: periodontolysis (*peri* around + *lysis* loosening)
			odontosis: periodontosis (*peri* around + *osis* condition)
			LEADING ROOT COMPOUND:
			odont:
			odontalgia (also called *odontodynia*) {odontalgic} (Latin *algos* pain; Greek *odyne* pain)
			odontectomy (*ektome* excision)
			odonterism (chattering of the teeth) (*erismos* quarrel)
			odontiasis (teething) (*iasis* condition)
			odontitis (also called *pulpitis*) (*itis* inflammation)
			odontoid (*eidos* form)
			odontodynia (also called *odontalgia*) (*odyne* pain)
			odontoma (*oma* tumor)
			odontonomy (also called *dentonomy*) (*onoma* name)
			odontosis (also called *odontogenesis*) (*osis* condition)
			odonto:
			odontoblast, odontoblastoma (*blastos* bud + *oma* tumor)
			odontodysplasia (*dys* abnormal + *plassein* to form)
			odontogen, odontogenesis (*genesis* origin)
			odontoiatria (dental therapeutics) (*iatrein* to heal)
			odontolith (dental calculus) (*lithos* stone)
			odontology (*logos* study)
			odontoloxia (or, odontoloxy; also called *odontoparallaxis*) (*loxos* slanting)
			odontolysis (also called *erosion*) (*lysis* dissolution)
			odontonosology (*nosos* disease + *logos* study)
			odontoparallaxis (also called *odontoloxia*) (*parallax* alternately)

Element	From	Meaning	Examples
odont (cont'd)		[tooth]	odontopathy {odontopathic} (*pathos* illness, disease)
			odontophobia ((*phobia* fear)
			odontoplasty (*plassein* to form)
			odontoprisis (*prisis* grinding)
			odontoptosis (*ptosis* a falling)
			odontorrhagia (*rhagia* bursting forth)
			odontoschism (fissure of a tooth) (*schisma* cleft)
			odontoscope, odontoscopy (*skopein* to examine)
			odontoseisis (looseness of the teeth) (*seiein* to shake)
			odontotheca (the dental sac) (*theke* case)
			odontotherapy (*therapy* treatment)
			odontotomy (*tomy* incision)
			odontotripsis (wearing away of the teeth) (*tripsis* rubbing)
			TRAILING ROOT COMPOUND:
			odont:
			anisodont (*aniso* unequal: *an* negative + *isos* equal)
			brachyodont (*brachys* short)
			cynodont (a canine tooth; a sharp-pointed tooth on either side of the upper jaw and lower jaw, between the incisors and the bicuspids, having a long narrow root) (*kynos* dog)
			odontia tooth condition:
			aerodontia (*aeros* air)
			allotriodontia (*allotrios* strange, foreign)
			gerodontia (*geros* old age)
			hypnodontia (or, hypnodontics) (*hypnos* sleep)
			leukodontia (*leukos* white)
			oligodontia (*oligos* few, scant)
			orthodontia (or, orthodontics) (*orthos* straight)
			pathodontia (also called *dental pathology*) (*pathos* disease)
			pediodontia (also called *pediatric dentistry*) (*paidos* child)
			prosthodontia (or, prosthodontics) (*prosthetic* artificial substitute)
			pseudoanodontia (*pseudes* false + anodontia)
			odontics:
			aerodontics (*aer* air)
			biodontics (an area of oral health) (*bios* life)
			ephebodontics (adolescent dentistry; related to *pedodontics*, children's dentistry) (*ephebe* young person)
			geriodontics (or, gerodontics) (*geras* old age)
			hypnodontics (*hypnos* sleep)
			implantodontics (implant)
			orthodontics (*orthos* straight)
			pedodontics (*paidos* child)
			periodontics (*peri* around)
			prosthodontics (branch of dentistry dealing with construction of artificial appliances for the mouth) (*prosthesis* artificial substitute)
			odontism: taurodontism (*taurus* bull)
			odontist:
			implantodontist (implant)
			orthodontist (a dentist who specializes in the prevention and correction of irregularities of the teeth and malocclusion) (*orthos* straight)
			pedodontist (*paidos* child)
			rhizodontropy (*rhiza* root + *tropein* to turn)
			odontoid: syndesmo-odontoid (*syndesis* bound together)

Element	From	Meaning	Examples
odont (cont'd)		[tooth]	*odontous*:
			leptodontous (*leptos* slender)
			xanthodontous (having yellowish teeth) (*xanthos* yellow)
			PREFIXED TRAILING ROOT COMPOUND:
			phyodont producing teeth:
			diphyodont (having two sets of teeth, as man) (*di* two)
			monophyodont (having only one set of teeth throughout life) (*monos* single)
			polyphyodont (developing several sets of teeth successively throughout life) (*polys* many)
			CROSS REFERENCE: dent
odyn	Greek *odyne*	pain, distress	PREFIXED ROOT:
			allodynia (pain that results from a noninjurious stimulus to the skin) (*allos* other)
			anodyne (a medication that relieves pain) (*an* negative)
			heterodyne (*heteros* other, different)
			LEADING ROOT COMPOUND:
			odyn: odynacusis (a condition in which noises cause pain in the ear) (*akouein* to hear)
			odyno:
			odynometer (also called *algesimeter*) (*metron* measure)
			odynophagia (pain on swallowing) (*phagein* to devour)
			odynophobia (*phobia* fear)
			odynophonia (pain on using the voice) (*phone* sound, voice)
			TRAILING ROOT COMPOUND:
			achillodynia (also called *achillobursitis*) (Achilles tendon)
			acrodynia (pain in the upper part of the body; also called *erythredema, polyneuropathy, pink disease*) (*akron* extremity)
			adenodynia (*adenos* gland)
			angiodynia (also called *angialgia*) (*angeion* blood vessel)
			arthrodynia (also called *arthralgia*) (*arthron* joint)
			calcaneodynia (or, calcodynia) (*calcaneus* heel)
			cardiodynia (also called *cardialgia*) (*kardia* heart)
			carotodynia (pain caused by pressure on the carotid artery)
			cephalodynia (headache) (*kephale* head)
			cervicodynia (also called *trachelodynia*) (*cervix* neck)
			chondrodynia (also called *chondralgia*) (*chondros* cartilage)
			coccygodynia (or, coccydynia; pain in the tail; also called *coccyalgia*)
			colpodynia (also called *vaginodynia*) (*kolpos* vagina)
			coxodynia (also called *coxalgia*) (*coxa* hip)
			crymodynia (*krymos* frost)
			cystodynia (also called *cystalgia*) (*kystis* bladder)
			dactylodynia (also called *dactylalgia*) (*daktylos* finger, toe)
			dermatodynia (also called *dermatalgia*) (*derma* skin)
			desmodynia (also called *desmalgia*) (*dein* to bind: ligament)
			diaphragmodynia (also called *diaphragmalgia*)
			dorsodynia (also called *dorsalgia*) (*dorsum* back)
			encephalodynia (or, cephalodynia; headache) (*kephalos* head)
			enterodynia (also called *enteralgia*) (*enteron* intestine)
			esophagodynia (also called *esophagalgia*)
			gastrodynia (also called *gastralgia*) (*gaster* stomach)
			glossodynia (also called *glossalgia*) (*glossa* tongue)
			gnathodynia (also called *gnathalgia*) (*gnathos* jaw)

Element	From	Meaning	Examples
odyn (cont'd)		[pain]	hepatodynia (also called *hepatalgia*) (*hepatos* liver)
			hysterodynia (also called *hysteralgia*) (*hystera* uterus)
			inguinodynia (*inguen* groin)
			ischiodynia (also called *ischialgia*) (*ischion* hip)
			lumbodynia (also called *lumbago*) (*lumbus* loin)
			mastodynia (also called *mastalgia, mazodynia*) (*mastos* breast)
			mazodynia (also called *mastodynia*) (*mazos* breast)
			metrodynia (also called *hysteralgia*) (*metra* uterus)
			myodynia (also called *myalgia*) (*myos* muscle)
			neurodynia (also called *neuralgia*) (*neuron* nerve)
			odontodynia (toothache; also called *dentalgia*) (*odontos* tooth)
			omodynia (also called *omalgia*) (*omos* shoulder)
			ophthalmodynia (also called *ophthalmalgia*) (*ophthalmos* eye)
			orchiodynia (also called *orchialgia*) (*orchis* testicle, testis)
			osteodynia (also called *ostealgia*) (*osteon* bone)
			otodynia (also called *otalgia*) (*otos* ear)
			parodynia (labor pains) (*parere* to beget)
			phallodynia (also called *phallalgia*) (*phallos* penis)
			pharyngodynia (also called *pharyngalgia*) (*pharynx* the throat)
			photodynia (also called *photalgia*) (*photos* light)
			phrenodynia (also called *phrenalgia*) (*phrenos* diaphragm)
			pleurodynia (also called *pleuralgia*) (*pleura* rib, side)
			pododynia (also called *podalgia*) (*podos* foot)
			proctodynia (also called *proctalgia*) (*proktos* anus, rectum)
			prostatodynia (also called *prostatalgia*)
			rachiodynia (also called *rachialgia*) (*rhachis* spine)
			rhinodynia (also called *rhinalgia*) (*rhinos* nose)
			sacrodynia (also called *sacralgia*) (*sacrum*)
			scapulodynia (also called *scapulalgia*) (*scapula* shoulder blade)
			splenodynia (also called *splenalgia*) (*splen* spleen)
			spondylodynia (also called *spondylalgia*) (*spondylos* vertebra)
			sternodynia (also called *sternalgia*) (*sternon* chest)
			stomachodynia (also called *gastrodynia*)
			stomatodynia (also called *stomatalgia*) (*stomatos* mouth)
			tenodynia (also called *tenalgia*) (*tenon* tendon)
			thoracodynia (also called *thoracalgia*) (*thorax* chest)
			trachelodynia (also called *cervicodynia*) (*trachelos* neck)
			urethrodynia (also called *urethralgia*)
			uterodynia (also called *hysteralgia*)
			vaginodynia (also called *colpodynia*)
			vulvodynia (*vulva* the external genitalia of the female)
			xiphodynia (*xiphos* sword: xiphoid process)
			CROSS REFERENCE: alg, path
-oid **-ode**	Greek *eidos* form	resembling	See Appendix C for examples of words ending in this suffix. Others are listed with the root to which it is attached. CROSS REFERENCE: eid
olecran	Greek *olene* ulna + *kranion* skull, head	elbow	SIMPLE ROOT: olecranon (the proximal bony projection of the ulna at the elbow, its anterior surface forming part of the trochlear notch) {olecranal} LEADING ROOT COMPOUND: olecranarthritis (*arthron* joint + *itis* inflammation) olecranarthropathy (*arthron* joint + *pathos* disease) olecranoid (*eidos* form) CROSS REFERENCE: ancon

Element	From	Meaning	Examples
olfact	Latin *olere* to smell + *facere* to make	to smell	SIMPLE ROOT: olfact (unit of odor), olfaction olfactism (a sensation of smell produced by other than olfactory stimuli), olfactory, olfactus (a unit of acuity of smell) LEADING ROOT COMPOUND: olfactology (also called *osmics*) (*logos* study) olfactometer {olfactometry} (*metron* measure) olfactophobia (*phobia* fear) CROSS REFERENCE: osm[1], osphr
olig	Greek *oligos* few	little, few, scanty	See Appendix B for examples of words with this element. Others are placed with the roots to which it is attached. CROSS REFERENCE: penia
olist	Greek *olisthanein*	to slip	SIMPLE ROOT: olisthe (or, olisthy; a slipping, as the slipping of the bones of a joint from their normal position in the joint) {olisthetic} PREFIXED ROOT: anterolisthesis (also called *spondylolisthesis*) (*anterior* front) retrolisthesis (also called *retrospondylolisthesis*) (*retro* back) TRAILING ROOT COMPOUND: hierolisthesis (displacement of the sacrum) (*hieros* sacral: sacrum) sacrolisthesis (also called *spondylolisthesis*) spondylolisthesis (also called *anterolisthesis*) (*spondylos* vertebra) CROSS REFERENCE: None
-oma	Greek suffix	tumor	See Appendix C for examples of words with this suffix. Others are listed with the root to which it is attached. CROSS REFERENCE: cel[2], gangli, onc, tub[2], tum
oment	Latin *omentum* fat skin	fat skin covering	SIMPLE ROOT: omentulum (also called *lesser omentum*) omentum (a fold of peritoneum extending from the stomach to adjacent organs in the abdominal cavity; pl., omenta) {omental} LEADING ROOT COMPOUND: *oment*: omentectomy (*ektome* excision) omentitis (*itis* inflammation) *omento*: omentofixation (also called *omentopexy*) (*figere* to fasten) omentopexy (also called *omentofixation*) (*pexis* fixation) omentoplasty (a procedure for using the greater omentum to cover or fill a defect) (*plassein* to form) omentoportography (radiography of the hepatic portal veins after injection of a contrast medium into the gastroepiploic vein in the base of the omentum) omentorrhaphy (suturing of the omentum) (*rhaphe* suture) omentotomy (*tomy* incision) omentovolvulus (*volvulus* intestinal obstruction) *omentum*: omentumectomy (or, omentectomy) (*ektome* excision) CROSS REFERENCE: epiplo
omo	Greek *omos*	shoulder	PREFIXED ROOT: supraomohyoid (*supra* above + omohyoid) LEADING ROOT COMPOUND: *om*: omacephalus (or, omocephalus; a fetus with no upper limbs and an incomplete head) (*a* privative + *kephale* head) omagra (gout in the shoulder) (*agra* seizure) omalgia (also called *omodynia*) (*algos* pain)

Element	From	Meaning	Examples
omo (cont'd)		[shoulder]	omarthritis (*arthron* joint + *itis* inflammation) omitis (*itis* inflammation) omodynia (also called *omalgia*) (*odyne* pain) *omo*: omocephalus (or, omacephalus) (*kephale* head) omoclavicular (clavicle) omohyoid (pertaining to the shoulder and the hyoid bone) omoplate (the shoulder blade, or scapula) omosternum (*sternum* the chest) TRAILING ROOT COMPOUND: acromion (the outer extremity of the spine of the shoulder blade, or scapula) (*akron* extremity) CROSS REFERENCE: None
omphal	Greek *omphalos*	navel, umbilicus	SIMPLE ROOT: omphalic (also called *umbilical*), omphalos PREFIXED ROOT: *omphalic*: paraomphalic (also called *paraumbilical*) (*para* alongside) periomphalic (also called *periumbilical*) (*peri* around) *omphalo*: paromphalocele (*para* beside + *kele* tumor) *omphalos*: exomphalos (also called *umbilical hernia*) (*ex* outside) *omphalus*: monomphalus (also called *omphalopagus*) (*monos* single) LEADING ROOT COMPOUND: *omphal*: omphalectomy (*ektome* excision) omphalelcosis (*helkosis* ulceration) [h of helkosis elided] omphalitis (*itis* inflammation) omphaloma (also called *omphaloncus*) (*oma* tumor) omphaloncus (also called *omphaloma*) (*onkos* mass) *omphalo*: omphaloangiopagus (*angeion* blood vessel + *pagos* fixed) omphalocele (congenital hernia of the navel) (*kele* hernia) omphalochorion (*chorion* membrane) omphalogenesis (*genesis* origin) omphalopagus (also called *monomphalus*) (*pagos* attached) omphalophlebitis (*phlebos* vein + *itis* inflammation) omphalorrhagia (*rhagia* bursting forth) omphalorrhea (*rhein* to flow) omphalorrhexis (*rhexis* rupture) omphalosite (*sitos* food) omphalospinous (spine) omphalotomy (cutting of the umbilical cord) (*tomy* incision) omphalotripsy (*tribein* to crush, rub) omphalovesical (also called *vesicoumbilical*) (*vesica* bladder) TRAILING ROOT COMPOUND: *omphalocele*: epiplomphalocele (*epiploon* omentum + *kele* hernia) *omphalos*: cirsomphalos (*kirsos* varix) hepatomphalos (*hepatos* liver) *omphalus*: acromphalus (abnormal projection of the umbilicus; center of the navel) (*akron* extremity) hydromphalus (*hydor* water) varicomphalus (*varix* varicose vein) CROSS REFERENCE: umbilic

Element	From	Meaning	Examples
onc, **onk**	Greek *onkos* mass	mass, bulk, tumor, swelling	PREFIXED ROOT: antioncogene (also called *tumor suppressor*) (*anti* against + *genesis* origin) hyperoncotic (*hyper* above) hypooncotic (*hypo* under) isoncotic (having the same oncotic pressure) (*isos* equal) polyoncosis (or, polyonchosis) (*polys* many + *osis* condition) LEADING ROOT COMPOUND: *onc*: oncoides (turgid swelling; intumescence) (*eidos* resemblance) oncoma (a swelling; tumor) (*oma* tumor) oncosis (a morbid condition characterized by the development of tumors) {oncotic} (*osis* condition) *onco*: oncocyte, oncocytoma (an oxyphilic granular cell adenoma of the parotid gland) (*kytos* cell + *oma* tumor) oncocytosis (*kytos* cell + *osis* condition) oncofetal (concerning tumors in the fetus) oncogenesis (the production or causation of tumors) {oncogenic, oncogenous}, oncogenicity (*genesis* origin) oncograph, oncography (*graphein* to write) oncology (*logos* study) oncolysis (the destruction of tumor cells) (*lyein* to loosen) oncometer {oncometric, oncometry} (*metron* measure) oncosphere (the larva of the tapeworm in the spherical stage; also called *hexacanth*) (*sphere* ball, globe) oncotherapy (*therapy* treatment) oncothlipsis (pressure caused by a tumor) (*thlipsis* pressure) oncotomy (*tomy* incision) oncotropic (*trepein* to turn) *onk*: onkinocele (a swollen condition of a tendon sheath) (*inos* fiber + *kele* tumor) TRAILING ROOT COMPOUND: *oncology*: neurooncology (*neuron* nerve + *logos* study) *oncus*: adenoncus (also called *adenomegaly*) (*adenos* gland) arthroncus (*arthron* joint) blepharoncus (*blepharon* eyelid) glossoncus (*glossa* tongue) gonyoncus (*gony* knee) iridoncus (*iridos* rainbow: iris) mastoncus (*mastos* breast, nipple) nymphoncus (*nymphe* labia minora) omphaloncus (*omphalos* navel) orchioncus (or, orchidoncus; also called *testicular tumor*) (*orchis* testicle) osteoncus (*osteon* bone) ovarioncus (*ovary* egg) phalloncus (*phallos* penis) splenoncus (also called *splenoma*) (*splen* spleen) staphyloncus (*staphyle* uvula) theloncus (a tumor of a nipple) (*thele* nipple) uroncus (also called *urinoma*) (*ouron* urine) CROSS REFERENCE: cel[2], gangli, mol, phyma

Element	From	Meaning	Examples
oneir, **onir**	Greek *oneiros*	dream	SIMPLE ROOT: oneiric (or, oniric; pertaining to dreams), oneirism (dreamlike hallucination in a waking state) PREFIXED ROOT: paroniria (dreaming of a terrifying nature) (*para* abnormal) LEADING ROOT COMPOUND: *oneir*: oneirodynia (bad dreams; nightmares) (*odyne* pain) oneirogmus (emission of semen accompanying erotic dreams; also called *nocturnal emission*) (*ogmus* effusion) oneiroid (resembling a dream) (*eidos* form) *oneiro*: oneirogenic (*genesis* origin) oneirology (the study of dreams and their content) (*logos* study) oneirophrenia (a state in which hallucinations occur, caused by prolonged deprivation of sleep, sensory isolation, and a variety of drugs) (*phren* mind) CROSS REFERENCE: None
onk			See onc- for *onkinocele*.
onom	Greek *onoma*	name	PREFIXED ROOT: anomia (inability to remember names of objects; also called *anomic aphasia*) (*an* privative) dysnomia (amnestic aphasia) (*dys* abnormal) paranomia (amnestic aphasia) (*para* abnormal) LEADING ROOT COMPOUND: onomatology (the science of names or of their classification) (*logos* study) onomatomania (irresistible preoccupation with specific words or names) (*mania* madness) onomatopoeia (or, onomatopoiesis) (*poiein* to make) CROSS REFERENCE: onym
onych, **onyx**	Greek *onyx*	nail of the finger, toe	SIMPLE ROOT: onychia (inflammation of the matrix of the nail resulting in the loss of the nail; also called *onychitis*) onyx (a fingernail or toenail; also, pus collection between the corneal layers of the eye), onyxis (ingrown nail) PREFIXED ROOT: *onychia* nail condition: anonychia (congenital absence of a nail or nails) (*an* privative) eponychia (in embryology, the modified outer layer of the epidermis that partially covers the fetal fingernails and toenails and that persists after birth as the cuticle; in anatomy, a thin, cuticular fold extending over the lunula of a nail) (*epi* upon) hyperonychia (also called *onychauxis*) (*hyper* over) megalonychia (also called *macronychia*) (*megalos* large) micronychia (*mikros* small) paronychia (acute or chronic infection of a marginal structure about the nail; also called *perionychia*) (*para* beside) perionychia (also called *paronychia*) (*peri* around) polyonychia (also called *polyunguia*) (*polys* many) synonychia (*syn* together) *onychial*: hyponychial (also called *subungual*) (*hypo* under) *onychium*: eponychium (also called *perionychium*) (*epi* upon) hyponychium (*hypo* under)

Element	From	Meaning	Examples
onych (cont'd)		[nail of the finger, toe]	perionychium (the epidermis forming the border around a fingernail or toenail; cuticle; also called *eponychium*; pl., perionychia) (*peri* around)
			onychon: hyponychon (subungual hemorrhage) (*hypo* under)
			onyx: perionyx (*peri* around)
			LEADING ROOT COMPOUND:
			onych:
			onychalgia (painful nails) (*algos* pain)
			onychatrophia (or, onychatrophy) (*a* negative + *trophein* to nourish)
			onychauxis (also called *hyperonychia*) (*auxein* to increase)
			onychectomy (*ektome* excision)
			onychitis (also called *onychia*) (*itis* inflammation)
			onychoid (*eidos* form)
			onychoma (*oma* tumor)
			onychosis (also called *onychopathy*) (*osis* condition)
			onycho:
			onychoclasis (breaking of the nails) (*klaein* to break)
			onychocryptosis (ingrown nail) (*kryptosis* hidden)
			onychodystrophy (*dystrophy* malnourishment)
			onychogram, onychograph (device for making record of capillary blood pressure under the fingernails) (*graphein* to write)
			onychogryposis (enlargement with increased thickening and curvature of the fingernails or toenails) (*gryposis* crooking, hooking)
			onychoheterotopia (*heteros* other + *topos* place)
			onycholysis (*lyein* to loosen)
			onychomadesis (complete shedding of the nails) (*madao* to fall off)
			onychomalacia (*malakos* soft)
			onychomycosis (*mykes* fungus + *osis* condition)
			onychopathy, onychopathology (*pathos* disease + *logos* study)
			onychophagy (the habit of biting the nails) (*phagein* to devour)
			onychophosis (*phos* light + *osis* condition)
			onychoptosis (dropping off of the nails) (*ptein* to fall)
			onychophyma (*phyma* tumor, growth)
			onychorrhexis (*rhexis* a breaking)
			onychoschizia (*schizein* to divide)
			onychstroma (also called *nail matrix*) (*stroma* bedding)
			onychotillomania (*tillein* to pluck + *mania* craze)
			onychotomy (*tomy* incision)
			onychotrophy (*trophein* to nourish)
			TRAILING ROOT COMPOUND:
			brachyonychia (nail condition in which the width of the nail plate is greater than the length) (*brachys* short)
			celonychia (also called *koilonychia, spoon nail*) (*koilos* hollowed)
			chromonychia (*chroma* color)
			hapalonychia (also called *eggshell nail*) (*hapalos* soft)
			koilonychia (also called *celonychia, spoon nail*) (*koilos* hollowed)
			leukonychia (*leukos* white)
			melanonychia (*melas* black, dark)
			pachyonychia (*pachys* thick)
			schizonychia (*schizein* to split)
			scleronychia (*skleros* hard)
			solenonychia (*solen* channel)
			trachyonychia (*trachys* rough)
			CROSS REFERENCE: None

Element	From	Meaning	Examples
onym	Greek *onyma*	name	PREFIXED ROOT: *onym*: synonym (a word or term that means the same or approximately the same as another word) (*syn* with) *onymous*: anonymous (nameless; also called *innominate*, as an innominate bone, a large flat bone formed by the fusion of the ilium, ischium, and pubis) (*an* negative) heteronymous (*heteros* different) homonymous (standing in the same relation) (*homos* same) metonymy (*meta* change) TRAILING ROOT COMPOUND: myonymy (nomenclature of the muscles) (*myos* muscle) toponym (the name of a region as distinguished from an organ) (*topos* place) CROSS REFERENCE: onom
onyx			See onych-.
oo	Greek *oon*	egg, ovum	SIMPLE ROOT: ootid (a ripe ovum) PREFIXED ROOT: perioothecitis (inflammation of the tissues surrounding the ovary; also called *perioophoritis, periovaritis*) (*peri* around + *theke* sheath + *itis* inflammation) LEADING ROOT COMPOUND: ooblast (*blastos* bud, germ, sprout) oocyesis (also called *ovarian pregnancy*) (*kyesis* pregnancy) oocyst (*kystis* bladder) oocyte (the early or primitive ovum before it has developed completely) (*kytos* cell) oogamy (also called *heterogamy*) (*gamos* reproduction) oogenesis (formation and development of the ovum; also called *ovigenesis, ovogenesis*) {oogenetic, oogenic} (*genesis* origin) oogonium (the primordial cell from which an oocyte develops; pl., oogonia) (*gone* seed) ookinesis (or, ookinesia; the mitotic movements of the egg during maturation and fertilization), ookinete (*kinein* to move) oolemma (plasma membrane of the oocyte) (*lemma* sheath) oomycosis (*mykes* fungus + *osis* condition) oophagia (or, oophagy; the habitual eating of eggs; subsisting largely on eggs) (*phagein* to devour) oophor (*pherein* to bear) [not a word itself; see separate entry: oophor-] oophyte (*phyton* plant: growth) ooplasm (*plassein* to form) oosome (*soma* body) oosperm (a fertilized ovum; recently fertilized oocyte) (*sperma* seed) oosphere (also called *oosporangium*) (*sphere* ball, sphere) oosporangium, oospore (*sporos* seed + *angeion* vessel) ootheca (*theke* a case) ootype (*typos* impression, type) CROSS REFERENCE: gon[1], lecith, oophor, ov
oophor	Greek *oo* egg + *pherein* to bear	egg-bearing (ovary)	SIMPLE ROOT: oophoron (also called *ovarium*) PREFIXED ROOT: epoophoron, epoophorectomy (*epi* upon + *ektome* excision) paroophoron, paroophoritis (*para* alongside + *itis* inflammation) perioophoritis (also called *periovaritis*) (*peri* around + *itis* inflammation) perioophorosalpingitis (*peri* around + oophorosalpingitis)

Element	From	Meaning	Examples
oophor (cont'd)		[bearing eggs]	LEADING ROOT COMPOUND: *oophor*: oophoralgia (also called *ovarialgia*) (*algos* pain) oophorectomy (also called *ovariectomy*) (*ektome* excision) oophoritis (also called *ovaritis*) (*itis* inflammation) oophoroma (also called *ovarioncus*) (*oma* tumor) oophorrhagia (*rhagia* bursting forth) *oophoro*: oophorocystectomy (*kystis* sac, bladder + *ektome* excision) oophorocystosis (*kystis* sac, bladder + *osis* condition) oophorogenous (*genesis* origin) oophorohysterectomy (*hystera* uterus + *ektome* excision) oophoropathy (also called *ovariopathy*) (*pathos* disease) oophoropeliopexy (also called *oophororrhaphy*) (*pellis* pelvis + *pexis* fixation) oophoropexy (also called *ovariopexy*) (*pexis* fixation) oophoroplasty (*plassein* to form) oophororrhaphy (also called *oophoropeliopexy*) (*rhaphe* suture) oophorosalpingectomy (also called *ovariosalpingectomy*) (*salpingos* tube + *ektome* excision) oophorosalpingitis (*salpingos* tube + *itis* inflammation) oophorostomy (*stoma* mouth, opening) oophorotomy (*tomy* incision) TRAILING ROOT COMPOUND: salpingo-oophorectomy (*salpinx* tube + *ektome* excision) sclero-oophoritis (*skleros* hard + *itis* inflammation) CROSS REFERENCE: oo, ov
op	Greek *ope* sight *opsis* vision	eye, vision; also, opening	PREFIXED ROOT: *opalgia*: hemiopalgia (pain in one eye, usually accompanied by hemicrania, or migraine) (*hemi* half + *algos* pain) *opia* vision condition: ambiopia (double vision; also called *diplopia*) (*ambi* both) diplopia (also called *ambiopia*) (*diploos* double) haplopia (*haplos* single) *opic*: metopic (lit., between the eyes, forehead; therefore, of the forehead; frontal) (*meta* between) *optric(s)*: catoptrics (*kata* down) catadioptric (pertaining to refraction and reflection of light simultaneously) (*kata* down + *dia* across) *opsia* vision disorder: anopsia (defect or loss of vision) (*an* privative) teleopsia (a visual disorder in which objects perceived in space have excessive depth or close objects seem far away) (*tele* afar) tetranopsia (also called *quadrantanopia*) (*tetra* four + *an* privative + *opsia* vision condition) *opy*: polyopy (or, polyopia) (*polys* many) LEADING ROOT COMPOUND: *opsio*: opsiometer (also called *optometer*) (*metron* measure) *opso*: opsoclonus (rapid, irregular, nonrhythmic movements of the eye in horizontal and vertical directions) (*klonos* turmoil) *opto*: optochiasmic (or, opticochiasmatic) (*chiasma* a cross) optogram (*graphein* to write)

Element	From	Meaning	Examples
op (cont'd)		[eye, vision]	optokinetic (pertaining to movement of the eyes in response to the movement of objects across the visual field) (*kinein* to move)
			optomeninx (*meninx* membrane)
			optometer, optometrist, optometry (*metron* measure)
			optomyometer (*myos* muscle + *metron* measure)
			optophone (*phone* sound, voice)
			TRAILING ROOT COMPOUND:
			opia vision condition:
			amblyopia (*amblys* dull)
			anisopia (*aniso* unequal, dissimilar: *an* negative + *isos* equal)
			argamblyopia (reduction in vision as a result of not using the eye) (*argos* idle + *amblys* dull, blunted)
			chloropia (a vision defect in which all things appear green; also called *chloropsia*) (*chloros* green)
			copiopia (*kopos* fatigue)
			erythropia (or, erythropsia) (*erythros* red)
			myopia (also called *nearsightedness*) (*myein* to shut)
			nyctalopia (also called *night blindness*) (*nyx* night + *alaos* blind)
			oxyopia (also called *oxyblepsia*) (*oxys* sharp)
			presbyopia {presbyopic} (*presbys* old age)
			protanopia (color blindness in which there is a defect in the perception of red, red being the first color in the spectrum) (*protos* first + *an* privative)
			quadrantanopia (*quadrant* fourth + *an* privative)
			scieropia (a defect of vision in which objects appear in a shadow) (*skieros* shady)
			triplopia (condition in which three images of the same object are seen) (*triple* threefold)
			opsia:
			chloropsia (*chloros* green)
			chromatopsia (*chromatos* color)
			cyanopsia (*kyanos* the color blue)
			erythropsia (or, erythropia) (*erythros* red)
			palinopsia (abnormally recurring visual stimulus) (*palin* again)
			phonopsia (*phone* sound)
			photopsia (*photos* light)
			pseudopsia (visual hallucinations or false perceptions; also called *pseudoblepsia*) (*pseudes* false)
			xanthopsia (or, xanthopia), xanthocyanopsia (*xanthos* yellow + *kyanos* blue)
			opsin: rhodopsin (visual purple, a pigment in outer segment of retinal rods) (*rhodos* red)
			opsis: stereopsis (also called *stereoscopic vision*) (*stereos* solid)
			opsy:
			biopsy {bioptic} (*bios* life)
			necropsy (also called *autopsy*) (*nekros* death)
			photopsy (or, photopsia) (*photos* light)
			opter: oxyopter (*oxys* sharp, acuity)
			PREFIXED TRAILING ROOT COMPOUND:
			opia vision condition:
			ametropia (*a* privative + *metron* measure)
			amphodiplopia (*ampho* both + *diploos* double)
			anorthopia (distorted vision in which straight lines appear bent or curved; also called *strabismus*) (*an* negative + *orthos* straight)

Element	From	Meaning	Examples
op (cont'd)		[eye, vision]	antimetropia (hypermetropia in one eye and myopia in the other) (*anti* against + *metron* measure)
			emmetropia {emmetropic} (*en* in + *metron* measure)
			heterometropia (*heteros* other + *metron* measure)
			opsia vision condition:
			achromatopsia (also called *monochromatic vision*) (*a* privative + *chromatos* color)
			dyschromatopsia (*dys* abnormal + *chromatos* color)
			hemiachromatopsia (*hemi* half + *chromatos* color)
			metamorphopsia (*meta* after + *morphe* shape)
			monochromatopsia (*monos* single + *chromatos* color)
			CROSS REFERENCE: ocul, ophthalm, optic
ophthalm	Greek *ophthal-mos*	eye	SIMPLE ROOT:
			ophthalmia (severe inflammation of the eye or of the conjunctiva; also called *ophthalmitis*) {ophthalmic}
			ophthalmiac (a person affected with ophthalmia)
			PREFIXED ROOT:
			ophthalmia eye condition:
			allophthalmia (also called *heterophthalmia*) (*allos* other)
			anophthalmia (or, anophthalmos; a developmental defect characterized by absence of all tissues of the eyes) (*an* privative)
			enophthalmia (or, enophthalmos) (*en* in)
			entophthalmia (also called *endophthalmitis*) (*enton* inside)
			exophthalmia (or, exophthalmos; abnormal protrusion of the eyeball; also called *ophthalmocele*) (*exo* outside)
			heterophthalmia (also called *allophthalmia*) (*heteros* other)
			macrophthalmia (also called *megalophthalmus*) (*makros* large)
			microphthalmia (or, microphthalmos) (*mikros* small)
			panophthalmia (purulent inflammation of all parts of the eye) (*pan* all)
			parophthalmia (*para* alongside, around)
			periophthalmia {periophthalmic} (*peri* around)
			synophthalmia (also called *cyclops*) (*syn* with, together)
			ophthalmic: periophthalmic (also called *circumocular*) (*peri* around)
			ophthalmitis inflammation of the eye:
			endophthalmitis (*endon* within)
			panophthalmitis (*pan* all)
			periophthalmitis (*peri* around)
			ophthalmos:
			anophthalmos (congenital absence of the eye or eyes) (*an* privative)
			exophthalmos (or, exophthalmia; abnormal protrusion of both eyes) {exophthalmic} (*ex* out)
			megalophthalmos (or, megalophthalmus) (*megalos* large)
			monophthalmos (*monos* single)
			tetranophthalmos (a fetus having four eyes) (*tetra* four)
			ophthalmus:
			megalophthalmus (or, megalophthalmos) (*megalos* large)
			monophthalmus (also called *cyclops*) (*monos* single)
			ophthaloncus: parophthalmoncus (*para* alongside + *onkos* mass)
			LEADING ROOT COMPOUND:
			ophthalm:
			ophthalmagra (a sudden attack of eye pain) (*agra* seizure)
			ophthalmalgia (also called *ophthalmodynia*) (*algos* pain)
			ophthalmatrophia (atrophy: *a* negative + *trephein* to nourish)

Element	From	Meaning	Examples
ophthalm (cont'd)		[eye]	ophthalmectomy (the surgical removal of an eye; enucleation of the eyeball) (*ektome* excision) ophthalmencephalon (*enkephalon* brain) ophthalmiatrics (*iatrien* to heal) ophthalmitis (also called *ophthalmia*) (*itis* inflammation) ophthalmodynia (also called *ophthalmalgia*) (*odyne* pain) *ophthalmo:* ophthalmoblennorrhea (purulent inflammation of the eye or conjunctiva) (*blennos* mucus + *rhein* to flow) ophthalmocele (also called *exophthalmos*) (*kele* hernia) ophthalmocopia (*kopos* weariness) ophthalmodesmitis (*desmitis* ligament inflammation) ophthalmodynamometer (*dynamis* power + *metron* measure) ophthalmolith (also called *dacryolith*) (*lithos* stone) ophthalmologist, ophthalmology (*logos* study) ophthalmomalacia (also called *ophthalmophthisis*) (*malakos* soft) ophthalmomelanosis (*melanosis* excessive pigmentation) ophthalmometer (also called *keratometer*) (*metron* measure) ophthalmomycosis (*mykes* fungus + *osis* condition) ophthalmomyiasis (infection of the conjunctival sac by fly larvae; also called *ocular myiasis*) (*myia* a fly + *iasis* condition) ophthalmomyositis (*myositis* muscle inflammation) ophthalmopathy (also called *oculopathy*) (*pathos* disease) ophthalmophthisis (also called *ophthalmomalacia*) (*phthisis* wasting away) ophthalmoplasty (*plassein* to form) ophthalmoplegia {ophthalmoplegic} (*plege* a blow, stroke) ophthalmoptosis (also called *exophthalmos*) (*ptosis* a falling) ophthalmorrhagia (*rhagia* bursting forth) ophthalmorrhea (*rhein* to flow) ophthalmorrhexis (*rhexis* rupture) ophthalmoscope {ophthalmoscopic}, ophthalmoscopy (*skopein* to examine) ophthalmosteresis (*steresis* loss, privation) ophthalmotomy (*tomy* incision) ophthalmovascular (*vas* blood vessel) ophthalmoxerosis (also called *xerophthalmia*) (*xerosis* dryness) TRAILING ROOT COMPOUND: *ophthalmia* eye condition: adenophthalmia (*adenos* gland) cirsophthalmia (*kirsos* varix) cryptophthalmia (*kryptos* hidden) echinophthalmia (*echinos* hedgehog: spiny) hemophthalmia (*haima* blood) hydrophthalmia (also called *congenital glaucoma*) (*hydor* water) nanophthalmia (*nanos* dwarf) photophthalmia (opthalmia caused by intense light or glare) (*photos* light) psorophthalmia (*psoros* itchy) pyophthalmia (also called *pyophthalmitis*) (*pyon* pus) scirrhophthalmia (*skirrhos* hard) sclerophthalmia (*skleros* hard: sclera of the eye) xenophthalmia (ophthalmia caused by a foreign body in the eye) (*xenos* strange, foreign)

Element	From	Meaning	Examples
ophthalm (cont'd)		[eye]	xerophthalmia (condition of dry eyes; also called *ophthalmoxerosis*) (*xeros* dry) *ophthalmitis*: periophthalmitis (*peri* around + *itis* inflammation) *ophthalmology*: neuroophthalmology (*neuron* nerve + *logos* study) *ophthalmos*: hydrophthalmos (also called *congenital glaucoma*) (*hydor* water) lagophthalmos (a condition in which the eye stands open, giving a peculiar staring appearance) (*lagos* hare, rabbit) nanophthalmos (*nanos* dwarf) CROSS REFERENCE: ocul, optic
opist	Greek *opisthen* behind; at the back	back of, behind, backward	SIMPLE ROOT: opisthe, opisthion (craniometric point at middle of lower border of the foramen magnum) LEADING ROOT COMPOUND: *opis*: opisthenar (back of the hand) (*thenar* palm) *opisth*: opisthotic (located behind the ear or in the interior ear) (*otos* ear) *opisthio*: opisthiobasial (basion; base) opisthionasial (*nasus* nose) *opistho*: opisthocheilia (or, opisthochilia) (*cheilos* lip) opisthocranion (*kranion* skull) opisthogenia (also called *retrognathism*) (*genys* jaw) opisthognathism (skull abnormality marked by a receding lower jaw; also called *retrognathism*) (*gnathos* jaw + *ismos* state of) opisthomastigote (*mastix* flagellus) opisthoporeia (involuntary walking backward due to loss of motor control; also called *retropulsion*) (*poreia* to walk) opisthotonos (*tonos* tension) CROSS REFERENCE: dors, noto, palin, retro
opo, opsi	Greek *ops*	face	LEADING ROOT COMPOUND: *opo*: opocephalus (a fetal monster with the ears fused, one orbit, no mouth, and no nose) (*kephale* head) opodidymus (conjoined twins with a single body having two fused heads fused at the back with partially separated facial regions; also called *opodymus*) (*didymos* twin) *opsi*: opsialgia (acute facial paralysis) (*algos* pain) TRAILING ROOT COMPOUND: iniops (a double-faced fetal monster with the posterior face incomplete) (*inion* occiput: back of head) platyopia (broadness of the face) {platyopic} (*platys* flat, broad) CROSS REFERENCE: faci, prosop
opson, opsin	Greek *opsonein* to purchase food	opsonin	SIMPLE ROOT: opsin (the protein portion of the rhodopsin molecule) opsonin (substance in blood serum which acts upon microorganisms and other cells, facilitating phagocytosis) {opsonic} opsonization (action of opsonins to facilitate phagocytosis) PREFIXED ROOT: antiopsonin (*anti* against) LEADING ROOT COMPOUND: *opsoni*: opsonification (effect of opsonins in rendering cells or bacteria phagocytized more readily) (*facere* to make) *opsino*: opsinogen (a substance that stimulates the formation of opsonin) (*genere* to begin)

A Thesaurus of Medical Word Roots

Element	From	Meaning	Examples
opson (cont'd)		[opsonin]	*opsono*: opsonocytophagic (*kytos* cell + *phagein* to devour) opsonometry (*metron* measure) opsonophilia {opsonophilic} (*philein* to love—have an affinity for) TRAILING ROOT COMPOUND: bacteriopsonin (bacteria) hemopsonin (*haima* blood) TERM: opsonic index (a measure of the resistance of a patient to bacterial invasion) CROSS REFERENCE: None
optic	Greek *optokos*	pertaining to sight	SIMPLE ROOT: optic (also called *ocular*), optical (also called *visual*), optician, opticianry, optics PREFIXED ROOT: *optic(s)*: entoptic (*enton* within) heteroptics (false or perverted vision) (*heteros* other) microptic (*mikros* small) panoptic (*pan* all) pleoptics (*pleon* more) preoptic (*pre* before) *opto*: perioptometry (*peri* around + *metron* measure) synoptophore (*syn* with + *phorein* to bear) LEADING ROOT COMPOUND: opticochiasmatic (or, optochiasmic) (*chiasma* a cross) opticociliary (relating to the optic and the ciliary nerves) opticonasion (*nasus* nose) opticopupillary (pupil of eye) TRAILING ROOT COMPOUND: orthoptic (pertaining to or producing binocular vision), orthoptics, orthoptist (*orthos* straight) CROSS REFERENCE: ocul, op, ophthalm
or, **os**	Latin *orare* to recite, to speak *os, oris* mouth	mouth, opening; speech	SIMPLE ROOT: *or*: ora (an edge or margin; also, the plural of *os*, bone; pl., orae) orad (toward the mouth), oral, orale, orality *os*: os (pl., ora), osculum (a small aperture or minute opening) ostium (a small opening, especially one into a tubular organ; pl., ostia) ostomate (one who has an ostomy), ostomy (an artificial opening) PREFIXED ROOT: *oral*: aboral (*ab* away) adoral (*ad* to, toward) circumoral (also called *perioral*) (*circum* around) extraoral (*extra* outside) intraoral (*intra* within) paraoral (*para* alongside) peroral (see *Pharmaceutical*) (*per* through) perioral (also called *circumoral*) (*peri* around) postoral (in the posterior part of the mouth) (*post* posterior) preoral (in front of the mouth) (*pre* before) *orality*: hyperorality (a condition characterized by insertion of inappropriate objects in the mouth) (*hyper* over)

Element	From	Meaning	Examples
or (cont'd)		[mouth, opening]	*orificial*: pluriorificial (pertaining to or affecting several orifices of the body) (*plus* more)
			os: inosculate (to unite or communicate by means of small openings or anastomoses), inosculation (*in* in)
			LEADING ROOT COMPOUND:
			ora: oralogy (also called *stomatology*) (*logos* study)
			ori: orifice (the entrance or outlet of a body cavity; also called *ostium, orificium*), orificium (pl., orificia) (*facere* to make)
			oro:
			orodigitofacial (*digit* finger + face)
			orofacial (relating to the mouth and the face)
			orolingual (*lingua* tongue)
			oromandibular (*mandible* lower jaw)
			oromaxillary (*maxilla* upper jaw)
			oronasal (*nasus* nose)
			oropharynx {oropharyngeal} (*pharynx* throat)
			orotracheal (*trachea* windpipe)
			PHARMACEUTICAL: per os, p.o. (by mouth)
			CROSS REFERENCE: for, op, stom
orb	Latin *orbis* circle	circle, eye socket	SIMPLE ROOT:
			orbicular (circular, or rounded), orbiculus (pl., orbiculi)
			orbit (also called *orbita*: the bony cavity that contains the eyeball), orbita (pl., orbitae) {orbital}, orbitale
			PREFIXED ROOT:
			orbicular: semiorbicular (also called *semicircular*) (*semi* half)
			orbita: periorbita (connective tissue covering the socket of the eye) {periorbital} (*peri* around)
			orbital:
			antorbital (*ante* before)
			biorbital (pertaining to both orbits) (*bi* two)
			circumorbital (also called *periorbital*) (*circum* around)
			infraorbital (lying under or on the floor of the orbit; also called *suborbital*) (*infra* below)
			interorbital (*inter* between)
			intraorbital (*intra* within)
			periorbital (also called *circumorbital*) (*peri* around)
			postorbital (behind the orbit) (*post* posterior)
			preorbital (*pre* before)
			suborbital (also called *infraorbital*) (*sub* below)
			supraorbital (situated above the orbit) (*supra* over)
			transorbital (*trans* across, through)
			LEADING ROOT COMPOUND:
			orbi: orbitonometer, orbitonometry (*tonos* tone + *metron* measure)
			orbito:
			orbitography (*graphein* to write)
			orbitonasal (*nasus* nose)
			orbitopagus (*pagus* thing fixed)
			orbitopathy (*pathos* disease)
			orbitosphenoid (*sphen* wedge: sphenoid bone)
			orbitotomy (*tomy* incision)
			TRAILING ROOT COMPOUND:
			sphenorbital (*sphenos* wedge: sphenoid bone)
			zygomaticoorbital (*zygon* yoke: zygomatic process)
			CROSS REFERENCE: an, cycl, gyr

Element	From	Meaning	Examples
orchi	Greek *orchis*	testicle	SIMPLE ROOT: orchic (or, orchidic), orchid (the flower, because of its roots being in the shape of testicles) orchidic (concerning or related to the testes; also called *testicular*) orchis (a testicle; the testis; pl., orchises) PREFIXED ROOT: *orchia*: anorchia (or, anorchism) {anorchic, anorchid} (*an* privative) monorchia (or, monorchism) (*monos* single) *orchid*: monorchid (*monos* single) triorchid (having three testes; also, an individual with three testes) (*tri* three) *orchidium*: parorchidium (misplacement of a testis or testes) (*para* abnormal) *orchidism*: hyperorchidism (abnormally increased testicular function) (*hyper* over, beyond) hypoorchidism (defective activity of the testes) (*hypo* below) macroorchidism (abnormal enlargement of the testis) (*makros* large) microorchidism (*mikros* small) polyorchidism (or, polyorchism) (*polys* more) synorchidism (or, synorchism) (*syn* together) *orchis*: parorchis (the epididymis) (*para* alongside) polyorchis (a person with more than two testes) (*polys* more) *orchism*: anorchism (congenital absence of the testes, which may occur uni-laterally or bilaterally) (*an* privative) polyorchism (or, polyorchidism) (*polys* many) synorchism (or, synorchidism; fusion of the two testes into one mass, which may be located in the scrotum or in the abdomen) (*syn* with) triorchism (*tri* three) *orchitis*: periorchitis (also called *perididymitis*) (*peri* around + *itis* inflammation) *orchium*: epiorchium (*epi* upon) mesorchium {mesorchial} (*mesos* middle) *orchous*: anorchous (having no testes) (*an* privative) LEADING ROOT COMPOUND: *orch*: orchalgia (also called *orchiodynia*) (*algos* pain) orchitis (or, orchiditis) {orchitic} (*itis* inflammation) *orcheo*: orcheoplasty (plastic repair of the testicle) (*plassein* to form) *orchi*: orchialgia (or, orchidalgia; also called *orchiodynia*, *testalgia*) (*algos* pain) orchichorea (involuntary rising and falling movements of the testis) (*choreia* dance) orchiectomy (or, orchidectomy) (*ektome* excision) orchiepididymitis (epididymis + *itis* inflammation) orchiodynia (also called *orchialgia*) (*odyne* pain) orchioncus (*onkos* mass, tumor)

Element	From	Meaning	Examples
orchi (cont'd)		[testicle]	*orchid*: orchidalgia (or, orchialgia) (*algos* pain) orchidectomy (or, orchiectomy) (*ektome* excision) orchiditis (or, orchitis) (*itis* inflammation) orchidoncus (also called *testicular tumor*) (*onkos* mass) *orchido*: orchidometer (*metron* measure) orchidopathy (or, orchiopathy) (*pathos* disease) orchidopexy (or, orchiopexy; also called *orchidorraphy*) (*pexis* fixation) orchidoplasty (or, orchioplasty) (*plassein* to form) orchidoptosis (the descending of the testicles) (*ptein* to fall) orchidorrhaphy (also called *orchidopexy*) (*rhaphe* suture) orchidotomy (or, orchiotomy) (*tomy* incision) *orchio*: orchioblastoma (also called *yolk sac tumor*) (*blastos* germ, cell + *oma* tumor) orchiocele (scrotal hernia) (*kele* hernia) orchioneuralgia (also called *orchialgia*) (*neuron* nerve + *algos* pain) orchiopathy (also called *testopathy*) (*pathos* disease) orchiopexy (also called *orchiorrhaphy*) (*pexis* fixation) orchioplasty (or, orchidoplasty) (*plassein* to form) orchiorrhaphy (also called *orchiopexy*) (*rhaphe* suture) orchiotherapy (*therapy* treatment) orchiotomy (or, orchidotomy) (*tomy* incision) *orcho*: orchotomy (or, orchiotomy) (*tomy* incision) TRAILING ROOT COMPOUND: cryptorchidism (also called *cryptorchism, undescended testis*) (*kryptein* to hide) CROSS REFERENCE: osche, test
orex	Greek *oregein* to stretch out for *orexis* appetite	appetite	SIMPLE ROOT: orexia (the affective aspects of an act, as opposed to the cognitive aspect) {orectic} PREFIXED ROOT: *orexia*: anorexia {anorectic, anoretic} (*an* negative) dysorexia (diminished or perverted appetite) (*dys* abnormal) hyperorexia (also called *bulimia nervosa*) (*hyper* above) parorexia (also called *pica*) (*para* abnormal) *orexigenic*: anorexigenic (*an* negative + orexigenic) LEADING ROOT COMPOUND: orexigenic (*genesis* origin) TRAILING ROOT COMPOUND: bulimarexia (an eating disorder, characterized by gorging large quantities of food followed by self-induced vomiting) (*bu* cow + *limos* hunger) cynorexia (a voracious appetite, like that of a starving dog) (*kyon* dog) xenorexia (the eating of strange or unusual objects) (*xenos* foreign) CROSS REFERENCE: None
organ	Greek *organon* from *ergon* work	implement, instrument	SIMPLE ROOT: organ (a part of the body having a special function) {organic} organelle (a specialized part of a cell which performs a definite function) organicism (the theory that all symptoms are due to organic disease), organicist organism (any individual living thing)

A Thesaurus of Medical Word Roots

Element	From	Meaning	Examples
organ (cont'd)		[implement, instrument]	organon (or, organum; an organ; pl., organa) PREFIXED ROOT: *organic*: anorganic (*an* privative) homorganic (*homos* same) inorganic (*in* negative) *organism*: ectorganism (also called *ectoparasite*) (*ektos* outside) entorganism (also called *endoparasite*) (*enton* inside) microorganism (*mikros* small) LEADING ROOT COMPOUND: *organ*: organoid (*eidos* form) organonymy (*onyma* name) *organo*: organoaxial (rotation around the long axis of the organ; a type of gastric volvulus) organofaction (also called *organogenesis*) (*facere* to make) organoferric (containing iron and some organic compound) (*ferrum* iron) organogenesis (or, organogeny) {organogenic} (*genesis* origin) organography (*graphein* to write) organoleptic (*lambanein* to seize) organomegaly (also called *visceromegaly*) (*megalos* large) organonomy (*nomos* law) organopathy (*pathos* disease) organopexy (or, organopexia) (*pexis* fixation) organophilicity {organophilic} (*philein* to love—have an affinity for) organotaxis (*taxis* arrangement) organotherapy (*therapy* treatment) organotrophic (*trophein* to nourish) organotropism {organotropic} (*trepein* to turn) CROSS REFERENCE: None
oro			See or- for *orofacial, orolingual*.
orth	Greek *orthos*	straight, normal, right	See Appendix B for examples of words with this element. Others are placed with the roots to which it is attached. CROSS REFERENCE: dextr, norm, rect
osche	Greek *osche*	scrotum	SIMPLE ROOT: oscheal (also called *scrotal*) PREFIXED ROOT: synoscheos (adhesion between the penis and scrotum) (*syn* with, together) LEADING ROOT COMPOUND: *osch*: oschelephantiasis (an enlargement or elephantiasis of the scrotum) *osche*: oscheitis (*itis* inflammation) oscheoma (*oma* tumor) oscheoncus (*onkos* mass) *oscheo*: oscheocele (a scrotal swelling or tumor) (*kele* tumor) oscheohydrocele (*hydor* water + *kele* tumor) oscheolith (*lithos* stone) oscheoplasty (*plassein* to form) CROSS REFERENCE: didym, orchi, scrot, test
osculum			See or-.

Element	From	Meaning	Examples
-osis	Greek suffix	condition	See Appendix C for examples of words with this suffix. Others are listed with the roots to which it is attached. CROSS REFERENCE: None
osm[1], **odm**	Greek *osme*, *odme* smell	smelling, odors	SIMPLE ROOT: osmatic (also called *olfactory*), osmesis (the act of smelling) osmics (the science of olfaction; also called *olfactology*) osmium (OsO_4; so named because of the odor of the vapor) PREFIXED ROOT: *odmia*: anodmia (also called *anosmia*) (*an* privative) *osmatic*: anosmatic (or, anosmic) (*an* privative) macrosmatic (*makros* large) microsmatic (*mikros* small) *osmia*: anosmia (also called *anodmia*) {anosmic} (*an* privative) autosmia (awareness of the odor of one's own body) (*autos* self) cacosmia (stench; a hallucination of unpleasant odor) (*kakos* bad) dysosmia (also called *parosmia*) (*dys* abnormal) euosmia (*eu* well, good) hemianosmia (anosmia in one of the nostrils) (*hemi* half + *anosmia*) heterosmia (a condition in which odors are incorrectly interpreted; also called *allotriosmia*) (*heteros* other) hyperosmia (also called *oxyosmia*) (*hyper* over, beyond) hyposmia (*hypo* under) kakosmia (or, cacosmia) (*kakos* bad) merosmia (*meros* part) microsmia (*mikros* small) paraosmia (or, parosmia; any disorder or perversion of the sense of smell; also called *dysosmia*) (*para* abnormal) phantosmia (*phantasia* imagination) LEADING ROOT COMPOUND: *osm*: osmesthesia (the ability to perceive and distinguish odors) (*esthesia* feeling, perception) osmidrosis (a condition in which the sweat has an unusually strong odor) (*hidros* perspiration) [h of hidros elided] *osmi*: osmification (treatment with osmium) (*facere* to make) *osmio*: osmiophobic (not readily stained with osmic acid) (*phobia* fear) *osmo*: osmoceptor (also called *osmoreceptor*) (*capere* to take, hold) osmodysphoria (an intense and abnormal dislike of certain odors) (*dys* abnormal + *pherein* to bear) osmology (also called *osphresiology*) (*logos* study) osmophobia (also called *olfactophobia*) (*phobia* fear of) osmophore (*pherein* to bear) osmoreceptor (olfactory receptor) [also listed under osm[2]] TRAILING ROOT COMPOUND: allotriosmia (incorrect recognition of odors; also called *heterosmia*) (*allotrios* strange, foreign) oxyosmia (also called *hyperosmia*) (*oxys* sharp) presbyosmia (the diminution or loss of the sense of smell associated with aging) (*presbys* old) CROSS REFERENCE: olfact, osphr

Element	From	Meaning	Examples
osm²	Greek *othein* to push	impulse; osmosis	SIMPLE ROOT: osmolality, osmolar (or, osmotic), osmolarity, osmole (the standard unit of osmotic pressure), osmose, osmosis {osmotic}, osmosity PREFIXED ROOT: *osmolality*: hyperosmolality (*hyper* above) hypo-osmolality (*hypo* under) *osmolarity*: hyperosmolarity (*hyper* above) hypo-osmolarity (*hypo* under) *osmosis*: endosmosis {endosmotic} (*endon* within) exosmosis (*exo* outside) hyposmosis (*hypo* under) *osmotic*: anisosmotic (*aniso* unequal: *an* negative + *isos* equal) hyperosmotic (*hyper* over, beyond) hyposmotic (*hypo* under) isosmotic (or, isoosmotic; having the same osmotic pressure) {is-osmoticity} (*isos* equal) LEADING ROOT COMPOUND: *osmo*: osmogen (*genesis* origin) osmology (*logos* study) osmolute (an osmotically active solute) (osmosis + solute) osmometer (*metron* measure) osmophil (or, osmophilic) (*philein* to love) osmoreceptor [also listed under osm¹] osmoregulation {osmoregulatory} osmotaxis (*tassein* to arrange) osmotherapy (*therapy* treatment) *osmoso*: osmosology (*logos* study) TRAILING ROOT COMPOUND: biosmosis (osmosis through a living membrane) (*bios* life) chemiosmosis (or, chemosmosis) {chemiosmotic} (chemical) poikilosmosis {poikilosmotic} (*poikilos* varied) zoosmosis (*zoos* living) CROSS REFERENCE: puls
osphr	Greek *osphresis*	smell, odor	SIMPLE ROOT: osphresis (also called *olfaction*) {osphretic; also called *olfactory*} PREFIXED ROOT: anosphresia (also called *anosmia*) (*an* privative) hyperosphresia (also called *hyperosmia*) (*hyper* over, beyond) hyposphresia (also called *hyposmia*) (*hypo* under) parosphresia (also called *dysosmia*) (*para* abnormal) LEADING ROOT COMPOUND: osphresiology (also called *osmology*) {osphresiologic} (*logos* study) osphresiophilia (an unusual interest in odors) (*philein* to love) osphresiophobia (also called *olfactophobia*) (*phobos* fear) TRAILING ROOT COMPOUND: oxyosphresia (abnormal acuity of the sense of smell) {oxyophretic} (*oxys* sharp) Note: There are an almost infinite number of odors, scents, smells. CROSS REFERENCE: olfact, osm¹

Element	From	Meaning	Examples
oss	Latin *osseus*	bone	SIMPLE ROOT: os (bone; pl., ossa) {osseous} ossature (the arrangement of bones in the body or in a part) ossein (the collagen of bone) ossicle (a small bone) {ossicular} ossiculum (ossicle; pl., ossicula) {ossicular} PREFIXED ROOT: *osseal*: interosseal (*inter* between) *osseous*: endosseous (*endon* within) extraosseous (*extra* outside) interosseous (*inter* between) intraosseous (also called *intraosteal*) (*intra* within) perosseous (*per* through) *osseus*: interosseus (pl., interossi) (*inter* between) *ossification* the making of bone: coossification (*co* with) deossification (*de* reversal) *ossify*: coossify (*co* with + ossify) LEADING ROOT COMPOUND: *osseo*: osseocartilaginous (cartilage) osseofibrous (*fibra* fiber) osseomucin, osseomucoid (mucus + *eidos* form) *ossi*: ossiferous (*ferre* to bear) ossific, ossification, ossify (*facere* to make) ossifluence (osteolysis or softening of the bone) (*fluere* to flow) ossiform (*forma* shape) ossiphone (*phone* sound) *ossicul*: ossiculectomy (*ektome* excision) *ossiculo*: ossiculotomy (*tomy* incision) TRAILING ROOT COMPOUND: fibro-osseous (*fibra* fiber) chondro-osseous (also called *osteochondrol*) (*chondros* cartilage) gingivo-osseous (*gingivae* gums) CROSS REFERENCE: ost(e)
ost(e)	Greek *osteon*	bone	SIMPLE ROOT: osteal (bony, osseous), ostein (or, osteine; also called *collagen*), osteon (or, osteone) PREFIXED ROOT: *ost*: periost (or, periosteum) (*peri* around) *osteal* pertaining to bone: ectosteal (*ektos* outside) endosteal (*endon* within) intraosteal (also called *intraosseous*) (*intra* within) parosteal (*para* alongside) periosteal (*peri* around) *ostectomy*: exostectomy (*exo* outside + *ektome* excision) *osteitis* inflammation of bone: endosteitis (or, endostitis) (*endon* within) panosteitis (*pan* all) parosteitis (*para* alongside) *osteo*: anosteoplasia (*an* privative + *plassein* to form)

Element	From	Meaning	Examples
ost(e) (cont'd)		[bone]	dysosteogenesis (*dys* abnormal + *genesis* production)
			hetero-osteoplasty (*heteros* other + *plassein* to mold, form)
			homeo-osteoplasty (*homeo* same, similar + *plassein* to mold, form)
			parosteosis (ossification of the tissues outside of the periosteum) (*para* alongside + *osis* condition)
			preosteoblast (*pre* before + *blastos* germ)
			synosteology (the sum of knowledge regarding the joints and articulations; also called *arthrology*) (*syn* with + *logos* study)
			synosteotomy (*syn* with + *tomy* incision)
			osteoma bone tumor:
			endosteoma (*endon* within)
			periosteoma (*peri* around
			osteosis bone condition:
			parosteosis (or, parostosis) (*para* abnormal)
			synosteosis (or, synostosis) (*syn* with)
			osteum:
			endosteum (*endon* within)
			periosteum (*peri* around) [see separate entry: periost-]
			ostitis inflammation of bone:
			parostitis (*para* beside)
			periostitis (*peri* around)
			polyperiostitis (*polys* many + periostitis)
			ostosis bone condition:
			anostosis (*an* privative)
			dysostosis (defective bone formation) (*dys* abnormal)
			ectostosis {exostotic} (*ektos* outside)
			enostosis (also called *entostosis*) (*en* in)
			endostosis (the formation of bone within cartilage) (*endon* within)
			entostosis (also called *enostosis*) (*entos* within)
			exostosis (also called *hyperostosis*; pl., exostoses) (*exo* outside)
			hyperostosis (hypertrophy of bone) {hyperostotic} (*hyper* above)
			hypostosis (deficient development of bone) (*hypo* under)
			inostosis (the re-formation of bony tissue to replace bone that has been destroyed) (uncertain meaning of prefix in-)
			parostosis {parostotic} (*para* beside, outside)
			synostosis {synostotic, or synosteotic} (*syn* with)
			ostotic pertaining to a bone condition:
			monostotic (*monos* single)
			polyostotic (*polys* many)
			LEADING ROOT COMPOUND:
			ost:
			ostalgia (or, ostealgia) (*algos* pain)
			ostarthritis (or, osteoarthritis) (*athron* joint + *itis* inflammation)
			ostectomy (or, osteoectomy) (*ektome* excision)
			ostembryon (also called *lithopedion*) (*embryon* fetus)
			ostemia (congestion of blood in the bone) (*emia* blood condition)
			ostempyesis (*empyesis* suppuration)
			osthexia (or, osthexy; excessive ossification, especially in abnormal places) (*hexia* condition)
			oste:
			ostealgia (or, ostalgia; also called *osteodynia*) (*algos* pain)
			osteanabrosis (*anabrosis* eating up)
			osteanagenesis (or, osteoanagenesis; regeneration of bone; also called *osteanaphysis*) (*anagenesis* regeneration)

Element	From	Meaning	Examples
ost(e) (cont'd)		[bone]	osteanaphysis (regeneration of bone; also called *osteoanagenesis*) (*anaphysis* a growing again)
			ostearthritis (*arthron* joint + *itis* inflammation)
			osteectopia (displacement of a bone) (*ektopia* displaced)
			osteitis {osteitic} (*itis* inflammation)
			ostempyesis (*empyesis* suppuration: *em* in + *pyon* pus)
			osteodynia (also called *ostealgia*) (*odyne* pain)
			osteoid (*eidos* form)
			osteoma, osteomatoid (*oma* tumor + *eidos* form)
			osteoncus (*onkos* mass, swelling)
			osteosis (*osis* condition)
			osteo:
			osteoacusis (bone conduction of sound) (*akouein* to hear)
			osteoanagenesis (or, osteanagenesis; also called *osteanaphysis*) (*anagenesis* regeneration: *ana* again + *genesis* beginning)
			osteoanesthesia (*an* negative + *esthesia* feeling)
			osteoaneurysm (aneurysm in a bone)
			osteoarthritis (*arthron* joint + *itis* inflammation)
			osteoarticular (*articular* pertaining to joints)
			osteoblast {osteoblastic}, osteoblastoma (*blastos* bud + *oma* tumor)
			osteocachexia (*cachexia* disorder: *kakos* bad + *hexis* habit)
			osteocalcin (calcium)
			osteocampsia (or, osteocampsis) (*kamptein* to bend)
			osteocartilaginous (also called *osseocartilaginous, osteochondrous*) (cartilage)
			osteochondrondritis (*chondros* cartilage + *itis* inflammation)
			osteoclasia (or, osteoclasis) (*klasis* a breaking)
			osteoclast (also called *osteophage*) {osteoclastic}, osteoclasty (*klastos* broken)
			osteoclastoma (also called *giant cell tumor of bone*) (*oma* tumor)
			osteocomma (*komma* fragment)
			osteocope {osteocopic} (*kopos* pain)
			osteocranium (*kranion* skull)
			osteocystoma (a bone cyst) (*kystis* sac + *oma* tumor)
			osteocyte (*kytos* cell)
			osteodentin (*dens* tooth)
			osteodermia (osteoma cutis) (*dermia* skin condition)
			osteodermatopoikilosis (*dermatos* skin + *poikilos* dappled + *osis* condition)
			osteodesmosis (*desmos* band, tendon + *osis* condition)
			osteodiastasis (*diastasis* a separation)
			osteodysplasty (*dysplasty* badly formed)
			osteodystrophia (or, osteodystrophy) (*dystrophia* badly nourished)
			osteoectasia (bowing of the bones) (*ectasia* dilatation)
			osteoectomy (*ektome* excision)
			osteoepiphysis (*epiphysis* an outgrowth or excrescence)
			osteofibroma (*fibroma* fibrous tumor)
			osteofibrosis (*fibrosis* fibrous condition)
			osteogen, osteogenesis {osteogenetic, osteogenous; also called *osteoplastic*} (*genesis* origin)
			osteography (*graphein* to write)
			osteohalisteresis (a condition of soft bone caused by a loss or deficiency of mineral elements) (*halos* salt + *steresis* deprivation)
			osteohypertrophy (*hyper* above + *trophein* to nourish)

Element	From	Meaning	Examples
ost(e) (cont'd)		[bone]	osteolipochondroma (*lipos* fat + *chondros* cartilage + *oma* tumor)
			osteology (*logos* study)
			osteolysis {osteolytic} (*lysis* dissolution)
			osteomalacia {osteomalacic} (*malakos* soft)
			osteomere (*meros* part)
			osteometry (*metron* measure)
			osteomiosis (*miosis* degeneration)
			osteomyelitis (*myelos* marrow + *itis* inflammation)
			osteomyelodysplasia (*myelos* marrow + dysplasia: *dys* abnormal + *plassein* to form)
			osteonecrosis (*nekrosis* death)
			osteopath (also called *osteopathic physician*), osteopathology, osteopathy (*pathos* disease + *logos* study)
			osteopenia (*penia* deficiency)
			osteoperiostitis (periosteum + *itis* inflammation)
			osteopetrosis {osteopetrotic} (*petra* stone + *osis* condition)
			osteophage (also called *osteoclast*) (*phagein* to eat, consume)
			osteophlebitis (*phlebos* vein + *itis* inflammation)
			osteophony (bone conduction of sound) (*phone* sound)
			osteophyma (also called *osteophyte*) (*phyma* tumor, growth)
			osteophyte (also called *osteophyma*) (*phyton* plant: growth)
			osteoplasty {osteoplastic; also called *osteogenic*} (*plassein* to form)
			osteopoikilosis (*poikilosis* dappled condition)
			osteoporosis {osteoporotic} (*porosis* porous condition)
			osteorrhagia (hemorrhage from bone) (*rhagia* bursting forth)
			osteorrhaphy (also called *osteosuture*) (*rhaphe* suture)
			osteosarcoma (*sarkos* flesh + *oma* tumor)
			osteosclerosis {osteosclerotic} (*sklerosis* hardening)
			osteoseptum (*septum* a dividing wall)
			osteospongioma (*spongos* sponge + *oma* tumor)
			osteosteatoma (*steatos* suet, fat + *oma* tumor)
			osteosuture (also called *osteorrhaphy*) (*suere* to sew)
			osteosynthesis (*synthesis* a putting together)
			osteothrombosis (*thrombosis* clotting condition)
			osteotome, osteotomy (*tomy* incision)
			osteotribe (or, osteotrite) (*tribein* to grind, rub)
			osteotrophy (*trophein* to nourish)
			osteotympanic (also called *otocranial*) (*tympanon* eardrum)
			TRAILING ROOT COMPOUND:
			osteitis: arthrosteitis (*arthron* joint + *itis* inflammation)
			osteoma bone tumor:
			chondrosteoma (*chondros* cartilage)
			fibro-osteoma (also called *ossifying fibroma*) (fiber)
			osteon: malacosteon (*malakos* soft)
			ostosis bone condition:
			acrodysostosis (*akron* extremity + *dys* abnormal)
			craniostosis (*kranion* the upper part of head: skull)
			dermostosis (ossification of the dermia, or skin) (*derma* skin)
			diclidostosis (*diklis* double door: valve)
			melorheostosis (*melos* limb + *rhein* to flow)
			necrosteosis (or, necrosteon) (*nekros* death)
			pyknodysostosis (*pyknos* thick + *dys* abnormal)
			rheostosis (a hypertrophying and condensing osteitis that tends to run in longitudinal streaks or columns) (*rheos* flow)

Element	From	Meaning	Examples
ost(e) (cont'd)		[bone]	sarcostosis (*sarkos* flesh)
			tenostosis (or, tenonostosis) (*tenon* sinew, tendon)
			osteomalacia: pseudoosteomalacia (*pseudes* false)
			ostotic: merostotic (pertaining to or affecting only a part of a bone) (*meros* part)
			CROSS REFERENCE: oss
ot	Greek *ous, otos*	ear	SIMPLE ROOT: otic (pertaining to the ear; aural)
			PREFIXED ROOT:
			otia:
			anotia (congenital absence of one or both external ears) (*an* privative)
			macrotia (abnormal enlargement of the pinna of the ear) (*makros* large) [pinna: the auricle, the external ear]
			microtia (*mikros* small)
			polyotia (the condition of having more than two ears) (*polys* many)
			synotia (*syn* with, together)
			otic:
			binotic (pertaining to both ears; also called *binaural*) (*bin* two)
			entotic (situated or arising within the ear) (*entos* inside)
			epiotic (situated on or above the ear) (*epi* upon)
			monotic (having only a single ear) (*monos* single)
			parotic (situated or occurring near the ear) (*para* beside)
			periotic (*peri* around)
			prootic (in front of the ear) (*pro* before)
			otid: parotid (*para* alongside) [see separate entry: parotid-]
			otitis: panotitis (*pan* all + *itis* inflammation)
			otus:
			anotus (an earless fetus) (*an* privative)
			tetraotus (or, tetrotus) (*tetra* four)
			triotus (*tri* three)
			LEADING ROOT COMPOUND:
			ot:
			otalgia (also called *otodynia*) {otalgic} (*algos* pain)
			otitis {otitic} (*itis* inflammation)
			otodynia (also called *otalgia*) (*odyne* pain)
			otosis (*osis* condition)
			otosteal (*osteon* bone)
			oto:
			otoacoustic (*akouein* to hear)
			otoantritis (*antrum* hollow + *itis* inflammation)
			otocephaly (*kephale* head)
			otocerebritis (also called *otoencephalitis*) (*cerebrum* brain + *itis* inflammation)
			otocyst (*kystis* sac)
			otoencephalitis (*enkephalon* brain + *itis* inflammation)
			otoganglion (also called *otic ganglion*) (*ganglion* knot)
			otogenic (or, otogenous) (*genesis* origin)
			otography (a description of the ear) (*graphein* to write)
			otolaryngology (larynx + *logos* study)
			otolite (or, otolith; also called *statoconium*) {otolithic} (*lithos* stone)
			otology {otologic} (*logos* study)
			otomastoiditis (mastoid + *itis* inflammation)
			otomyasthenia (*myasthenia* muscle weakness)
			otomycosis (*mykes* fungus + *osis* condition)

Element	From	Meaning	Examples
ot (cont'd)		[ear]	otoneuralgia (*neuron* nerve + *algos* pain)
			otopalatodigital (palate + *digitus* finger)
			otopathy (*pathos* disease)
			otopharyngeal (*pharynx* throat)
			otoplasty (*plassein* to form)
			otorhinology (*rhinos* nose + *logos* study)
			otorrhagia (*rhagia* bursting forth)
			otorhinolaryngology (*rhinos* nose + larynx + *logos* study)
			otorrhea (*rhein* to flow)
			otosalpinx (*salpinx* trumpet, tube)
			otosclerosis {otosclerotic} (*sklerosis* a hardening)
			otoscope {otoscopy} (*skopein* to examine)
			ototomy (*tomy* incision)
			ototoxic, ototoxicity (*toxikon* poison)
			TRAILING ROOT COMPOUND:
			otia:
			cryptotia (*kryptos* hidden)
			melotia (*melon* cheek)
			pachyotia (*pachys* thick)
			pleonotia (*pleon* more)
			otic: opisthotic (*opisthein* behind)
			otitis inflammation of ear:
			aerotitis (also called *barotitis*) (*aer* air)
			barotitis (also called *aerotitis*) (*baros* weight)
			parotitis (the parotid gland)
			otology: neurootology (or, neurotology; a medical specialty that combines neurology and otology, dealing especially with portions of the nervous system of the ear) (*neuron* nerve + *logos* study)
			CROSS REFERENCE: aur, parotid
oulo, ul	Greek *oulon*	gums	PREFIXED ROOT:
			epulis (gumboil; any growth on the gingiva; pl. epulides)
			epulofibroma (a fibroma of the gingiva) (*epi* upon + fibroma)
			epuloid (*epi* upon + *eidos* form, resembling)
			parulis (also called *gumboil, gingival abscess*) (*para* beside)
			LEADING ROOT COMPOUND:
			oul:
			oulectomy (also called *ulectomy, gingivectomy*) (*ektome* excision)
			oulitis (also called *gingivitis*) (*itis* inflammation)
			ul:
			ulaganactesis (itching of the gingiva) (*aganaktesis* irritation)
			ulalgia (*algos* pain)
			ulatrophia (shrinkage of the gums; gum recession) (*a* negative + *trephein* to nourish) [see atroph-]
			ulectomy (removal of gum tissue) (*ektome* excision)
			ulemorrhagia (*hemo* blood + *rhagia* bursting forth) [h of hemo elided]
			ulitis (also called *gingivitis*) (*itis* inflammation)
			ulo:
			ulocarcinoma (*karkinos* cancer + *oma* tumor)
			uloglossitis (*glossa* tongue + *itis* inflammation)
			ulorrhagia (discharge of blood from the gums) (*rhagia* bursting forth)
			ulorrhea (an oozing of blood from the gingivae) (*rhein* to flow)
			ulotomy (*tomy* incision) [another *ulotomy* is listed under ule-]
			ulotripsis (revitalizing of the gingivae by massage) (*tribein* to rub)
			CROSS REFERENCE: gingiv

Element	From	Meaning	Examples
ov	Latin *ovum*	egg, ovum	SIMPLE ROOT:
			oval, ovarium (pl., ovaria), ovary (or, ovarium; one of two glands that produce the reproductive cell, the ovum, and two hormones)
			ovulation {ovulatory}, ovule {ovular}, ovum (pl., ova)
			PREFIXED ROOT:
			ovarial: transovarial (*trans* across)
			ovarian:
			intraovarian (*intra* within)
			mesovarian (*mesos* middle)
			paraovarian (or, parovarian) (*para* alongside)
			ovarianism:
			anovarianism (or, anovarism) (*an* privative)
			hyperovarianism (also called *precocious puberty*) (*hyper* over)
			hypoovarianism (or, hypovarianism) (*hypo* under)
			ovaritomy: parovariotomy (*para* alongside + *tomy* incision)
			ovarism:
			anovarism (absence of the ovaries) (*an* privative)
			hyperovarism (*hyper* above, beyond)
			hypovarianism (*hypo* below)
			ovaritis inflammation of the ovaries:
			parovaritis (*para* beside)
			periovaritis (also called *perioophoritis*) (*peri* around)
			ovarium:
			mesovarium (pl., mesovaria) (*mesos* middle)
			parovarium (also called *epoöphoron*) (*para* alongside)
			ovia: synovia [see separate entry: synov-]
			ovular:
			anovular (also called *anovulatory*) (*an* privative)
			biovular (or, binovular; also called *diovular*) (*bi* two)
			binovular (or, biovular, diovular) (*bin* two)
			diovular (also called *biovular*) (*di* two)
			extraovular (*extra* outside)
			hetero-ovular (*heteros* other)
			intraovular (*intra* within)
			monovular (also called *uniovular*) (*monos* one, single)
			periovular (*peri* around)
			polyovular {polyovulatory} (*polys* many)
			uniovular (or, unioval; arising from one ovum: said of certain twin pregnancies; also called *monovular*) (*uni* one)
			ovulation:
			anovulation (absence of ovulation) (*an* privative)
			polyovulation (*polys* many)
			superovulation (*super* above)
			ovulatory:
			anovulatory (also called *anovular*) (*an* privative)
			antiovulatory (*anti* against)
			LEADING ROOT COMPOUND:
			ovar: ovaritis (*itis* inflammation)
			ovari:
			ovarialgia (also called *oophoralgia*) (*algos* pain)
			ovariectomy (also called *oophorectomy*) (*ektome* excision)
			ovarioncus (also called *oophoroma*) (*onkos* mass)
			ovario:
			ovariocele (*kele* hernia)

Element	From	Meaning	Examples
ov (cont'd)		[egg]	ovariocentesis (*kentesis* puncture)
			ovariocyesis (also called *ovarian pregnancy*) (*kyesis* pregnancy)
			ovariodysneuria (*dys* bad + *neuria* nerve condition)
			ovariogenic (*genesis* origin)
			ovariolytic (*lysis* dissolution)
			ovariopathy (also called *oophoropathy*) (*pathos* disease)
			ovariopexy (also called *oophoropexy*) (*pexis* fixation)
			ovariorrhexis (*rhexis* rupture)
			ovariosalpingectomy (*salpingos* tube + *ektome* excision)
			ovariosalpingitis (*salpingos* tube + *itis* inflammation)
			ovariosteresis (also called *ovariectomy*) (*steresis* privation, loss)
			ovariostomy (*stoma* mouth, opening)
			ovariotestis (also called *ovotestis*) (*testis* testicle)
			ovariotomy (*tomy* incision)
			ovi:
			ovicidal (*caedere* to kill*)*
			oviduct {oviducal, oviductal} (*ducere* to lead)
			oviferous (also called *ovigerous*) (*ferre* to bear)
			oviform (also called *ovoid*) (*forma* shape)
			ovigenesis (also called *oogenesis*) (*genere* to produce)
			ovigerous (also called *oviferous*) (*gerere* to bear)
			oviparous (producing eggs which hatch without further attention from the bearer; opposed to *ovoviviparous*) (*parere* to bear)
			oviposition, ovipositor (*position* place)
			ovisac (*sac* sack, pouch)
			ovo:
			ovocyte (also called *oocyte*) (*kytos* cell)
			ovoflavin (riboflavin found in eggs) (*flavus* yellow)
			ovogenesis (also called *oogenesis*) (*genesis* origin)
			ovoglobulin (globulin in the white of an egg)
			ovolytic (*lyein* to dissolve)
			ovoplasm (*plassein* to form)
			ovotestis (also called *ovariotestis*) (*testis* testicle)
			ovoviviparous (*vivere* to live + *parere* to bear)
			ovulo: ovulogenous (*genere* to produce)
			TRAILING ROOT COMPOUND:
			ovari: tuboovariectomy (also called *salpingo-oophorectomy*)
			ovarian:
			lactovarian (also called *ovolactarian*; a vegetarian whose diet includes dairy products and eggs) (*lactis* milk)
			pyo-ovarian (presence of purulent material in the ovary; an ovarian abscess) (*pyon* pus)
			tubo-ovarian (relating to the uterine tube and the ovary) (*tubus* tube)
			ovarium: hydrovarium (a collection of serous fluid in an ovary) (*hydor* water)
			ovaritis: tubo-ovaritis (*tubus* tube + *itis* inflammation)
			CROSS REFERENCE: lecith, oo, oophor
ox	Greek *oxnein* to sharpen; *oxys* sour, sharp, keen	sharp, quick, sour the presence of oxygen in a compound	SIMPLE ROOT:
			oxalate (a salt of oxalic acid), oxalism
			oxidant, oxidation, oxide
			oxidize (to combine or cause an element or radical to combine with oxygen or to lose electrons), oxime
			oxonium (containing tetravalent basic oxygen)
			oxyntic (acid-forming, as the parietal cells of gastric glands)

Element	From	Meaning	Examples
ox (cont'd)		[sharp]	PREFIXED ROOT:

oxaluria: hyperoxaluria (*hyper* over + *uria* urine condition)

oxemia oxygenous blood condition:

anoxemia (also called *hypoxemia*) (*an* privative)

hyperoxemia (*hyper* over)

hypoxemia (also called *anoxemia*) (*hypo* under)

oxia:

anoxia (*an* privative)

hyperoxia {hyperoxic} (*hyper* over)

hypoxia {hypoxic} (*hypo* under)

normoxia (*norma* normal)

oxidant: antioxidant (*anti* against)

oxidation:

antioxidation (*anti* against)

autoxidation (*autos* self)

deoxidation (*de* reversal)

hyperoxidation (*hyper* above)

suboxidation (*sub* under)

oxidize: deoxidize (*de* reversal)

oxidosis: hypoxidosis (*hypo* under + *osis* condition)

oxide:

suboxide (*sub* below)

superoxide (*super* over)

monoxide (an oxide with one atom of oxygen in each molecule) (*monos* one, single)

peroxide (*per* through)

suboxide (also called *protoxide*) (*sub* under)

oxygen:

antioxygen (or, antioxidant) (*anti* against)

preoxygenation (*pre* before)

oxysm:

interparoxysmal (*inter* between + paroxysm)

paroxysm (a sudden attack, or intensification, of the symptoms of a disease) {paroxysmal} (*para* alongside)

LEADING ROOT COMPOUND:

oxal (from *oxalate*):

oxalemia (*emia* blood condition)

oxalosis (*osis* condition)

oxaluria (*uria* urine condition)

oxi: oximeter, oximetry (determination of the oxygen saturation of arterial blood using an oximeter) (*metron* measure)

oxid: oxidosis (also called *acidosis*) (*osis* condition)

oxy:

oxyacoia (or, oxyakoia; also called *hyperacusis*) (*akouein* to hear)

oxyaphia (also called *hyperaphia*) (*haphe* touch) [h of haphe elided]

oxyblepsia (also called *oxyopia*) (*blepsis* vision)

oxycephalia (or, oxycephaly) {oxycephalic} (*kephale* head)

oxychromatic (staining with acid dyes) (*chroma* color)

oxycinesia (also called *kinesialgia*) (*kinein* to move)

oxygen, oxygenate, oxygenator (*genere* to produce)

oxygeusia (unusual acuteness of the sense of taste; also called *hypergeusia*) (*geusis* taste)

oxyopia (acuteness of vision; also called *oxyblepsia*) (*opia* vision condition)

Element	From	Meaning	Examples
ox (cont'd)		[sharp]	oxyopter (*opter* observer)
			oxyosmia (also called *hyperosmia*) (*osme* smell)
			oxyphilic (stainable with an acid dye; also called *acidophilic*) (*philein* to love—have an affinity for)
			oxyphonia (a sharp quality to the voice) (*phone* sound)
			oxyplasm (*plassein* to form)
			oxyrhine (*rhis* nose)
			oxytocia {oxytocic} (rapid labor) (*tokos* childbirth)
			CROSS REFERENCE: None
oz	Greek *ozein* to smell	stench	SIMPLE ROOT:
			ozena (a fetid polypus in the nose) {ozenous}
			ozonator, ozone, ozonide, ozonize (to convert into ozone, as oxygen), ozonizer
			LEADING ROOT COMPOUND:
			ozo:
			ozochrotia (strong odor of the skin; also called *bromidrosis*) (*chroa* skin)
			ozokerite (or, ozocerite) (*keros* wax)
			ozostomia (also called *halitosis*, *bad breath*) (*stoma* mouth)
			ozono:
			ozonolysis (*lysis* dissolution)
			ozonometer (*metron* measure)
			ozonoscope (*skopein* to examine)
			CROSS REFERENCE: brom

Element	From	Meaning	Examples
pachy(n)	Greek *pachys* thick, clotted	thick	SIMPLE ROOT: pachynsis {pachyntic} See Appendix B for examples of words beginning with this combining form. Others are listed with the roots to which it is attached. CROSS REFERENCE: pykn
pact, pag	Latin *pangere*	to strike, fix, attach	PREFIXED ROOT: *pact*: compaction (packing together as in twin births when both fetuses engage in the pelvis at the same time) (*com* with, together) disimpaction (*dis* reversal + impaction) impact (a sudden and forcible collision) impacted (pressed tightly together; wedged in: said especially of a tooth unable to erupt properly because of its abnormal position, lack of space, etc.), impaction (*in* in) *pagat*: propagate (to reproduce; to generate, propagation (reproduction) {propagative} (*pro* before) *pages*: compages (a joining together or that which is joined together) (*com* with, together) *pagus*: diplopagus (a double fetal monster in which the component parts are equal to and the symmetrical equivalents of one another) (*diploos* two-fold) ectopagus (conjoined twins in which the bodies are joined laterally) (*ektos* outside) hemipagus (*hemi* half) heteropagus [a twin fetal monster in which one component (the parasite) is much smaller than and dependent on the other (the autosite)] (*heteros* other) TRAILING ROOT COMPOUND: cephalopagus (also called *craniopagus*) (*kephale* head) craniopagus (also called *cephalopagus*) (*kranion* top of head) gastropagus (*gaster* stomach, abdomen) iliopagus (symmetrical conjoined twins united in the iliac region) (*ilium*) iniopagus (also called *iniodymus*) (*inion* occiput: back of head) ischiopagus (*ischion* hip joint) lecanopagus (also called *ischiodidymus*) (*lekane* basin) metopagus (or, metopopagus) (*metopon* forehead) omphalopagus (*omphalos* navel) orbitopagus (*orbita* eyeball) palatopagus (*palatum* palate—roof of mouth) prosopopagus (*prosopon* face) pygopagus (*pyge* rump) rachiopagus (*rhachis* spine) somatopagus (*somatos* body) sphenopagus (*sphenos* wedge: base of skull) sternopagus (also called *thoracopagus*) (*sternum* breastbone) thoracopagus (also called *thoracodidymus*) (*thorax* chest) xiphopagus (*xiphos* sword; xiphoid process) CROSS REFERENCE: cuss, fix, pex

Element	From	Meaning	Examples
palat	Latin *palatum*	palate: roof of mouth	SIMPLE ROOT: palate (or, palatum; the partition separating the nasal and oral cavities; pl., palati) {palatal, palatine} PREFIXED ROOT: postpalatine (*post* posterior) prepalatal (*pre* before) transpalatal (*trans* through) LEADING ROOT COMPOUND: *palat*: palatitis (*itis* inflammation) *palato*: palatoglossal (*glossa* tongue) palatognathous (*gnathos* jaw) palatogram, palatograph (*graphein* to write) palatomaxillary (*maxilla* upper jaw) palatomyograph (*myos* muscle + *graphein* to write) palatonasal (also called *nasopalatine*) (*nasus* nose) palatopagus (symmetrical twins joined at the palate) (*pagus* fixed) palatopharyngeal (*pharynx* the throat) palatopharyngoplasty (*pharynx* the throat + *plassein* to form) palatopharyngorrhaphy (surgical repair of defects in the uvulam soft palate, and pharynx; also called *staphylopharyngorrhaphy*) (*pharynx* the throat+ *rhaphe* suture) palatoplasty (*plassein* to form) palatoplegia (*plessein* to strike; paralysis) palatorrhaphy (also called *uranorrhaphy*) (*rhaphe* suture) palatoschisis (also called *cleft palate*) (*schisis* fissure) TRAILING ROOT COMPOUND: glossopalatine (also called *palatoglossal*) (*glossa* tongue) labiopalatine (*labium* lip) nasopalatine (also called *palatonasal*) (*nasus* nose) pterygopalatine (pertaining to the pterygoid process and the palatine bone) (*pterygion* wing) sphenopalatine (*sphenos* wedge: sphenoid bones) CROSS REFERENCE: uran
palin	Greek *palin*	backward, again	SIMPLE ROOT: palinal (moved or moving backward) PREFIXED ROOT: propalinal (back and forth; denoting a forward and backward movement) (*pro* before) See Appendix B for examples of words with this combining form. Others are listed with the roots to which it is attached. CROSS REFERENCE: opist, re-, retro-
palp	Latin *palpare* to touch	stroke, touch	SIMPLE ROOT: palpable (perceptible, especially by touch) palpate (to examine by touch; to feel), palpation palpitation (forcible or irregular pulsation of the heart) PREFIXED ROOT: impalpable (*in* negative) LEADING ROOT COMPOUND: palpatometry (measurement of the amount of pressure that can be borne without causing pain) (*metron* measure) palpatopercussion (palpation combined with percussion) TRAILING ROOT COMPOUND: galvanopalpation (testing of nerves of the skin by a galvanic current) sphygmopalpation (*sphygmos* pulse) thermopalpation (*therme* heat) CROSS REFERENCE: crot, hapt, ict, sphygmo

Element	From	Meaning	Examples
palpebr	Latin *palpebra*	eyelid	SIMPLE ROOT: palpebra (pl., palpebrae) {palpebral} palpebrate (as a verb, to wink; as an adjective, having eyelids) PREFIXED ROOT: interpalpebral (*inter* between) subpalpebral (*sub* under) LEADING ROOT COMPOUND: palpebritis (inflammation of the eyelid; also called *blepharitis*) (*itis* inflammation) TRAILING ROOT COMPOUND: auriculopalpetral (*auris* ear) CROSS REFERENCE: blephar, cili
pan-	Greek *pantos* all, every, universal	all, every	PREFIXED ROOT: diapason (lit., through all the pitches of sound; a tuning fork: used in the diagnosis of certain ear ailments) (*dia* across) See Appendix B for examples of words with this prefix. Others are placed with the roots to which it is attached. CROSS REFERENCE: hol
pancrea	Greek *pan* all + *kreas* flesh	pancreas	SIMPLE ROOT: pancreas (a long, elongated racemose gland behind the stomach; pl., pancreata) {pancreatic} PREFIXED ROOT: *pancrea*: hemipancreatectomy (*hemi* half + *ektome* excision) *pancreatic*: apancreatic (*a* privative) extrapancreatic (*extra* outside) intrapancreatic (*intra* within) parapancreatic (*para* alongside) *pancreatism*: eupancreatism (*eu* well) heteropancreatism (an irregular condition of functioning on the part of the pancreas) (*heteros* other) hypopancreatism (*hypo* below) *pancreorrhea* flowing of the pancreas: hyperpancreorrhea (*hyper* above) hypopancreorrhea (*hypo* below) *pancreatitis*: peripancreatitis (*peri* around + *itis* inflammation) LEADING ROOT COMPOUND: *pancrea*: pancreatomy (or, pancreatotomy) (*tomy* incision) *pancreat*: pancreatalgia (pain in the pancreas) (*algos* pain) pancreatectomy (or, pancreectomy) (*ektome* excision) pancreatemphraxis (*emphraxis* stoppage, obstruction) pancreatitis (*itis* inflammation) *pancreatico*: pancreaticoduodenal (duodenum) pancreaticoduodenectomy (duodenum + *ektome* excision) pancreaticoenterostomy (*enteron* intestine + *stoma* mouth, opening) *pancreato*: pancreatoduodenostomy (duodenum + *stoma* mouth, opening) pancreatogenic (or, pancreatogenous) (*genesis* origin) pancreatogram, pancreatography (*graphein* to write) pancreatojejunostomy (jejunum + *stoma* mouth, opening) pancreatolithectomy (*lithos* stone + *ektome* excision) pancreatolithiasis (*lithos* stone + *iasis* condition) pancreatolithotomy (*lithos* stone + *tomy* incision)

A Thesaurus of Medical Word Roots

Element	From	Meaning	Examples
pancreat (cont'd)		[pancreas]	pancreatolysis {pancreatolytic} (*lysis* dissolution) pancreatomegaly (*megalos* large) pancreatopathy (or, pancreopathy) (*pathos* disease) pancreatoscopy (*skopein* to examine) pancreatotomy (or, pancreatomy) (*tomy* incision) *pancreo*: pancreolith (also called *pancreatic calculus*) (*lithos* stone) pancreolysis {pancreolytic} (*lyein* to dissolve) pancreopathy (or, pancreatopathy) (*pathos* disease) TRAILING ROOT COMPOUND: bronchopancreatic (*bronchos* windpipe) gastroenteropancreatic (*gaster* stomach, belly + *enteron* intestine) hepatopancreatic (*hepatos* liver) lienopancreatic (also called *splenopancreatic*) (*lien* spleen) splenopancreatic (also called *lienopancreatic*) (spleen) CROSS REFERENCE: None
papill	Latin *papilla*	nipple	SIMPLE ROOT: papilla (a small nipplelike protuberance, structure, or elevation; also called *teat*; pl., papillae) {papillary} papillary (or, papillate: marked by nipplelike elevations) papillula (a small papilla; pl., papillulae) PREFIXED ROOT: *papillary*: extrapapillary (*extra* outside) peripapillary (*peri* around) subpapillary (*sub* below) *papilloma*: polypapilloma (*polys* many + *oma* tumor) LEADING ROOT COMPOUND: *papill*: papillectomy (*ektome* excision) papilledema (*edema* swelling) papillitis (*itis* inflammation) papilloma, papillomatosis (*oma* tumor + *osis* condition) *papilli*: papilliferous (*ferre* to bear) papilliform (*forma* shape) *papillo*: papilloadenocystoma (*aden* gland + *kystis* sac + *oma* tumor) papillocarcinoma (*karkinos* cancer + *oma* tumor) papilloretinitis (*rete* net, retina + *itis* inflammation) papillotomy (*tomy* incision) TRAILING ROOT COMPOUND: fibropapilloma (*fibra* fiber + *oma* tumor) myxopapilloma (*myxa* mucus + *oma* tumor) stomatopapilloma (*stomatos* mouth + *oma* tumor) CROSS REFERENCE: mamm, thel
papul	Latin *papula*	pimple, papule	SIMPLE ROOT: papulation, papule (a small circumscribed, solid elevation of the skin) {papular} PREFIXED ROOT: subpapular (*sub* below) LEADING ROOT COMPOUND: *papul*: papuloid (*eidos* form) papulosis (*osis* condition)

Element	From	Meaning	Examples
papul (cont'd)		[pimple]	*papuli*: papuliferous (*ferre* to bear)
			papulo:
			papuloerythematous (*erythros* red)
			papulopustular (pustule — a small pus-filled pimple)
			papulosquamous (*squama* scale, scaly)
			papulovesicle (*vesicle* blister)
			TRAILING ROOT COMPOUND:
			lenticulopapular (*lenticula* lens)
			maculopapular (*macula* spot)
			vesiculopapular (*vesicula* small sac)
			CROSS REFERENCE: None
par	Latin *parere* to beget; to appear *parenunos* lying with	give birth to; to produce; childbirth; labor	SIMPLE ROOT:
			parent, parentage, parity (the state of having given birth)
			parous (having borne one or more viable offspring)
			parturient (giving birth, or pertaining to childbirth)
			parturition (childbirth) {partal}
			PREFIXED ROOT:
			par: transparent (*trans* across)
			para:
			multipara (also called *pluripara*) (*multus* many)
			secundipara (*secundus* second)
			octipara (*octo* eight)
			pluripara (also called *multipara*), pluriparity (*plus* more)
			quadripara (*quattuor* four)
			septipara (*septum* seven)
			sextipara (a woman who has had six pregnancies which resulted in viable offspring; written *Para VI*, or *VI para*) (*sexti* six)
			tripara (also called *tertipara*) (*tri* three)
			unipara (also called *primipara*), uniparous (*uni* one)
			pareunia sexual intercourse: [*eune* as in *eunuch* means "bed"]
			apareunia (inability to accomplish sexual intercourse) (*a* privative)
			dyspareunia (difficult or painful sexual intercourse) (*dys* abnormal)
			parity:
			multiparity (*multus* many)
			semelparity (the state in an individual organism of reproducing only once in a lifetime) (*semel* once)
			parous:
			biparous (producing two ova or offspring at a time) (*bi* two)
			multiparous (*multus* many)
			partal:
			antepartal (or, antepartum; also called *prepartal*) (*ante* before)
			intrapartal (or, intrapartum) (*intra* within)
			postpartal (or, postpartum) (*post* after)
			prepartal (or, prepartum; also called *antepartal*) (*pre* before)
			partum:
			antepartum (*ante* before)
			intrapartum (occurring during childbirth) (*intra* within)
			peripartum (*peri* around)
			postpartum (occurring after childbirth, or after delivery, with reference to the mother) (*post* after)
			parturient: preparturient (*pre* before)
			LEADING ROOT COMPOUND:
			parto: partogram (also called *labor curve*) (*graphein* to write)

Element	From	Meaning	Examples
par (cont'd)		[give birth to; produce]	*parturi*: parturifacient (inducing or easing labor in childbirth) (*facere* to make) *parturio*: parturiometer (a device used in measuring the expulsive power of the uterus) (*metron* measure) TRAILING ROOT COMPOUND: *para*: gemellipara (a woman who has given birth to twins) (*gemelli* twins) primipara (*primus* first) *parous*: dentiparous (bearing teeth) (*dens* tooth) fissiparous (produced by fission) (*findere* to split) muciparous (secreting mucus) oviparous (*ovum* egg) ovoviviparous (*ovum* egg + *vivere* to live) primiparous (*primus* first) sebiparous (also called *sebiferous*) (*sebum* suet) sporiparous (also called *sporogenous*) (*sporos* seed) sudoriparous (*sudor* perspiration, sweat) synoviparous (synovial: *syn* with + *oon* egg) viviparous (*vivere* to live) CROSS REFERENCE: gen, nat, toc
para-	Greek prefix	alongside; sometimes, abnormal	See Appendix B for examples of words with this prefix. Others are placed with the roots to which it is attached. CROSS REFERENCE: meta-
paraly	Greek *para* alongside + *lyein* to loosen	paralysis	SIMPLE ROOT: paralysis (loss or impairment of motor function in a part due to lesion of the neural or muscular mechanism) {paralytic}, paralyze, paralyzer PREFIXED ROOT: *paralysis*: hemiparalysis (also called *hemiplegia*) (*hemi* half) *paralytic*: aparalytic (without paralysis; not causing paralysis) (*a* negative) antiparalytic (*anti* against) postparalytic (*post* after) subparalytic (*sub* under) TRAILING ROOT COMPOUND: acroparalysis (*akros* extremity) angioparalysis (*angeion* blood vessel) cystoparalysis (also called *cystoplegia*) (*kystis* bladder) gastroparalysis (also called *gastroparesis*) (*gaster* stomach, belly) iridoparalysis (also called *iridoplegia*) (iris—of the eye) isthmoparalysis (also called *isthmoplegia*) (isthmus) laryngoparalysis (larynx) metroparalysis (*metra* uterus) myeloparalysis (also called *spinal paralysis*) (*myelos* marrow) myoparalysis (*myos* muscle) neuroparalysis {neuroparalytic} (*neuron* nerve) pharyngoparalysis (pharynx) proctoparalysis (also called *proctoplegia*) (*proktos* anus) pseudoparalysis (*pseudes* false) stethoparalysis (paralysis of the respiratory muscles) (*stethos* chest) taboparalysis (also called *taboparesis*) (*tabes* wasting away) vasoparalysis (*vas* vessel: blood vessel) CROSS REFERENCE: pares, pleg

Element	From	Meaning	Examples
parasit	Greek *para* alongside + *sitos* food	parasite	SIMPLE ROOT: parasite (a plant or animal that lives upon or within another living organism at whose expense it obtains some advantage) {parasitic}, parasitism, parasitization PREFIXED ROOT: *parasite*: antiparasite (*anti* against) ectoparasite (also called *ectozoon*) (*ektos* outside) endoparasite (*endon* within) hyperparasite (a parasite that preys on another parasite) (*hyper* over) macroparasite (*makros* large) microparasite (*mikros* small) semiparasite (*semi* half) superparasite (*super* over, above) *parasitic*: antiparasitic (*anti* against) hyperparasitic (*hyper* over) *parasitism*: biparasitism (also called *hyperparasitism*) (*bi* two) hyperparasitism (also called *biparasitism*) (*hyper* over) polyparasitism (*polys* many) superparasitism (*super* over, above) LEADING ROOT COMPOUND: *parasit*: parasitemia (*emia* blood condition) parasitoid (*eidos* form) parasitome (*oma* mass) parasitosis (*osis* condition) *parasiti*: parasiticide {parasiticidal} (*caedere* to kill) parasitifer (*ferre* to bear) *parasito*: parasitogenic (*genere* to produce) parasitology (*logos* study) parasitophobia (*phobia* fear) parasitotropism {parasitotropic} (*trepein* to turn) TRAILING ROOT COMPOUND: cleptoparasite (or, kleptoparasite) (*kleptein* to steal) erythroparasite (*erythros* red) hemoparasite (*haima* blood) necroparasite (*nekros* death) phytoparasite (*phyton* plant) nosoparasite (*nosos* disease) pseudoparasite (*pseudes* false) xenoparasite (*xenos* foreign: stranger) zooparasite (*zoon* animal) CROSS REFERENCE: None
pares	Greek *para* beside + *hienai* to set in motion	relaxation, weakness, partial paralysis	SIMPLE ROOT: paresis (partial or slight paralysis) {paretic} PREFIXED ROOT: hemiparesis {hemiparetic} (*hemi* half) monoparesis (paralysis of a single limb) (*monos* single) paraparesis {paraparetic} (*para* alongside) quadriparesis (also called *tetraparesis*) (*quadri* four) tetraparesis (also called *quadriparesis*) (*tetra* four)

Element	From	Meaning	Examples
pares (cont'd)		[relaxation]	TRAILING ROOT COMPOUND: angioparesis (also called *vasoparesis*) (*angeion* blood vessel) cystoparesis (also called *cystoplegia*) (*kystis* bladder) enteroparesis (*enteron* intestine) gastroparesis (weakness of the stomach) (*gaster* stomach) myoparesis (muscle weakness) (*myos* muscle) ophthalmoparesis (also called *ophthalmoplegia*) (*ophthalmos* eye) pseudoparesis (*pseudes* false) taboparesis (also called *taboparalysis*) (*tabescere* to waste away) vasoparesis (also called *angioparesis*) (*vas* vessel—blood vessel) CROSS REFERENCE: asthen, chalas, paraly, pleg
parie	Latin *paries*	wall	SIMPLE ROOT: paries (wall of an organ or body cavity; pl., parietes) parietal (pertaining to the wall of a cavity; pertaining to the parietal bone) PREFIXED ROOT: anteroparietal (*anterior* front) biparietal (*bi* two) interparietal (*inter* between) intraparietal (*intra* within) transparietal (*trans* across) LEADING ROOT COMPOUND: *pariet*: parietitis (*itis* inflammation) *parieto*: parietofrontal (pertaining to the parietal and frontal bones) parietography (*graphein* to write) parietomastoid (mastoid process) parieto-occipital (*occiput* back of head: *ob* against + *caput* head) parietosphenoid (pertaining to the parietal and sphenoid bones) parietosplanchnic (also called *parietovisceral*) (*splanchnos* viscus) parietosquamosal (*squama* plate) parietovisceral (also called *parietosplanchnic*) (*viscera* internal organs) TRAILING ROOT COMPOUND: frontoparietal (also called *parietofrontal*) (*frontis* front) gastroparietal (*gaster* stomach, belly) mastoparietal (*mastos* breast) occipitoparietal (*occiput* back of head: *ob* against + *caput* head) sphenoparietal (*sphenos* wedge) squamoparietal (*squama* plate) uteroparietal (uterus) visceroparietal (*viscera* internal organs) CROSS REFERENCE: diaphragm, sept[1]
parotid	Greek *para* beside + *otos* ear	parotid	SIMPLE ROOT: parotid (situated or occurring near the ear, as the parotid gland) {parotic} LEADING ROOT COMPOUND: *parotid*: parotidectomy (*ektome* excision) parotiditis (or, parotitis) (*itis* inflammation) *parotido*: parotidoauricularis (*auricle* external ear) parotidoscirrhus (*skirrhos* hard) CROSS REFERENCE: ot

Element	From	Meaning	Examples
patell	Latin *patina* a shallow pan	knee cap	SIMPLE ROOT: patella (a lens-shaped bone situated in front of the knee in the tendon of the quadriceps femoris muscle) {patellar} PREFIXED ROOT: infrapatellar (also called *subpatellar*) (*infra* below, beneath) peripatellar (*peri* around) prepatellar (in front of the patella) (*pre* before) subpatellar (also called *infrapatellar*) (*sub* below) suprapatellar (*super* above) LEADING ROOT COMPOUND: *patell*: patellalgia (*algos* pain) patellectomy (*ektome* excision) *patelli*: patelliform (*forma* shape) *patello*: patellofemoral (concerning the patella and the femur) TERM: prepatellar bursitis (inflammation of the bursa in front of the patella; also called *housemaid's knee*) CROSS REFERENCE: geni², gon³
pas			See pan- for *diapason*.
path	Greek *pathos*	suffering, feeling, disease	SIMPLE ROOT: pathema (obsolete term for a disease or morbid condition), pathetic (pertaining to the trochlear nerve; denoting that which arouses sorrow or pity) PREFIXED ROOT: *path*: amphipath {amphipathic} (*amphi* both) *pathetic*: apathetic (indifferent; undemonstrative), apathy (*a* privative) apopathetic (describing the behavior in which an individual adapts his or her actions to the presence of other persons) (*apo* from) sympathetic (or sympathic; concerning the sympathetic nervous system) (*syn* with) [see separate entry: sympath-] *pathia*: hyperpathia (*hyper* over) polypathia (*polys* many) *pathic*: protopathic (*protos* first) *pathism*: apathism (sluggish of response to stimuli) (*a* negative) *pathology* study of disease: macropathology (*makros* large) micropathology (*mikros* small) *pathy*: apathy (*a* privative) allopathy (also called *heteropathy*) (*allos* other) empathy {empathic} (*em* in) exopathy (a disease having its cause or source outside the body) {exopathic} (*exo* outside) haplopathy (an uncomplicated disease) (*haplos* simple) heteropathy (also called *allopathy, hyperesthesia*) (*heteros* other) isopathy (*isos* equal) monopathy {monopathic} (*monos* single) sympathy (*syn* with) [see separate entry: sympath-] telepathy (*tele* afar) LEADING ROOT COMPOUND: *path*: pathergy (or, pathergia) {pathergic} (*ergon* work) pathodontia (also called *dental pathology*) (*odontos* tooth)

A Thesaurus of Medical Word Roots

Element	From	Meaning	Examples
path (cont'd)		[disease, suffering]	pathosis (also called *disease*) (*osis* condition) *patho*: pathobiology (also called *pathology*) (*bios* life + *logos* study) pathogen, pathogenesis {pathogenetic, pathogenic} (*genere* to produce) pathognomy (the science of the signs and symptoms of disease) {pathognomic} (*gnome* knowledge) pathology {pathological} (*logos* study) pathomimesis (intentional imitation of a disease, particularly malingering) (*mimein* to imitate) pathomorphism (*morphe* form) pathonomia (or, pathonomy) (*nomos* law) pathophobia (also called *nosophobia*) (*phobia* fear) pathopoiesis (*poiein* to make, produce) pathopsychology (the psychology of mental disease) (*psyche* mind + *logos* study) pathopsychosis (*psyche* mind + *osis* condition) pathotropism (attraction of drugs toward diseased structures) (*tropein* to turn) TRAILING ROOT COMPOUND: *pathia*: leukopathia (any disease of the leukocytes) (*leukos* white) naupathia (seasickness) (*naus* ship) neuropathia {neuropathic} (*neuron* nerve) osteopathia (*osteon* bone) *pathogenesis* origin of pain or disease: cytopathogenesis (*kytos* cell) enteropathogenesis (*enteron* intestine) histopathogenesis (*histos* web, tissue) immunopathogenesis (immune system) neuropathogenesis (*neuron* nerve) *pathologic*: anatomicopathologic (anatomy + *logos* study) *pathology* study of disease: acropathology (*akros* extremities) arthropathology (*arthron* a joint) cytopathology (also called *cellular pathology*) (*kytos* cell) dermatopathology (*dermatos* skin) etiopathology (*aitia* cause) hemopathology (*haima* blood) histopathology (also called *pathologic histology*) (*histos* tissue) immunopathology (immunity) mycopathology (*mykes* fungus) neuropathology (*neuron* nerve) onychopathology (*onychos* nail) osteopathology (*osteon* bone) paleopathology (*paleos* old, ancient) physiopathology (also called *pathologic physiology*) (*physis* nature) psychopathology (*psyche* mind) radiopathology (radiation) *pathy*: acropathy (any disease of the extremities) (*akron* extremity) adenopathy (also called *adenomegaly*) (*adenos* gland) adrenopathy (or, adrenalopathy) (adrenal glands)

Element	From	Meaning	Examples
path (cont'd)		[disease, suffering]	andropathy (*andros* man)
			angioneuropathy (any neuropathy affecting primarily the blood vessels) {angioneuropathic} (*angeion* vessel + *neuron* nerve)
			angiopathy (*angeion* blood vessel)
			aortopathy (aorta)
			arteriolopathy (small artery)
			arteriopathy (artery)
			arthropathy (*arthron* joint)
			axonopathy (*axon* axle)
			bronchopathy (*bronchos* windpipe)
			bursopathy (*bursa* sac, pouch)
			cardiomyopathy (*kardia* heart + *myos* muscle)
			cardiopathy {cardiopathic} (*kardia* heart)
			celiopathy (*koilia* belly)
			cenesthopathy (a general feeling of discomfort not referable to any particular part of the body) (*koinos* common)
			cephalopathy (*kephale* head)
			cerebropathy (*cerebrum* brain)
			chondropathy (*chondros* cartilage)
			coagulopathy (coagulation, clot)
			colopathy (or, colonopathy) (colon)
			craniopathy (*kranion* skull)
			cryopathy (*kryos* cold)
			cytopathy (*kytos* cell)
			dermopathy (also called *dermatosis*) (*derma* skin)
			desmopathy (*desmos* band: ligament)
			deuteropathy {deuteropathic} (*deuteros* second)
			discopathy (*diskos* disk)
			echopathy (also called *echolalia, echopraxia*)
			elastopathy (elastic tissue)
			embryopathy (embryo)
			encephalopathy (*enkephalon* brain)
			enteropathy (*enteron* intestine)
			erotopathy (*eros* sexual love)
			fetopathy (fetus)
			gastropathy (also called *gastrosis*) (*gaster* stomach)
			glossopathy (*glossa* tongue)
			gynecopathy (*gyne* woman, female)
			hemopathy (*haima* blood)
			hepatopathy (*hepatos* liver)
			histopathology (also called *pathologic histology*) (*histos* web)
			hysteropathy (*hystera* uterus)
			idiopathy (*idios* one's own)
			keratopathy (*keratos* horn: cornea)
			leukopathy (also called *leukoderma*) (*leukos* white)
			mastopathy (*mastos* breast, nipple)
			melanopathy (*melanos* black, dark)
			meningopathy (*meningos* membrane)
			metropathy (also called *hysteropathy*) (*metra* uterus)
			myelinopathy (myelin)
			myelopathy {myelopathic} (*myelos* marrow)
			myocardiopathy (also called *cardiomyopathy*) (*myos* muscle + *kardia* heart)

Element	From	Meaning	Examples
path (cont'd)		[disease, suffering]	myopathy {myopathic} (*myos* muscle)
			naprapathy (Czech *napravit* to correct)
			naturopathy (nature)
			necropathy (*nekros* death)
			nephropathy (also called *nephrosis, renopathy*) (*nephros* kidney)
			neuropathy (*neuron* nerve)
			oculopathy (also called *ophthalmopathy*) (*oculus* eye)
			odontopathy {odontopathic} (*odontos* tooth)
			onychopathy (also called *onychosis*) (*onychos* nail)
			oophoropathy (also called *ovariopathy*) (*oophoros* ovary duct)
			ophthalmopathy (also called *oculopathy*) (*ophthalmos* eye)
			orbitopathy (*orbita* eye socket)
			orchidopathy (or, orchiopathy; also called *testopathy*) (*orchis* testicle)
			organopathy (also called *organic disease*) (*organon* organ)
			osteopathy (*osteon* bone)
			ovariopathy (also called *oophoropathy*) (ovary)
			pancreatopathy (or, pancreopathy) (pancreas)
			pedopathy (*pedis* foot)
			peritoneopathy (peritoneuem)
			pharyngopathy (*pharynx* the throat)
			phonopathy (*phone* sound, voice)
			photopathy (*photos* light)
			pinealopathy (pineal gland)
			placentopathy (placenta)
			plexopathy (*plexus* network)
			pneumonopathy (also called *pneumonosis*) (*pneumon* lung)
			psychopath {psychopathic}, psychopathy (*psyche* mind)
			pyelopathy (*pyelos* pelvis)
			rachiopathy (also called *spondylopathy*) (*rhachis* spine)
			renopathy (also called *nephrosis, nephropathy*) (*ren* kidney)
			retinopathy (retina)
			rhinopathy (*rhinos* nose)
			sexopathy (also called *paraphilia*) (sex)
			somatopathy (*somatos* body)
			somnipathy (*somnus* sleep)
			spermatopathy (also called *dysspermia*) (*spermatos* seed)
			splanchnopathy (*splanchnos* viscus)
			splenopathy (*splen* spleen)
			spondylopathy (also called *rachiopathy*) (*spondylos* vertebra)
			stomatopathy (*stomatos* mouth)
			testopathy (also called *orchiopathy*) (*testis* testicle)
			thoracopathy (*thorakos* chest)
			thrombopathy (also called *thrombocytopathy*) (*thrombos* clot)
			thymopathy (thymus)
			thyropathy (thyroid gland)
			tonsillopathy (tonsil)
			toxicopathy (or, toxipathy; also called *toxicosis*) (*toxikon* poison)
			tracheopathy (*trachea* windpipe)
			traumatopathy (*traumatos* wound, injury)
			trichopathy (also called *trichonosis*) (*trichos* hair)
			trophopathy (*trophein* to nourish)
			tubulopathy (*tubulus* tube; renal tubules)

Element	From	Meaning	Examples
path (cont'd)		[disease, suffering]	ureteropathy (ureter) uropathy (*ouron* urine: urinary tract) vaginopathy (vagina) vasculopathy (*vas* vessel—blood vessel) vulvopathy (vulva) CROSS REFERENCE: alg, esthes, noso, sens
pect	Latin *pectus, pectoris*	breast, chest, thorax	SIMPLE ROOT: pectoral (or, pectoralis; pertaining to the breast or chest; also called *thoracic*) pectus (the front of the chest; pl., pectora) PREFIXED ROOT: ectopectoralis (*ektos* outside) expectorant, expectorate, expectoration (spitting) (*ex* out) subpectoral (*sub* below) LEADING ROOT COMPOUND: *pector*: pectoralgia (*algos* pain) *pectori*: pectoriloquy (also called *pectorophony*) (*loqui* to speak) TRAILING ROOT COMPOUND: clavipectoral (*clavis* clavicle, collarbone) genupectoral (*genus* knee) CROSS REFERENCE: mast, stern, steth, thora
pecten, pectin, pectun	Latin *pectinare* to comb; *pecten* comb	comb-like	SIMPLE ROOT: *pecten*: pecten (applied to certain anatomical structures because of a fancied resemblance to a comb; e.g., the pubic bone, middle portion of the anal canal; pl., pectines) *pectin*: pectinate (having toothlike projections, like those on a comb; also called *pectiniform*), pectineal (pertaining to the os pubis) *pectun*: pectunculus (pl., pectunculi) LEADING ROOT COMPOUND: *pecten*: pectenitis (inflammation of the pectin of the anus) (*itis* inflammation) pectenosis (stenosis of the anal canal caused by a rigid ring of tissue between the anal canal groove and the anal crypts, producing pain on defecation, bleeding, and anal irritation) (*osis* condition) *pecteno*: pectenotomy (*tomy* incision) *pectini*: pectiniform (also called *pectinate*) (*forma* shape) CROSS REFERENCE: None
ped[1]	Greek *pais, paidos*	child	LEADING ROOT COMPOUND: *ped*: pedarthrocace (carious condition of the joints of children) (*arthron* joint + *kakos* bad) pedatrophia (nutrition deficiency chiefly in the first year of life; also called *marasmus*) (atrophy: *a* privative + *trephein* to nourish) pederast (lit., sexual lover of children), pederasty (anal intercourse between a man and a boy) (*eros* love) pediatrician, pediatrics (*iatrein* to heal) pedodontics (or, pediadontia) (*odontos* tooth) *pedo*: pedomorphism (retention of juvenile characteristics in the adult) (*morphe* form) pedophilia (abnormal fondness for children) (*philein* to love) pedophobia (*phobia* fear)

Element	From	Meaning	Examples
ped[1] (cont'd)		[child]	TRAILING ROOT COMPOUND: lithopedion (also called *calcified fetus*) (*lithos* stone) logopedics (or, logopedia) (*logos* word + ortho*pedics*) misopedia (or, misopedy) (*misein* to hate) orthopedics (orig., the practice of straightening children's bones; now, the correction or prevention of skeletal deformities) (*orthos* straight) CROSS REFERENCE: puer
ped[2], **pes**	Latin *pes,* *pedalis,* *pedis*	foot	SIMPLE ROOT: *ped*: pedal (concerning the foot or feet) pedicel (also called *footplate*), pedicellate (or, pediculate), pedicellation (the development of a pedicle) pedicle (a footlike or stemlike part; also called *pediculus*) pediculate (or, pedunculate; provided with a pedicle), pediculation [also listed under pedicul-], pediculus (a footlike part; pl., pediculi) peduncle (or, pedunculus; a stemlike process) {peduncular, pedunculated}, pedunculus (pl., pedunculi) *pes*: pes (the foot, or a footlike structure; pl., pedes) PREFIXED ROOT: impedance (the opposition to the flow of an alternating current which is the vector sum of ohmic resistance plus additional resistance, if any, due to induction, capacity, or both) (*in* negative) interpediculate, interpeduncular (*inter* between) subpeduncular (situated below a peduncle) (*sub* below) LEADING ROOT COMPOUND: *pedi*: pedialgia (pain of the foot; also called *podalgia*) (*algos* pain) pedicure (care of the feet) (*cura* care) pediphalanx (a phalanx of the foot, distinguished from *maniphalanx,* phalanx of the hand) *pedion*: pedionalgia (neuralgic pain in the sole of the foot) (*algos* pain) [pedion: metatarsus] *pedo*: pedodynamometer (*dynamis* force + *metron* measure) pedograph, pedography (*graphein* to write) pedometer (*metron* measure) pedopathy (*pathos* disease) TRAILING ROOT COMPOUND: longipedate (having long feet) (*longus* long) sinistropedal (*sinister* left) taliped (*talus* ankle) CROSS REFERENCE: pod
pelli			See pelvi- for *brachypellic*, and others.
pelvi, **pelli**	Latin *pelvis* cup	pelvis	SIMPLE ROOT: pelvis (the lower portion of the trunk of the body, bounded anteriorly and laterally by the two hip bones and posteriorly by the sacrum and the coccyx; pl., pelves) {pelvic} PREFIXED ROOT: *pelv*: hemipelvectomy (*hemi* half + *ektome* excision) *pelvi*: subpelviperitoneal (*sub* under + peritoneum) *pelvic*: endopelvic (also called *intrapelvic*) (*endon* within) extrapelvic (*extra* outside)

A Thesaurus of Medical Word Roots

Element	From	Meaning	Examples
pelvi (cont'd)		[pelvis]	intrapelvic (also called *endopelvic*) (*intra* within)
			peripelvic (*peri* around)
			suprapelvic (*supra* above)
			LEADING ROOT COMPOUND:
			pelvi:
			pelvicalyceal (or, pelvicaliceal) (*kalyx* cup)
			pelvicephalography (roentgenographic measurement of the fetal head and of the birth canal) (*kephale* head + *graphein* to write)
			pelvicephalometry (*kephale* head + *metron* measure)
			pelvifemoral (femur)
			pelvifixation (*fixare* to fix)
			pelvilithotomy (or, pelviolithotomy) (*lithos* stone + *tomy* incision)
			pelvimeter, pelvimetry (*metron* measure)
			pelvirectal (rectum)
			pelvisacrum {pelvisacral} (sacrum)
			pelviscope, pelviscopy (*skopein* to examine)
			pelvisternum (*sternon* breastbone)
			pelvitherm (an instrument for applying heat to the pelvic organs) (*therme* heat)
			pelviureteral (also called *ureteropelvic*) (ureter)
			pelvio:
			pelviography (*graphein* to write)
			pelviolithotomy (also called *pyelolithotomy*) (*lithos* stone + *tomy* incision)
			pelvioperitonitis (also called *pelvic peritonitis*) (peritoneum + *itis* inflammation)
			pelvioplasty (*plassein* to form)
			pelvioscopy (or, pelviscopy) (*skopein* to examine)
			pelviotomy (*tomy* incision)
			TRAILING ROOT COMPOUND:
			pellic:
			brachypellic (also called *brachypelvic*) (*brachys* short)
			dolichopellic (or, dolichopelvic) (*dolichos* long)
			leptopellic (having a narrow pelvis) (*leptos* slender)
			mesatipellic (having a moderate size pelvis with a pelvic index between 90 and 95) (*mesatos* medium)
			platypellic (*platys* broad, flat)
			pelvic:
			abdominopelvic (relating to the abdomen and pelvis, especially the abdominal and pelvic cavities)
			brachypelvic (denoting a transverse oval pelvis) (*brachys* short)
			cephalopelvic (*kephale* head)
			dolichopelvic (or, dolichopellic) (*dolichos* long)
			iliopelvic (ileum)
			mesatipelvic (or, mesatipellic) (*mesatos* medium)
			renipelvic (also called *pyelic*) (*ren* kidney)
			ureteropelvic (also called *pelviureteral*) (ureter)
			uteropelvic (uterus)
			pelvis:
			acanthopelvis (a pelvis with the crest of the pubes sharp) (*akantha* thorn)
			tortipelvis (*tortus* twisted)
			CROSS REFERENCE: pyel

Element	From	Meaning	Examples
peni	Latin *penis* tail	tail, penis	SIMPLE ROOT: penicillate, penicillin, penicillium, penicillus (pl., penicilli) penile (or, penial; pertaining to the penis) penis (male organ of copulation and urination; pl., penes, penises) LEADING ROOT COMPOUND: *pen*: penectomy (also called *phallectomy*) (*ektome* excision) penitis (also called *phallitis*) (*itis* inflammation) *peni*: penischisis (*schisis* fissure) *peno*: penoscrotal (*scrotum* bag: testicle pouch) CROSS REFERENCE: balano, phall
penia	Greek *penia* poverty	deficiency; lack of	PREFIXED ROOT: monopenia (also called *monocytopenia*) (*monos* single) TRAILING ROOT COMPOUND: basopenia (also called *basophilic leukopenia*) calcipenia (also called *hypocalcia*) (*calcis* lime, calcium) cytopenia (also called *hematocytopenia*) (*kytos* cell) ductopenia (*ductus* duct) eosinopenia (also called *hypoeosinophilia*) (*eos* dawn: rose-colored) erythrocytopenia (also called *erythropenia*) (*erythros* red + *kytos* cell) esterapenia (estrus) glucopenia (also called *glycopenia*) (*glykys* sweet) granulopenia (also called *granulocytopenia, agranulocytosis*) (*granule* small grain) hematopenia (*haima* blood) hydropenia (*hydor* water) kaliopenia (also called *hypokalemia*) (*kalium* potassium) leukopenia (also called *aleukia*) (*leukos* white—blood cells) lipopenia (*lipos* fat) lymphopenia (also called *lymphocytopenia*) (*lympha* fluid) neuroglycopenia (*neuron* nerve + *glykys* sweet) neutropenia (diminished number of neutrophils in the blood) osteopenia {osteopenic} (*osteon* bone) reticulopenia (also called *reticulocytopenia*) (*reticulum* network) sarcopenia (*sarkos* flesh) sideropenia (*sideros* iron) thrombopenia (also called *thrombocytopenia*) (*thrombos* clot) uropenia (also called *oliguria*) (*ouron* urine) CROSS REFERENCE: olig
pept, peps	Greek *peptein*	to cook, digest	SIMPLE ROOT: pepsin (the chief enzyme of gastric juice which converts proteins into proteoses and peptones), pepsinate, pepsinia peptic, peptide, peptization, peptone {peptonic}, peptonization PREFIXED ROOT: *pepsia* digestive condition: anapepsia (complete absence of pepsin from the stomach secretion) (*ana* completely) dyspepsia {dyspeptic} (*dys* abnormal) eupepsia (or, eupepsy) {eupeptic} (*eu* good, well) hyperpepsia (abnormally rapid digestion; also called *hyperchlorhydria*) (*hyper* above) hypopepsia (also called *oligopepsia*) (*hypo* below)

A Thesaurus of Medical Word Roots

Element	From	Meaning	Examples
pept (cont'd)		[to cook, digest]	*pepsin*: depepsinized (*de* reversal) hypopepsinia (*hypo* below) *peptid(o)*: eupeptide (*eu* well) hexapeptide (*hex* six) polypeptide, polypeptidemia (*polys* many + *emia* blood condition) polypeptidorrhachia (*polys* many + *rhachis* spine) transpeptidation (*trans* across) *peptone*: antipeptone (*anti* against) hemipeptone (*hemi* half) LEADING ROOT COMPOUND: *pepsin*: pepsinuria (the presence of pepsin in the urine) (*uria* urine condition) *pepsini*: pepsiniferous (*ferre* to bear) *pepsino*: pepsinogen (*genesis* origin) *pept*: peptoid (*eidos* form) *peptid*: peptidergic (having an action resembling that of a peptide hormone) (*ergon* work) *peptido*: peptidolytic (*lysis* dissolving, loosening) *pepto*: peptogenic (or, peptogenous) (*genesis* origin) peptolysis {peptolytic} (*lyein* to loosen) peptotoxin (*toxon* poison) *pepton*: peptonemia (*emia* blood condition) peptonuria (*uria* urine condition) TRAILING ROOT COMPOUND: bradypepsia (*bradys* slow) colodyspepsia (colon + dyspepsia) oligopepsia (also called *hypopepsia*) (*oligos* little, scant) proteopepsis (protein) CROSS REFERENCE: None
per-	Latin prefix	through; extremely	See Appendix B for examples of words with this prefix. Others are placed with the roots to which it is attached. CROSS REFERENCE: dia-, trans-
peri-	Greek prefix	around	See Appendix B for examples of words with this prefix. Others are placed with the roots to which it is attached. CROSS REFERENCE: circ-
pericard	Greek *peri* around + *kardia* heart	pericardium	SIMPLE ROOT: pericardium (the fibroserous sac that surrounds the heart; pl., pericardia) {pericardiac, pericardial} PREFIXED ROOT: *pericardial*: endopericardial (*endon* within) epipericardial (upon or about the pericardium) (*epi* upon) intrapericardial (*intra* within) subpericardial (*sub* under) *pericarditis*: endopericarditis (*endon* within + *itis* inflammation) LEADING ROOT COMPOUND: *pericard*: pericardectomy (or, pericardiectomy) (*ektome* excision) pericarditis {pericarditic} (*itis* inflammation)

Element	From	Meaning	Examples
pericard (cont'd)		[pericardium]	*pericardi*: pericardicentesis (or, pericardiocentesis) (*kentesis* puncture) pericardiectomy (or, pericardectomy) (*ektome* excision) *pericardio*: pericardiology (*logos* study) pericardiolysis (*lysis* loosening) pericardiomediastinitis (*mediastinum* septum + *itis* inflammation) pericardioperitoneal (peritoneum) pericardiophrenic (*phren* diaphragm) pericardiopleural (*pleura* rib, side) pericardiorrhaphy (*rhaphe* suture) pericardiostomy (*stoma* mouth, opening) pericardiotomy (or, pericardotomy) (*tomy* incision) TRAILING ROOT COMPOUND: *pericardial*: peritoneopericardial (peritoneum) pleuropericardial (*pleura* side, rib) sternopericardial (*sternon* chest, breast) *pericarditis* inflammation of the pericardium: cardiopericarditis (*kardia* heart) hydropericarditis (*hydor* water) myopericarditis (*myos* muscle) pleuropericarditis (*pleura* rib, side: pleura) pseudopericarditis (*pseudes* false) pyopercarditis (*pyon* pus) reticulopericarditis (*reticulum*) *pericardium*: chylopericardium (*chylos* juice) hemopericardium (*haima* blood) hydropericardium (*hydor* water) pneumohydropericardium (*pneuma* air + *hydor* water) pneumoparicardium (*pneuma* air) pyopericardium (*pyon* pus) CROSS REFERENCE: None
perine	Greek *peri* around + *inein* to discharge, to defecate	perineum	SIMPLE ROOT: perineum (the region of the body between the thighs; specifically, the small area between the anus and the vulva in the female, or between the anus and the scrotum in the male) {perineal} PREFIXED ROOT: extraperineal (*extra* outside) intraperineal (*intra* within) LEADING ROOT COMPOUND: perineocele (*kele* hernia) perineoplasty (*plassein* to form) perineorrhaphy (*rhaphe* suture) perineoscrotal (*scrotum* bag: testicle pouch) perineotomy (*tomy* incision) perineovaginal, perineovaginorectal (vagina + rectum) perineovulvar (vulva) TRAILING ROOT COMPOUND: abdominoperineal (abdomen) anoperineal (anus) episioperineoplasty (*epision* vulva + *plassein* to form)

Element	From	Meaning	Examples
perine (cont'd)		[perineum]	episioperineorrhaphy (*epision* vulva + *rhaphe* suture) ischioperineal (ischium) rectoperineal (rectum) sacroperineal (sacrum) urethroperineal (urethra) vaginoperineal (vagina) vesicoperineal (*vesica* bladder) CROSS REFERENCE: None
periost	Greek *peri-* around + *osteon* bone	periosteum	SIMPLE ROOT: periosteum (the membrane of tough, fibrous connective tissue covering all bones except at the joints) {periosteal, periosteous} PREFIXED ROOT: extraperiosteal (*extra* outside) subperiosteal (*sub* under) LEADING ROOT COMPOUND: *periost*: periostitis (or, periosteitis) (*itis* inflammation) periostoma (or, periosteoma) (*oma* tumor) periostosis (*osis* condition) *perioste*: periosteitis (or, periostitis) (*itis* inflammation) periosteoma (*oma* tumor) *periosteo*: periosteoedema (or, periosteodema) (*edema* swelling) periosteomedullitis (also called *periosteomyelitis*) (*medulla* marrow + *itis* inflammation) periosteomyelitis (*myelos* marrow + *itis* inflammation) periosteopathy (*pathos* disease) periosteophyte (*phytos* plant: growth) periosteotome, periosteotomy (*tomy* incision) *periosto*: periostomedullitis (*medulla* marrow + *itis* inflammation) periostotome (*temnein* to cut; *tome* a cutting instrument) *periostoste*: periostosteitis (also called *osteoperiostitis*) (*itis* inflammation) TRAILING ROOT COMPOUND: osteoperiostitis (*osteon* bone + *itis* inflammation) pachyperiostitis (*pachys* thick + *itis* inflammation) CROSS REFERENCE: None
peristol	Greek *peri* around + *stello* to contract	contraction	SIMPLE ROOT: peristole (the tonic activity of the walls of the stomach whereby the organ contracts around its contents) TRAILING ROOT COMPOUND: pharyngoperistole (pharynx) CROSS REFERENCE: diastol, systol
periton	Greek *peri-* around + *teinein* to stretch	peritoneum	SIMPLE ROOT: peritonealize (to cover with peritoneum) peritoneum (the membrane lining the abdominopelvic walls; pl., peritonea) {peritoneal} peritonism, peritonization, peritonize PREFIXED ROOT: *peritoneal*: ectoperitoneal (*ektos* outside) endoperitoneal (*endon* within) extraperitoneal (*extra* outside)

Element	From	Meaning	Examples

periton
(cont'd)
		[peritoneum]	intraperitoneal (*intra* within)
			paraperitoneal (*para* alongside)
			preperitoneal (or, properitoneal) (*pre* before)
			subperitoneal (*sub* under)
			symperitoneal (*sym* with, together)
			transperitoneal (*trans* across)
			peritoneo:
			subperitoneoabdominal (*sub* under + abdomen)
			subperitoneopelvic (*sub* under + pelvis)
			peritoneum: retroperitoneum {retroperitoneal} (*retro* behind)
			peritonitis inflammation of the peritoneum:
			ectoperitonitis (*ektos* outside)
			endoperitonitis (*endon* within)
			retroperitonitis (*retro* behind)
			LEADING ROOT COMPOUND:
			periton: peritonitis {peritonitic} (*itis* inflammation)
			peritone: peritonealgia (*algos* pain)
			peritoneo:
			peritoneocentesis (*kentein* to puncture)
			peritoneoclysis (*klyzein* to cleanse)
			peritoneography (*graphein* to write)
			peritoneomuscular
			peritoneopathy (*pathos* disease)
			peritoneopericardial (pericardium)
			peritoneopexy (*pexis* fixation)
			peritoneoplasty (*plassein* to form)
			peritoneoscope (also called *laparoscope*), peritoneoscopy (also called
			   laparoscopy) (*skopein* to examine)
			peritoneotomy (also called *celotomy*) (*tomy* incision)
			peritoneovenous (*vena* vein)
			TRAILING ROOT COMPOUND:
			peritoneal:
			pleuroperitoneal (*pleura* rib, side: pleura)
			tuboperitoneal (*tubus* tube—uterine, or Fallopian tube)
			visceroperitoneal (*viscera* internal organs)
			peritoneum:
			aeroperitoneum (also called *pneumoperitoneum*) (*aer* air)
			choleperitoneum (*chole* bile)
			chyloperitoneum (also called *chyliform ascites*) (*chylus* juice)
			hematoperitoneum (or, hemoperitoneum) (*hematos* blood)
			hydraeroperitoneum (*hydor* water + *aer* air)
			hydroperitoneum (*hydor* water)
			pneumoperitoneum (the presence of air or gas in the peritoneal cav-
			   ity, usually as a result of disease) (*pneuma* air, gas)
			pyoperitoneum (an accumulation of pus in the peritoneal cavity)
			   (*pyon* pus)
			peritonitis inflammation of the peritoneum:
			choleperitonitis (*chole* bile)
			metroperitonitis (*metra* uterus)
			myoperitonitis (*myos* muscle)
			pachyperitonitis (*pachys* thick)
			pelviperitonitis (pelvis)
			CROSS REFERENCE: None

A Thesaurus of Medical Word Roots

Element	From	Meaning	Examples
pero	Greek *peros*	maimed	SIMPLE ROOT: peronia (a developmental malformation or mutilation) See Appendix B for examples of words with this combining form. Others are placed with the roots to which it is attached. CROSS REFERENCE: None
petr	Latin *petra* stone Greek *petros*	stone [part of the temporal bone]	SIMPLE ROOT: petrosa (the petrous part of the temporal bone) {petrosal} petrous (resembling a rock; hard) PREFIXED ROOT: subpetrosal (*sub* under) superpetrosal (*super* above) LEADING ROOT COMPOUND: *petri*: petrifaction (*facere* to make) *petro*: petromastoid (also called *otocranium*) (*mastos* breast + *eidos* form) petro-occipital (*occiput* back of head: *ob* against + *caput* head) petrosphenoid (*sphenos* wedge + *eidos* form) petrosquamous (or, petrosquamosal) (*squama* scale) petrotympanic (*tympanon* eardrum) *petros*: petrosectomy (*ektome* excision) petrositis (*itis* inflammation) TRAILING ROOT COMPOUND: sphenopetrosal (*sphenos* wedge: sphenoid bone) squamopetrosal (*squama* plate, scale) CROSS REFERENCE: calc, lith
pex	Greek *pexis* fixation	attached, fixed	SIMPLE ROOT: pex (to fix or fasten), pexia (or, pexis; the fixation of matter by a tissue) {pexic} PREFIXED ROOT: hyperpexia (or, hyperpexy) (*hyper* more, above) hypopexia (or, hypopexy) (*hypo* below) TRAILING ROOT COMPOUND: *pexia*: inopexia (*inos* fiber) *pexis*: adipopexis {adipopectic} (*adeps* fat) glycopexis (*glykys* sweet) hydropexis (or, hydropexia) {hydropexic} (*hydor* water) toxicopexis (*toxikon* poison) viropexis (*virus* poison) *pexy*: aortopexy (aorta) calcipexy (calcium) cecopexy (*cecum* blind gut) cervicopexy (*cervix* neck of the uterus) chromopexy (or, chromatopexy) {chromopectic} (*chroma* color) colopexy (or, colopexia) (colon) colpopexy (*kolpos* vagina) cordopexy (or, chordopexy) (*chorda* cord) corepexy (*kore* pupil of eye) cryopexy (*kryos* cold) cystopexy (*kystis* bladder) enteropexy (*enteron* intestine) epiplopexy (also called *omentopexy*) (*epiploon* omentum)

Element	From	Meaning	Examples
pex (cont'd)		[attached, fixed]	galactopexy (*galaktos* milk)
			gastropexy (*gaster* stomach, belly)
			glossopexy (lip-tongue adhesion) (*glossa* tongue)
			hepatopexy (*hepar* liver)
			hysteropexy (*hystera* womb, uterus)
			ligamentopexy (ligament)
			mastopexy (also called *mazopexy*) (*mastos* breast, nipple)
			meniscopexy (also called *meniscorrhaphy*) (meniscus)
			mesenteriopexy (also called *mesopexy*) (*mesentery* membranous fold)
			nephropexy (*nephros* kidney)
			omentopexy (*omentum* fat skin)
			oophoropexy (also called *ovariopexy*) (*oophor* egg bearer)
			orchiopexy (or, orchidopexy) (*orchis* testicle)
			organopexy (*organum* organ)
			ovariopexy (also called *oophoropexy*) (*ovarium* ovary)
			peritoneopexy (peritoneum: *peri* around + *teinein* to stretch)
			pneumonopexy (or, pneumopexy) (*pneumon* lung)
			proctopexy (also called *rectopexy*) (*proktos* anus, rectum)
			proteopexy (protein)
			rectopexy (also called *proctopexy*) (rectum, anus)
			retinopexy (retina)
			rheopexy (*rheos* flow)
			salpingopexy (*salpingos* tube: uterine tube)
			scapulopexy (*scapula* shoulder blade)
			sigmoidopexy (the sigmoid colon)
			splenopexy (*splen* spleen)
			syndesmopexy (*syndesis* bound together: ligament)
			trachelopexy (also called *cervicopexy*) (*trachelos* neck—of uterus)
			typhlopexy (*typhlon* cecum: blind gut)
			urethropexy (also called *bladder neck suspension*) (urethra)
			uteropexy (also called *hysteropexy*) (uterus)
			vaginopexy (also called *colpopexy*) (vagina)
			CROSS REFERENCE: fix, pact
phac, phak	Greek *phakos* lentil	lens of the eye	PREFIXED ROOT:
			phac: periphacitis (*peri* around + *itis* inflammation)
			phak:
			aphakia (congenital absence of the lens of the eye) (*a* privative)
			microphakia (*mikros* small)
			periphakitis (or, periphacitis) (*peri* around + *itis* inflammation)
			LEADING ROOT COMPOUND:
			phac:
			phacitis (also called *phakitis*) (*itis* inflammation)
			phacoid, phacoiditis (also called *phakitis*) (*eidos* form + *itis* inflammation)
			phacoma, phacomatosis (*oma* tumor + *osis* condition)
			phaco:
			phacoanaphylaxis (*anaphylaxis* sensitivity)
			phacocele (*kele* tumor, swelling)
			phacocyst, phacocystectomy (*kystis* sac + *ektome* excision)
			phacocystitis (inflammation of the capsule of the eye lens; also called *phacohymenitis*) (*kystis* sac + *itis* inflammation)
			phacodonesis (*donein* to shake)

Element	From	Meaning	Examples
phac (cont'd)		[lens]	phacoemulsification (*emulgere* to milk out + *facere* to make) phacoerysis (*erysis* dragging away, or drawing off) phacofragmentation (*frangere* to break) phacoglaucoma (*glaukos* gray + *oma* tumor) phacohymenitis (also called *phacocystitis*) (*hymen* membrane + *itis* inflammation) phacolysis (or, phakolysis) {phacolytic} (*lyein* to loosen) phacomalacia (*malakos* soft) phacometer (also called *lensometer*) (*metron* measure) phacoplanesis (abnormal mobility of the crystalline lens) (*planan* to wander) phacoscope, phacoscopy (*skopein* to examine) phacosclerosis (*sklerosis* hardening) phacoscope (also called *phacoidoscope*) (*skopein* to examine) phacoscotasmus (*skotasmos* a clouding) phacotoxic (*toxic* poisonous) *phak*: phakitis (*itis* inflammation) phakoma (or, phacoma) (*oma* tumor) TRAILING ROOT COMPOUND: erysiphake (an instrument for removing the lens in cataract by suction; also called *erisophake*) (*erysis* suction: a drawing) keratophakia (*keratos* horn: cornea) pseudophakia (*pseudes* false) spherophakia (*sphere* ball, globe) CROSS REFERENCE: lens
phag	Greek *phagein* to devour	to eat, swallow; consume	SIMPLE ROOT: phage (also called *bacteriophage*), phagedena (a canker; rapidly spreading destructive ulceration of soft tissue) {phagedenic} PREFIXED ROOT: *phage*: macrophage {macrophagic} (*makros* large) microphage (also called *microphagocyte*) {microphagic} (*mikros* small) prophage (also called *probacteriophage*) (*pro* before) *phagia*: aphagia (abstention from eating; inability to swallow) (*a* privative) autophagia (or, autophagy) {autophagic} (*autos* self) dysphagia (or, dysphagy; also called *aphagopraxia*) {dysphagic} (*dys* abnormal) hyperphagia (also called *polyphagia*) (*hyper* over, beyond) polyphagia (excessive eating; gluttony) (*polys* many) *phagism*: monophagism (*monos* single) *phago*: aphagopraxia (loss of the ability to swallow; also called *dysphagia*) (*a* privative + *praxis* action) antiphagocytic (*anti* against + *kytos* cell) dysphagocytosis (*dys* abnormal + *kytos* cell + *osis* condition) macrophagocyte (*makros* large + *kytos* cell) microphagocyte (*mikros* small + *kytos* cell) *phagy*: heterophagy (*heteros* other) isophagy (also called *autolysis*) (*isos* equal)

Element	From	Meaning	Examples
phag (cont'd)		[to devour]	LEADING ROOT COMPOUND: phagocyte (*kytos* cell) phagolysis (also called *phagocytolysis*) {phagolytic} (*lyein* to loosen) phagomania (an insatiable craving for food) (*mania* craze) phagophobia (irrational fear of eating) (*phobia* fear) phagosome (*soma* body) phagotype (*typos* type) TRAILING ROOT COMPOUND: *phage*: bacteriophage {bacteriophagic} (*bakterion* little rod) erythrophage (a phagocyte that ingests blood pigment) (*erythros* red) melanophage (*melanos* dark) mycophage (*mykes* fungus) myelophage (*myelos* marrow) myophage (*myos* muscle) siderophage (*sideros* iron) *phagia*: aerophagia (*aer* air) allotriophagy (*allotrios* strange) amylophagia (*amyle* starch) bradyphagia (*bradys* slow) erythrophagia (also called *erythrophagocytosis*) (*erythros* red) geophagia (*geo* earth) hemophagia (or, hematophagia; also called *hemoposia*; the drinking of blood, as by parasites) (*haima* blood) hyalophagia (*hyalos* glass) lipophagia (also called *lipolysis*) {lipophagic} (*lipos* fat) neuronophagia (*neuron* nerve) odynophagia (pain in swallowing) (*odyne* pain) omophagia (the eating of raw food) (*omos* raw) onychophagia (nail-biting; biting of the nails) (*onychos* nail) oophagia (*oon* egg, ovum) pyophagia (swallowing of pus) (*pyon* pus) tachyphagia (*tachys* rapid) trichophagia (*trichos* hair) *phagous* pertaining to eating or consumption: biophagous (*bios* life) galactophagous (also called *lactivorous*) (*galactos* milk) ichthyophagous (*ichthys* fish) necrophagous (*nekros* death) *phagy*: coprophagy (or, coprophagia; also called *scatophagy*) (*kopros* dung, feces) creophagy (or, creophagism) (*kreas* meat, flesh) crinophagy (the disposal of excess secretory granules by lysomes) (*krinein* to separate) cytophagy {cytophagic} (*kytos* cell) mycophagy (*mykes* fungus: mushroom) onychophagy (the habit of nail biting) (*onyx* nail) sialoaerophagy (*sialon* saliva + *aer* air) CROSS REFERENCE: None

Element	From	Meaning	Examples
phalang, **phalanx**	Greek *phalanx* closely knit row	phalanx, row	SIMPLE ROOT: phalangette (the distal phalanx of a digit), phalangization phalanx [any of the bones of the fingers or toes; one of a set of plates formed of phalangeal cells (inner and outer) forming the reticular membrane of the organ of Corti; pl., phalanges] {phalangeal} [organ of Corti: spiral organ in the inner ear] PREFIXED ROOT: *phalang*: hemiphalangectomy (*hemi* half + *ektome* excision) interphalangeal (*inter* between) *phylangia*: aphalangia (*a* privative) hyperphalangia (*hyper* over) polyphalangia (*polys* many) symphalangia (*sym* with, together) triphalangia (malformation in which three phalanges are present in the thumb or great toe) (*tri* three) *phalangism*: hyperphalangism (*hyper* over) hypophalangism (*hypo* under) polyphalangism (*polys* many) triphalangism (*tri* three) *phalangy*: symphalangy (also called *syndactyly*) (*syn* together) LEADING ROOT COMPOUND: phalangectomy (*ektome* excision) phalangitis (*itis* inflammation) phalangosis (a condition in which the eyelashes grow in rows) (*osis* condition) TRAILING ROOT COMPOUND: *phalangeal*: carpophalangeal (*carpus* wrist) tarsophalangeal (*tarsus* ankle) *phalangia*: brachyphalangia (*brachys* short) ectrophalangia (congenital absence of one or more phalanges of a digit—a finger or toe) (*ektrosis* congenitally absent) *phalanx*: maniphalanx (*manus* hand) pediphalanx (*pes* foot) CROSS REFERENCE: None
phall	Greek *phallos*	penis, phallus	SIMPLE ROOT: phallicism (or, phallism; worship of the male genitalia) phallus (pl., phalli) {phallic; relating to the penis; also called *penile*; in psychoanalysis, relating to the penis, especially during the phases of infantile psychosexuality} PREFIXED ROOT: *phallic*: polyphallic (pertaining to the fantasy of possessing multiple penises) (*polys* many) *phallus*: diphallus (also called *bifid penis, double penis*) (*di* two) macrophallus (also called *macropenis, megalopenis, megalophallus*) (*makros* large) megalophallus (also called *macropenis*) (*megalos* large)

Element	From	Meaning	Examples
phall (cont'd)		[penis]	microphallus (also called *micropenis*) (*mikros* small) LEADING ROOT COMPOUND: *phall*: phallalgia (also called *phallodynia*) (*algos* pain) phallanastrophe (upward distortion of the penis) (*ana* upward + *strephein* to turn) phallaneurysm (*aneurysm* a widening) phallectomy (also called *penectomy*) (*ektome* to excise) phallitis (also called *penitis*) (*itis* inflammation) phallodynia (also called *phallalgia*) (*odyne* pain) phalloid (similar to a penis; also called *phalliform*) (*eidos* form) phalloncus (morbid swelling or tumor of the penis) (*onkos* mass) *phalli*: phalliform (also called *phalloid*) (*forma* shape) *phallo*: phallocampsis (curvature of the penis when erect) (*kampsis* a bending) phallocrypsis (retraction of the penis) (*kryptein* to hide) phalloplasty (surgical reconstruction of the penis) (*plassein* to form) phallorrhagia (*rhagia* bursting forth) phallotomy (*tomy* incision) TRAILING ROOT COMPOUND: dolichophallic (having a long penis) (*dolichos* long) CROSS REFERENCE: balano, peni
phan, **phas**, **phen**, **fan**	Greek *phanein* to appear	to show, appear	SIMPLE ROOT: *phan*: phantasia, phantasm (or, phantom), phantasy (or, fantasy), phantom *phas*: phase (a stage of development) {phasic} *phen*: phenomenon (any sign or objective symptom; any observable occurrence or fact; pl., phenomena) PREFIXED ROOT: *phan*: diaphane (a minute electric lamp for use in transillumination) diaphaneity (transparent), diaphanography (transillumination of the breast, with photography of the transilluminated light on an infrared-sensitive film) (*graphein* to write) diaphanous (extremely thin and transparent) (*dia* through) *phano*: diaphanoscope, diaphanoscopy (also called *transillumination*) (*dia* across, through + *skopein* to examine) *phase*: anaphase (stage in miosis and mitosis) (*ana* again) antephase (*ante* before) diplophase (*diploos* double) interphase (between two successive cell divisions) (*inter* between) metaphase (the stage in mitosis in which the duplicated chromosomes lie on the equatorial plane of the spindle) (*meta* after) polyphase (having many phases; containing colloids of several types) (*polys* many) prometaphase (*pro* before + metaphase) prophase (first phase of indirect cell division) (*pro* before) telophase (the last of four stages of mitosis and of the two divisions of meiosis (*telos* end) *phasic*: diphasic (*di* two)

Element	From	Meaning	Examples
phan (cont'd)		[to show, appear]	polyphasic (*polys* many) triphasic (*tri* three) *phen*: epiphenomenon (an accessory, exceptional, or accidental occurrence in the course of an attack of any disease) (*epi* upon) euphenics (*eu* well) polyphenic (also called *pleiotropic*), polyphenism (*polys* many) LEADING ROOT COMPOUND: *phaner*: phanerosis (the process of becoming visible) (*osis* condition) *phanero*: phanerogenetic (or, phanerogenic; having a known cause) (*genere* to produce) phaneroscope (*skopein* to examine) *phant*: phantosmia (*osme* smell) *phantasmato*: phantasmatomoria (childishness or dementia with absurd delusions) (*moria* folly) *phantasmo*: phantasmology (*logos* study) phantasmoscopia (the delusion of seeing phantoms) (*skopein* to examine) *phanto*: phantogeusia (*geusis* taste) *pheno*: phenology (a study of the effects of climate upon the life and health of living organisms) (*logos* study) phenoscopy (*skopein* to examine) phenotype {phenotypic} (*typos* type) *phenomeno*: phenomenology (*logos* study) TRAILING ROOT COMPOUND: *phan*: menophania (first appearance of the menses at puberty) (*mene* month: menstruation) *phen*: phosphene (a luminous appearance caused by pressing on the eyeball) (*phos* light) CROSS REFERENCE: ide
pharyn	Greek *pharynx* throat	throat	SIMPLE ROOT: pharynx (passageway for air from the nasal cavity to the larynx and for food from the mouth to the esophagus; pl., pharynges) {pharyngeal, pharyngeus} pharyngism (or, pharyngismus; also called *pharyngospasm*) PREFIXED ROOT: *pharyng*: epipharyngeal, epipharyngitis (also called *nasopharyngitis*) (*epi* upon + *itis* inflammation) hypopharyngeal, hypopharyngoscopy (*hypo* under + *skopein* to examine) parapharyngeal (*para* alongside) peripharyngeal (*peri* around) postpharyngeal (*post* posterior) retropharyngeal, retropharyngitis (*retro* behind + *itis* inflammation) subpharyngeal (*sub* below) *pharynx*: epipharynx (also called *nasopharynx*) (*epi* upon) hypopharynx (*hypo* under)

Element	From	Meaning	Examples
pharyn (cont'd)		[throat]	retropharynx (*retro* back, backward) LEADING ROOT COMPOUND: *pharyng*: pharyngalgia (also called *pharyngodynia*) (*algos* pain) pharyngectasia (also called *pharyngocele*) (*ektasis* dilatation) pharyngectomy (*ektome* excision) pharyngemphraxis (*emphraxis* stoppage, obstruction) pharyngitis (also called *sore throat*) {pharyngitic} (*itis* inflamma- tion) pharyngodynia (also called *pharyngalgia*) (*odyne* pain) *pharyngo*: pharyngocele (also called *pharyngectasia*) (*kele* hernia) pharyngoepiglottic (epiglottis) pharyngoesophageal, pharynoesophagoplasty (plastic surgery of the pharynx and the esophagus) (esophagus + *plassein* to form) pharyngoglossal (also called *glossopharyngeal*) (*glossa* tongue) pharyngokeratosis (also called *keratosis pharyngea*) (*keras* horn: hard + *osis* condition) pharyngolaryngeal, pharyngolaryngitis (also called *laryngopharyn- gitis*) (larynx + *itis* inflammation) pharyngolith (a concretion in the pharynx; also called *pharyngeal calculus*) (*lithos* stone) pharyngolysis (also called *pharyngoparalysis*) (*lyein* to loosen) pharyngomaxillary (*maxilla* upper jaw) pharyngomycosis (*mykes* fungus + *osis* condition) pharyngonasal (*nasus* nose) pharyngo-oral (also called *oropharyngeal*) (*os, ora* mouth) pharyngopalatine (palate) pharyngoparalysis (*paralysis* a loosening at the side) pharyngopathy (*pathos* disease) pharyngoperistole (also called *pharyngostenosis*) (*peristole* contrac- ture) pharyngoplasty (*plassein* to form) pharyngoplegia (also called *pharyngoparalysis*) (*plessein* to strike) pharyngorhinitis (*rhinos* nose + *itis* inflammation) pharyngorhinoscopy (*rhinos* nose + *skopein* to examine) pharyngorrhea (mucous discharge from the pharynx) (*rhein* to flow) pharyngoscope, pharyngoscopy (*skopein* to examine) pharyngospasm (also called *pharyngism*) (*spasmos* contraction) pharyngostenosis (also called *pharyngoperistole*) (*stenosis* narrow) pharyngostoma (*stoma* mouth, opening) pharyngotome, pharyngotomy (*tomy* incision) pharyngotonsillitis (tonsil + *itis* inflammation) pharyngoxerosis (*xerosis* dryness) TRAILING ROOT COMPOUND: *phagyneal*: buccopharyngeal (*bucca* cheek, mouth) craniopharyngeal (*kranion* skull) glossopharyngeal (*glossa* tongue) maxillopharyngeal (*maxilla* upper jaw) mylopharyngeal (*mylai* molar teeth) nasopharyngeal (*nasus* nose) oropharyngeal (also called *pharyngo-oral*) (*oris* mouth)

Element	From	Meaning	Examples
pharyn (cont'd)		[throat]	otopharyngeal (*otos* ear) palatopharyngeal (palate: roof of mouth) tracheopharyngeal (*trachea* windpipe) *pharyngitis* inflammation of the pharynx: adenopharyngitis (*adenos* gland) laryngopharyngitis (larynx) nasopharyngitis (*nasus* nose) rhinopharyngitis (also called *nasopharyngitis*) (*rhinos* nose) tonsillopharyngitis (tonsils) *pharyngo*: staphylopharyngorrhaphy (*staphyle* uvula + *rhaphy* to suture) CROSS REFERENCE: None
phas			See phan- for *phase, phasmophobia*.
phas	Greek *phanai*	to speak, say	PREFIXED ROOT: aphasia (absence or impairment of the ability to communicate through speech) (*a* privative) bradyphasia (also called *bradylalia, bradyphemia*) (*bradys* slow) cataphasia (a speech disorder in which the patient constantly or repeatedly utters the same word or phrase; also called *verbigeration*) (*kata* down) dysphasia (also called *dysphrasia*) (*dys* abnormal) heterophasia (or, heterophasis; the uttering of words other than those intended by the speaker) (*heteros* other) paraphasia (partial aphasia; also called *paraphemia, paraphrasia*) {paraphasic} (*para* abnormal + aphasia) tachyphasia (also called *logorrhea*) (*tachys* swift) TRAILING ROOT COMPOUND: ataxiaphasia (a type of agrammatism in which some necessary elements for coherent sentences are lacking; also called *syntactical aphasia*) (*ataxia* disorder; *a* negative + *taxos* order) dactylophasia (communication between individuals, especially, the deaf, using signs made with the hands and fingers; also called *signing, cheirology, dactylology*) (*dactyl* finger) schizophasia (also called *word salad*) (*schizein* to split) tonaphasia (tone + aphasia) CROSS REFERENCE: lal, logo, or, phem, phras
phem	Greek *pheme*	voice	PREFIXED ROOT: *phem*: aphemesthesia (failure of word perception; word blindness) (*a* privative + *esthesia* perception) *phemia*: bradyphemia (also called *bradyphasia*) (*bradys* slow) dysphemia (an old term for stuttering or other disorder of psychogenic origin) (*dys* abnormal) heterophemia (also called *heterophasia*) (*heteros* other) paraphemia (aphasia marked by the employment of the wrong words; also called *paraphrasia*) (*para* alongside) tachyphemia (also called *tachyphasia*) (*tachys* swift) TRAILING ROOT COMPOUND: ataxiophemia (also called *dysarthria*) (*ataxia* disorder: *a* negative + *taxis* order) CROSS REFERENCE: phas, phon[1]
phen			See phan- for *phenology, phenoscopy*.
pher			See phor- for *periphery*.
pheresis			See apheres- for *cytapheresis*, and others.

A Thesaurus of Medical Word Roots

Element	From	Meaning	Examples
phil	Greek *philein* to love	loving, love of; have an affinity for	SIMPLE ROOT: philtrum (a philter or love potion; pl., philtra) PREFIXED ROOT: amphophil {amphophilic, amphophilous} (*ampho* both, around) heterophil (or, heterophile) {heterophilic} (*heteros* other, different) homophil {homophilic} (*homos* same) mesophil {mesophilic} (*mesos* middle) paraphilia {paraphiliac} (*para* abnormal) LEADING ROOT COMPOUND: *phil*: philiater (a person interested in medical science; particularly, a medical student) (*iatreia* healing) *philo*: philomimesia (a morbid impulse to mimic) (*mimesis* imitation) philoprogenitive (procreative; producing offspring) (*pro* before + *genere* to produce) TRAILING ROOT COMPOUND: *phil*: chromatophil {chromatophilic} (*chromatos* color) eosinophil (*eos* dawn: rose-colored) erythrophil (*erythros* red) *phile*: cryophile (also called *psychrophile*) {cryophilic} (*kryos* cold) thermophile (*therme* heat) *philia*: calciphilia (calcium) eosinophilia (*eos* dawn: rose-colored) gerontophilia (*gerontos* old age) glycophilia (*glykys* sweet) hydrophilia (*hydor* water) lipophilia (*lipos* fat) mysophilia (*mysos* uncleanness) necrophilia (or, necrophilism) (*nekros* dead body, corpse) opsonophilia (attraction for opsonins) pharmacophilia (*pharmikos* medicine, drug) thrombophilia (*thrombos* clot) *philiac*: hemophiliac (*haima* blood) *philic*: acidophilic (also called *oxyphilic*) (*acidus* sharp) aerophilic (*aer* air) anthropophilic (preferring humans, as parasites) (*anthropos* human beings) barophilic (*baros* weight*)* basophilic (basis) coprophilic (*kopros* dung, filth) crymophilic (also called *psychrophilic*) (*krymos* frost) cryophilic (also called *psychrophilic*) (*kryos* cold) cytophilic (*kytos* cell) eosinophilic (*eos* dawn: rose-colored) halophilic (*hals* salt) hemophilic (*haima* blood) hydrophilic (*hydor* water) lipophilic (*lipos* fat) lyophilic (*lyein* to dissolve) necrophilic (*nekros* dead body, corpse)

Element	From	Meaning	Examples
phil (cont'd)		[love of]	neurophilic (also called *neurotropic*) (*neuron* nerve) nucelophilic (nucleus) organophilic (attraction for certain organs) osmophilic (osmosis) oxyphilic (also called *acidophilic*) (*oxys* sharp) photophilic (*photos* light) psychrophilic (also called *crymophilic*) (*psychros* cold) serophilic (*serum* whey) toxophilic (*toxikon* poison) *philous*: aerophilous (*aer* air) saprophilous (*sapros* rotten) siderophilous (*sideros* iron) CROSS REFERENCE: None
phleb	Greek *phleps, phlebos* blood vessel	vein	SIMPLE ROOT: phlebismus (obstruction and consequent dilation of veins) PREFIXED ROOT: *phlebitis* inflammation of a vein or veins: endophlebitis (also called *endovenitis*) (*endon* within) mesophlebitis (*mesos* middle) periphlebitis {periphlebitic} (*peri* around) LEADING ROOT COMPOUND: *phleb*: phlebalgia (pain originating in a vein) (*algos* pain) phlebanesthesia (also called *phlebonarcosis*) (*an* negative + *esthesia* feeling) phlebangioma (*angeion* blood vessel + *oma* tumor) phlebarteriectasia (*arteria* artery + *ektasis* dilatation) phlebectasis (also called *varicosity*) (*ektasis* dilatation) phlebectomy (*ektome* excision) phlebectopia (*ektopia* displacement) phlebemphraxis (*emphraxis* obstruction) phlebitis {phlebitic} (*itis* inflammation) phleboid (*eidos* form) phlebosis (*osis* condition) *phlebo*: phleboclysis (*klysis* injection) phlebodynamics (*dynamis* power) phlebofibrosis (*fibra* fiber + *osis* condition) phlebogenous (*genere* to originate) phlebogram, phlebography (*graphein* to write) phlebolite (or, phlebolith), phlebolithiasis (*lithos* stone + *iasis* condition) phlebology (*logos* study) phlebomanometer (*manos* thin + *metron* measure) phlebometritis (*metra* uterus + *itis* inflammation) phlebomyomatosis (myoma + *osis* condition) phlebonarcosis (narcosis produced by intravenous injections) phlebophlebostomy (operative anastomosis of vein to vein) (*stoma* mouth, opening) phlebopiezometry (*piesis* pressure + *metron* measure) phleboplasty (*plassein* to form) phleborrhaphy (also called *venisuture*) (*rhaphe* suture)

Element	From	Meaning	Examples
phleb (cont'd)		[vein]	phleborrhexis (*rhexis* rupture)
			phlebosclerosis (also called *phlebofibrosis, venosclerosis*) (*sklerosis* hardening)
			phlebostasis (*stasis* a standing still)
			phlebostenosis (*stenosis* constriction, narrow)
			phlebothrombosis (*thrombosis* a clotting)
			phlebotomy (*tomy* incision)
			TRAILING ROOT COMPOUND:
			phleb: pylephlebectasis (dilatation of the portal vein) (*pyle* gate + *ektasis* dilatation)
			phlebitis inflammation of a vein:
			celophlebitis (also called *cavitis*) (*koilos* hollow)
			dermophlebitis (*derma* skin)
			galactophlebitis (*galaktos* milk)
			hepatophlebitis (*hepatos* liver)
			metrophlebitis (*metra* uterus)
			omphalophlebitis (*omphalos* navel)
			osteophlebitis (*osteon* bone)
			pyelophlebitis (*pyelos* pelvis)
			pylephlebitis (*pyle* gate, portal vein)
			thrombophlebitis (*thrombos* clot)
			varicophlebitis (*varix* varicose veins)
			PREFIXED TRAILING ROOT COMPOUND: peripylephlebitis (*peri* around + *pyle* gate + phlebitis)
			CROSS REFERENCE: cirs, vari, ven
phleg, phlog	Greek *phlegein* to burn	flame, fever; inflammation	SIMPLE ROOT:
			phleg:
			phlegm (as a single word, *phlegm* has come to mean "body moisture," thought by the early Greeks to be caused by inflammation) {phlegmatic: calm, apathetic, unexcitable}
			phlegmasia (also called *phlegmonosis*), phlegmon, phlegmonous
			phlog: phlogistic, phlogiston, phlogotic (inflammatory)
			PREFIXED ROOT:
			phleg: apophlegmatic (causing a discharge of mucus; expectorant) (*apo* from)
			phlog: antiphlogistic (counteracting both inflammation and fever) (*anti* against)
			LEADING ROOT COMPOUND:
			phlegmon: phlegmonosis (also called *phlegmasia*) (*osis* condition)
			phlog: phlogosis (inflammation of the external parts of the body) (*osis* condition)
			phlogo:
			phlogogenic (or, phlogogenous) (*genere* to originate)
			phlogotherapy (also called *nonspecific therapy*)
			TRAILING ROOT COMPOUND: adenophlegmon (phlegmonous adenitis) (*adenos* gland)
			CROSS REFERENCE: caum, itis, pyr, therm
phlog			See phlegm-.
phob	Greek *phobos* fear, flight	morbid fear; dislike of	SIMPLE ROOT: phobia, phobiac, phobic
			TRAILING ROOT COMPOUND:
			[Phobias are listed with the roots to which they are attached.]
			[Phobias listed by that which is feared. Because there are hundreds of phobias, those listed pertain only to medical issues.]
			air (aerophobia)

Element	From	Meaning	Examples
phob (cont'd)		[morbid fear; dislike of]	all (omniphobia)
			bleeding, blood (hematophobia, hemophobia)
			blushing (ereuthophobia, erythrophobia)
			brain disease (meningitophobia)
			cadaver (necrophobia)
			cancer (cancerophobia, carcinomatophobia, carcinophobia)
			childbirth (maieusiophobia, parturiphobia, tocophobia)
			choking (anginophobia, pnigophobia)
			contamination (molysmophobia)
			corpse (necrophobia)
			death (necrophobia, thanatophobia)
			deformed infant, bearing a (teratophobia)
			deformity (dysmorphophobia)
			diabetes (diabetophobia)
			disease (nosophobia, pathophobia)
			drugs (pharmacophobia)
			eating (phagophobia, sitophobia)
			eyes (ommatophobia)
			feces (coprophobia)
			female sex (gynephobia)
			fever (febriphobia, pyrexiophobia)
			food (cibophobia, sitophobia)
			heart disease (cardiophobia)
			homosexual behavior, homosexuals (homophobia)
			infection (molysmophobia)
			injury (traumatophobia)
			insanity (lyssophobia, maniaphobia)
			insects (entomophobia)
			marriage (gamophobia)
			meningitis (meningitophobia)
			microorganisms (microphobia)
			nudity (gymnophobia, nudophobia)
			old people (gerontophobia)
			pain (algophobia, odynophobia, ponophobia)
			parasites (parasitophobia, phthiriophobia)
			pointed objects (aichurophobia, belonepobia)
			protein food (proteinophobia)
			rectal disease (proctophobia, rectophobia)
			sex and sexuality (erotophobia, genophobia)
			sexual intercourse (coitophobia)
			skin diseases (dermatosiophobia)
			skin irritations, skin lesions (dermatophobia)
			sleep, falling to (hypnophobia)
			solitude (autophobia, eremophobia, monophobia)
			speaking, or hearing one's own voice (glossophobia, laliophobia, lalophobia, phonophobia)
			spiders (arachnephobia, arachnophobia)
			trauma (traumatophobia)
			tuberculosis (phthisiophobia)
			venereal disease (venereophobia)
			vomiting (emetophobia)
			women (gynephobia)
			CROSS REFERENCE: None

Element	From	Meaning	Examples
phon	Greek *phone* sound	sound; sound of the voice	SIMPLE ROOT: phon (a unit of the subjective loudness of sound) phonal, phonation {phonatory} phoneme {phonemic}, phonetic, phonetics (also called *phonology*) phonic (relating to the voice or to sound) PREFIXED ROOT: *phonia*: aphonia (inability to produce speech sounds from the larynx; also called *dysphonia, mutism*) {aphonic, aphonous} (*a* privative) diphonia (also called *double voice*) (*di* two) diplophonia (also called *diphthongia*) (*diploos* double) dysphonia {dysphonic} (*dys* abnormal) heterophonia (*heteros* other) hyperphonia (*hyper* above) hypophonia (also called *leptophonia, microphonia*) (*hypo* below) microphonia (also called *hypophonia, leptophonia*) (*mikros* small) paraphonia (morbid alteration of the voice) (*para* abnormal) *phono*: aphonogelia (inability to laugh aloud) (*a* privative + *gelos* laughter) microphonoscope (*mikros* small + *skopein* to examine) *phony*: autophony (also called *tympanophony*) (*autos* self) dysphony (*dys* abnormal) microphony (*mikros* small) orthophony (*orthos* straight) LEADING ROOT COMPOUND: *phon*: phonacoscopy (*akouein* to listen + *skopein* to examine) phonasthenia (*a* negative + *sthenos* strength: weakness) phonendoscope (a stethoscope that intensifies sound) (*endon* within + *skopein* to examine) phoniatrics (*iatrein* to heal) phonopsia (the subjective perception of color sensations upon hearing certain sounds) (*opsia* vision condition) *phono*: phonoangiography (*angeion* blood vessel + *graphein* to write) phonocardiogram, phonocardiograph, phonocardiography (*kardia* heart + *graphein* to write) phonocatheter (catheter: *kata* down + *hienai* to send) phonogram (*graphein* to write) phonometer (*metron* measure) phonomyoclonus (*myos* muscle + *klonos* tumult) phonomyogram (a tracing of the sound produced by muscle action), phonomyography (*myos* muscle + *graphein* to write) phonopathy (*pathos* disease) phonophobia (*phobia* fear) phonophore (an ossicle of the ear; also, a kind of stethoscope that renders the sounds more audible) (*pherein* to carry) phonoscope, phonoscopy (*skopein* to examine) TRAILING ROOT COMPOUND: *phone*: cardiophone (*kardia* heart) myophone (*myos* muscle)

A Thesaurus of Medical Word Roots

Element	From	Meaning	Examples
phon (cont'd)		[sound]	optophone (*optos* sight) ossiphone (*ossis* bone) siderophone (*sideros* iron) *phonia*: leptophonia (also called *hypophonia, microphonia*) (*leptos* thin) misophonia (*misein* to hate) mogiphonia (also called *dysphonia*) (*mogis* with difficulty) neurophonia (*neuron* nerve) nyctaphonia (elective mutism with loss of voice during the night) (*nyctos* night + aphonia) nyctophonia (elective mutism with loss of voice during the day but not at night) (*nyctos* night) odynophonia (*odyne* pain) olophonia (*oloos* destroyed, lost) oxyphonia (a sharp quality to the voice) (*oxys* sharp, keen) plegaphonia (*plessein* to strike + aphonia) pneumophonia (*pneuma* breath) rhinophonia (also called *rhinism, rhinolalia*) (*rhinos* nose) trachyphonia (also called *hoarseness*) (*trachys* rough) tragophonia (also called *egophony*) (*tragos* goat) xenophonia (*xenos* strange, foreign) *phono*: stethophonometer (*stethos* chest + *metron* measure) *phony*: bronchophony (*bronchos* windpipe) echophony (*echo* a returned sound) egophony (also called *tragophonia*) (*aix* goat) gutturophony (*guttur* throat) osteophony (*osteon* bone) pectorophony (also called *pectoriloquy*) (*pectus* chest) tracheophony (*trachea* windpipe) tragophony (also called *egophony*) (*tragos* goat) tympanophony (also called *autophony*) (*tympanon* drum) CROSS REFERENCE: phem, son
phor, **pher**	Greek *pherein*	to carry, to bear	SIMPLE ROOT: pheresis (a procedure in which blood is removed from a donor) phoresis (or, phoresy; also called *electrophoresis*) PREFIXED ROOT: *pher*: apheresis (*a* reversal) [see separate listing: apheres-] peripherad (in the direction of the periphery) peripherocentral (both peripheral and central) periphery (outer part or surface of the body; the part away from the center) {peripheral, peripheric} (*peri* around) *phora*: cataphora (semicoma) (*kata* down) epiphora (an abnormal overflow of tears down the cheek, mainly due to stricture of the lacrimal passages; also called *illacrimation*) (*epi* upon) paraphora (a slight mental disorder) (*para* abnormal) *phoresis*: adiaphoresis (deficiency or absence of sweat; also called *anhidrosis*) (*a* privative + diaphoresis) anaphoresis (diminished activity of the sweat glands) (*ana* up)

Element	From	Meaning	Examples
phor (cont'd)		[to carry]	cataphoresis (cataphoretic} (*kata* down)

diaphoresis (lit., to carry through; perspiration, especially when pro-
   fuse; also called *sudoresis*) {diaphoretic} (*dia* across)

eudiaphoresis (*eu* well + diaphoresis)

hemidiaphoresis (also called *hemihyperidrosis*) (*hemi* half + diaphoresis)

phoria:

adiaphoria (*a* negative + *dia* through)

anaphoria (a tendency for the visual axes of both eyes to divert above
   the horizontal plane) (*ana* again)

anisophoria (*aniso* unequal: *an* negative + *isos* equal)

anophoria (also called *hyperphoria*) (*ano* upward)

cataphoria (or, katophoria) (*kata* down)

dysphoria {dysphoric} (*dys* abnormal)

esophoria (deviation of a visual axis toward that of the other eye when
   fusion is prevented) {esophoric} (*eso* inward)

euphoria (exaggerated feeling of well-being) {euphoretic, euphoric,
   euphoristic}, euphorigenic (*eu* well + *genere* to produce)

exophoria (deviation of a visual axis away from that of the other eye)
   {exophoric} (*exo* outside)

heterophoria {heterophoric} (*heteros* other)

hyperesophoria (*hyper* above + esophoria)

hyperexophoria (*hyper* above + exophoria)

hyperphoria (also called *anophoria*) (*hyper* above)

hypoesophoria (*hypo* under + esophoria)

hypoexophoria (*hypo* under + exophoria)

hypophoria (*hypo* under)

incyclophoria (*in* in + *kyklos* circle)

isophoria (equality in the tension of the vertical muscles of each eye)
   (*isos* equal)

periphoria (tendency of the axis of the eye to deviate from the normal due to the weakness of oblique muscles; also called *cyclo-
   phoria*) (*peri* around)

phorize: ecphorize (a bringing back of the effect of a psychic experience in an attempt to experience it again in memory) (*ek* out)

phorous: adiaphorous (neutral or indifferent; in medicine, neither
   harmful nor helpful) (*a* negative + *dia* across)

LEADING ROOT COMPOUND:

phero: pheromone (hormone)

phor: phoront (*ontos* being)

phoro:

phoroblast (also called *fibroblast*) (*blastos* bud, shoot, germ)

phorocyte (a connective tissue cell), phorocytosis (proliferation of
   connective tissue cells) (*kytos* cell + *osis* condition)

phorometer, phorometry (*metron* measure)

phoroscope (*skopein* to examine)

phorotone (device for exercising eye muscles) (*tonos* tension)

TRAILING ROOT COMPOUND:

phore:

chromophore (*chroma* color)

melanophore (*melas* dark, black)

oophore [not a word itself; see separate entry: oophor-]

ozonophore (*ozein* to smell)

Element	From	Meaning	Examples
phor (cont'd)		[to carry]	siderophore (*sideros* iron)
			spermatophore (*spermatos* seed, sperm)
			sporophore (*sporos* seed, spore)
			thermophore (*therme* heat)
			toxophore (*toxikon* poison)
			xanthophore (*xanthos* yellow)
			phoria:
			cyclophoria (also called *periphoria*) (*kyklos* circle)
			orthophoria {orthophoric} (*orthos* straight)
			phoric:
			chylophoric (also called *chyliferous*) (*chylus* juice)
			chromophoric (*chroma* color)
			phorous:
			adenophorous (*adenos* gland)
			calcophorous (also called *calciferous*) (calcium)
			cystophorous (*kystis* sac, bladder)
			galactophorous (*galaktos* milk)
			phosphorus {phosphorous} (*phos* light)
			CROSS REFERENCE: fer, ger[1]
phos, **phot**	Greek *phos, photos*	light	SIMPLE ROOT:
			phose (any subjective visual sensation, as of light or color)
			phosis (the production of a phose)
			photic (relating to light), photism
			photon (a corpuscle of energy or particle of light)
			PREFIXED ROOT:
			aphose {aphotic} (*a* privative)
			aphotesthesia (*a* privative + *esthesia* perception)
			LEADING ROOT COMPOUND:
			phos:
			phosgenic (producing light) (*genesis* origin)
			phosphene (*phanein* to show)
			phosphorous (*phorein* to bear) [see separate entry: phosphor-]
			phot:
			photalgia (also called *photodynia, photophobia*) (*algos* pain)
			photaugiaphobia (morbid fear of, or overreaction to, a glare of light)
			photerythrous (also called *deuteranopic*) (*erythros* red)
			photesthesis (or, photesthesia) (*esthesis* feeling, sensation)
			photodynia (also called *photalgia*) (*odyne* pain)
			photophthalmia (*ophthalmia* eye condition)
			photopia (also called *photopic vision, day vision*) (*opia* vision condition)
			photopsia (or, photopsy) (*opsia* vision condition)
			photo:
			photoactinic (*aktis* ray)
			photoautotroph {photoautotrophic} (*autos* self + *trophein* to nourish)
			photobiotic (*bios* life + *osis* condition)
			photocatalysis (the promotion or stimulation of a reaction by light)
			photocutaneous (*cutis* skin)
			photodermatitis (*dermatos* skin + *itis* inflammation)
			photodromy (*dromos* running)
			photodynamic (*dynamis* power)
			photodysphoria (*dys* abnormal + *phorein* to bear)

Element	From	Meaning	Examples
phos (cont'd)		[light]	photoerythema (*erythema* blush)
			photoesthetic (*esthesis* sensation, feeling)
			photofluorography (*fluor* a flow + *graphein* to write)
			photogastroscope (*gaster* stomach, belly + *skopein* to examine)
			photogen, photogenesis {photogenic, photogeneous} (*genere* to produce)
			photography (*graphein* to write)
			photohemotachometer (*haima* blood + *tachos* speed + *metron* measure)
			photoheterotroph {photoheterotrophic} (*heteros* other + *trophein* to nourish)
			photokinesis {photokinetic} (*kinein* to move)
			photokymograph (*kyma* wave + *graphein* to write)
			photolithotroph (*lithos* stone, mineral + *trophein* to nourish)
			photoluminescent (*lumen* light)
			photolysis {photolytic} (*lyein* to dissolve)
			photomacrography (*makros* large + *graphein* to write)
			photomania (*mania* frenzy, craze)
			photometer {photometry} (*metron* measure)
			photomicrograph (*mikros* small + *graphein* to write)
			photomyoclonus (*myos* muscle + *klonus* turmoil)
			photopathy (*pathos* disease)
			photoperceptive (*per* through + *capere* to hold)
			photophilic (*philein* to love—have an affinity for)
			photophobia (also called *photalgia*) (*phobia* fear)
			photophore (*phorein* to bear)
			photopigment (*pingere* to paint: color)
			photoptarmosis (*ptarmosis* sneezing condition)
			photoradiation (also called *photochemotherapy*)
			photoretinopathy (retina + *pathos* suffering, disease)
			photoscope (a kind of fluoroscope), photoscopy (*skopein* to examine)
			photostethoscope (*sthethos* chest + *skopein* to examine)
			photosynthesis (*synthesis* a putting together)
			phototaxis {phototactic} (*taxis* arrangement)
			phototherapy (*therapy* treatment)
			photothermal (*therme* heat)
			phototoxicity {phototoxic} (*toxic* poisonous)
			phototrophic (*trophe* nourishment)
			phototropism {phototropic} (*trepein* to turn)
			TRAILING ROOT COMPOUND:
			antrophose (*antrum* sinus)
			centrophose (*kentron* point, center)
			chromophose (*chroma* color)
			cyanophose (*kyanos* blue)
			erythrophose (*erythros* red)
			CROSS REFERENCE: lum
phosphor	Greek *phos* light + *pherein* to bear	phosphorus	SIMPLE ROOT:
			phosphorism (also called *chronic phosphorus poisoning*)
			phosphorated (charged or combined with phosphorus)
			phosphoresence (the emission of light without appreciable heat) {phosphorescent}
			phosphorus (a nonmetallic element not found in a free state but in combination with alkalies) {phosphorous}

A Thesaurus of Medical Word Roots

Element	From	Meaning	Examples
phosphor (cont'd)		[phosphorus]	LEADING ROOT COMPOUND: *phosph*: phosphuria (or, phosphoruria) (*uria* urine condition) *phospho*: phospholipid, phospholipidemia (*lipos* fat + *emia* blood condition) phosphonecrosis (also called *phosphorous necrosis, phossy jaw*) (*nekros* dead + *osis* condition) phosphopenia (or, phosphorpenia) (*penia* deficiency) *phosphor*: phosphorhidrosis (or, phosphoridrosis; the secretion of luminous sweat) (*hidrosis* perspiration) phosphorpenia (or, phosphopenia) (*penia* deficiency) phosphoruria (or, phosphuria) (*uria* urine condition) CROSS REFERENCE: None
phot			See phos- for *photalgia*.
phragm, phrax	Greek *phragmos*	enclosure; wall off; stop up	PREFIXED ROOT: *phragm*: diaphragm, diaphragma [see separate entry: diaphragm] mesophragma (*mesos* middle) *phrax*: emphraxis (*en* in) [see separate entry: emphrax-] LEADING ROOT COMPOUND: phragmoplast (the barrel-shaped spindle within which the midbody forms in mitosis) (*plassein* to form) TRAILING ROOT COMPOUND: inophragma (*inos* fiber) telophragma (*telos* the end) CROSS REFERENCE: diaphragm, phren[1], sept
phras	Greek *phrazein* to show, explain, speak	speech; to speak	PREFIXED ROOT: aphrasia (inability to speak or understand phrases) (*a* privative) dysphrasia (also called *dysphasia*) (*dys* abnormal) hyperphrasia (also called *logorrhea*) (*hyper* over, above) hypophrasia (slowness or lack of speech associated with a psychosis or brain injury) (*hypo* under) palinphrasia (or, paliphrasia) (*palin* again, backward) paraphrasia (partial aphrasia; speech defect marked by disorderly arrangement of spoken words; also called *paraphasia*) (*para* abnormal) polyphrasia (also called *logorrhea*) (*polys* much) pyknophrasia (thickness of speech) (*pyknos* thick) tachyphrasia (also called *logorrhea*) (*tachys* swift) TRAILING ROOT COMPOUND: bradyphrasia (also called *bradylalia, bradyphrenia*) (*bradys* slow) echophrasia (a stereotyped repetition, or echoing of another person's words or phrases; also called *echolalia*) embolophrasia (the interpolation of meaningless words into speech; also called *embololalia*) (*emballein* to throw in) CROSS REFERENCE: lingu, or, phas
phrax			See phragm- for *emphraxis*.
phren[1]	Greek *phrenicus*	diaphragm	SIMPLE ROOT: phren {phrenic; also called *diaphragmatic*} [The *phrenic nerve* is the nerve chiefly supplying the diaphragm.] *Phrenic* is also listed under phren[2]. PREFIXED ROOT: *phrenal*: epiphrenal (or, epiphrenic) (*epi* upon) *phrenia*: paraphrenia {paraphrenic} (*para* alongside)

Element	From	Meaning	Examples
phren[1] (cont'd)		[diaphragm]	*phrenic*:

phrenic:
epiphrenic (or, epiphrenal) (*epi* upon)
hypophrenic (also called *subphrenic, hypodiaphragmatic, subdiaphragmatic*) (*hypo* below)
subphrenic (situated inferior to the diaphragm; also called *hypophrenic, hypodiaphragmatic, subdiaphragmatic*) (*sub* below)
phrenitis inflammation of the diaphragm:
paraphrenitis (inflammation of the tissues around the diaphragm; also called *periphrenitis*) (*para* beside)
periphrenitis (inflammation of the diaphragm and the structures around it; also called *paraphrenitis*) (*peri* around)
LEADING ROOT COMPOUND:
phren:
phrenalgia (also called *diaphragmalgia, phrenodynia*) (*algos* pain) [another is listed under phren[2]]
phrenectomy (or, phreniectomy; exsection of a portion of the phrenic nerve, to prevent reunion such as may follow phrenicotomy) (*ektome* excision)
phrenemphraxis (crushing of the phrenic nerve with a clamp; also called *phreniclasia*) (*emphraxis* stoppage)
phrenitis (*itis* inflammation)
phrenodynia (also called *phrenalgia, diaphragmalgia*) (*odyne* pain)
phreni: phreniclasia (or, phreniclasis; crushing of the phrenic nerve with a clamp; also called *phrenicotripsy*) (*klaein* to break)
phrenic: phrenicectomy (*ektome* excision)
phrenico:
phrenicocolic (or, phrenocolic) (colon)
phrenicoexeresis (excision of part of the phrenic nerve; also called *phrenectomy*) (*exeresis* taking out)
phrenicogastric (or, phrenogastric) (*gaster* stomach, belly)
phrenicoglottic (*glossa* tongue)
phrenicohepatic (*hepatos* liver)
phreniconeurectomy (*neuron* nerve + *ektome* excision)
phrenicosplenic (spleen)
phrenicotomy (surgical division of the phrenic nerve) (*tomy* incision)
phrenicotripsy (crushing of the phrenic nerve; also called *phreniclasia*) (*tribein* to crush)
phreno:
phrenocolic (or, phrenicocolic) (colon)
phrenogastric (or, phrenicogastric) (*gaster* stomach, belly)
phrenoglottic (*glossa* tongue)
phrenograph (*graphein* to write)
phrenohepatic (or, phrenicohepatic) (*hepatos* liver)
phrenoplegia (also called *diaphragmatic paralysis*) (*plessein* to strike)
phrenoptosia (*ptein* to fall)
phrenospasm (*spasmos* contraction)
phrenosplenic (*splen* spleen)
phrenotropic (*tropic* turning)
TRAILING ROOT COMPOUND:
phrenia: cardiophrenia (also called *phrenocardia*) (*kardia* heart)
phrenic:
cardiophrenic (*kardia* heart)

Element	From	Meaning	Examples
phren[1] (cont'd)		[diaphragm]	costophrenic (*costa* rib) electrophrenic gastrophrenic (*gaster* stomach, belly) musculophrenic (muscle) pericardiophrenic (pericardium) splenophrenic (*splen* spleen) CROSS REFERENCE: diaphragm, phragm
phren[2]	Greek *phren*	mind, brain	SIMPLE ROOT: phren {phrenetic; or, frenetic; phrenic} *Phrenic is* also listed under phren[1]. PREFIXED ROOT: hyperphrenia (excessive mental activity) (*hyper* over, above) hypophrenia {hypophrenic} (*hypo* below) paraphrenia {paraphrenic} (*para* alongside) LEADING ROOT COMPOUND: phrenalgia (*algos* pain) [another is listed under phren[1]] phrenocardia (also called *cardiophrenia*) (*kardia* heart) phrenology (*logos* study) phrenotropic (*trope* a turning) TRAILING ROOT COMPOUND: *phrenia*: bradyphrenia (*bradys* slow) hebephrenia {hebephrenic} (*hebe* youth) oligophrenia (defective mental development) (*oligos* little) orthophrenia (soundness of mind) (*orthos* straight) presbyophrenia (*presbys* old age) schizophrenia {schizophrenic} (*schizein* to split) somatophrenia (*somatos* body) *phrenic*: idiophrenic (relating to, or originating in, the mind or brain alone, not reflex or secondary) (*idios* one's own) CROSS REFERENCE: cerebr, psych, thym[2]
phthis	Greek *phthiein* to decay	wasting away	SIMPLE ROOT: phthisis (a wasting away of the body or a part of the body; old name for *pulmonary tuberculosis*) PREFIXED ROOT: antiphthisic (*anti* against) TRAILING ROOT COMPOUND: gastrophthisis (emaciation due to abdominal disease) (*gaster* stomach, belly) laryngophthisis (also called *laryngeal tuberculosis*) (larynx) limophthisis (also called *inanition*) (*limos* hunger) myelophthisis (also called *bone marrow suppression*) {myelophthisic} (*myelos* marrow) nephrophthisis (*nephros* kidney) ophthalmophthisis (also called *ophthalmomalacia*) (*ophthalmos* eye) PREFIXED TRAILING ROOT COMPOUND: panmyelophthisis (also called *aplastic anema*) (*pan* all + *myelos* marrow) CROSS REFERENCE: atroph
phylax, **phylact**	Greek *phylassein* to guard	prevention, guard against, ward off	SIMPLE ROOT: phylaxis (the active defense of the body against infection) {phylactic} PREFIXED ROOT: *phylactic*: anaphylactic (pertaining to anaphylaxis) (*ana* completely) prophylactic (a condom, that which is designed to prevent sexually transmittable diseases; as an adjective, that which is preventative, as *prophylactic medicine, prophylactic dentistry*) (*pro* before)

Element	From	Meaning	Examples
phylax (cont'd)		[prevention]	*phylacto*: anaphylactogenesis (*ana* completely + *genere* to produce) anaphylatoxin (*ana* completely + *toxin* poison) *phylaxia*: dysphylaxia (a type of insomnia marked by awakening too early) (*dys* abnormal) *phylaxis*: aphylaxis (also called *nonimmunity*) {aphylactic} (*a* privative) ananaphylaxis (the reduction or abolition of allergic sensitivity or reactions to the specific antigen, or allergen; also called *antianaphylaxis*) (*an* negative + *ana* again) anaphylaxis (systemic or generalized anaphylactic shock) {anaphylactic} (*ana* completely) apophylaxis (decrease of the phylactic power of the blood) (*apo* from, away) cataphylaxis (the process of carrying antibodies and leukocytes to the site of an infection) (*kata* down) epiphylaxis (increase or reinforcement of normal phylaxis, as seen in the positive phase by opsonic or vaccine therapy) (*epi* upon) miniprophylaxis (*mini* small + prophylaxis) prophylaxis (the prevention of or protective treatment for disease; in dentistry, cleaning the teeth's surface; pl., prophylaxes) (*pro* before) LEADING ROOT COMPOUND: phylacagogic (stimulating the production of protective antibodies) (*agein* to lead) TRAILING ROOT COMPOUND: *phylactic*: calciphylactic (calcium) crymophylactic (also called *cryophylactic*) (*krymos* frost) cryophylactic (also called *crymophylactic*) (*kryos* cold) pyophylactic (providng protection against purulent infections, such as administering an antibiotic before the onset of an infection) (*pyon* pus) *phylaxis*: biophylaxis {biophylactic} (*bios* life) calciphylaxis (*calx, calcis* lime, calcium) chemoprophylaxis (disease prevention by use of chemicals or drugs) cytophylaxis (also called *cytoprotection*) {cytophylactic} (*kytos* cell) dermatophylaxis (*dermatos* skin) pseudoanaphylaxis (*pseudes* false + anaphylaxis) psychoprophylaxis (*psyche* mind + prophylaxis) radiophylaxis (radium) tachyphylaxis (a swiftly developed tolerance to a drug achieved through repeated exposure to minute doses) (*tachys* rapid) CROSS REFERENCE: None
phyma	Greek *phyein* to grow	tumor, growth	SIMPLE ROOT: phyma (a small, rounded skin tumor; pl., phymata) PREFIXED ROOT: ecphyma (a warty growth or protuberance) (*ek* out) LEADING ROOT COMPOUND: *phymat*: phymatoid (resembling a tumor or a phyma) (*eidos* form) phymatosis (*osis* condition) *phymato*: phymatology (*logos* study)

Element	From	Meaning	Examples
phyma (cont'd)		[tumor]	phymatorrhysin (or, phymatorhusin; a dark pigment from hair and melanotic tumors) (*rhysis* flow) TRAILING ROOT COMPOUND: arthrophyma (the swelling of a joint) (*arthron* joint) hepatophyma (*hepatos* liver) onychophyma (swelling or hypertrophy of the nails) (*onychos* nail) osteophyma (also called *osteophyte*) (*osteon* bone) rhinophyma (*rhinos* nose) tenontophyma (*tenontos* tendon) trachelophyma (*trachelos* neck) urethrophyma (urethra) CROSS REFERENCE: cel^2, gangli, oma, onc, tub^2, tum
phys^1	Greek *phyein* to grow, produce	nature, growth, physical	SIMPLE ROOT: physeal (pertaining to growth, or to the segment of tubular bone which is concerned mainly with growth) physic, physical, physician, physicist, physics, physique physis (the segment of tubular bone concerned with the growth in length of the bone) {physial} PREFIXED ROOT: *phyodont* tooth growth or development: diphyodont (having two dentitions, a primary and a permanent one) (*di* two) monophyodont (*monos* single) polyphyodont (developing several sets of teeth successively throughout life) (*polys* many) *physio*: extraphysiologic (*extra* outside + *logos* study) *physis*: apophysis (*apo* from) [see separate listing: apophys-] diaphysis (the portion of a long bone between the ends or extremities; pl., diaphyses) {diaphysial}, diaphysisitis (*dia* across + *itis* inflammation) epiphysis (pl., epiphyses) (*epi* upon) [see separate entry: epiphys-] hypophysis (lit., undergrowth; the pituitary gland of the body) {hypophysial; also called *pituitary*} (*hypo* under) metaphysis (pl., metaphyses) {metaphyseal} (*meta* after) paraphysis (also called *paraphyseal body*; pl., paraphases) {paraphyseal, paraphysial} (*para* alongside) prehypophysis {prehypophysial} (*pre* before + hypophysis) symphysis (lit., a growing together; natural junction; pl., symphyses) (*syn* with, together) *physitis*: metaphysitis (*meta* after + *itis* inflammation) LEADING ROOT COMPOUND: *phys*: physiatrics (the curing of disease by natural methods, especially physical therapy), physiatrician, physiatrist, physiatry (also called *physical medicine*) (*iatrein* to cure) *physio*: physiogenesis (embryology) {physiogenic} (*genesis* origin) physiognosis (or, physiognomy; diagnosis determined from one's physical features) (*gnosis* knowledge) physiology {physiologic, physiological} (*logos* study) physiolysis (*lysis* dissolution) physiopathology {physiopathologic} (*pathos* disease + *logos* study) physiophyly (*phylon* tribe)

Element	From	Meaning	Examples
phys[1] (cont'd)		[nature, growth, physical]	physiopsychic (*psyche* mind) physiopyrexia (*pyrexis* feverishness) physiotherapy {physiotherapeutic} (*therapy* treatment) TRAILING ROOT COMPOUND: *physiology* study of living organisms: biophysiology (*bios* life) histophysiology (*histos* web, tissue) neurophysiology (*neuron* nerve) pathophysiology (*pathos* pain, disease) psychophysiology (*psyche* mind) CROSS REFERENCE: aug, embryo, phyt
phys[2]	Greek *physaein* to blow, inflate *physa* air	gas, air, bubble	SIMPLE ROOT: physalis (a vacuole cavity found in certain cells, such as the giant cells of sarcoma or chordoma; pl., physalides) physallization (the formation of a permanent froth when a liquid is shaken together with a gas) PREFIXED ROOT: emphysema (an inflation; a pathological condition of air in tissues or organs) {emphysematous} (*em* in) LEADING ROOT COMPOUND: *physali*: physaliferous (having bubbles or vacuoles; also called *physaliphorous*) (*ferre* to bear) physaliform (resembling bubbles) (*forma* form) physaliphorous (also called *physaliferous*) (*pherein* to bear) *physo*: physocele (a tumor filled with gas) (*kele* tumor) physocephaly (swelling of the head resulting from introduction of air into the subcutaneous tissues) (*kephale* head) physohematometra (*hematos* blood + *metra* uterus) physohydrometra (*hydor* water + *metra* uterus) physometra (air or gas in the uterine cavity) (*metra* uterus) physopyosalpinx (pus and gas in the fallopian tube) (*pyon* pus + *salpinx* tube) TRAILING ROOT COMPOUND: pyophysometra (*pyon* pus + *metra* uterus) CROSS REFERENCE: aer, pneuma, spir[1]
phyt	Greek *phyton* a plant	a growth; that which grows	PREFIXED ROOT: autophyte (a organism lacking the power of motility) (*autos* self) ectophyte {also called *epiphyte*} (*ektos* outside) endophyte (also called *entophyte*) {endophytic} (*endon* within) entophyte (a parasitic plant organism living within the body of its host; also called *endophyte*) (*entos* within) epiphyte (also called *ectophyte*) {epiphytic} (*epi* upon) exophyte {exophytic} (*exo* outside) microphyte (*mikros* small) LEADING ROOT COMPOUND: *phyt*: phytalbumin (an albumin found in plants and vegetables) phytoid (*eidos* form) phytosis (any disease caused by a phytoparasite) (*osis* condition) *phyto*: phytobezoar (a mass composed of vegetable matter found in the stomach) (Persian *badzahr* concretion)

Element	From	Meaning	Examples
phyt (cont'd)		[a growth]	phytodermatitis (*dermatos* skin + *itis* inflammation)
			phytogenesis (the origin and development of plants) {phytogenous} (*genesis* origin)
			phytonosis (*nosos* disease)
			phytoparasite (parasite: *para* alongside + *sitos* food)
			phytopathogenic (*pathos* disease + *genesis* origin)
			phytophagous (plant-eating; vegetarian) (*phagein* to devour)
			phytotoxin {phytotoxic} (*toxin* poison)
			TRAILING ROOT COMPOUND:
			arthrophyte (an abnormal growth in a joint cavity) (*arthron* joint)
			chondrophyte (*chondros* cartilage)
			dermatophyte (*dermatos* skin)
			gametophyte (the haploid or sexual stage in the antithetic alternations of generations) (*gamos* reproduction)
			nosophyte (*nosos* disease)
			osteophyte (*osteon* bone)
			periosteophyte (periosteum)
			saprophyte (*sapros* rotten)
			sporophyte (*sporos* seed)
			syndesmophyte (*syndesis* bound together: ligament)
			tenophyte (tendon)
			trichophytosis (*trichos* hair + *osis* condition)
			phytosis: dermatophytosis (*dermatos* skin + *osis* condition)
			CROSS REFERENCE: phys[1]
pia	Latin *pia*	tender, soft (membrane)	SIMPLE ROOT: pia (tender; soft; the pia mater) {pial}
			PREFIXED ROOT:
			epipia {epipial; situated upon the pia mater} (*epi* upon)
			interpial (*inter* between)
			intrapial (*intra* within)
			subpial (situated below the pia mater) (*sub* below)
			LEADING ROOT COMPOUND:
			pi:
			piarachnitis (inflammation of the arachnoid and pia mater; also called *leptomeningitis*) (*arachne* spider + *itis* inflammation)
			piarachnoid (the pia mater and arachnoid membranes regarded as one structure; also called *leptomeninges*) (*eidos* form)
			piitis (inflammation of the pia mater) (*itis* inflammation)
			pia:
			pia-glia (a membrane formed by the fusion of the pia mater and the membrana limitans; it constitutes one of the layers of the pia-arachnoid) (*glia* glue)
			pia mater (the innermost of the three membranes covering the brain and the spinal cord) {piamatral} (*mater* mother)
			CROSS REFERENCE: malac, membran
pies, piez	Greek *piezein* to press	pressure	SIMPLE ROOT: piesis (blood pressure)
			PREFIXED ROOT:
			anisopiesis (difference in blood pressure recorded in corresponding arteries on either side of the body) (*aniso* unequal)
			hyperpiesis (also called *hypertension*) {hyperpietic} (*hyper* above)
			hypopiesis (also called *hypotension*) {hypopietic} (*hypo* under)
			LEADING ROOT COMPOUND:
			pies: piesesthesia (pressure sensibility; the sense by which pressure stimuli are felt) (*esthesia* perception)

Element	From	Meaning	Examples
pies (cont'd)		[pressure]	*piesi*: piesimeter (or, piezometer) (*metron* measure) *piez*: piezallochromy (change of color of a substance caused by crushing) (*allos* other + *chroma* color) piezesthesia (or, piesesthesia) (*esthesia* perception, feeling) *piezo*: piezogenic (*genere* to produce) piezometer (or, piesimeter) (*metron* measure) TRAILING ROOT COMPOUND: *pies(o)*: aeropiesotherapy (treatment of disease by compressed air) (*aer* air + *therapy* treatment) retinopiesis (retina) *piezo*: phlebopiezometry (*phlebos* vein + *metron* measure) CROSS REFERENCE: bar
pimel	Greek *pimele*	fat	LEADING ROOT COMPOUND: *pimel*: pimelitis (inflammation of adipose tissue) (*itis* inflammation) pimeloma (also called *lipoma*) (*oma* tumor) pimelorthopnea (difficulty in breathing while lying down, due to excessive fatness; also called *piorthopnea*) (*orthos* straight + *pnein* to breathe) pimelosis (*osis* condition) pimeluria (*uria* urine condition) *pimelo*: pimelopterygium (a fatty outgrowth of the conjunctiva) (*pterygion* wing) pimelorrhea (also called *fatty diarrhea*) (*rhein* to flow) CROSS REFERENCE: adip, ather, lip, stear
pine	Latin *pinea* pine cone	cone; pineal body	SIMPLE ROOT: pineal (pertaining to the pineal body: a glandlike structure in the brain, shaped like a pine cone), pinealism (disorder caused by abnormal secretion of the pineal body) PREFIXED ROOT: *pineal*: parapineal (*para* alongside) subpineal (*sub* under) *pinealism*: apinealism (acquired absence of the pineal gland) (*a* privative) hypopinealism (*hypo* below) LEADING ROOT COMPOUND: *pineal*: pinealectomy (*ektome* excision) pinealoma (*oma* tumor) *pinealo*: pinealoblastoma (also called *pinealoma*) (*blastos* bud + *oma* tumor) pinealocyte, pinealocytoma (a tumor arising in the pineal gland that resembles normal pineal parenchyma) (*kytos* cell + *oma* tumor) pinealopathy (*pathos* disease) *pineo*: pineoblastoma (also called *pinealoblastoma*) (*blastos* germ + *oma* tumor) pineocytoma (also called *pinealoma*) (*kytos* cell + *oma* tumor) CROSS REFERENCE: None

A Thesaurus of Medical Word Roots

Element	From	Meaning	Examples
pituit	Latin *pituita*	phlegm, rheum	SIMPLE ROOT: pituita (a glutinous mucus) {pituitous} pituitarism (disorder of pituitary function) pituitary (or, pituitarium; concerning phlegm; the pituitary body or gland) [see Term] pituitous (pertaining to mucus or characterized by its secretion) PREFIXED ROOT: apituitarism (*a* privative) dyspituitarism (*dys* abnormal) hyperpituitarism (*hyper* over, beyond) hypopituitarism (*hypo* below) LEADING ROOT COMPOUND: pituicyte, pituicytoma (*kytos* cell + *oma* tumor) pituitectomy (also called *hypophysectomy*) (*ektome* excision) TERM: pituitary gland (a small, gray, rounded body attached to the base of the brain; it secretes a number of hormones which regulate growth, reproduction, and various metabolic activities) CROSS REFERENCE: None
placent	Greek *plax* a flat cake	placenta; also, flat, as a plate	SIMPLE ROOT: placenta (a cakelike mass; pl., placentas, placentae) {placental}, placentation PREFIXED ROOT: *placenta*: hemiplacenta (*hemi* half) subplacenta (the decidua basalis) {subplacental} (*sub* under) [decidua basalis: an area of the endometrium] *placental*: aplacental (having no placenta) (*a* privative) diaplacental (passing through or across the placenta) (*dia* through) ectoplacental (outside, beyond, or surrounding the placenta) (*ektos* outside) extraplacental (outside of or independent of the placenta) (*extra* outside) intraplacental (*intra* within) preplacental (before formation of a placenta) (*pre* before) retroplacental (behind the placenta, or behind both the placenta and the uterine wall) (*retro* behind) subplacental (*sub* under) transplacental (*trans* through) LEADING ROOT COMPOUND: *plac*: placode (a platelike structure from which a sense organ develops) (*eidos* form) placoid (*eidos* form) *placent*: placentitis (*itis* inflammation) placentoid (*eidos* form, shape) placentoma (*oma* tumor) *placento*: placentogenesis (*genere* to produce) placentogram, placentography (*graphein* to write) placentology (*logos* study) placentopathy (*pathos* disease) placentotherapy (*therapy* treatment)

Element	From	Meaning	Examples
placent (cont'd)		[placenta]	TRAILING ROOT COMPOUND: chorioplacental (*chorion* membrane) fetoplacental (pertaining to the fetus and the placenta) uteroplacental (pertaining to the uterus and the placenta) CROSS REFERENCE: None
plak, plat, plax	Greek *plax*	plate	SIMPLE ROOT: platelet (a disk-shaped structure) PREFIXED ROOT: antiplatelet (*anti* against) TRAILING ROOT COMPOUND: *plakia*: erythroplakia (*erythros* red) leucoplakia (or, leukoplakia) (*leukos* white) malacoplakia (or, malakoplakia) (*malakos* soft) melanoplakia (the formation of pigmented patches on the mucous membrane of the mouth in certain diseases, as stomatitis, jaundice, etc.) (*melanos* black, dark) *platelet*: protoplatelet (*protos* first) pseudoplatelet (*pseudes* false) *plaxia*: spiloplaxia (a red spot seen in cases of leprosy or pellagra) (*spilos* spot) FRENCH: plaque (a patch on the skin or on a mucous surface; a blood platelet) TERM: dental plaque (a gummy mass of microorganisms which grows on the crowns and spreads along the roots of the teeth) CROSS REFERENCE: cort, lam, squam
plan[1]	Latin *planare* to flatten	a plane; sole of the foot	SIMPLE ROOT: plane (or, planum; a flat or relatively smooth surface) planta (the sole of the foot) {plantar}, plantaris (also called *plantar*) planula (pl., planulae), planum (pl., plana) PREFIXED ROOT: *plan*: applanation (abnormal flattening, esp. of the corneal surface) (*ad* to) microplania (decreased horizontal diameter of erythrocytes) (*mikros* small) *plant*: implant (*im* in) interplant (*inter* between) isotransplantation (*isos* equal + transplantation) reimplantation (*re* again + implantation) transplant (also called *graft*), transplantation (*trans* across) *plantar*: transplantar (across the sole of the foot) (*trans* across) LEADING ROOT COMPOUND: *plani*: planigram (also called *tomogram*) (*gramma* a writing) planigraphy (also called *tomography*) (*graphein* to write) planimeter (*metron* measure) planithorax (a diagram of the front and back of the chest) *plano*: planocellular (*cella* cell) planoconvex (flat on one side and convex on the other) *plant*: plantalgia (pain in the sole of the foot) (*algos* pain) *planti*: plantigrade (*gradi* to walk) CROSS REFERENCE: None

Element	From	Meaning	Examples
plan²	Greek *planan*	to wander	SIMPLE ROOT: *plan*: planula (a larval coelenterate; something resembling such an animal; pl., planulae) *plank*: plankter (any type of plankton), plankton (minute, usually microscopic, free-floating organisms that float or drift in natural waters) {planktonic} PREFIXED ROOT: aplanatism (freedom from spherical aberration and coma: said of a lens) {aplanatic} (*a* negative) LEADING ROOT COMPOUND: *plan*: planuria (the voiding of urine from an abnormal passage of the body) (*uria* urine condition) *plano*: planocyte (a wandering cell) (*kytos* cell) planomania (morbid desire to wander and to be free of social restraints) (*mania* madness) planotopokinesia (loss of orientation in space) (*topos* place + *kinein* to move) TRAILING ROOT COMPOUND: *planesis*: phacoplanesis (*phakos* lens) *plania*: arterioplania (*arteria* artery) choloplania (*chole* bile) galactoplania (also called *galactometastasis*) (*galaktos* milk) leukocytoplania (wandering of leukocytes; passage of leukocytes through a membrane) (*leukos* white + *kytos* cell) menoplania (vicarious menstruation) (*men* month: menses) pyoplania (*pyon* pus) uroplania (*ouron* urine) CROSS REFERENCE: helc, noma, rad¹, vag
plas	Greek *plassein*	to mold, form, shape	SIMPLE ROOT: plasma (or, plasm; the liquid part of the lymph and of the blood; also called *blood*) {plasmatic, plasmic} plasmid, plasmon (the total of the extrachromosonal genetic properties of the eukaryotic cell cytoplasm) plasson (primitive protoplasm in cytode or non-nucleated cell stage) plaster, plastic (capable of being molded; contributing to building tissues), plasticity, plastid, plastinate {plastination} PREFIXED ROOT: *plasia*: aplasia (failure of any organ or tissue to develop normally) {aplastic} (*a* privative) adysplasia (severe form of dysplasia in which an organ or part is shrunken and sometimes ectopic, and initially appears to be absent) (*a* privative + dysplasia) alloplasia (also called *heteroplasia*) (*allos* other) anaplasia (*ana* again) cataplasia (or, cataplasis; a change in cells or tissues, characterized by reversion to an earlier stage) (*kata* negative) dysplasia (*dys* abnormal) [see separate entry: dysplas-] euplasia (*eu* good, well) hemiaplasia (*hemi* half + aplasia) hemihyperplasia (*hemi* half + hyperplasia) hemihypoplasia (*hemi* half + hypoplasia)

A Thesaurus of Medical Word Roots

Element	From	Meaning	Examples
plas (cont'd)		[to mold, form, shape]	heterometaplasia (*heteros* other + metaplasia)
			heteroplasia (also called *alloplasia*) {heteroplastic} (*heteros* other)
			hypermetaplasia (increased metaplasia) (*hyper* above, over)
			hyperplasia {hyperplastic} (*hyper* over, beyond)
			hypoplasia (incomplete development or underdevelopment of an organ or tissue) {hypoplastic} (*hypo* under)
			macroplasia (excessive growth of a part or tissue) (*makros* large)
			metaplasia (*meta* after, change)
			microplasia (dwarfism) (*mikros* small)
			polydysplasia (*polys* many + dysplasia)
			proplasia (*pro* before)
			protoplasia (*protos* first)
			retroplasia (*retro* backward)
			plasm:
			deuteroplasm (*deuteros* second)
			ectoplasm (distinguished from *endoplasm*) (*ektos* outside)
			endoplasm (distinguished from *ectoplasm*) {endoplasmic} (*endon* within)
			exoplasm (or, ectoplasm) (*exo* outside)
			heteroplasm (*heteros* other)
			metaplasm (also called *deuteroplasm*) (*meta* after)
			neoplasm (*neos* new)
			paraplasm (an abnormal growth) {paraplasmic} (*para* abnormal)
			periplasm {periplasmic} (*peri* around)
			protoplasm {protoplasmatic, protoplasmic} (*protos* first)
			symplasm (*sym* together)
			plasmacyte: proplasmacyte (*pro* before + *kytos* cell)
			plasmatic:
			alloplasmatic (*allos* other)
			ectoplasmatic (*ektos* outside)
			monoplasmatic (*monos* single)
			protoplasmatic (*protos* first)
			symplasmatic (*sym* together)
			plasmia:
			apoplasmia (deficiency of the blood plasm) (*apo* away, from)
			hyperplasmia (*hyper* over, beyond)
			plasmic: protoplasmic (*protos* first)
			plasmin: antiplasmin (*anti* against)
			plasmolysis:
			deplasmolysis (*de* reversal + *lyein* to dissolve)
			protoplasmolysis (*protos* first + plasmolysis)
			plast:
			alloplast (*allos* other)
			autoplast (*autos* self)
			ectoplast {ectoplastic} (*ektos* outside)
			protoplast (*protos* first)
			symplast (*sym* together)
			plastia: macroplastia (or, macroplasia) (*makros* large)
			plastic:
			aplastic (characterized by aplasia) (*a* privative)
			anaplastic (characterized by anaplasia) (*ana* backward)
			antiplastic (unfavorable to the healing process; an agent that impoverishes the blood) (*anti* against)

Element	From	Meaning	Examples
plas (cont'd)		[to mold, form, shape]	autoplastic (*autos* self)
			cacoplastic (*kakos* bad)
			dysplastic (*dys* abnormal)
			emplastic (adhesive or glutinous; a constipating medicine) (*em* in)
			euplastic (adapted to the formation of tissue, as in embryonic development or wound healing) (*eu* well)
			homoplastic (*homos* same)
			isoplastic (taken from another animal of the same species: said of tissue transplants or grafts; also called *syngeneic*) (*isos* equal)
			metaplastic (*meta* after)
			nonneoplastic (*non* negative + neoplastic)
			paraplastic (*para* abnormal)
			polyplastic (*polys* many)
			plasty:
			alloplasty (*allos* other)
			autoplasty {autoplastic} (*autos* self)
			heteroplasty (plastic surgery in which tissue from one individual is transferred onto another) (*heteros* other)
			homoplasty (*homos* same)
			LEADING ROOT COMPOUND:
			plasm:
			plasmapheresis {plasmapheretic} (*apheresis* removal)
			plasmodium (a multinucleate continuous mass of protoplasm; pl., plasmodia) {plasmodial} (*eidos* form)
			plasmoid (*eidos* form)
			plasma:
			plasmablast (*blastos* cell, germ, sprout)
			plasmacrit (*krinein* to separate)
			plasmacyte (*kytos* cell)
			plasmagene (*genere* to produce)
			plasmalemma (*lemma* membrane)
			plasmarrhexis (*rhexis* rupture)
			plasmato:
			plasmatogamy (or, plasmogamy) (*gamy* reproduction)
			plasmatorrhexis (or, plasmorrhexis) (*rhexis* rupture)
			plasmo:
			plasmocyte (a plasma cell) (*kytos* cell)
			plasmogamy (also called *plastogamy*) (*gamos* reproduction)
			plasmogen (also called *protoplasm*) (*genere* to produce)
			plasmolysis {plasmolytic}, plasmolyze (*lyein* to loosen)
			plasmorrhexis (or, plasmatorrhexis; dissolution of the cytoplasm) (*rhexis* rupture)
			plasmoschisis (the splitting of a cell) (*schisis* fissure)
			plasmotomy (mitosis in which the cytoplasm divides into two or more masses) (*tomy* incision)
			plasmotropism {plasmotropic} (*tropein* to turn)
			plasmotype (also called *plasmon*) (type)
			plasto:
			plastogamy (also called *plasmogamy*) (*gamy* reproduction)
			plastogel (a gel possessing great plasticity)
			TRAILING ROOT COMPOUND:
			plasia:
			bioplasia (*bios* life)

A Thesaurus of Medical Word Roots

Element	From	Meaning	Examples
plas (cont'd)		[to mold, form, shape]	chondroplasia (*chondros* cartilage)
			erythroplasia (*erythros* red)
			fibroplasia, fibrodysplasia (*fibra* fiber + dysplasia)
			homeoplasia (*homeos* same, similar)
			leukoplasia (also called *leukoplakia*) (*leukos* white)
			mammiplasia (or, mammoplasia) (*mamma* breast)
			mastoplasia (also called *mammoplasia*) (*mastos* breast, nipple)
			mazoplasia (*mazos* breast, nipple)
			neoplasia (*neos* new)
			tarsoplasia (also called *blepharoplasty*) (*tarsos* eyelid)
			plasm:
			cytoplasm (*kytos* cell)
			morphoplasm (*morphe* form, shape)
			myoplasm (*myos* muscle)
			neoplasm (*neos* new)
			ooplasm (also called *ovoplasm*) (*oon* egg, ovum)
			ovoplasm (also called *ooplasm*) (*ovum* egg)
			oxyplasm (*oxys* sharp)
			phagoplasm (*phagein* to consume)
			phaneroplasm (*phaneros* visible)
			phytoplasm (vegetable protoplasm) (*phyton* plant)
			pseudoplasm (*pseudes* false)
			sarcoplasm (*sarkos* flesh)
			somatoplasm (*somatos* body)
			spermoplasm (*spermatos* seed)
			spongioplasm (*spongia* sponge)
			sporoplasm (*sporos* seed, spore)
			stereoplasm (*stereos* solid)
			viroplasm (*virus* poison)
			plasson: pyknoplasson (the protoplasm of a non-nucleated cell in its unexpended form) (*pyknos* thick)
			plast:
			chloroplast (*chloros* green)
			chondroplast (*chondros* cartilage)
			chromoplast (*chroma* color)
			cytoplast (*kytos* cell)
			eleoplast (a globular body made up of granular protoplasm and containing drops of oil) (*elaion* oil)
			gymnoplast (a mass of protoplasm without an enclosing wall) (*gymnos* nude)
			leucoplast (*leukos* white)
			myeloplast (*myelos* marrow)
			protoplast (*protos* first)
			trophoplast (*trophe* nourishment)
			plastic:
			desmoplastic (*dein* to bind: ligament)
			fibroplastic (*fibra* fiber)
			neoplastic (*neo* new)
			seroplastic (*serum* whey)
			thromboplastic (*thrombos* clot)
			plasty:
			abdominoplasty (abdomen)
			acromioplasty (*acromion* high point of shoulder)

Element	From	Meaning	Examples
plas (cont'd)		[to mold, form, shape]	angioplasty (*angeion* blood vessel)
			annuloplasty (*annulus* ringlike structure)
			anoplasty (anus)
			aortoplasty (aorta)
			arterioplasty (*arteria* artery)
			arthroplasty (*arthron* joint)
			balanoplasty (*balanos* glans penis—head of penis)
			blepharoplasty (also called *tarsoplasty*) (*blepharon* eyelid)
			bronchoplasty (*bronchos* windpipe)
			canthoplasty (*kanthos* corner of the eye)
			capsuloplasty (capsule—of a joint)
			cardioplasty (*kardia* heart)
			cervicoplasty (also called *tracheloplasty*) (*cervix* neck, or cervix uteri)
			cheiloplasty (also called *labioplasty*) (*cheilos* lip)
			chiroplasty (or, cheiroplasty) (*cheir* hand)
			chondroplasty (*chondros* cartilage)
			cineplasty (also called *kineplasty*) (*kinein* to move)
			clitoroplasty (clitoris)
			colpoplasty (*kolpos* vagina)
			cranioplasty (*kranion* skull)
			cystoplasty (*kystis* bladder)
			dermatoplasty (*dermatos* skin)
			enteroplasty (*enteron* intestine)
			episioplasty (*epision* vulva)
			esophagoplasty (esophagus)
			facioplasty (*facies* face)
			fascioplasty (*fascia* band)
			flexorplasty (flexor muscle)
			frenoplasty (*frenum* bridle, curb)
			gastroplasty (*gaster* stomach, belly)
			genioplasty (see *mentoplasty*) (*geneion* chin)
			genitoplasty (genital organs)
			hernioplasty (*hernia* protrusion)
			keratoplasty (*keratos* cornea)
			kineplasty (or, cineplasty) (*kinein* to move)
			labioplasty (also called *cheiloplasty*) (*labium* lip)
			lipoplasty (*lipos* fat)
			mammaplasty (or, mammoplasty) (*mamma* breast)
			meloplasty (*melon* cheek)
			mentoplasty (see *genioplasty*) (*mentum* chin)
			metroplasty (also called *uteroplasty*) (*metra* uterus)
			myoplasty (*myos* muscle)
			myringoplasty (*myringa* membane—tympanic)
			neuroplasty (*neuron* nerve)
			odontoplasty (*odontos* tooth)
			omentoplasty (*omentum* fat skin)
			oophoroplasty (*oophor* egg bearer)
			ophthalmoplasty (*ophthalmos* eye)
			orchioplasty (or, orchidoplasty) (*orchis* testicle)
			oscheoplasty (also called *scrotoplasty*) (*osche* scrotum)
			osteoplasty (*osteon* bone)
			otoplasty (*otos* ear)

A Thesaurus of Medical Word Roots

Element	From	Meaning	Examples
plas (cont'd)		[to mold, form, shape]	palatoplasty (palate—roof of mouth)
			pelvioplasty (pelvis)
			perineoplasty (perineum)
			peritoneoplasty (peritoneum)
			phalloplasty (*phallos* penis)
			pharyngoplasty (pharynx)
			phleboplasty (*phlebos* vein)
			proctoplasty (also called *rectoplasty*) (*proktos* anus, rectum)
			pubioplasty (*pubes* genitals)
			pyeloplasty (*pyelos* pelvis)
			pyloroplasty (pyloros)
			rectoplasty (also called *proctoplasty*) (rectum)
			rhinoplasty (*rhinos* nose)
			rhytidoplasty (also called *rhytidectomy*) (*rhytidos* wrinkle)
			salpingoplasty (also called *tuboplasty*) (*salpingos* tube)
			scleroplasty (*skleros* hard)
			scrotoplasty (also called *oscheoplasty*) (*scrotum* bag: testicle pouch)
			septoplasty (*septum* wall, partition)
			septorhinoplasty (*septum* partition + *rhinos* nose)
			staphyloplasty (*staphyle* uvula)
			stomatoplasty (*stomatos* mouth)
			syndesmoplasty (*syndesis* bound together: ligament)
			tarsoplasty (also called *blepharoplasty*) (*tarsus* eyelid)
			tendoplasty (or, tendinoplasty, tenoplasty) (tendon)
			tenomyoplasty (tendon + *myos* muscle)
			trabeculoplasty (*trabecula* little beam)
			tracheloplasty (also called *cervicoplasty*) (*trachelos* neck of uterus)
			tracheoplasty (*trachea* windpipe)
			tuboplasty (also called *salpingoplasty*) (*tubus* tube)
			tympanoplasty (*tympanon* eardrum)
			ureteroplasty (ureter)
			uteroplasty (uterus)
			vaginoplasty (vagina)
			valvuloplasty (valve, especially of the heart)
			vertebroplasty (vertebra)
			PREFIXED TRAILING ROOT COMPOUND:
			amyoplasia (*a* privative + *myos* muscle)
			anangioplasia (*an* privative + *angeion* blood vessel)
			anerythroplasia (*an* privative + *erythros* red)
			anosteoplasia (*an* privative + *osteon* bone)
			FRENCH: plastron (orig., a metal breastplate worn under a coat of mail; the sternum and attached cartilages)
			CROSS REFERENCE: eid, form, ide, morph
plat(y), **plate**	Greek *platys*	flat, broad	SIMPLE ROOT:
			plate:
			plate (a thin flattened part or portion, such as a flattened process of a bone; also called *lamella*, *lamina*)
			platelet (also called *thrombocyte*)
			platys: platysma (a platelike muscle) {platysmal}
			PREFIXED ROOT: antiplatelet (*anti* against)
			See Appendix B for examples of words with this initial combining form. Others are listed with the roots to which it is attached.
			CROSS REFERENCE: eury, lam, plan[1]

Element	From	Meaning	Examples
plax			See plak-.
pleg, **plect**, **pless**, **plex** -**plegia** (see Appendix C)	Greek *plessein* to strike *plektron* anything to strike with	stroke (medical), paralysis	SIMPLE ROOT: *plectr*: plectron (or, plektron; the hammer form assumed by certain bacilli during sporulation) *pless*: plessor (also called *plexor*) *plex*: plexor (a hammer used in performing percussion) PREFIXED ROOT: *plectic*: antapoplectic (relieving or preventing stroke; an agent that alleviates strokes; also spelled *antiapoplectic*) (*anti* against + *apo* away) cataplectic (coming on suddenly and overwhelmingly) (*kata* down) paraplectic (also called *paraplegic*) (*para* alongside) *plegia*: diplegia (bilateral paralysis; paralysis affecting like parts on both sides of the body) {diplegic} (*di* two) hemiplegia (also called *semiplegia*) {hemiplegic} (*hemi* half) hemiparaplegia (*hemi* half + paraplegia) monoplegia (paralysis of but a single part; different varieties are distinguished according to the part affected or the site of the lesion producing the disease, such as brachial, facial; central, peripheral) (*monos* one) paraplegia (paralysis of the legs and lower part of the body, both motion and sensation being affected) {paraplegic; also called *paraplectic*}, paraplegiform (*para* alongside + *forma* shape) posthemiplegic (*post* after + hemiplegic) quadriplegia (also called *tetraplegia*) (*quattuor* four) semiplegia (also called *hemiplegia*) (*semi* half) tetraplegia (also called *quadriplegia*) (tetra four) triplegia (hemiplegia with paralysis of one limb on the other side of the body) (*tri* three) *plexis*: cataplexis (or, cataplexy) {cataplectic} (*kata* down) *plexy*: apoplexy (*apo* from) [see separate entry: apoplec-] LEADING ROOT COMPOUND: *pleg*: plegaphonia (a sound produced in percussion of the larynx when the glottis is open during auscultation of the chest) (*a* privative + *phone* sound) *pless*: plessesthesia (palpatory percussion) (*esthesia* feeling) *plessi*: plessigraph (*graphein* to write) plessimeter (also called *pleximeter*) {plessimetric} (*metron* measure) *plex*: pleximeter (also called *plessimeter*) (*metron* measure) TRAILING ROOT COMPOUND: *plegia*: blepharoplegia (*blepharon* eyelid) bronchoplegia (*bronchos* windpipe) cardioplegia (*kardia* heart) cephaloplegia (*kephale* head) colicoplegia (*kolikos* colic condition) cycloplegia (paralysis of ciliary muscle) (*kyklos* circle) cystoplegia (also called *cystoparesis, cystoparalysis*) (*kystis* bladder) enteroplegia (also called *adynamic ileus*) (*enteron* intestine) gastroplegia (*gaster* stomach, belly) glossoplegia (*glossa* tongue)

A Thesaurus of Medical Word Roots

Element	From	Meaning	Examples
pleg (cont'd)		[stroke]	iridoplegia (also called *iridoparalysis*) (iris—of eye)
			isthmoplegia (paralysis of the isthmus of the fauces, or throat)
			laloplegia (also called *logoplegia*) (*lalein* to speak)
			laryngoplegia (larynx)
			logoplegia (also called *laloplegia*) (*logos* word)
			myeloplegia (also called *spinal paralysis*) (*myelos* marrow)
			ophthalmoplegia (*ophthalmos* eye)
			palatoplegia (*palate* roof of mouth)
			pharyngoplegia (also called *pharyngoparalysis*) (*pharyngos* throat)
			phrenoplegia (*phren* diaphragm)
			proctoplegia (also called *proctoparalysis*) (*proktos* anus)
			prosopoplegia (also called *facioplegia*) (*prosopon* face)
			pseudoplegia (*pseudes* false)
			pupilloplegia (also called *tonic pupil*)
			rachioplegia (paralysis due to a lesion in the spinal cord; also called *spinal paralysis*) (*rhachis* spine)
			stauroplegia (also called *alternate hemiplegia*) (*stauros* cross)
			plegic:
			cardioplegic (*kardia* heart)
			cycloplegic (*kyklos* circle)
			facioplegia (also called *facial paralysis*) (*facies* face)
			ganglioplegic (drugs or other agents that block transmission of impulses through the sympathetic and parasympathetic ganglia) (*ganglion* knot, swelling)
			psychoplegic (*psyche* mind)
			CROSS REFERENCE: pares
plei, **pleo**	Greek *pleion,* *pleon*	more	SIMPLE ROOT: pleonasm (an excess in number of parts)
			LEADING ROOT COMPOUND:
			ple:
			pleoptics (*optikos* pertaining to vision)
			pleoptophor (*optos* visible + *phorein* to bear)
			pleio:
			pleiochloruria (an excess of chlorides in the urine) (*uria* urine condition)
			pleiotropy (or, pleiotropia; the ability of a gene to manifest itself in more than one way; the control of a single gene of several seemingly unrelated effects) {pleiotropic} (*trepein* to turn)
			pleo:
			pleochroic (also called *pleochromatic*) (*chroa* color)
			pleochromatism (exhibiting different colors under different circumstances) {pleochromatic; also called *pleochroic*} (*chroma* color)
			pleocytosis (presence of a greater than normal number of cells in the cerebrospinal fluid) (*kytos* cell + *osis* condition)
			pleomastia (or, pleomazia; the state of having more than two mammae; also called *polymastia*) {pleomastic} (*mastos* breast)
			pleomorphic (or, pleomorphous; occurring in various distinct forms), pleomorphism (also called *polymorphic*) (*morphe* form)
			pleon:
			pleonexia (greediness) (*echein* to have)
			pleonosteosis (*osteosis* bone condition)
			pleonotia (a developmental anomaly characterized by the presence of a supernumerary ear located on the neck) (*otos* ear)
			CROSS REFERENCE: pler, pluri

Element	From	Meaning	Examples
pless			See pleg- for *plessesthesia, plessimeter*.
pleur	Greek *pleura*	rib, side	SIMPLE ROOT: pleura (serous membrane that enfolds both lungs; pl., pleurae) {pleural} pleurisy (inflammation of the pleura; also called *pleuritis*) {pleuritic} PREFIXED ROOT: *pleural*: epipleural (*epi* upon) extrapleural (*extra* outside) interpleural (*inter* between) intrapleural (*intra* within) peripleural (*peri* around) subpleural (*sub* beneath) transpleural (*trans* across) *pleuria*: apleuria (absence of one or more ribs) (*a* privative) *pleuritis* inflammation of the pleura: parapleuritis (*para* alongside) peripleuritis (*peri* around) LEADING ROOT COMPOUND: *pleur*: pleuralgia (rarely used term for *pleurodynia*) (*algos* pain) pleuramnion (*amnion* membrane) pleurapophysis (*apophysis* outgrowth, offshoot) pleurectomy (*ektome* excision) pleuritis (also called *pleurisy*) {pleuritic} (*itis* inflammation) pleurodynia (also called *costalgia, pleuralgia*) (*odyne* pain) *pleura*: pleuracentesis (also called *thoracentesis*) (*kentesis* puncture) *pleurito*: pleuritogenous (*genous* producing) *pleuro*: pleurobronchitis (*bronchos* windpipe + *itis* inflammation) pleurocele (also called *pneumonocele*) (*kele* hernia) pleurocentesis (also called *thoracentesis*) (*kentesis* puncture) pleurocentrum (*kentron* point, center) pleurocholecystitis (*chole* bile + *kystis* bladder + *itis* inflammation) pleuroclysis (*klysis* a washing out) pleurocutaneous (*cutis* skin) pleurodesis (*desis* a binding together) pleuroesophagus {pleuroesophageal} (esophagus) pleurogenic (or, pleurogenous) (*genere* to produce) pleurography (x-ray examination of the lungs and pleura) (*graphein* to write) pleurohepatitis (*hepatos* liver + *itis* inflammation) pleurolith (a calculus in the pleura) (*lithos* stone) pleurolysis (*lyein* to loosen) pleuromelus (*melos* limb) pleuropericardial (pericardium: *peri* around + *kardia* heart) pleuropneumonia (pleurisy complicated with pneumonia) pleuropulmonary (*pulmo* lung) pleurorrhea (*rhein* to flow) pleuroscopy (also called *thoracoscopy*) (*skopein* to examine) pleurosoma (or, pleurosomus) (*soma* body) pleurotomy (also called *thoracotomy*) (*tomy* incision)

Element	From	Meaning	Examples
pleur (cont'd)		[rib, side]	pleurotyphoid (acute pleurisy followed by and complicated with typhoid fever)
			pleurovisceral (*viscera* inner organs)
			TRAILING ROOT COMPOUND:
			pleura:
			chylopleura (also called *chylothorax, chylous pleurisy*) (*chylus* juice)
			hemopleura (a pleural effusion containing blood; also called *hemathorax*) (*haima* blood)
			pleural:
			bronchopleural (*bronchos* windpipe)
			costopleural (*costa* rib)
			hepatopleural (*hepatos* liver)
			pericardiopleural (pericardium: *peri* around + *kardia* heart)
			visceropleural (*viscera* internal organs)
			pleure:
			somatopleure {somatopleural} (*somatos* body)
			splanchnopleure {splanchnopleural} (*splanchnos* viscus)
			pleuritis inflammation of the pleura:
			corticopleuritis (also called *pulmonary pleurisy*) (*cortex* outer layer)
			pachypleuritis (*pachys* thick)
			pneumonopleuritis (also called *pleuropneumonia*)
			CROSS REFERENCE: canth, cost, later
plex			See pleg- for *apoplexy*.
ploid	Greek *plasios*	fold	NOTE: This root is often combined with *di* two; thus, double, or twofold; see dipl-. The suffix formed from this root is –ploid(y).
			PREFIXED ROOT:
			aneuploid, aneuploidy (*an* negative + euploid)
			diploid (*di* two)
			endopolyploidy (*endon* within + polyploidy)
			euploid, euploidy (*eu* well)
			haploidy (*haplous* single)
			heteroploid, heteroploidy (*heteros* other)
			hexaploidy (also called *polyploidy*) (*hex* six)
			hyperploid, hyperploidy (*hyper* over)
			hypoploidy (*hypo* under)
			monoploid (*monos* single)
			octaploid, octaploidy (*okto* eight)
			polyploid, polyploidy (*polys* many)
			tetraploid (*tetra* four)
			CROSS REFERENCE: None
pluri-	Latin *pluris*	more	See Appendix B for examples of words using this initial combining form. Others are listed with the roots to which it is attached.
			CROSS REFERENCE: plei, poly
pnea	Greek *pnein* to breathe	breath, breathing	PREFIXED ROOT:
			apnea (the transient cessation of the breathing impulse that follows forced breathing) (*a* privative)
			anapnea (respiration; regaining the breath), anapnoic (relieving dyspnea; also, pertaining to respiration), anapnotherapy (*ana* again + *therapy* treatment)
			dyspnea {dyspneic} (*dys* abnormal)
			eupnea {eupneic} (*eu* well)
			hyperpnea (also called *polypnea*) {hyperpneic} (*hyper* above)
			hypopnea {hypopneic} (*hypo* under)

Element	From	Meaning	Examples
pnea (cont'd)		[breath]	polypnea (very rapid breathing; also called *hyperpnea*) {polypneic; also called *hyperpneic*} (*polys* many)
			LEADING ROOT COMPOUND:
			pneogram (also called *spirogram*), pneograph (*graphein* to write)
			pneometer (also called *spirometer*) (*metron* measure)
			TRAILING ROOT COMPOUND:
			bathypnea (deep breathing) (*bathys* deep)
			bradypnea (*bradys* slow)
			bromopnea (also called *halitosis; bad breath*) (*bromos* stench)
			oligopnea (also called *hypopnea*) (*oligos* scant, little)
			orthopnea (inability to breathe except in upright position; (opposite of *platypnea*) (*orthos* straight)
			piorthopnea (also called *pimelorthopnea*) (*pion* fat + *orthos* straight)
			platypnea (opposite of *orthopnea*) (*platys* flat)
			tachypnea (*tachys* swift)
			thermopolypnea (quickened breathing due to high body temperature or great environmental heat) (*therme* heat + *poly* much)
			traumatopnea (a condition of partial asphyxia with collapse caused by traumatic opening of the pleura) (*trauma* wound)
			CROSS REFERENCE: pneumat
pneumat	Greek *pneumatos* air from *pnein* to breathe	air, gas, respiration, breath	SIMPLE ROOT:
			pneumatic (of, or pertaining to air or gas, or to respiration)
			pneumatics, pneumatization
			pneumatized (filled with air; containing pneumatic cells)
			PREFIXED ROOT:
			pneum: apneumatic (free from air; done with the exclusion of air) (*a* negative)
			pneus: apneusis (an abnormal respiratory pattern) (*a* negative)
			LEADING ROOT COMPOUND:
			pneum:
			pneumarthrogram, pneumarthrography (*arthron* joint + *graphein* to write)
			pneumarthrosis (*arthron* joint + *osis* condition)
			pneumat:
			pneumatosis (*osis* condition)
			pneumaturia (*ouron* urine)
			pneumato:
			pneumatocardia (the presence of air in the heart) (*kardia* heart)
			pneumatocele (a tumor or cyst formed by air or other gas filling an adventitious pouch, such as a laryngocele, tracheocele, or gaseous swelling of the scrotum) (*kele* tumor)
			pneumatocephalus (or, pneumocephalus) (*kephale* head)
			pneumatoenteric (also called *celomic bay*) (*enteron* intestine)
			pneumatogram (also called *spirogram*), pneumatograph (*graphein* to write)
			pneumatohemia (*hemia* blood condition)
			pneumatorrhachis (or, pneumorrhachis) (*rhachis* spine)
			pneumo:
			pneumocephalus (*kephale* head)
			pneumocholecystitis (*cholecyst* gallbladder + *itis* inflammation)
			TRAILING ROOT COMPOUND: hydropneumatosis (*hydor* water + *osis* condition)
			CROSS REFERENCE: aer, phys, pnea

A Thesaurus of Medical Word Roots

Element	From	Meaning	Examples
pneumo	Greek *pneumon* lung; from *pnein* to breathe	lung, air, respiration, pneumonia	SIMPLE ROOT: pneumal (pertaining to the lungs) pneumonia (inflammation of the lungs with consolidation) PREFIXED ROOT: apneumia (congenital absence of the lungs) (*a* privative) mesopneumonium (*mesos* middle) metapneumonic (following pneumonia) (*meta* after) parapneumonia (resembling pneumonia) (*para* resembling) peripneumonia (also called *pleuropneumonia*) (*peri* around) postpneumonia (*post* after) synpneumonic (*syn* with, together) LEADING ROOT COMPOUND: *pneumo*: pneumobacillus (*bacillus* rod-shaped bacterium) pneumobulbar (*bulbus* bulb) pneumocardial (also called *cardiopulmonary*) (*kardia* heart) pneumocele (or, pneumonocele) (*kele* hernia) pneumocentesis (*kentein* to puncture) pneumocephalus (the presence of air in the intracranial cavity) (*kephale* head) pneumococcus (*kokkos* berry-shaped bacterium) pneumocolon (the presence of air in the colon) pneumoconiosis (*konos* dust + *osis* condition) pneumocranium (*kranion* skull) pneumocystography (*kystis* bladder + *graphein* to write) pneumoderma (also called *subcutaneous emphysema*) (*derma* skin) pneumodynamics (*dynamis* power) pneumoencephalography (*enkephale* brain + *graphein* to write) pneumogastric, pneumogastrography (*gaster* stomach, belly + *graphein* to write) pneumogram, pneumograph (*graphein* to write) pneumohemia (*hemia* blood condition) pnumohydrometra (*hydor* water + *metra* uterus) pneumohypoderma (or, pneumoderma; also called *subcutaneous emphysema*) (*hypo* beneath + *derma* skin) pneumolith (also called *pulmolith*), pneumolithiasis (*lithos* stone + *iasis* condition) pneumology (*logos* study) pneumolysis (or, pneumonolysis) (*lysis* loosening) pneumomalacia (*malakos* soft) pneumomassage pneumomediastinum pneumomelanosis (*melanosis* blackening) pneumomycosis (*mycosis* fungal disease) pneumomyelography (*myelos* marrow + *graphein* to write) pneumopathy (*pathos* disease) pneumopericardium (pericardium: *peri* around + *kardia* heart) pneumoperitoneum, pneumoperitonitis (peritoneum + *itis* inflammation) pneumophagia (also called *aerophagia*) (*phagein* to consume) pneumophonia (*phone* voice, sound) pneumopleuritis (*pleura* side + *itis* inflammation) pneumopyelography (*pyelos* pelvis + *graphein* to write)

Element	From	Meaning	Examples
pneumo (cont'd)		[lung, air, respiration]	pneumopyothorax (also called *pyopneumothorax*) (*pyon* pus + *thorax* chest)
			pneumoresection (excision of part of a lung)
			pneumorrhachis (*rhachis* spinal column)
			pneumosclerosis (fibrosis of the lungs) (*sklerosis* hardening)
			pneumoscrotum (air or gas in the scrotum, the testicle pouch)
			pneumotachograph (*tachys* swift + *graphein* to write)
			pneumotaxic (*taxis* arrangement)
			pneumotherapy (*therapy* treatment)
			pneumothermomassage (*therme* heat + massage)
			pneumothorax (*thorax* the chest)
			pneumotomy (*tomy* incision)
			pneumotropic (*tropein* to turn)
			pneumoventricle (air in the ventricular system of the brain)
			pneumon:
			pneumonectomy (*ektome* excision)
			pneumonitis (*itis* inflammation)
			pneumono:
			pneumonocele (or, pneumocele; also called *pleurocele*) (*kele* hernia)
			pneumonocentesis (or, pneumocentesis) (*kentesis* puncture)
			pneumonococcus (or, pneumococcus) (*kokkos* berry-shaped bacterium)
			pneumonocyte (alveolar cell) (*kytos* cell)
			pneumonography (or, pneumography) (*graphein* to write)
			pneumonolysis (or, pneumolysis) (*lyein* to loosen)
			pneumonopathy (also called *pneumonosis*) (*pathos* disease)
			pneumonopexy (or, pneumopexy) (*pexis* fixation)
			pneumopleuritis (also called *pleuritic pneumonia*) (*pleura* side + *itis* inflammation)
			pneumonorrhagia (pulmonary hemorrhage) (*rhagia* bursting forth)
			pneumonorrhaphy (suture of the lung) (*rhaphe* suture)
			pneumonotomy (*tomy* incision)
			TRAILING ROOT COMPOUND: pleuropneumonia (pleurisy complicated with pneumonia), pleuropneumonectomy (*pleura* side, rib + *ektome* excision)
			CROSS REFERENCE: pulmo(n)
pod, pus	Greek *pous* foot	foot	SIMPLE ROOT: podalic (relating to the foot), podismus (also called *podospasm*)
			PREFIXED ROOT:
			podag: antipodagric (*anti* against + *agra* seizure)
			podal: heteropodal (having branches or processes of different kinds: said of neurons) (*heteros* other)
			pode: antipode {antipodal; located at opposite positions; diametrically opposed} (*anti* against)
			podia:
			apodia {apodal} (*a* privative)
			dipodia (a developmental anomaly involving complete or incomplete duplication of a foot) (*di* two)
			diplopodia (duplication of digits of the foot) (*diploos* double)
			macropodia (also called *megalopodia*) (*makros* large)
			megalopodia (also called *macropodia*) (*megalos* large)
			micropodia (*mikros* small)
			monopodia (*monos* single)

A Thesaurus of Medical Word Roots

Element	From	Meaning	Examples
pod (cont'd)		[foot]	sympodia (also called *symmelia*; a developmental anomaly characterized by apparent fusion of the lower limbs) (*syn* with)
			tripodia (also called *symmelia, sympodia*) (*tri* three)
			*polyp [a morbid excrescence (the final letter retains the first letter of the root under consideration)] (*polys* many) [see separate entry]
			pus:
			apus (an individual exhibiting apodia; also called *sirenomelus*) (*a* privative)
			dipus (conjoined twins with only two feet) (*di* two)
			micropus (a person with abnormally small feet) (*mikros* small)
			polypus (a polyp) (*polys* many) [see separate entry: polyp]
			sympus (a malformed fetus in which the lower extremities are completely fused or rotated and genitalia are defective) (*sym* with, together)
			tetrapus (a person with four feet) (*tetra* four)
			LEADING ROOT COMPOUND:
			pod:
			podagra (gouty pain in the great toe) {podagral, podagric, podagrous} (*agra* seizure)
			podalgia (also called *pedialgia, pododynia*) (*algos* pain)
			podarthritis (*arthron* joint + *itis* inflammation)
			podiatrist, podiatry {podiatric} (*iatrein* to heal)
			poditis (*itis* inflammation)
			pododynia (also called *pedialgia, podalgia*) (*odyne* pain)
			podo:
			podobromidrosis (foul-smelling perspiration of the feet) (*bromos* stench + *hidros* sweat + *osis* condition) [h of hidros elided]
			podocyte (*kytos* cell)
			pododynamometer (*dynamis* power + *metron* measure)
			podogram, podograph (*graphein* to write)
			podology (also called *podiatry*) (*logos* study)
			podometer (also called *pedometer*) (*metron* measure)
			podospasm (also called *podismus*) (*spasm* contraction)
			TRAILING ROOT COMPOUND:
			podia:
			cryptopodia (*kryptos* concealed)
			filopodia (plural of *filopodium*: a thin protrusion from a cell, usually supported by microfilaments) (filament)
			leptopodia (*leptos* slender)
			platypodia (*platys* flat)
			podist: chiropodist (also called *podiatrist*) (*cheir* hand)
			podous: pachypodous (having large thick feet) (*pachys* thick)
			pody:
			chiropody (also called *podiatry*) (*cheir* hand)
			ectropody (*ektrosis* congenitally absent)
			pus: peropus (*peros* maimed)
			PREFIXED TRAILING ROOT COMPOUND:
			acephalopodia (congenital absence of the head and feet) (*a* privative + *kephale* head)
			acheiropodia (congenital absence of hands and feet) (*a* privative + *cheiros* hand)
			atelopodia (*atelos* incomplete: *a* negative + *telos* end)
			CROSS REFERENCE: ped[2]

Element	From	Meaning	Examples
poie	Greek *poiein*	to make, produce	PREFIXED ROOT: dyspoiesis (also called *dysgenesis, dyshematopoiesis*) (*dys* abnormal) monopoiesis (also called *monocytopoiesis*) (*monos* single) TRAILING ROOT COMPOUND: *poiesis*: angiopoiesis (also called *angiogenesis*) (*angeion* blood vessel) biopoiesis (the origin of life from inorganic matter) (*bios* life) cholanopoiesis (*chole* bile + *ano* upward) cholepoiesis (or, cholopoiesis) (*chole* bile) chylopoiesis (also called *chylifaction, chylification*) (*chylus* juice) chymopoiesis (also called *chymification*) (*chymos* juice) colpopoiesis (the creation of a vagina by plastic surgery) (*kolpos* vagina) cytopoiesis (*kytos* cell) erythropoiesis (also called *erythrocytopoiesis*) (*erythros* red) galactopoiesis (also called *lactogenesis*) (*galaktos* milk) gonepoiesis (*gone* seed, semen) granulopoiesis (also called *granulocytopoiesis*) (*granula* small grain) hematopoiesis (or, hemopoiesis) (*haima* blood) hidropoiesis (*hidros* sweat) hormonopoiesis (also called *hormonogenesis*) (*hormaein* to excite) leukopoiesis (also called *leukocytogenesis, leukocytopoiesis*) (*leukos* white) lymphopoiesis (also called *lymphocytopoiesis*) (*lympha* fluid) myelopoiesis (also called *myelogenesis*) (*myelos* marrow) myxopoiesis (*myxa* mucus) onomatopoiesis (or, onomatopoeia) (*onoma* name) pyopoiesis (also called *pyogenesis, suppuration*) (*pyon* pus) thrombocytopoiesis (*thrombos* clot + *kytos* cell) thrombopoiesis (also called *thrombogenesis*) (*thrombos* clot) ureapoiesis (also called *ureagenesis*) (*urea*) uropoiesis (also called *urogenesis*) (*ouron* urine) *poietic*: angiopoietic (*angeion* vessel—blood vessel) cholepoietic (*chole* bile) gonepoietic (*gone* seed, sperm) hematopoietic (also called *sanguinopoietic*) (*hematos* blood) hormonopoietic (hormone: *hormaein* to excite) leukopoietic (*leukos* white) myelopoietic (*myelos* marrow) nephropoietic (also called *nephrogenic*) (*nephros* kidney) nosopoietic (also called *pathogenic*) (*nosos* disease) sanguinopoietic (also called *hematopoietic*) (*sanguis* blood) sarcopoietic (forming muscle or flesh) (*sarkos* flesh) spermatopoietic (also called *spermatogenic*) (*spermatos* seed) PREFIXED TRAILING ROOT COMPOUND: anerythropoiesis (also called *erythropenia*) (*an* negative + *erythros* red) dyserythropoiesis (*dys* abnormal + *erythros* red) dyshematopoiesis (*dys* abnormal + *hematos* blood) dysmyelopoiesis (*dys* abnormal + *myelos* marrow) CROSS REFERENCE: fac, fer, gen

A Thesaurus of Medical Word Roots

Element	From	Meaning	Examples
poikilo	Greek *poikilos*	varied, mottled, irregular	See Appendix B for examples of words with this initial combining form. Others are listed with the roots to which it is attached. CROSS REFERENCE: None
polio	Greek *polios*	gray [gray matter of the nervous system]	LEADING ROOT COMPOUND: *poli*: poliosis (whiteness of the hair) (*osis* condition) *polio*: poliocidal (*caedere* to kill) polioclastic (*klaein* to break) poliodystrophy (or, poliodystrophia) (*dys* abnormal + *trophein* to nourish) polioencephalitis (*enkephalos* brain + *itis* inflammation) poliomyelitis (*myelos* marrow + *itis* inflammation) poliovirus (*virus* poison) CROSS REFERENCE: tephr
poly-	Greek *polys*	many, much; diverse	See Appendix B for examples of words with this prefix. Others are listed with the roots to which it is attached. CROSS REFERENCE: pluri-
polyp	Greek *polys* many + *podos* foot	polyp	SIMPLE ROOT: polyp (a morbid excrescence, or protruding growth, from a mucous membrane; originally applied to the mucous membrane of the nose) {polypous}, polypus (a polyp; pl., polypi) LEADING ROOT COMPOUND: *polyp*: polypectomy (*ektome* excision) polypoid (also called *polypoidosis, polypiform*) (*eidos* form) polyposis (*osis* condition) *polypo*: polypotome (*tome* a cutting instrument) polypotrite (an instrument for crushing polyps) (*terere* to crush) TRAILING ROOT COMPOUND: otopolypus (*otos* ear) proctopolypus (*proktos* anus, rectum) pseudopolyp (*pseudes* false) CROSS REFERENCE: None
por	Greek *poreia* journey, passage	passage, pore	SIMPLE ROOT: pore (or, porus) {poral, porous, porion (pl., poria), porosity porus (also called *pore, sweat pore*; pl., pori) PREFIXED ROOT: hypoporosis (deficient callus formation after bone fracture) (*hypo* under + *osis* condition) micropore (*mikros* small) periporitis (*peri* around + *itis* inflammation) polyporous (*polys* many) LEADING ROOT COMPOUND: *por*: poradenitis (also called *poradenia*) (*adenos* gland + *itis* inflammation) porencephalia (or, porencephaly) {porencephalic, porencephalous}, porencephalitis (*enkephalon* brain + *itis* inflammation) porosis (cavity formation) {porosity, porotic} (*osis* condition) *poro*: poroconidium (also called *porospore*) (*konis* dust) porokeratosis (*keras* horn + *osis* condition) poroplastic (both porous and plastic) (*plassein* to form)

A Thesaurus of Medical Word Roots

Element	From	Meaning	Examples
por (cont'd)		[pore]	porospore (also called *poroconidium*) (*sporos* seed) porotomy (also called *meatotomy*) (*tomy* incision) TRAILING ROOT COMPOUND: *pore*: blastopore (*blastos* bud, shoot, germ) myelopore (*myelos* marrow) neuropore (*neuron* nerve) *porosis* pore condition: chondroporosis (*chondros* cartilage) osteoporosis (*osteon* bone) CROSS REFERENCE: for, meat, tub[1]
post-	Latin prefix	after, beyond	See Appendix B for examples of words with this prefix. Others are placed with the roots to which it is attached. CROSS REFERENCE: meta-, ultra-
posth	Greek *posthe*	foreskin, prepuce (of the penis or clitoris)	PREFIXED ROOT: aposthia (congenital absence of the prepuce) (*a* privative) LEADING ROOT COMPOUND: *posth*: posthitis (*itis* inflammation) *posthe*: posthetomy (surgical removal of the foreskin; circumcision) (*tomy* incision) *posthio*: posthioplasty (plastic surgery of the prepuce; also called *preputioplasty*) (*plassein* to form) *postho*: postholith (a preputial concretion or calculus) (*lithos* stone) TRAILING ROOT COMPOUND: acroposthitis (inflammation of the prepuce of the penis; also called *acrobystitis*) (*akron* extremity + *itis* inflammation) balanoposthitis (inflammation of the glans penis and the prepuce) (*balanos* acorn: head of penis) CROSS REFERENCE: None
prac, prag			See prax- for *eupractic, dyspragia*.
prax, prac, prag	Greek *praxis*	action, exercise	SIMPLE ROOT: *prac*: practice (the exercise of the profession of medicine or one of the allied health professions), practitioner *prag*: pragmatics, pragmatism (a belief that the practical application of a principle should be the determining factor), pragmatist *prax*: praxis (the doing or performance of an action) PREFIXED ROOT: *prac*: malpractice (*malus* bad) *pragia*: dyspragia (painful performance of any function; impairment of the ability to execute purposeful, voluntary movement) (*dys* abnor- mal) miopragia (diminished functional activity in a part) (*meion* less) *pragic*: hyperpragic (characterized by excessive mental activity) (*hyper* above) *pragmasy*: polypragmasy (also called *polypharmacy*) (*polys* many) *praxia*: apraxia (inability to perform purposive movements) {apraxic, aprac- tic} (*a* privative) dyspraxia (partial loss of ability to perform coordinated acts) (*dys* abnormal) eupraxia (intactness of reproduction of acquired, skillful movements) {eupraxic} (*eu* well)

Element	From	Meaning	Examples
prax (cont'd)		[action]	hemiapraxia (affecting only one side of the body) (*hemi* half + apraxia) hyperpraxia (excessive activity; restlessness) (*hyper* over) hypopraxia (*hypo* under) parapraxia (or, parapraxis; disturbed mental processes producing inaccuracy, forgetfulness, and tendency to misplace things and make slips of speech or in writing) (*para* abnormal) LEADING ROOT COMPOUND: *pragmat*: pragmatagnosia (inability to recognize objects once familiar; also called *agnosia*) (agnosia: *a* privative + *gnosis* knowledge) pragmatamnesia (inability to recall the appearance of an object; also called *visual agnosia*) (*amnesia* forgetfulness) *praxio*: praxiology (the study of behavior or conduct, rather than of thought or consciousness) (*logos* study) TRAILING ROOT COMPOUND: *pract*: chiropractic, chiropractor (*cheir* hand) *pragia*: bradypragia (slowness of action) (*bradys* slow) *praxia*: axonapraxia (also called *neurapraxia*) (*axon* axle, axis + apraxia) copropraxia (the involuntary display of unacceptable or obscene gestures) (*kopros* dung, filth) echopraxia (imitation of the movements of another person) neurapraxia (also called *axonapraxia*) (*neuron* nerve + apraxia) pseudoapraxia (*pseudes* false + apraxia) *praxis*: orthopraxis (or, orthopraxy) (*orthos* straight, correct) *praxy*: corepraxy (also called *corepexy*) (*kore* pupil—of eye) PREFIXED TRAILING ROOT COMPOUND: aphagopraxia (also called *dysphagia*) (*a* privative + *phagein* to devour) CROSS REFERENCE: None
pre-	Latin prefix	before	See Appendix B for examples of words with this prefix. Others are placed with the roots to which it is attached. CROSS REFERENCE: ante-, pro-
presby	Greek *presbys* old	old age	See Appendix B for examples of words with this initial combining form. Others are listed with the roots to which it is attached. CROSS REFERENCE: ger[2]
priv	Latin *privare*	to remove, deprive	PREFIXED ROOT: deprivation (loss or absence of parts, organs, powers, or things that are needed) (*de* intensive) TRAILING ROOT COMPOUND: *prival*: renoprival (*renes* kidney) thymyoprival (thymus) thyroprival (also called *hypothyroid*) *privia*: calciprivia (deprivation or loss of calcium; also called *hypocalcemia*) hormonoprivia (hormone: *hormaein* to excite) thyroprivia (also called *hypothyroidism*) *privic*: calciprivic (calcium) chloroprivic (also called *hypochloremic*) (chlorine) thymoprivic (or, thymoprivous) (thymus) CROSS REFERENCE: apheres, steres

A Thesaurus of Medical Word Roots

Element	From	Meaning	Examples
pro-	Greek prefix	before	See Appendix B for examples of words with this prefix. Others are placed with the roots to which it is attached. CROSS REFERENCE: ante-, pre-
proct	Greek *proktos* anus	rectum, anus	PREFIXED ROOT: *proctia*: aproctia (congenital absence or imperforation of the anus) (*a* privative) *proctitis* inflammation of the anus: paraproctitis (compare *periproctitis*) (*para* alongside) periproctitis (also called *perirectitis*) {periproctic} (*peri* around) *proctium*: paraproctium (pl., paraproctia) (*para* alongside) LEADING ROOT COMPOUND: *proct*: proctalgia (also called *proctodynia*) (*algos* pain) proctatresia (imperforation of the anus) (*a* negative + *tresis* hole) proctectasia (*ektasis* dilatation) proctectomy (*ektome* excision) procteurynter (a baglike device used in dilating the rectum) (*eurys* wide) proctitis (*itis* inflammation) proctodeum (pl., proctodea) (*hodaios* a way) [h of hodaios elided] proctodynia (also called *proctalgia*) (*odyne* pain) *procto*: proctocele (also called *rectocele*) (*kele* hernia) proctoclysis (slow introduction of large quantities of liquid into the rectum) (*klysis* a drenching) proctococcypexia (or, proctococcypexy; suture of rectum to the coccyx; also called *rectococcypexy*) (*kokkyx* coccyx + *pexis* fixation) proctocolectomy (colon + *ektome* excision) proctocolitis (also called *coloproctitis*) (colon + *itis* inflammation) proctocolonoscopy (colon + *skopein* to examine) proctocolpoplasty (*kolpos* vagina + *plassein* to form) proctocystocele (*kystis* bladder + *kele* hernia) proctocystoplasty (*kytis* bladder + *plassein* to form) proctocystotomy (*kystis* bladder + *tomy* incision) proctogenic (*genere* to produce) proctography (*graphein* to write) proctology {proctologic} (*logos* study) proctoparalysis (also called *proctoplegia*) proctoperineoplasty (perineum + *plassein* to form) proctoperitoneoplasty (peritoneum + *plassein* to form) proctopexy (also called *rectopexy*) (*pexis* fixation) proctophobia (a morbid fear of rectal disease) (*phobia* fear) proctoplasty (also called *rectoplasty*) (*plassein* to form) proctoplegia (also called *proctoparalysis*) (*plege* stroke) proctopolypus (polypus) proctoptosis (prolapse of the rectum and the anus) (*ptein* to fall) proctorrhagia (*rhagia* bursting forth) proctorrhaphy (also called *rectorrhaphy*) (*rhaphe* suture) proctorrhea (a mucous discharge from the rectum) (*rhein* to flow) proctoscope, proctoscopy (*skopein* to examine) proctosigmoiditis (sigmoid colon + *itis* inflammation) proctospasm (*spasmos* contraction) proctostasis (*stasis* stagnation)

A Thesaurus of Medical Word Roots

Element	From	Meaning	Examples
proct (cont'd)		[rectum, anus]	proctostenosis (also called *rectostenosis*) (*stenosis* a narrowing) proctostomy (*stoma* mouth, opening) proctotomy (*tomy* incision) proctotresia (*tresis* a boring: an opening) proctovalvotomy (valve + *tomy* incision) TRAILING ROOT COMPOUND: coloproctitis (also called *proctocolitis*) (colon + *itis* inflammation) hemoproctia (hemorrhage from the rectum) (*haima* blood) ureteroproctostomy (also called *ureterorectostomy*) (ureter + *stoma* surgical opening) CROSS REFERENCE: an
prosop	Greek *prosopon* from *pros* near + *ops* eye	face	PREFIXED ROOT: aprosopia (*a* privative) diprosopus (*di* two) heteroprosopus (see *janiceps*, under capit-) (*heteros* other) hypereuryprosopic (*hyper* above + *eurys* wide) macroprosopia (also called *megaprosopis*) (*makros* large) megaprosopous (also called *macroprosopia*) (*mega* large) mesoprosopic (*mesos* middle) microprosopia (*mikros* small) triprosopus (*tri* three) LEADING ROOT COMPOUND: *prosop*: prosopagnosia (agnosia: *a* privative + *gnosis* knowledge) prosopalgia (facial pain) (*algos* pain) prosopantritis (*antron* cavity + *itis* inflammation) prosopectasia (oversize of the face) (*ektasis* dilatation) *prosopo*: prosopoanoschisis (oblique facial cleft) (*ana* up + *schisis* fissure) prosopodiplegia (*di* two + *plessein* to strike) prosopopagus (asymmetrical conjoined twins in which the parasite is attached to the face elsewhere than at the jaw) (*pagus* thing fixed) prosopoplegia (facial paralysis) (*plessein* to strike) prosoposchisis (*schisis* fissure) prosopospasm (*spasmos* contraction) prosoposternodymus (conjoined twins face to face and sternum to sternum) TRAILING ROOT COMPOUND: ateloprosopia (*ateles* incomplete) brachyprosopopic (also called *brachyfacial*) (*brachys* short) chamaeprosopy (*chamai* low) dolichoprosopic (also called *dolichofacial*) (*dolichos* long) leptoprosopia (*leptos* slender, thin) schistoprosopia (also known as *facial cleft*) (*schistos* split) schizoprosopia (also known as *facial cleft*) (*schizein* to split) CROSS REFERENCE: faci, opo
prostat	Greek *pro* before + *histanai* to stand	prostate gland	SIMPLE ROOT: prostate (or, prostata; a gland which surrounds the neck of the bladder and the urethra in the male) {prostatic}, prostatism (or, prostatism) PREFIXED ROOT: *prostatic* pertaining to the prostate: extraprostatic (*extra* outside)

Element	From	Meaning	Examples
prostat (cont'd)		[prostate]	intraprostatic (*intra* within)
			periprostatic (*peri* around)
			prostatitis inflammation of the prostate:
			anteprostatitis (*ante* before)
			paraprostatitis (*para* alongside)
			periprostatitis (*peri* around)
			LEADING ROOT COMPOUND:
			prosta: prostatomy (or, prostatotomy) (*tomy* incision)
			prostat:
			prostatalgia (also called *prostatodynia*) (*algos* pain)
			prostatauxe (enlargement of the prostate; also called *prostatomegaly*) (*auxe* increase)
			prostatectomy (*ektome* excision)
			prostatelcosis (*helcosis* ulceration) [h of helcosis elided]
			prostatitis {prostatitic} (*itis* inflammation)
			prostatodynia (also called *prostatalgia*) (*odyne* pain)
			prostatico: prostaticovesical (*vesica* bladder)
			prostato:
			prostatocystitis (*kystis* bladder + *itis* inflammation)
			prostatocystotomy (*kystis* bladder + *tomy* incision)
			prostatography (*graphein* to write)
			prostatolith, prostatolithotomy (*lithos* stone + *tomy* incision)
			prostatomegaly (*megalos* large)
			prostatometer (*metron* measure)
			prostatorrhea (a discharge from the prostate) (*rhein* to flow)
			prostatotomy (or, prostatomy) (*tomy* incision)
			prostatovesiculectomy (*vesica* bladder + *ektome* excision)
			prostatovesiculitis (*vesica* bladder + *itis* inflammation)
			TRAILING ROOT COMPOUND:
			puboprostatic (pubic bone)
			urethroprostatic (urethra)
			vesicoprostatic (*vesica* bladder)
			vesiculoprostatitis (*vesicula* small bladder + *itis* inflammation)
			CROSS REFERENCE: None
prot	Greek *protos* (see NB)	first	SIMPLE ROOT:
			protal (existing from time of birth or before; also called *congenital*)
			protein [see separate entry]
			protium, proton
			PREFIXED ROOT: intraprotoplasmic (*intra* within + *plassein* to form)
			LEADING ROOT COMPOUND:
			prot:
			protanopia (or, protanopsia; color blindness in which there is a defect in the perception of red, red being the first color in the spectrum) {protanopic} (*a* privative + *opia* vision condition)
			protoxide (*oxys* sharp)
			proto:
			protoactinium (or, protactinium) (*aktinos* ray of light)
			protoalbumose (albumin)
			protobiology (the study of bacteriophages) (*bios* life + *logos* study)
			protoblast {protoblastic} (*blastos* bud, shoot, germ)
			protobrochal (denoting the first stage in the development of an ovary) (*brochos* mesh)

A Thesaurus of Medical Word Roots

Element	From	Meaning	Examples
prot (cont'd)		[first]	protocaryon (*karyon* nucleus)
			protochondrium {protochondrial} (*chondros* cartilage)
			protocol (a clinical report from notes first taken; minutes of a meeting; description of steps to be taken in an experiment (*kolla* glue) [orig., the first leaf glued to a manuscript, describing its contents]
			protocone (*konos* cone)
			protoderm (*derma* skin)
			protoduodenum
			protogaster (also called *archenteron*) (*gaster* stomach)
			protonephros (or, protonephron) (*nephros* kidney)
			protopathic (*pathos* disease)
			protoplasia, protoplasm {protoplasmic}, protoplast (*plassein* to form)
			prototroph {prototrophic} (*trephein* to nourish)
			prototype (the original type or form after which other types or forms are developed) (*typos* type)
			protozoon (pl., protozoa) {protozoal} (*zoion* animal)
			NB: *Proteus* is not related to this family. In mythology, he was a sea god who could change his own form or appearance at will; in lower case, *proteus* is a person who changes his or her appearance or principles easily; *protean* is the adjective describing such a person; in medicine, *protean* means having the power to change body form, such as the amoeba.
			CROSS REFERENCE: arch
protein	Greek *protos* first	protein	SIMPLE ROOT:
			protein (any one of a group of complex organic compounds, widely distributed in plants and animals and which form the principal constituents of the cell protoplasm) {proteinaceous, proteinic}
			proteinase (any enzyme that splits native proteins)
			proteome, proteomics, proteose
			PREFIXED ROOT:
			protein:
			metaprotein (*meta* after)
			paraprotein (*para* alongside)
			preprotein (*pre* before)
			proprotein (*pro* before)
			proteinemia condition of protein in the blood:
			dysproteinemia {dysproteinemic} (*dys* abnormal)
			hyperproteinemia (*hyper* above)
			hypoproteinemia (*hypo* below)
			paraproteinemia (also called *plasma cell dyscrasia*) (*para* abnormal)
			proteinosis protein condition:
			hyperproteosis (*hyper* above)
			hypoproteinosis (*hypo* below)
			LEADING ROOT COMPOUND:
			prote: proteuria (or, proteinuria) (*uria* urine condition)
			protein:
			proteinemia (an excess of protein in the blood; also called *albuminuria*) (*emia* blood condition)
			proteinoids (*eidos* form)
			proteinosis (*osis* condition)
			proteinuria (or, proteuria; also called *albuminuria*) (*uria* urine condition)
			proteino:
			proteinochrome (*chroma* color)
			proteinogenous (*genere* to produce)

A Thesaurus of Medical Word Roots

Element	From	Meaning	Examples
protein (cont'd)		[protein]	*proteo*: proteoclastic (*klasis* breakage) proteogenic (*genere* to produce) proteolipids (*lipos* fat) proteolysis {proteolytic} (*lyein* to dissolve) proteometabolism {proteometabolic} proteopepsis {proteopeptic} (*peptein* to digest) proteopexis {proteopectic} (*pexis* fixation) proteosome (*soma* body) *proteos*: proteosuria (*uria* urine condition) TRAILING ROOT COMPOUND: *protein*: lipoprotein (*lipos* fat) myoprotein (*myos* muscle) *proteinosis* protein condition: glycoproteinosis (*glykys* sweet) lipoproteinosis (*lipos* fat) silicoproteinosis (*silex* silica) PREFIXED TRAILING ROOT COMPOUND: *lipoproteinemia* condition of fat protein in the blood: dyslipoproteinemia (*dys* abnormal) hypolipoproteinemia (*hypo* under) CROSS REFERENCE: arch, prot
pseud	Greek *pseudein* to lie, cheat	false	See Appendix B for examples of words with this initial combining form. Others are listed with the roots to which it is attached. CROSS REFERENCE: None
psor	Greek *psora*	itch, scabies	SIMPLE ROOT: psora (an itching disease of the skin) {psoriasic} PREFIXED ROOT: antipsoriatic (also called *antipruritic*) (*anti* against) parapsoriasis (*para* resembling, similar to) LEADING ROOT COMPOUND: *psor*: psorelcosis (*helkosis* ulceration) [h of helcosis elided] psorenteritis (*enteron* intestine + *itis* inflammation) psoroid (resembling scabies) (*eidos* form) psorophthalmia (*ophthalmos* eye) *psoriasi*: psoriasiform (*forma* shape) CROSS REFERENCE: None
psych	Greek *psychein* to breathe, blow, to make cold	mind, spirit, soul	SIMPLE ROOT: psyche (from Psyche, a maiden in Greek and Roman mythology, who personifies the soul) {psychic} PREFIXED ROOT: *psychic*: allopsychic (related mentally to the outside world) (*allos* other) autopsychic (*autos* self) extrapsychic (*extra* outside, beyond) infrapsychic (*infra* below, beneath) intrapsychic (*intra* within) *psychology* study of the mind: metapsychology (*meta* beyond) parapsychology (*para* beside) *psychotic*: antipsychotic (*anti* against) prepsychotic (*pre* before)

A Thesaurus of Medical Word Roots

Element	From	Meaning	Examples
psych (cont'd)		[the mind]	LEADING ROOT COMPOUND:
			psych:
			psychalgia (pain of emotional origin) {psychalgic} (*algos* pain)
			psychanopsia (*an* privative + *opsia* vision condition)
			psychasthenia (*a* privative + *sthenos* strength: weakness)
			psychataxia (*a* privative + *tassein* to arrange)
			psychiatrist, psychiatry {psychiatric} (*iatrein* to heal)
			psychodometry (*hodos* way + *metron* measure) [h of hodos elided]
			psychosis (pl., psychoses) {psychotic} (*osis* condition)
			psyche: psychedelic (*deloun* to make manifest)
			psycho:
			psychoacoustics (*akouein* to hear)
			psychobiology (*bios* life + *logos* study)
			psychocatharsis (*katharos* pure)
			psychochrome, psychochromesthesia (*chroma* color + *esthesia* sensation, feeling)
			psychocortical (pertaining to the mind and to the cortex of the brain) (*cortex* rind: outer covering)
			psychocutaneous (*cutis* skin)
			psychodermatology (*dermatos* skin + *logos* study)
			psychogenesis (*genere* to produce)
			psychogeusic (*geusis* taste)
			psychogogic (*agein* to lead)
			psychogram, psychograph (*graphein* to write)
			psychohormonal (*horme* impulse)
			psychokinesis (*kinein* to move)
			psycholinguistics (*lingua* tongue)
			psychology (*logos* study)
			psychometry (*metron* measure)
			psychomotor (*movere* to move)
			psychoneurosis {psychoneurotic} (*neuron* nerve + *osis* condition)
			psychonosology (*nosos* disease + *logos* study)
			psychonoxious (*noxious* harmful)
			psychopath {psychopathic}, psychopathy (*pathos* disease)
			psychopharmaceuticals, psychopharmacology (*pharmakos* drug + *logos* study)
			psychophysiology (*physein* to grow + *logos* study)
			psychoplegic (an agent that lessens cerebral activity or excitability) (*plege* a blow, stroke)
			psychoprophylaxis (*prophylaxis* guarding against)
			psychosedation, psychosedative (*sedare* to settle, calm)
			psychosensory (*sentire* to feel)
			psychosexual (pertaining to the mental aspects of sex)
			psychosomatic (also called *psychophysiologic*) (*soma* body)
			psychostimulant (*stimulus* goad, incentive)
			psychosurgery (surgical intervention for mental disorders, especially for certain types of violent or antisocial behavior)
			psychotherapy (*therapy* treatment)
			TRAILING ROOT COMPOUND:
			biopsychic (*bios* life)
			bradypsychia (*bradys* slow)
			cenopsychic (*kainos* new, fresh, recent)
			neuropsychic (*neuron* nerve)

Element	From	Meaning	Examples
psych (cont'd)		[the mind]	physiopsychic (pertaining to both mind and body) (*physis* nature) somatopsychic (*somatos* body) visuopsychic (*videre* to see) CROSS REFERENCE: ment, phren², thym²
pto	Greek *ptein* to fall *ptoma* corpse	to fall	SIMPLE ROOT: ptosis (also called *prolapse*; also, *blepharoptosis*; pl., ptoses) {ptosed, ptotic} PREFIXED ROOT: *ptom*: proptometer (also called *exophthalmometer*) (*pro* forward + *metron* measure) symptom (lit., that which falls together; a sign) (*sym* together) *ptosis*: apoptosis (apoptotic} (*apo* away) panoptosis (general prolapse of the abdominal organs) (*pano* all) proptosis (forward displacement of an organ, such as the eyeball; also called *exophthalmos*) {proptotic} (*pro* forward) symptosis (gradual wasting of the whole body or of any organ) (*syn* with) TRAILING ROOT COMPOUND: *ptosia*: aortoptosia (aorta) cardioptosia (or, cardioptosis) (*kardia* heart) enteroptosia (or, enteroptosis) (*enteron* intestine) hysteroptosia (or, hysteroptosis) (*hystera* uterus) nephroptosia (or, nephroptosis) (*nephros* kidney) phrenoptosia (abnormal downward placement of the diaphragm) proctoptosia (or, proctoptosis) (*proktos* anus, rectum) pyloroptosia (downward displacement of the pyloric end of the stomach) splanchnoptosia (or, splanchnoptosis; also called *visceroptosis*) (*splanchnos* viscera: internal organs) splenoptosia (or, splenoptosis) (*splen* spleen) staphyloptosia (or, staphyloptosis) (*staphyle* uvula) ventroptosia (also called *gastroptosis*) (*venter* belly) *ptosis*: blepharoptosis (also called *ptosis*) (*blepharon* eyelid) cardioptosis (or, cardioptosia) (*kardia* heart) carpoptosis (also called *wristdrop*, *drop hand*) (*carpus* wrist) coleoptosis (*koleos* sheath: vagina) coloptosis (colon) colpoptosis (also called *vaginocele*) (*kolpos* vagina) cystoptosis (*kystis* bladder) dacryocystoptosis (*dacyrocyst* lacrimal sac) esophagoptosis (esophagus) gastroptosis (*gaster* stomach, belly) glossoptosis (*glossa* tongue) hepatoptosis (*hepar* liver) iridoptosis (iris—of eye) laryngoptosis (larynx) mastoptosis (pendulous breasts) (*mastos* breast) metroptosis (*metra* uterus) nephroptosis (or, nephroptosia) (*nephros* kidney) odontoptosis (*odontos* tooth)

Element	From	Meaning	Examples
pto (cont'd)		[to fall]	onychoptosis (dropping off of the nails) (*onychos* nail) ophthalmoptosis (also called *exophthalmos*) (*ophthalmos* eye) orchidoptosis (the descending of the testicles) (*orchis* testicle) phrenoptosis (*phren* diaphragm) pseudoptosis (apparent ptosis of the eyelid) (*pseudes* false) pyloroptosis (pylorus) spondyloptosis (also called *spondylolisthesis*) (*spondylos* vertebra) tarsoptosis (also called *flatfoot*) (*tarsus* broad surface) thyroptosis (thyroid gland) uvuloptosis (also called *staphyloptosis*) (uvula) visceroptosis (*viscera* internal organs) CROSS REFERENCE: None
ptyal, ptys	Greek *ptyalon* spittle *ptysis* spitting	spittle, saliva	SIMPLE ROOT: *ptyal*: ptyalin, ptyalism (excessive flow of saliva; also called *hyperptyalism, hypersalivation, polysialia, ptyalorrhea, salivation, sialism, sialismus, sialorrhea*), ptyalize *ptys*: ptysis (spitting; the ejection of saliva from the mouth) PREFIXED ROOT: aptyalism (or, aptyalia; also called *xerostomia*) (*a* privative) hyperptyalism (also called *ptyalism*) (*hyper* above) hypoptyalism (also called *hyposalivation*) (*hypo* under) oligoptyalism (also called *oligosialia*) (*oligos* little, few) LEADING ROOT COMPOUND: *ptya*: ptyalith (a salivary calculus) (*lithos* stone) *ptyal*: ptyalagogue (also called *sialagogue*) (*agein* to lead) ptyalectasis (operative dilatation of a salivary duct; also called *sialectasis*) (*ektasis* dilatation) *ptyalo*: ptyalocele (a salivary cystic tumor or cystic dilatation of a salivary duct; also called *ranula*) (*kele* hernia) ptyalogenic (formed from or by the action of saliva) (*genere* to produce) ptyalography (also called *sialography*) (*graphein* to write) ptyalolith, ptyalolithiasis (also called *sialolithiasis*) (*lithos* stone + *iasis* condition) ptyalolithotomy (also called *sialolithotomy*) (*lithos* stone + *tomy* incision) ptyalorrhea (also called *ptyalism*) (*rhein* to flow) *ptysm*: ptysmagogue (*agein* to lead) TRAILING ROOT COMPOUND: glycoptyalism (*glykos* sweet) melitoptyalism (*melitos* honey) pyoptysis (*pyon* pus) CROSS REFERENCE: sial
pub	Latin *puber*	adult, grown up; becoming an adult	SIMPLE ROOT: puber (one at the onset of puberty), puberal (or, pubertal) pubertas (or, puberty), puberty (period in life at which one of either sex becomes functionally capable of reproduction) pubes (the hair growing over the pubic region), pubescence pubescent (reaching puberty; covered with downy hair) pubic (pertaining to the pubes, or pubic bones) pubis (the os pubis; pl., pubes), pubisure (the pubic hair)

A Thesaurus of Medical Word Roots

Element	From	Meaning	Examples
pub (cont'd)		[becoming an adult]	PREFIXED ROOT: *puberal*: impuberal (destitute of pubic hairs; immature) (*im* negative) postpuberal (or, postpubertal) (*post* after) prepuberal (or, prepubertal) (*pre* before) *puberty*: postpuberty (*post* after) *pubes*: postpubescent (also called *postpuberal*) (*post* following) prepubescence (also called *prepuberty*) (*pre* before) *pubic*: interpubic (between the pubic bones) (*inter* between) retropubic (posterior to the pubic arch) (*retro* behind) subpubic (inferior to the pubic arch) (*sub* under) suprapubic (*supra* above) transpubic (*trans* across) LEADING ROOT COMPOUND: *pub*: pubarche (the beginning of puberty, marked by growth of pubic hair) (*archein* to begin) *puber*: puberphonia (continued use of a high-pitched voice by a male after puberty) (*phone* sound) *pubio*: pubioplasty (a plastic operation on the pubes) (*plassein* to form) pubiotomy (*tomy* incision) *pubo*: pubocapsular (relating to the pubis and the capsule of the hip joint) pubococcygeal (pertaining to the pubis and the coccyx) pubofemoral (pertaining to the os pubis and the femur) puboprostatic (pertaining to the os pubis and the prostate) puborectal (rectum) pubotibial (tibia) pubovesical (also called *vesicopubic*) (*vesica* bladder) TRAILING ROOT COMPOUND: *puberty*: pseudopuberty (*pseudes* false) *pubic*: cotylopubic (relating to both the acetabulum and the os pubis) (*kotyledon* socket) iliopubic (also called *iliopectineal*) (ileum) ischiopubic (of or relating to the ischium and the pubic bone) (*ischion* hip) vesicopubic (pertaining to the bladder and the pubic area; also called *pubovesical*) (*vesica* bladder) TERM: pubertas praecox (puberty at an early age) CROSS REFERENCE: puer
puer	Latin *puer* child	child, childish	SIMPLE ROOT: puerile (pertaining to childhood or to children; childish), puerilism (a condition in which the patient's mind seems to return to its state when a child) LEADING ROOT COMPOUND: puerpera (or, puerperant; a woman who has just given birth; pl., puerperae) {puerperal} puerperalism (pathological condition accompanying childbirth) puerperium (the period or state of confinement after childbirth; pl., puerperia) {puerperal} (*parere* to bring forth, to bear) CROSS REFERENCE: ped[1], pub

A Thesaurus of Medical Word Roots

Element	From	Meaning	Examples
pulmo(n)	Latin *pulmo*	lung	SIMPLE ROOT: pulmo (pl., pulmones) {pulmonal, pulmonary, pulmonic} PREFIXED ROOT: extrapulmonary (not connected with the lungs) (*extra* outside) intrapulmonary (*intra* within) juxtapulmonary (also called *parapulmonary*) (*juxta* near) parapulmonary (also called *juxtapulmonary*) (*para* alongside) subpulmonary (*sub* below) LEADING ROOT COMPOUND: *pulmo*: pulmoaortic (also called *aorticopulmonary*) (aorta) pulmolith (also called *pneumolith*) (*lithos* stone) pulmometer (*metron* measure) *pulmon*: pulmonectomy (also called *pneumonectomy*) (*ektome* excision) pulmonitis (*itis* inflammation) *pulmono*: pulmonohepatic (also called *hepatopulmonary*) (*hepatos* liver) pulmonology (*logos* study) pulmonoperitoneal (peritoneum) TRAILING ROOT COMPOUND: aorticopulmonary (or, aortopulmonary) (aorta) bronchopulmonary (*bronchos* windpipe) cardiopulmonary (also called *pneumocardial*) (*kardia* heart) gastropulmonary (also called *pneumongastric*) (*gaster* stomach) hepaticopulmonary (also called *hepatopneumonic*) (*hepatos* liver) pleuropulmonary (*pleura* side, rib) renopulmonary (*renes* kidney) sinopulmonary (sinus) CROSS REFERENCE: pneumon
puls	Latin *pellere* to beat	to drive, push	SIMPLE ROOT: pulsate (to throb or beat in rhythm) pulsatile (also called *throbbing, beating*) pulsation (a throb or rhythmical beat, as of the heart) pulsator (an apparatus for maintaining respiration) pulse (the expansion and contraction of an artery which may be felt with the finger; also called *pulsus*) pulsellum (a posterior flagellum constituting the organ of locomotion of certain protozoa) pulsion (a pushing forward, or outward or to either side) pulsus (or, pulse) PREFIXED ROOT: compulsion {compulsive} (*com* with) expulsive (tending to expel) (*ex* out) impulse {impulsive}, impulsion (*in* in) propulsion (a tendency to push or fall forward in walking; also called *festination*) (*pro* forward) repulsion (act of driving back; the force of one body on another to cause separation; opposite of *attraction*) (*re* back) retropulsion (pushing back of any part) (*retro* back) LEADING ROOT COMPOUND: pulsimeter (or, pulsometer; a sphygmograph) (*metron* measure) CROSS REFERENCE: crot, sphygm

Element	From	Meaning	Examples
punct, **pung,** **point**	Latin *pungere* to pierce	prick, pierce, spot; point	**SIMPLE ROOT:** *point*: point (a sharp end or apex), pointing (preparing to open spontaneously, as an abscess or boil) *punct*: punctate (having pinpoint punctures or depressions on the surface; marked with dots) punctum (pl., puncta), puncture *pung*: pungent (sharp or biting; somewhat acrid) **PREFIXED ROOT:** counterpuncture (also called *counteropening*) (*contra* against) micropuncture (*mikros* small) **LEADING ROOT COMPOUND:** *puncti*: punctiform (in bacteriology, referring to pinpoint colonies of less than 1mm in diameter) (*forma* shape) *puncto*: punctograph (*graphein* to write) *punctu*: punctumeter (*metron* measure) **TRAILING ROOT COMPOUND:** acupuncture (*acus* needle) aquapuncture (*aqua* water) colipuncture (or, colopuncture; also called *colocentesis*) (colon) craniopuncture (also called *cephalocentesis*) (*kranion* skull) encephalopuncture (*enkephalon* brain) funipuncture (also called *cordocentesis*) (*funis* cord) goniopuncture (an operation for congenital glaucoma) (*gonia* angle) herniopuncture (hernia) ignipuncture (*ignis* fire) vasopuncture (also called *vasotomy*) (*vas* vessel) venipuncture (or, venepuncture; also called *phlebotomy*) (*vena* vein) **FRENCH:** pointillage (a massage manipulation with the tips of the fingers) **CROSS REFERENCE:** cente, macul, nyx
pupil	Latin *pupilla* girl, doll	opening at the center of the iris	**SIMPLE ROOT:** pupil (or, pupilla; the opening at the center of the iris of the eye for the transmission of light) pupilla (or, pupil; pl., pupillae), pupillary (concerning the pupil) **PREFIXED ROOT:** interpupillary (*inter* between) **LEADING ROOT COMPOUND:** *pupill*: pupillatonia (failure of the pupil to react to light; also called *tonic pupil*) (*a* privative + *tonos* tension) *pupillo*: pupillography (*graphein* to write) pupillometer {pupillometry} (*metron* measure) pupillomotor (*movere* to move) pupilloplegia (*plessein* to strike) pupilloscope, pupilloscopy (also called *retinoscopy*) (*skopein* to examine) pupillostatometer (*statos* placed, standing + *metron* measure) **TRAILING ROOT COMPOUND:** iridopupillary (iris of the eye) oculopupillary (pertaining to the pupil and the eye) (*oculus* eye) opticopupillary (pertaining to the optic nerve and the pupil) (*optokos* sight) **CROSS REFERENCE:** cor[2]

Element	From	Meaning	Examples
pur, **pus**	Latin *pus*; *puris* (genitive)	pus	SIMPLE ROOT: *pur*: purulence (or, purulency; also called *suppuration*), purulent *pus*: pus (pl., pura), pustula, pustular, pustulation, pustule PREFIXED ROOT: depurant, depurate {depurative}, depurator (*de* intensive) nonpurulent (not containing pus) (*non* negative) presuppuration (*pre* before + suppuration) suppuration (the formation of pus; the act of becoming converted into and discharging pus) {suppurant, suppurative} (*sub* under) LEADING ROOT COMPOUND: *puri*: puriform (resembling pus; pyoid) (*forma* form) *puro*: purohepatitis (also called *hepatic abscess*) (*hepatos* liver + *itis* inflammation) puromucous (consisting of or containing pus and mucus; also called *mucopurulent*) *pustul*: pustulosis (*osis* condition) *pustuli*: pustuliform (*forma* shape) *pustulo*: pustulocrustaceous (marked by the presence of both pustules and crusts) TRAILING ROOT COMPOUND: *purulent*: fibropurulent (fiber) mucopurulent (also called *puromucous*) sanguinopurulent (*sanguis* blood) saniopurulent (partly sanious and partly purulent) seropurulent (both serous and purulent) *pus*: seropus (purulent serum) (*serum* whey) *pustule*: pseudopustule (*pseudes* false) vesicopustule (*vesica* bladder) CROSS REFERENCE: py
pus			See pod- for *apus*.
pus			See pur- for *pustule*.
py	Greek *pyon*	pus	SIMPLE ROOT: pyesis (suppuration; also called *pyosis*) {pyic} PREFIXED ROOT: apyetous (nonsuppurative; nonpurulent), apyogenic (*a* negative + *genere* to produce) antipyogenic (also called *pyostatic*) (*anti* against + *genere* to produce) diapyesis (suppuration) {diapyetic} (*dia* through) empyectomy (*em* in + *ektome* excision) empyema (abscess) {empyemic}, empyesis (*em* in) empyocele (a collection of pus at the umbilicus) (*em* in + *kele* tumor) hypopyon (an accumulation of pus in the anterior chamber of the eye) (*hypo* under) LEADING ROOT COMPOUND: *py*: pyarthrosis (also called *acute suppurative arthritis*) (*arthron* joint + *osis* condition) pyecchysis (*ec* out + *chein* to pour) pyemesis (vomiting of purulent matter) (*emein* to vomit)

Element	From	Meaning	Examples
py (cont'd)		[pus]	pyemia (also called *metastatic infection*) (*emia* blood condition)
			pyencephalus (or, pyocephalus; also called *brain abscess*) (*enkephalon* brain)
			pyoid (*eidos* form)
			pyophthalmitis (*ophthalmos* eye + *itis* inflammation)
			pyosis (also called *pyesis*) (*osis* condition)
			pyuria (pus in the urine; evidence of renal disease) (*uria* urine condition)
			pyo:
			pyoblennorrhea (*blennos* mucus + *rhein* to flow)
			pyocalix (the presence of pus in a calix of the renal pelvis) (*kalyx* cup)
			pyocele (a hernia or distended cavity containing pus) (*kele* hernia)
			pyocelia (pus in the abdominal cavity) (*koilia* cavity)
			pyocephalus (also called *brain abscess*) (*kephale* head)
			pyochezia (also called *pyofecia*) (*chezein* to defecate)
			pyococcus (*kokkus* a bacterial cell)
			pyocolpos, pyocolpocele (*kolpos* vagina + *kele* hernia)
			pyocyanic, pyocyanogenic (*kyanos* blue + *genic* producing)
			pyocyst, pyocystis (*kystis* sac, bladder)
			pyocyte (also called *pus corpuscle*) (*kytos* cell)
			pyoderma (or, pyodermia) (*derma* skin)
			pyogenesis (also called *pyopoiesis*) {pyogenic} (*genesis* origin)
			pyohemia (also called *pyemia*) (*hemia* blood condition)
			pyohemothorax (*haima* blood + *thorax* chest)
			pyometra, pyometritis (*metra* uterus + *itis* inflammation)
			pyomyoma (*myoma* muscle tumor)
			pyomyositis (*myositis* muscle inflammation)
			pyonephritis (*nephritis* kidney inflammation)
			pyonephrolithiasis (*nephros* kidney + *lithos* stone + *iasis* condition)
			pyonephrosis (also called *nephropyosis*) (*nephros* kidney + *osis* condition)
			pyo-ovarian (ovary)
			pyoperitoneum (peritoneum)
			pyophagia (the swallowing of pus) (*phagein* to devour, consume)
			pyoplania (wandering of pus from one part to another) (*planan* to wander)
			pyopoiesis (also called *pyogenesis, suppuration*) {pyopoietic} (*poiein* to produce)
			pyoptysis (*ptysis* spitting)
			pyopyelectasis (*pyelos* pelvis + *ektasis* a stretching)
			pyorrhea (also called *periodontitis*) {pyorrheal} (*rhein* to flow)
			pyosalpingitis (*salpingos* tube + *itis* inflammation)
			pyosalpingo-oophoritis (*salpingo* tube + oophoritis)
			pyosalpingo-oothecitis (*salpingos* tube + *ootheca* ovary capsule + *itis* inflammation)
			pyosclerosis (*sklerosis* a hardening)
			pyosemia (also called *pyospermia*) (*semia* semen condition)
			pyosepticemia (*septikos* putrefying + *emia* blood condition)
			pyospermia (also called *pyosemia*) (*sperma* seed, sperm)
			pyostatic (*statikos* causing to stand)
			pyostomatitis (*stoma* mouth + *itis* inflammation)
			pyothorax (*thorax* chest)

Element	From	Meaning	Examples
py (cont'd)		[pus]	pyoumbilicus (*umbilicus* navel)
			pyourachus (*urachus* urinary canal of a fetus)
			pyoureter (ureter)
			pyovesiculosis (an accumulation of pus in the seminal vesicles)
			TRAILING ROOT COMPOUND:
			empyema: typhloempyema (*typhlon* blind gut)
			empyesis condition of pus in a part:
			arthroempyesis (also called *arthropyosis*) (*arthron* joint)
			ostempyesis (suppuration within a bone) (*osteon* bone)
			pyo: physopyosalpinx (pus and gas in the Fallopian tube) (*physa* air + *salpinx* tube)
			pyorrhea flowing of pus:
			blepharopyorrhea (also called *purulent ophthalmia*) (*blepharon* eyelid)
			dacryopyorrhea (*dakryon* teardrop)
			otopyorrhea (*otos* ear)
			pyosis condition of pus:
			arthropyosis (also called *arthroempyesis*) (*arthron* joint)
			dacryopyosis (*dakryon* teardrop)
			encephalopyosis (*enkephalon* brain)
			nephropyosis (*nephros* kidney)
			spondylopyosis (*spondylos* vertebra)
			tracheopyosis (trachea)
			ureteropyosis (also called *pyoureter*) (ureter)
			CROSS REFERENCE: pur
pyel	Greek *pyelos* trough, basin	pelvis	SIMPLE ROOT: pyelic (pertaining to the pelvis)
			LEADING ROOT COMPOUND:
			pyel:
			pyelectasia (or, pyelectasis) (*ektasis* dilatation)
			pyelitis {pyelitic} (*itis* inflammation)
			pyelo:
			pyelocaliceal (or, pyelocalyceal; pertaining to the renal pelves and calices; also called *pelvicaliceal, pelvicalyceal*) (*kalyx* cup)
			pyelocaliectasis (*kalyx* cup + *ektasis* dilatation)
			pyelocutaneous (*cutis* skin)
			pyelocystitis (also called *cystopyelitis*) (*kystis* bladder + *itis* inflammation)
			pyelogram, pyelograph {pyelography} (*graphein* to write)
			pyelolithotomy (*lithos* stone + *tomy* incision)
			pyelolymphatic (*lympha* fluid)
			pyelonephritis (*nephritis* kidney inflammation)
			pyelonephrosis (*nephrosis* kidney condition)
			pyelopathy (*pathos* disease)
			pyelophlebitis (*phlebitis* vein inflammation)
			pyeloplasty (*plassein* to form)
			pyeloplication (*plicare* to fold)
			pyeloscopy (*skopein* to examine)
			pyelostomy (*stoma* mouth, opening)
			pyelotomy (incision of renal pelvis) (*tomy* incision)
			pyeloureterectasis (ureter + *ektasis* a stretching)
			pyelovenous (denoting the phenomenon of drainage from the renal pelvis into the venous system because of back pressure) (*vena* vein)

Element	From	Meaning	Examples
pyel (cont'd)		[pelvis]	TRAILING ROOT COMPOUND: *pyelitis* inflammation of the pelvis: cystopyelitis (*kystis* bladder) nephropyelitis (*nephros* kidney) ureteropyelitis (ureter) CROSS REFERENCE: pelvi
pyg	Greek *pyge*	rump, buttocks	SIMPLE ROOT: pygal (also called *natal*, *gluteal*) PREFIXED ROOT: dipygus (a fetus with a double pelvis) (*di* two) epipygus (a fetus with a supernumerary limb or limbs attached to or near the buttock; also called *pygomelus*) (*epi* upon) LEADING ROOT COMPOUND: *pyg*: pygalgia (*algos* pain) *pygo*: pygoamorphus (*a* privative + *morphe* form) pygodidymus (a fetal monster with double hips and pelvis) (*didymos* twin) pygomelus (a fetus with a supernumerary limb or limbs attached to or near the buttocks) (*melos* limb) pygopagus {pygopagy} (*pagos* something fixed) TRAILING ROOT COMPOUND: steatopygia (excessive fatness of the buttocks, usually seen in women) {steatopygous} (*steatos* fat) CROSS REFERENCE: glut[1]
pykn, **pycn**	Greek *pyknos* thick, dense	compact, thick, dense	SIMPLE ROOT: pyknic (having a short, thick, stocky build) PREFIXED ROOT: apyknomorphous (not pyknomorphous; not having the stainable cell elements compactly placed: said of certain nerve cells) (*a* negative + *morphe* form) heteropyknosis (the quality of showing variations in density throughout) {heteropyknotic} (*heteros* other + *osis* condition) isopyknic (*isos* equal) parapyknomorphous (*para* alongside + *morphe* form) postpyknotic (*post* following + *osis* condition) LEADING ROOT COMPOUND: *pykn*: pyknosis {pyknotic} (*osis* condition) *pykno*: pyknocytosis (or, erythropyknosis) (*kytos* cell + *osis* condition) pyknodysostosis (*dys* abnormal + *ostosis* bone condition) pyknometer (an instrument for determining the specific gravity of fluids) {pyknometry} (*metron* measure) pyknomorphic (or, pyknomorphous) (*morphe* form) pyknophrasia (*phrazein* to speak) TRAILING ROOT COMPOUND: *pyknosis* a thickened condition: erythropyknosis (also called *pyknocytosis*) (*erythros* red) karyopyknosis (*karyon* nut, kernel) CROSS REFERENCE: pachy
pyl	Greek *pyle* gate, portal	door, orifice, esp. that of the portal vein	SIMPLE ROOT: pylic (porta, an opening) pylon (a simple prosthesis, usually for a lower limb amputation) pylorus [see separate entry: pylor-] PREFIXED ROOT: micropyle (a minute opening) (*mikros* small)

Element	From	Meaning	Examples
pyl (cont'd)		[orifice]	parapyle (*para* alongside) peripylic (*peri* around) peripylephlebitis (*peri* around + *phlebos* vein + *itis* inflammation) LEADING ROOT COMPOUND: pylephlebectasis (*phlebos* vein + *ektasis* dilatation) pylephlebitis (*phlebos* vein + *itis* inflammation) pylethrombosis (*thrombos* a clot + *osis* condition) CROSS REFERENCE: for, pylor, stom

pylor	Greek
	pyle
	gate +
	ouros
	guard
		pylorus	SIMPLE ROOT: pylorus (lit., gatekeeper; the lower orifice of the
			    stomach opening into the duodenum; pl., pylori) {pyloric}
			PREFIXED ROOT:
			hemipylorectomy (*hemi* half + *ektome* excision)
			juxtapyloric (*juxta* near, close by)
			peripyloric (*peri* around)
			prepyloric (*pre* before)
			LEADING ROOT COMPOUND:
			pylor:
			pyloralgia (rarely used term for pain in the pyloric regions of the
			    stomach) (*algos* pain)
			pylorectomy (*ektome* excision)
			pyloritis (*itis* inflammation)
			pylori: pyloristenosis (*stenos* narrow + *osis* condition)
			pyloro:
			pylorodiosis (*diosis* pushing asunder)
			pyloroduodenal, pyloroduodenitis (duodenum + *itis* inflammation)
			pylorogastrectomy (*gaster* stomach, belly + *ektome* excision)
			pyloromyotomy (*myos* muscle + *tomy* incision)
			pyloroplasty (*plassein* to form)
			pyloroptosis (or, pyloroptosia) (*ptosis* a falling)
			pyloroscopy (*skopein* to examine)
			pylorospasm (*spasmos* contraction)
			pylorostenosis (*stenos* narrow + *osis* condition)
			pylorostomy (*stoma* mouth, opening)
			pylorotomy (*tomy* incision)
			CROSS REFERENCE: pyl

pyr	Greek *pyr* fire	fever, burn	SIMPLE ROOT: pyrectic (or, pyretic; also called *febrile, pyrogen*) pyrexia (fever; pl., pyrexiae) {pyrexial} PREFIXED ROOT: *pyresis*: antipyresis (*anti* against) *pyretic*: apyretic (having no fever; also called *afebrile*) (*a* negative) antepyretic (before the development of fever) (*ante* before) antipyretic (also called *antifebrile, antithermic, febrifugal*) (*anti* against) hyperpyretic (*hyper* above) intrapyretic (also called *intrafebrile*) (*intra* within) metapyretic (also called *postfebrile*) (*meta* after) *pyreuma*: empyreuma (*em* in) *pyrexia*: apyrexia (*a* negative) eupyrexia (*eu* well) hyperpyrexia {hyperpyrexial, hyperpyretic} (*hyper* above)

Element	From	Meaning	Examples
pyr (cont'd)		[fever]	*pyrogenic*: apyrogenic (*a* negative + *genere* to produce) *pyrotic*: antipyrotic (therapeutically effective against burns) (*anti* against) LEADING ROOT COMPOUND: *pyr*: pyrosis (heartburn) {pyrotic} (*osis* condition) *pyreto*: pyretogen, pyretogenesis {pyretogenous} (*genere* to produce) pyretology (*logos* study) pyretolysis (*lyein* to loosen) pyretotyphosis (*tyhposis* delirium) *pyrexio*: pyrexiogenic (*genere* to produce) pyrexiophobia (*phobia* fear) *pyro*: pyrogen (or, pyretogen) {pyrogenic} (*genere* to produce) pyroligneous (relating to or produced by the dry distillation of wood) (*lignum* wood) pyrolysis (*lysis* dissolution) pyromania {pyromaniac} (*mania* craze) pyrometer (*metron* measure) pyrophobia (*phobia* fear) pyroscope (*skopein* to examine) pyrotherapy (also called *fever therapy, therapeutic fever, pyrotherapy*) (*therapy* treatment) TRAILING ROOT COMPOUND: alexipyretic (reducing fever; that which reduces fever) (*alexein* to ward off) galactopyra (milk fever) (*gala* milk) lechopyra (puerperal fever) (*lecho* parturient woman) CROSS REFERENCE: caum, phleg
pyren	Greek *pyren* fruit stone	nucleus	PREFIXED ROOT: apyrene (having no nucleus or nuclear material) (*a* privative) amphipyrenin (*amphi* both) LEADING ROOT COMPOUND: pyrenemia (the presence of nucleated red corpuscles in the blood) (*emia* blood condition) pyrenoid (*eidos* form) CROSS REFERENCE: karyo, nuc(le)

Q

Element	From	Meaning	Examples
quadr, **quat**	Latin *quattuor* four	four, fourth; forty, fortieth	SIMPLE ROOT: *quad*: quadrant (the quarter or fourth of a circle; one of four corresponding regions, as of the abdomen, divided for descriptive and diagnostic purposes), quadrate (or, quadratus) *quat*: quaternary (fourth in order) LEADING ROOT COMPOUND: *quadr*: quadrangular (having four angles) *quadrant*: quadrantanopia (loss of sight in approximately one fourth of the vision field) (*an* privative + *opia* vision condition) *quadri*: quadriceps (four-headed; possessing four heads; a particular muscle; pl., quadriceps, quadricepses) (*caput* head) quadricepsplasty (quadriceps + *plassein* to form) quadricuspid (*cuspis* point) quadridentate (having four coordinate covalent bonds in a chelate) (*dens* tooth) [chelate: a chemical compound] quadridigitate (also called *tetradactylous*) (*digit* finger, toe) quadrigeminus (quadruplet) (*geminus* twin) quadrilateral (*laterus* side) quadrilocular (*loculus* a small space) quadripara (also called *quartipara*) (*parere* to bear young) quadriparesis (also called *tetraparesis*) (*paresis* paralysis) quadripartite (*partire* to divide) quadriplegia (paralysis of all four extremities; also called *tetraplegia*) {quadriplegic} (*plessein* to strike) quadripolar (having four poles, as a cell) quadrisect, quadrisection (*sectare* to cut) quadritubercular (having four tubercles or cusps, as a molar tooth) (*tubercule* a small swelling) quadrivalent (also called *tetravalent*) (*valere* to be strong) *quadru*: quadruped (a four-footed animal) (*pes* foot) quadruplet (also called *quadrigeminus*) CROSS REFERENCE: quart, tetra
quart	Latin *quartus*	fourth	SIMPLE ROOT: quart, quartan (recurring every fourth day), quarter quartile (one fourth of the distribution of scores) LEADING ROOT COMPOUND: quartipara (also called *quadripara*) (*parere* to bear) quartisect (*sectere* to cut) quartisternal (sternum) PRESCRIPTION TERM: quarter in die (four times a day; abbreviated q.i.d.) CROSS REFERENCE: quadr

R

Element	From	Meaning	Examples
rachi, **rhachi**	Greek *rhachis* spine	spine, backbone; also, rickets	SIMPLE ROOT: rachial (or, rachidial, rachidian; also called *spinal*) rachis (or, rhachis; the spinal column; pl., rachises) rachitism PREFIXED ROOT: *rachidian*: intrarachidian (also called *intraspinal*) (*intra* within) *rachis*: endorrhachis (also called *spinal dura mater*) (*endon* within) *rachitic*: antirachitic (effective against rickets) (*anti* against) *rachischisis* spine fissure: hemirachischisis (*hemi* half) holorachischisis (fissure of the entire spinal cord; also called *rachischisis totalis*) (*holos* whole, entire) LEADING ROOT COMPOUND: *rach*: rachitis (rickets; also called *spondylitis*) (*itis* inflammation) *rachi*: rachialgia (also called *rachiodynia*) (*algos* pain) rachianesthesia (anesthesia: *an* negative + *esthesia* feeling) rachicentesis (or, rachiocentesis; also called *lumbar puncture*) (*kentein* to puncture) rachigraph (*graphein* to write) rachilysis (*lyein* to loosen) rachiodynia (also called *rachialgia*) (*odyne* pain) rachischisis (also called *spina bifida*) (*schisis* fissure) rachitome (or, rachiotome; a cutting instrument for opening the spinal canal) (*temnein* to cut) *rachio*: rachiocampsis (*kampis* curve) rachiocentesis (or, rachicentesis) (*kentein* to puncture) rachiochysis (the effusion of a fluid within the vertebral canal) (*chein* to pour) rachiocyphosis (also called *kyphosis*) (*kyphosis* humpback) rachiometer (an instrument for measuring the curvature of the spine) (*metron* measure) rachiomyelitis (also called *myelitis*) (*myelos* marrow + *itis* inflammation) rachiopagus (twins united at the back) (*pagos* thing fixed) rachiopathy (also called *spondylopathy*) (*pathos* disease) rachioplegia (spinal paralysis) (*plessein* to strike) rachioscoliosis (*skoliosis* bending) rachiotome (or, rachitome), rachiotomy (*tomy* incision) *rachito*: rachitogenic (causing rickets) (*genere* to produce) TRAILING ROOT COMPOUND: atelorachidia (*ateles* incomplete: *a* negative + *telos* complete) cerebrorachidian (also called *cerebrospinal*) (*cerebrum* brain) encephalorachidian (also called *cerebrospinal*) (*enkephalon* brain) meningorachidian (*meningos* membrane) merorachischisis (*meros* part, share) schistorachis (*schistos* split) scoliorachitic (*skolios* twisted) CROSS REFERENCE: dors, noto, spin, spondyl, vertebr

A Thesaurus of Medical Word Roots

Element	From	Meaning	Examples
rad[1]	Latin *radius* ray, spoke of wheel	ray; spread out; radium	SIMPLE ROOT: radiability, radiable, radiad (toward the radius or radial side of the forearm) radial, radialis, radian, radiant (diverging from the common center; emitting radiation or heat; transmitted by radiation) radiate, radiation, radium (Ra), radius (pl., radii) PREFIXED ROOT: *radial*: interradial (situated between rays) (*inter* between) transradial (through the radial artery; across the radius) (*trans* across, through) triradial (also called *triradiate*) (*tri* three) *radiation*: antiradiation (*anti* against) diradiation (the emission and diffusion of rays of light) (*dis* away) irradiation (also called *radiotherapy*) (*in* in) triradiation (*tri* three) *radiograph*: microradiography (*mikros* small + *graphein* to write) LEADING ROOT COMPOUND: *radi*: radiferous (containing radium) (*ferre* to bear) *radio*: radioactive, radioactivity (*agere* to do, act) radiobicipital (pertaining to the radius and the biceps) radiocarpus {radiocarpal} (*karpos* wrist) radiogenesis (*genere* to produce) radiology (*logos* study) radiometer (*metron* measure) radiomutation (*mutare* to change) radiophobia (*phobia* fear) radiophylaxis (*phylaxis* protection) radioscopy (*skopein* to examine) radiotherapy (also called *irradiation*) (*therapy* treatment) TRAILING ROOT COMPOUND: brachioradial (muscle used to rotate the hand) (*brachium* arm) cubitoradial (*cubitalis* elbow) dorsoradial (relating to the radial, or outer, side of the back of the forearm, wrist, hand, or fingers) (*dorsum* back) humeroradial (humerus) ulnoradial (*ulna* the arm) CROSS REFERENCE: actin, helc, noma, plan[2]
rad[2]	Latin *radix, radicis*	root	SIMPLE ROOT: radical, radicle (or, radicula; also called *ramulus*) radix (pl., radices) {radicular} PREFIXED ROOT: interradicular (*inter* between) periradicular (*peri* around) LEADING ROOT COMPOUND: *radi*: radiectomy (or, radectomy; also called *root amputation*) (*ektome* excision) *radici*: radiciform (*forma* shape) *radico*: radicotomy (also called *rhizotomy*) (*tomy* incision) *radicul*: radiculalgia (*algos* pain) radiculectomy (excision of a rootlet) (*ektome* excision)

Element	From	Meaning	Examples
rad[2] (cont'd)		[root]	radiculitis (also called *radiculopathy*) (*itis* inflammation)
			radiculo:
			radiculoganglionitis (*ganglion* knot + *itis* inflammation)
			radiculography (*graphein* to write)
			radiculomedullary (*medulla* marrow)
			radiculomeningomyelitis (*meningos* membrane + *myelos* marrow + *itis* inflammation)
			radiculoneuritis (*neuron* nerve + *itis* inflammation)
			radiculoneuropathy (*neuron* nerve + *pathos* disease)
			radiculopathy (also called *radiculitis*) (*pathos* disease)
			TRAILING ROOT COMPOUND:
			radiculitis root inflammation:
			encephaloradiculitis (*enkephalon* brain)
			meningoradiculitis (*meningos* membrane)
			myeloradiculitis (*myelos* marrow)
			radiculo: myeloradiculopathy (*myelos* marrow + *pathos* disease)
			CROSS REFERENCE: rhiz
raphe			See rhaph-.
re-	Latin prefix	back, again	See Appendix B for examples of words with this prefix. Others are placed with the roots to which it is attached.
			CROSS REFERENCE: ana-, retro-
rect, reg	Latin *regere* to be straight; *rectum* straight; *regula* rule	to be straight; rectum	SIMPLE ROOT:
			rect: rectum (the terminal portion of the large intestine; pl., rectums, recta) {rectal}, rectus (straight; not crooked)
			reg: regimen (a strictly regulated scheme of diet, exercise, or other activity designed to achieve certain ends)
			PREFIXED ROOT:
			rect:
			arrector (raising, or that which raises; pl., arrectores) (*ad* to)
			correction {corrective; also called *corrigent*) (*com* with, together)
			erectile, erection (the condition of being made rigid and elevated)
			erector (that which or one who erects, such as a muscle which raises or holds up a part) (*ex* out)
			rectal:
			intrarectal (*intra* within)
			pararectal (*para* beside)
			perirectal (*peri* around)
			prerectal (*pre* before)
			subrectal (*sub* below)
			rectum:
			megarectum (*mega* large: dilated)
			mesorectum {mesorectal} (*mesos* middle)
			LEADING ROOT COMPOUND:
			rect:
			rectalgia (also called *proctalgia*) (*algos* pain)
			rectectomy (also called *proctectomy*) (*ektome* excision)
			rectischiac (*ischion* hip)
			rectitis (also called *proctitis*) (*itis* inflammation)
			recto:
			rectoabdominal (abdomen)
			rectocele (also called *proctocele*) (*kele* hernia)
			rectoclysis (also called *proctoclysis*) (*klysis* a drenching)
			rectococcypexy (fixation of rectum by suturing it to coccyx; also called *proctococcypexy*) (coccyx + *pexis* fixation)

Element	From	Meaning	Examples
rect (cont'd)		[to be straight; rectum]	rectocolitis (also called *proctocolitis, coloproctitis*) (colon + *itis* inflammation)
			rectocutaneous (*cutis* skin)
			rectocystotomy (incision of the bladder through rectum, usually to remove a calculus; also called *proctocystotomy*) (*kystis* bladder + *tomy* incision)
			rectoclysis (also called *proctoclysis*) (*klysis* a washing out)
			rectoperineal (perineum)
			rectopexy (also called *proctopexy*) (*pexis* fixation)
			rectophobia (also called *proctophobia*) (*phobia* fear)
			rectoplasty (also called *proctoplasty*) (*plassein* to form)
			rectorrhaphy (also called *proctorrhaphy*) (*rhaphe* suture)
			rectoscope (also called *proctoscope*) (*skopein* to examine)
			rectosigmoid (sigmoid process)
			rectostenosis (also called *proctostenosis*) (*stenosis* narrow)
			rectostomy (also called *proctostomy*) (*stoma* mouth, opening)
			rectotome, rectotomy (also called *proctotomy*) (*tomy* incision)
			rectourethral (also called *urethrorectal*) (urethra)
			rectouterine (also called *uterorectal*) (uterus)
			rectovaginal (vagina)
			rectovesical (also called *vesicorectal*) (*vesica* bladder)
			rectovestibular (pertaining to the rectum and the vestibule of the vagina)
			rectovulvar (also called *vulvorectal*) (*vulvae* external female genitals)
			TRAILING ROOT COMPOUND:
			rectal:
			ileorectal (ileum)
			ischiorectal (*ischion* hip)
			pelvirectal (pelvis)
			puborectal (pubic bone)
			ureterorectal (ureter)
			urethrorectal (also called *rectourethral*) (urethra)
			urorectal (relating to the urinary tract and rectum) (*ouron* urine)
			uterorectal (also called *rectouterine*) (uterus)
			vesicorectal (also called *rectovesical*) (*vesica* bladder)
			vulvorectal (also called *rectovulvar*) (vulva)
			rectum:
			anorectum (the anus and the rectum considered together as a single unit) {anorectal}
			colorectum {colorectal}, colorectitis (also called *coloproctitis*) (colon + *itis* inflammation)
			TERM: per rectum (by way of the rectum)
			FRENCH: redressement (a second or repeated dressing; correction of a deformity)
			CROSS REFERENCE: orth (straight); an, proct (rectum)
reg			See rect- for *regimen*.
ren	Latin *ren*	kidney	SIMPLE ROOT:
			ren (pl., renes), renal (also called *nephric*)
			renculus (also called *cortical lobules of kidney*)
			reniculus (pl., reniculi), renin, reninism
			renule, renunculus (renal lobe)
			PREFIXED ROOT:
			renal:
			adrenal (*ad* to) [see separate entry: adren-]

Element	From	Meaning	Examples
ren (cont'd)		[kidney]	circumrenal (also called *perinephric*) (*circum* around)
			extrarenal (*extra* outside)
			infrarenal (*infra* below)
			interrenal (*inter* between)
			intrarenal (*intra* within)
			nonrenal (not resulting from dysfunction of the kidneys)
			pararenal (also called *paranephric*) (*para* alongside)
			perirenal (also called *perinephric*) (*peri* around)
			postrenal (*post* after, behind)
			prerenal (*pre* before)
			suprarenal (*supra* above)
			renalism: hyposuprarenalism (also called *adrenal insufficiency*) (*hypo* under + *supra* over)
			reninemia condition of renin in the blood:
			hyperreninemia {hyperreninemic} (*hyper* above)
			hyporeninemia {hyporeninemic} (*hypo* under)
			LEADING ROOT COMPOUND:
			reni:
			renicapsule (the capsule of the kidney)
			renicardiac (also called *cardiorenal*) (*kardia* heart)
			reniform (*forma* shape)
			reniportal (*porta* gate)
			renin: reninoma (*oma* tumor)
			reno:
			renocortical (*cortex* covering)
			renocutaneous (also called *nephrocutaneous*) (*cutis* skin)
			renocystogram (also called *renogram*) (*kystis* bladder + *graphein* to write)
			renogastric (*gaster* stomach, belly)
			renogram, renography (*graphein* to write)
			renointestinal (also called *enterorenal*)
			renomedullary (*medulla* marrow)
			renopathy (also called *nephropathy*) (*pathos* disease)
			renoprival (*privare* to deprive, excise)
			renopulmonary (*pulmon* lung)
			renoscopy (*skopein* to examine)
			renotrophic (having the ability to increase kidney size, due mainly to hypertrophy of the convoluted tubules) (*trephein* to nourish)
			renotropic (*trepein* to turn)
			renovascular (*vas* blood vessel)
			TRAILING ROOT COMPOUND:
			renal:
			aorticorenal (aorta)
			arteriorenal (artery)
			cardiorenal (*kardia* heart)
			enterorenal (also called *renointestinal*) (*enteron* intestine)
			gastrorenal (also called *renogastric*) (*gaster* stomach)
			hepatorenal (also called *hepatoneprhic*) (*hepatos* liver)
			lienorenal (also called *splenorenal*) (*lien* spleen)
			splenorenal (also called *lienorenal*) (*splen* spleen)
			vesicorenal (pertaining to the urinary bladder and the kidney) (*vesica* bladder)
			renism: primaryreninism (*primary* first, foremost)
			CROSS REFERENCE: nephr

Element	From	Meaning	Examples
ret	Latin *rete* net	net, retina	SIMPLE ROOT: rete (pl., retia) {retial} reticulated (or, reticular; netlike; pertaining to a reticulum) reticulum (a network, especially a protoplasmic network in cells; pl., reticula) retina (innermost or third tunic of the eye which receives images formed by the lens and is the immediate instrument of vision) {retinal} retinaculum (the structure that retains an organ or tissue in place; pl., retinacula) PREFIXED ROOT: *reticular*: antireticular (*anti* against) *retina*: ectoretina (also called *pigmented layer of retina*) (*ektos* outside) entoretina (*enton* within) *retinal*: epiretinal (*epi* upon) intraretinal (*intra* within) panretinal (*pan* all) preretinal (*pre* before) subretinal (*sub* below) LEADING ROOT COMPOUND: *reti*: retiform (*forma* shape) *reticul*: reticulitis (*itis* inflammation) reticuloid (*eidos* form) reticulosis (*osis* condition) *reticulo*: reticulocyte, reticulocytogenic (*kytos* cell + *genere* to produce) reticulocytosis (*kytos* cell + *osis* condition) reticulocytopenia (or, reticulopenia) (*kytos* cell + *penia* deficiency) reticulopodium (also called *rhizopodium*) (*pous* foot) *retin*: retinectomy (*ektome* excision) retinitis (*itis* inflammation) retinoid (*eidos* form) retinoma (also called *retinocytoma*) (*oma* tumor) retinosis (*osis* condition) *retino*: retinoblastoma (*blastos* germ, cell + *oma* tumor) retinochoroiditis (choroid + *itis* inflammation) retinocytoma (also called *retinoma*) (*kytos* cell + *oma* tumor) retinodialysis (*dialysis* separation) retinograph, retinography (*graphein* to write) retinomalacia (*malakos* soft) retinopapillitis (*papilla* nipple-like process + *itis* inflammation) retinopathy (*pathos* disease) retinopexy (*pexis* fixation) retinopiesis (*piesis* pressure) retinoschisis (a congenital cleft of the retina) (*schisis* fissure) retinoscopy (also called *koroscopy*) (*skopein* to examine) *reto*: retoperithelium (*peri* around + *thele* papilla, nipple) retothelium {retothelial} (*thele* papilla, nipple)

A Thesaurus of Medical Word Roots

Element	From	Meaning	Examples
ret (cont'd)		[net, retina]	TRAILING ROOT COMPOUND: *reticulate*: fibroreticulate (fiber) *retinal*: chorioretinal (*chorion* membrane—enclosing the fetus) idioretinal (pertaining to the retina alone) (*idios* one's own) tapetoretinal (*tapetum* membranous covering) *retinitis* inflammation of the retina: chorioretinitis (*chorion* membrane—enclosing the fetus) neuroretinitis (*neuron* optic nerve) papilloretinitis (*papilla* nipple-shaped projection) photoretinitis (*phos* light) *retinogram*: electroretinogram (elektron + *graphein* to write) *retinograph*: electroretinograph (elektron + *graphein* to write) *retinopathy* disease of the retina: chorioretinopathy (*chorion* membrane—enclosing the fetus) neuroretinopathy (*neuron* optic disk) tapetoretinopathy (*tapetum* membranous layer) CROSS REFERENCE: None
retro-	Latin prefix	back, backward	See Appendix B for examples of words with this prefix. Others are placed with the roots to which it is attached. CROSS REFERENCE: opist, re-
rhabd	Greek *rhabdos*	rod, stick	LEADING ROOT COMPOUND: *rhabd*: rhabdoid (resembling a rod; rod-shaped) (*eidos* shape) *rhabdo*: rhabdomyo [not a word itself: see separate entry] rhabdovirus (any of a group of rod-shaped RNA viruses with one important member, the rabies virus, pathogenic to man) (*virus* poison) CROSS REFERENCE: bac, bacteri
rhabdomyo	Greek *rhabdos* rod + *myos* muscle	rod-shaped muscle	LEADING ROOT COMPOUND: rhabdomyoblast {rhabdomyoblastic}, rhabdomyoblastoma (*blastos* germ + *oma* tumor) rhabdomyochondroma (*chondros* cartilage + *oma* tumor) rhabdomyolysis (*lyein* to loosen) rhabdomyoma (*oma* tumor) rhabdomyomyxoma (*myxa* mucus + *oma* tumor) rhabdomyosarcoma (*sarkos* flesh + *oma* tumor) CROSS REFERENCE: None
rhaph, **rrhaph**, **raphe**	Greek *rhaphein* to stitch together	to suture, sew, stitch; seam, ridge	SIMPLE ROOT: rhaphe (or, raphe; a seam or ridge) PREFIXED ROOT: *raph*: dysraphism (or, dysraphia) (*dys* abnormal) *rraphy*: autorrhaphy (wound enclosure by using strands of tissue taken from edges of the wound) (*autos* self) encatarrhaphy (lit., to sew in; the operation of burying a structure by suturing the sides of the tissues surrounding it) (*en* in + *kata* down) mesorrhaphy (also called *mesenteriorrhaphy*) (*mesos* middle) prorrhaphy (*pro* before) TRAILING ROOT COMPOUND: achillorrhaphy (suture of the Achilles tendon) aneurysmorrhaphy (*aneurysm* a widening) angiorrhaphy (*angeion* blood vessel) annulorrhaphy (*anulus* ringlike structure)

A Thesaurus of Medical Word Roots

Element	From	Meaning	Examples
rhaph (cont'd)		[to suture]	aortorrhaphy (aorta)
			arteriorrhaphy (artery)
			blepharorrhaphy (also called *tarsorrhaphy*) (*blepharon* eyelid)
			bronchorrhaphy (*bronchus* windpipe)
			canthorrhaphy (*canthus* angle of the eye)
			cardiorrhaphy (*kardia* heart)
			cecorrhaphy (*cecum* blind gut)
			celiorrhaphy (also called *laparorrhaphy*) (*koilia* belly)
			cheilorrhaphy (*cheilos* lip)
			colorrhaphy (colon)
			colporrhaphy (*kolpos* vagina)
			cystorrhaphy (*kystis* bladder)
			duodenorrhaphy (duodenum)
			enterorrhaphy (*enteron* intestine)
			episiorrhaphy (*epision* pubic region: vulva)
			fasciorrhaphy (*fascia* band of tissue)
			gastrorrhaphy (*gaster* stomach, belly)
			glossorrhaphy (*glossa* tongue)
			hepatorrhaphy (*hepatos* liver)
			herniorrhaphy (*hernia* rupture: protrusion)
			hymenorrhaphy (*hymen* membrane)
			hysterorrhaphy (*hystera* uterus)
			ileorrhaphy (*eilein* to roll up: *ileum* lower abdomen, intestines)
			jejunorrhaphy (*jejunum* empty: portion of the small intestine)
			laparorrhaphy (also called *celiorrhaphy*) (*lapara* flank, loin)
			laryngorrhaphy (larynx)
			meatorrhaphy (*meatus* passage)
			meningeorrhaphy (*meningos* membrane)
			mesenteriorrhaphy (also called *mesorrhaphy*) (*mesentery* membranous fold)
			myelorrhaphy (*myelos* spinal cord)
			myocardiorrhaphy (*myos* muscle + *kardia* heart: myocardium)
			myorrhaphy (also called *myosuture*) (*myos* muscle)
			nephrorrhaphy (*nephros* kidney)
			neurorrhaphy (also called *neurosuture*) (*neuron* nerve)
			omentorrhaphy (*omentum* fat skin)
			orchiorrhaphy (also called *orchiopexy*) (*orchis* testicle, testis)
			osteorrhaphy (*osteon* bone)
			palatorrhaphy (also called *uranorrhaphy*) (*palatum* roof of mouth)
			pericardiorrhaphy (pericardium)
			perineorrhaphy (perineum)
			phleborrhaphy (also called *venorrhaphy*) (*phlebos* vein)
			pneumonorrhaphy (*pneumon* lung)
			proctorrhaphy (also called *rectorrhaphy*) (*proktos* anus)
			rectorrhaphy (also called *proctorrhaphy*) (rectum)
			rhinorrhaphy (*rhinos* nose)
			salpingorrhaphy (*salpingos* tube)
			splenorrhaphy (also called *splenopexy*) (spleen)
			staphylorrhaphy (*staphyle* uvula)
			syndesmorrhaphy (*syndesis* bound together: ligament)
			tarsorrhaphy (also called *blepharorrhaphy*) (*tarsos* eyelid)
			tenorrhaphy (also called *tenosuture*) (tendon)
			trachelorrhaphy (suture of the uterine cervix) (*trachelos* neck)
			tracheorrhaphy (*trachea* windpipe)

Element	From	Meaning	Examples
rhaph (cont'd)		[to suture]	typhlorrhaphy (also called *cecorrhaphy*) (*typhlon* blind gut)
			ureterorrhaphy (ureter)
			urethrorrhaphy (urethra)
			CROSS REFERENCE: None
rhe, **rrhe**	Greek *rhein* to flow	to run, flow	PREFIXED ROOT:
			diarrhea (also called *enterorrhea*) (*dia* across, through)
			dysmenorrhea (painful menstruation) (*dys* abnormal + menses)
			hyporrhea (slight hemorrhage) (*hypo* below)
			isorrhea {isorrheic} (*isos* equal)
			polyrrhea (*polys* much)
			LEADING ROOT COMPOUND:
			rhe: rheostosis (*osteon* bone + *osis* condition)
			rheo:
			rheobase (*baein* to go)
			rheography (*graphein* to write)
			rheology (the science of the deformation and flow of matter, such as the flow of blood through the heart and blood vessels) (*logos* study)
			rheometer (*metron* measure)
			rheonome (*nemein* to distribute)
			rheophore (*pherein* to bear)
			rheostat (*statikos* standing)
			rheotachygraphy (*tachys* swift, rapid + *graphein* to write)
			rheotaxis (also called *rheotropism*) (*tassein* to arrange)
			rheotropism (also called *rheotaxis*) (*trepein* to turn)
			TRAILING ROOT COMPOUND:
			albuminorrhea (albumin)
			amniorrhea (the escape of amniotic fluid) (*amnion* membrane)
			amylorrhea (the presence of excessive or undigested starch in the stools) (*amylon* starch)
			azotorrhea (discharged of excessive quantities of nitrogenous matter in the stools) (*azote* nitrogen)
			blennorrhea (a mucous discharge, especially from the urethra or vagina; also called *blennorrhagia, myxorrhea*) (*blenna* mucus)
			blepharopyorrhea (also called *purulent ophthalmia*) (*blepharon* eyelid + *pyon* pus)
			bronchorrhea (*bronchos* windpipe)
			cholororrhea (excessive secretion of bile) (*chole* bile)
			chylorrhea (*chylus* gastric juice)
			chymorrhea (*chymos* juice)
			colorrhea (colon)
			colostrorrhea (the thin, yellow, milky fluid secreted by the mammary gland before or after parturition) (colostrum)
			creatorrhea (*kreas* flesh, meat)
			cystorrhea (*kystis* sac, bladder)
			dacryorrhea (*dakyron* teardrop)
			enterorrhea (also called *diarrhea*) (*enteron* intestine)
			fibrinorrhea (*fibra* fiber)
			galactorrhea (also called *lactorrhea*) (*galaktos* milk)
			gastrorrhea (*gaster* stomach, belly)
			glycorrhea (*glykys* sweet)
			gonorrhea (*gone* a seed: genitalia)
			graphorrhea (*graphein* to write)
			hepatorrhea (*hepatos* liver)

Element	From	Meaning	Examples
rhe (cont'd)		[to run, flow]	hydrorrhea (*hydor* water)
			ichorrhea (*ichor* fluid from a sore)
			lactorrhea (also called *galactorrhea*) (*lactis* milk)
			lalorrhea (also called *logorrhea*) (*lalein* to babble)
			laryngorrhea (larynx)
			leukorrhea (also called *leukorrhagia*) (*leukos* white)
			lochiorrhea (*lochia* vaginal discharge after childbirth)
			logorrhea (a ceaseless flow of words; also called *agitophasia, tachylalia, verbomania*) (*logos* word)
			lymphorrhea (*lympha* water, fluid)
			melanorrhea (passage of dark-colored tarry stools, due to the presence of blood altered by the intestinal juices; also called *melena*) (*melanos* dark)
			meningorrhea (also called *meningorrhagia*) (*meningos* membrane)
			menorrhea (normal menstrual flow; also, *profuse* menstruation) (*mene* month: menstruation)
			metrorrhea (*metra* uterus)
			omphalorrhea (*omphalos* navel)
			ophthalmorrhea (*ophthalmos* eye)
			otorrhea (*otos* ear)
			pharyngorrhea (pharynx)
			pimelorrhea (also called *fatty diarrhea*) (*pimele* fat)
			pleurorrhea (*pleura* side, rib)
			proctorrhea (*proktos* anus)
			prostatorrhea (prostate)
			ptyalorrhea (also called *pytalism, sialorrhea*) (*ptyalon* saliva)
			pyorrhea (also called *periodontitis*) (*pyon* pus)
			rhinorrhea (*rhis* nose)
			seborrhea (also called *hypersteatosis*) (*sebum* suet)
			sialorrhea (also called *ptyalism, ptyalorrhea*) (*sialon* saliva)
			spermatorrhea (*spermatos* seed, sperm)
			steatorrhea (an excessive amount of fat in the stool) (*steatos* fat)
			sudorrhea (*sudor* perspiration, sweat)
			tuborrhea (a fluid discharge from the auditory tube)
			ulorrhea (*oulon* gums)
			urethrorrhea (urethra)
			PREFIXED TRAILING ROOT COMPOUND:
			agalorrhea (*a* privative + *gala* milk)
			amenorrhea (also called *amenia*) (*a* privative + menses)
			amyxorrhea (*a* privative + *myxa* mucus)
			CROSS REFERENCE: drom, rheum, rrhag
rheum	Greek *rheuma*	flux (excessive flow)	SIMPLE ROOT:
			rheum (any watery or catarrhal discharge) {rheumic}
			rheumatic, rheumatism (lit., suffering from a flux)
			PREFIXED ROOT: antirheumatic (*anti* against)
			LEADING ROOT COMPOUND:
			rheumat:
			rheumatalgia (*algos* pain)
			rheumatoid (*eidos* form)
			rheumatosis (*osis* condition)
			rheumato:
			rheumatogenic (*genere* to produce)
			rheumatologist, rheumatology (*logos* study)
			CROSS REFERENCE: rhe

Element	From	Meaning	Examples
rhex, **rrhex**	Greek *rhexis*	breaking forth, bursting, rupture	SIMPLE ROOT: rhexis (the rupture of an organ or vessel) PREFIXED ROOT: anarrhexis (the operation of refracturing a bone) (*ana* again) TRAILING ROOT COMPOUND: amniorrhexis (*amnion* membrane) arteriorrhexis (artery) capsulorrhexis (capsule of the lens) cardiorrhexis (*kardia* heart) colporrhexis (*kolpos* vagina) dermatorrhexis (*dermatos* skin) desmorrhexis (*desmos* ligament) elastorrhexis (elastic fibers) enterorrhexis (*enteron* intestine) erythrorrhexis (also called *erythrocytorrhexis*) (*erythros* red) gastrorrhexis (*gaster* stomach, belly) hepatorrhexis (*hepatos* liver) historrhexis (*histos* web, tissue) hysterorrhexis (also called *metrorrhexis*) (*hystera* uterus) karyorrhexis (*karyon* nut: nucleus) keratorrhexis (or, keratorhexis) (*keratos* horn: cornea) metrorrhexis (*metra* uterus) myorrhexis (*myos* muscle) nucleorrhexis (nucleus of a cell) omphalorrhexis (*omphalos* navel, umbilicus) onychorrhexis (*onychos* nail) ophthalmorrhexis (*ophthalmos* eye) ovariorrhexis (ovary) phleborrhexis (*phlebos* vein) plasmorrhexis (or, plasmatorrhexis; the bursting of a cell due to the pressure exerted from the pressure of the protoplasm) (*plassein* to form) trichorrhexis (*trichos* hair) tubulorrhexis (renal tubes) CROSS REFERENCE: hern
rhin, **rrhin**	Greek *rhis*	nose	SIMPLE ROOT: rhinal (also called *nasal*), rhinion (lower end of the suture between nasal bones; a craniometric point) rhinism (also called *rhinolalia*) PREFIXED ROOT: *rhinal*: entorhinal (*enton* within) perirhinal (*peri* around) *rhine*: errhine (promoting a nasal discharge; an agent that promotes nasal discharge or secretion) (*en* in) mesorhine (*mesos* middle) *rhinia*: arhinia (or, arrhinia) (*a* privative) macrorhinia (excessive size of nose, either congenital or pathological) (*makros* large) microrhinia (*mikros* small) *rhinic*: dirhinic (*di* two) monorhinic (having only one nasal passage) (*monos* single)

Element	From	Meaning	Examples
rhin (cont'd)		[nose]	*rrhin*:
			arrhinia (or, arhinia; congenital anomaly characterized by absence of the nose) (*an* privative)
			catarrhine (having a slender nose with the nostrils spaced close together; as a noun, a catarrhine creature, as man or certain other primates; distinguished from *platyrrhine*, flat-nosed) (*kata* down)
			leptorrhine (*leptos* thin, slender)
			platyrrhine (*platys* flat, broad)
			LEADING ROOT COMPOUND:
			rhin:
			rhinalgia (also called *rhinodynia*) (*algos* pain)
			rhinallergosis (also called *allergic rhinitis*) (allergy + *osis* condition)
			rhinedema (*edema* swelling)
			rhinencephalon (*enkephalon* brain)
			rhinenchysis (a nasal douche) (*enchysis* a pouring in)
			rhinitis (*itis* inflammation)
			rhinodynia (also called *rhinalgia*) (*odyne* pain)
			rhino:
			rhinoanemometer (also called *rhinomanometer*) (*anemos* wind + *metron* measure)
			rhinoantritis (also called *nasoantritis*) (*antron* cavity + *itis* inflammation)
			rhinobyon (a nasal tampon or plug) (*byein* to plug)
			rhinocele (or, rhinocoele; the ventricle of the olfactory lobe of the brain) (*koilia* cavity, hollow)
			rhinocephaly (or, rhinocephalia) (*kephale* head)
			rhinocheiloplasty (*cheilos* lip + *plassein* to form)
			rhinocleisis (also called *rhinostenosis*) (*kleisis* a closure)
			rhinodymia (duplication of the nose on an otherwise normal face) (*dymos* fold)
			rhinogenous (arising in the nose) (*genere* to produce)
			rhinokyphosis (*kyphosis* humped condition)
			rhinolalia (also called *rhinism, rhinophonia*) (*lalein* to speak)
			rhinolaryngitis (larynx + *itis* inflammation)
			rhinoliquorrhea (*liquor* fluid + *rhein* to flow)
			rhinolith, rhinolithiasis (*lithos* stone + *iasis* condition)
			rhinologist (a medical doctor specializing in problems of the nose), rhinology (*logos* study)
			rhinomanometry (*manos* thin + *metron* measure)
			rhinometer (*metron* measure)
			rhinomycosis (*mykes* fungus + *osis* condition)
			rhinonecrosis (necrosis of the bones of the nose) (*nekrosis* deadness)
			rhinopathy (*pathos* disease)
			rhinopharyngeal (also called *nasopharyngeal*), rhinopharyngolith (pharynx + *lithos* stone, calculus)
			rhinopharynx (also called *nasopharynx*)
			rhinophonia (also called *rhinolalia*) (*phone* sound, voice)
			rhinophyma (*phyma* tumor, growth)
			rhinoplasty (*plassein* to form)
			rhinopneumonitis (*pneumon* lung + *itis* inflammation)
			rhinorrhagia (hemorrhage from the nose; also called *epistaxis*)
			rhinorrhaphy (*rhaphe* suture)
			rhinorrhea (runny nose) (*rhein* to flow)
			rhinosalpingitis (*salpingos* tube + *itis* inflammation)

Element	From	Meaning	Examples
rhin (cont'd)		[nose]	rhinoscleroma (a chronic granulomatous condition involving the nose, upper lip, mouth, and upper air passages that is possibly caused by a bacterium) (*skleros* hard + *oma* tumor) rhinoscope, rhinoscopy {rhinoscopic—for both} (*skopein* to examine) rhinosinusitis (also called *nasosinusitis*) (sinus + *itis* inflammation) rhinostenosis (also called *rhinocleisis*) (*stenosis* narrow) rhinotillexomania (compulsive nose-picking) (*tillexein* to pluck + *mania* craze) rhinotomy (*tomy* incision) rhinotracheitis (*trachea* windpipe + *itis* inflammation) TRAILING ROOT COMPOUND: basirhinal (pertaining to the base of the brain and to the nose) brachyrhinia (abnormal shortness of the nose) (*brachys* short) dacryorhinocystotomy (also called *dacryocystorhinostomy*) (*dakryon* teardrop + *kystis* sac + *tomy* incision) otorhinolaryngology (*otos* ear + *larynx* throat + *logos* study) otorhinology (*otos* ear + *logos* study) oxyrhine (having a sharp-pointed nose) (*oxys* sharp) pharyngorhinitis (pharynx + *itis* inflammation) pharyngorhinoscopy (pharynx + *skopein* to examine) platyrrhine (characterized by a nose of large width in proportion to its length) (*platys* flat) CROSS REFERENCE: nari, nas
rhiz	Greek *rhiza*	root	PREFIXED ROOT: perirhizoclasia (inflammatory destruction of tissues around the root of a tooth) (*peri* around + *klasis* destruction) LEADING ROOT COMPOUND: *rhiz*: rhizoid (a filamentous rootlike structure of fungi and certain algae that extends into the substrate) (*eidos* resembling) rhizodontropy (process of attaching an artificial crown upon the root of a tooth) (*odontos* tooth + *tropein* to turn) rhizodontrypy (*odontos* tooth + trephination) [trephine: a small crown saw used in surgery] *rhizo*: rhizoblast (flagellar rootlet) (*blastos* germ, shoot) rhizomelic (pertaining to or involving the hip joint and shoulder joint—the roots and the limbs) (*melos* limb) rhizoplast (*plassein* to form) rhizotomy (also called *radicotomy*) (*tomy* incision) CROSS REFERENCE: rad²
rhomb	Greek *rhembein*	to turn	SIMPLE ROOT: rhombic (or, rhomboid; relating to the rhombencephalon) LEADING ROOT COMPOUND: *rhomb*: rhombencephalon (the most caudal of the three primary vesicles of the embryonic brain) (*enkephalon* brain) rhomboid (*eidos* form) *rhombo*: rhombocoele (or, rhombocele) (*koilia* cavity) rhombomere (also called *neuromere*) (*meros* part) NOTE: A non-medical word is *rhombus*, an equilateral parallelogram; literally, an object that can be turned. CROSS REFERENCE: spir, trop

Element	From	Meaning	Examples
rhythm	Greek *rhythmos*	rhythm	SIMPLE ROOT: rhythm {rhythmical}, rhythmeur (a device for making rhythmic interruptions of the current in an x-ray machine), rhythmicity (also called *automaticity*) PREFIXED ROOT: allorhythmia {allorhythmic} (*allos* other) anisorrhythmia (*aniso* unequal: *an* negative + *isos* equal) arrhythmia {arrhythmic} (*an* negative) cacorhythmic (ill-modulated, as a pulse) (*kakos* bad, abnormal) dysrhythmia (defective rhythm) (*dys* abnormal) eurhythmia (*eu* well) hypsarrhythmia (*hypsos* high + arrhythmia) pararrhythmia (*para* abnormal + arrhythmia) proarrhythmia {proarrhythmic} (*pro* before + arrhythmia) TRAILING ROOT COMPOUND: biorhythm (also called *biological rhythm*) (*bios* life) bradyarrhythmia (*bradys* slow + arrhythmia) tachyrhythmia (*tachys* swift, rapid) CROSS REFERENCE: None
rhytid, rutid	Greek *rhytis*	wrinkle	SIMPLE ROOT: rhytide (a skin wrinkle) LEADING ROOT COMPOUND: *rhytid*: rhytidectomy (face-lift; also called *rhytidoplasty*) (*ektome* excision) rhytidosis (a wrinkling of the cornea; one of the signs of approaching death; also called *rutidosis*) (*osis* condition) *rhytido*: rhytidoplasty (also called *rhytidectomy*) (*plassein* to form) *rutid*: rutidosis (also called *rhytidosis*) (*osis* condition) CROSS REFERENCE: None
rrhag	Greek *rhegnynai* to burst forth	excessive flow	TRAILING ROOT COMPOUND: balanorrhagia (*balanos* glans penis: the head of the penis) blennorrhagia (*blenna* mucus) bronchorrhagia (*bronchos* windpipe) cholerrhagia (*chole* bile) colonorrhagia (*kolon* colon) colporrhagia (*kolpos* vagina) cystorrhagia (*kystis* bladder) dermatorrhagia (*dermatos* skin) encephalorrhagia (*enkephalon* brain) enterorrhagia (*enteron* intestine) gastrorrhagia (*gaster* stomach, belly) hemorrhage {hemorrhagic} (*haima* blood) hepatorrhagia (*hepatos* liver) laryngorrhagia (larynx) leukorrhagia (profuse leukorrhea) (*leukos* white) lochiorrhagia (*lochia* vaginal discharge) lymphorrhagia (also called *lymphorrhea*) (*lymph* water, fluid) mastorrhagia (*mastos* breast, nipple) melanorrhagia (the free and frequent discharge of feces darkened with blood pigments; also called *melena*) (*melanos* dark) meningorrhagia (also called *meningorrhea*) (*meningos* membrane) menorrhagia (also called *hypermenorrhea*) (*mene* menstruation) metrorrhagia (*metra* uterus) myelorrhagia (also called *hematomyelia*) (*myelos* marrow) nephrorrhagia (also called *renal hemorrhage*) (*nephros* kidney) odontorrhagia (*odontos* tooth)

A Thesaurus of Medical Word Roots

Element	From	Meaning	Examples
rrhag (cont'd)		[excessive flow]	omphalorrhagia (*omphalos* navel)
			oophorrhagia (ovarian hemorrhage)
			ophthalmorrhagia (*ophthalmos* eye)
			osteorrhagia (*osteon* bone)
			otorrhagia (*otos* ear)
			phallorrhagia (*phallos* penis)
			pharyngorrhagia (pharynx)
			pneumonorrhagia (also called *pulmonary hemorrhage*) (*pneumon* lung)
			proctorrhagia (*proktos* anus, rectum)
			rhinorrhagia (also called *epistaxis*) (*rhinos* nose)
			salpingorrhagia (*salpingos* tube—Fallopian tube)
			splenorrhagia (*splen* spleen)
			stomatorrhagia (*stomatos* mouth)
			thelorrhagia (*thele* nipple)
			tracheorrhagia (*trachea* windpipe)
			ulorrhagia (*oulon* gums, gingivae)
			ureterorrhagia (*ureter* urine tube)
			urethrorrhagia (*urethra* urine canal)
			CROSS REFERENCE: rhe
rrhea			See melan- for *melanorrhea*; rhe- for *diarrhea*.
rrhex			See rhex- for *cardiorrhexis*.
rrhin			See rhin- for *catarrhine*.
rub(r)	Latin *rubeus*	red, measles	SIMPLE ROOT:
			rubedo (temporary redness of the skin; blushing)
			rubella (German measles), rubeola (measles), rubescent
			rubidium (from the red lines in its spectrum; Rb)
			rubiginous (or, rubiginose; rust-colored; reddish-brown)
			rubor (redness, one of the cardinal signs of inflammation)
			rubric (pertaining to the red nucleus)
			PREFIXED ROOT: erubescence (a reddening of the skin) (*e* out)
			LEADING ROOT COMPOUND:
			rube: rubefacient (causing redness; any external application causing redness of skin), rubefaction (*facere* to make)
			rubeosis (reddish discoloration, as of the skin) (*osis* condition)
			rubr: rubruria {ruburic} (*uria* urine condition)
			rubri:
			rubriblast (also called *proerythroblast, pronormoblast*) (*blastos* bud germ, shoot)
			rubricyte (also called *polychromatic normoblast*) (*kytos* cell)
			rubro:
			rubrospinal (pertaining to the red nucleus and the spinal cord) (*spina* spine)
			rubrothalamic (thalamus)
			TRAILING ROOT COMPOUND: bilirubin (*bilis* bile)
			CROSS REFERENCE: erythr, rhod

S

Element	From	Meaning	Examples
sacchar	Sanskrit *sarkara* sugar	sugar, sucrose	SIMPLE ROOT: saccharide, saccharin, saccharine (sugary) saccharose (also called *sucrose*) saccharum (sugar, especially cane sugar, or sucrose) PREFIXED ROOT: disaccharide (a sugar such as sucrose, which is made up of two mono-saccharides) (*di* two) heterosaccharide (*heteros* other) monosaccharide (*monos* single) polysaccharide (*polys* many) LEADING ROOT COMPOUND: *acchari*: sacchariferous (producing sugar) (*ferre* to carry) saccharification (*facere* to make) saccharimeter (*metron* measure) *saccharo*: saccharolytic (*lyein* to dissolve) saccharomycetolysis (*mykes* fungus + *lysis* dissolution) CROSS REFERENCE: glyc
sacr	Latin *sacrum* holy, sacred	sacrum	NOTE: A thick bone, the *os sacrum* (from Greek *hieron osteon*, or sacred bone), was that part of a body not consumed in a ritual sacrifice. SIMPLE ROOT: sacrad (toward the sacrum, or sacral aspect) sacralization (anomalous fusion of the fifth lumbar vertebra with the first segment of the sacrum) sacrum (the triangular-shaped bone formed usually by five fused vertebrae that are wedged dorsally between the two hip bones; pl., sacra) {sacral} PREFIXED ROOT: *sacral*: parasacral (*para* alongside) postsacral (referring to the coccyx) (*post* posterior) presacral (*pre* before) subsacral (*sub* under) transsacral (*trans* across) *sacralization*: hemisacralization (fusion of the last lumbar vertebra to the first segment of the sacrum on one side) (*hemi* half) LEADING ROOT COMPOUND: *sacr*: sacralgia (also called *sacrodynia*) (*algos* pain) sacrarthrogenic (*arthron* joint + *genere* to produce) sacrectomy (*ektome* excision) sacrodynia (also called *sacralgia*) (*odyne* pain) *sacro*: sacroanterior (the position of the fetus in utero when its back is directed toward the anterior abdominal wall of the mother) (*anterior* forward) sacrococcyx (the sacrum and coccyx together)

A Thesaurus of Medical Word Roots

Element	From	Meaning	Examples
sacr (cont'd)		[sacrum]	sacrocoxalgia (*coxa* hip + *algos* pain)
			sacrocoxitis (*coxa* hip + *itis* inflammation)
			sacroiliac, sacroiliitis (*ileum* hipbone + *itis* inflammation)
			sacrolumbar (*lumbus* loin)
			sacroperineal (perineum)
			sacroposterior (*posterior* backward)
			sacropromontory (the promontory of the sacrum)
			sacrosciatic (*sciatic* ischial)
			sacrospinal (*spina* spine)
			sacrotomy (*tomy* incision)
			sacrouterine (*uterus* womb)
			sacrovertebral (vertebra)
			TRAILING ROOT COMPOUND:
			cotylosacral (*cotyledon* cup: acetabulum)
			craniosacral (*kranion* skull)
			iliosacral (ilium)
			ischiosacral (ischium)
			lumbosacral (*lumbus* loin)
			pelvisacral (pelvis)
			uterosacral (uterus)
			vertebrosacral (vertebra)
			CROSS REFERENCE: None
salping, salpinx	Greek *salpinx, salpingos* tube	tube, trumpet	SIMPLE ROOT:
			salpingian (relating to either the uterine, or Fallopian, tube or the auditory tube; also called *tubal*), salpingion
			salpinx (a tube; also called *tuba uterine*; pl. salpinges)
			PREFIXED ROOT:
			salpingiosis: endosalpingiosis (*endon* within + *osis* condition)
			salpingitis inflammation of a tube:
			endosalpingitis (*endon* within)
			parasalpingitis (*para* beside)
			perisalpingitis (*peri* around)
			salpingo: perisalpingoovaritis (inflammation of peritoneal tissues surrounding the Fallopian tubes and ovaries; also called *perio-ophorsalpingitis*) (*peri* around + ovary + *itis* inflammation)
			salpingoma: endosalpingoma (*endon* within + *oma* tumor)
			salpinx:
			endosalpinx (*endon* within)
			mesosalpinx (*mesos* middle)
			perisalpinx (*peri* around)
			LEADING ROOT COMPOUND:
			salping:
			salpingectomy (surgical removal of the uterine tube; also called *tubectomy*) (*ektome* excision)
			salpingemphraxis (*emphraxis* stoppage, obstruction)
			salpingitis {salpingitic} (*itis* inflammation)
			salpingo:
			salpingocele (hernial protrusion of a fallopian tube) (*kele* hernia)
			salpingocyesis (*kyesis* pregnancy)
			salpingography (radiography of the Fallopian tubes after the injection of a radiopaque contrast medium) (*graphein* to write)
			salpingolithiasis (*lithos* stone + *iasis* condition)
			salpingolysis (surgical lysis of adhesions involving the uterine tubes) (*lyein* to loosen)

A Thesaurus of Medical Word Roots

Element	From	Meaning	Examples
salping (cont'd)		[tube]	salpingoneostomy (*neos* new + *stoma* mouth, opening) salpingo-oophorectomy (*oophor* egg-bearer + *ektome* excision) salpingo-oophoritis (*oophor* egg-bearer + *itis* inflammation) salpingoperitonitis (peritoneum + *itis* inflammation) salpingopexy (*pexis* fixation) salpingopharyngeal (pharynx) salpingoplasty (*plassein* to form) salpingorrhagia (*rhagia* bursting forth) salpingorrhaphy (*rhaphe* suture) salpingoscopy (*skopein* to examine) salpingostomatomy (*stoma* mouth, opening + *tomy* incision) salpingotomy (*tomy* incision) TRAILING ROOT COMPOUND: *salpingitis* inflammation of a tube: adenosalpingitis (*adenos* gland) metrosalpingitis (*metra* uterus) myosalpingitis (*myos* muscle) oophorosalpingitis (*oophoro* egg-bearer) pachysalpingitis (*pachys* thick) pyosalpingitis (*pyon* pus) rhinosalpingitis (*rhinos* nose) CROSS REFERENCE: fistul, syring, tub[1]
sangui	Latin *sanguis*	blood	SIMPLE ROOT: sanguine (or, sanguineous; abounding in blood; also called *plethoric*), sanguinolent (of a bloody tinge), sanguis PREFIXED ROOT: consanguineous (lit., of the same blood; having the same ancestor), consanguinity (*con* with) exsanguinate, exsanguination, exsanguine, exsanguineous (destitute of blood) (*ex* out) LEADING ROOT COMPOUND: *sangui*: sanguicolous (living in the blood, as certain parasites) (*colere* to dwell) sanguifacient (also called *hemopoietic*) (*facere* to make) sanguiferous (also called *circulatory*) (*ferre* to carry) sanguification (also called *hemopoiesis*) (*facere* to make) sanguivorous (also called *hematophagous*) (*vorare* to eat, consume) *sanguino*: sanguinopoietic (also called *hematopoietic*) (*poiein* to produce) sanguinopurulent (containing both blood and pus) (*puris* pus) TRAILING ROOT COMPOUND: mucosanguineous (mucus) serosanguineous (*serum* whey) CROSS REFERENCE: hem
sapr	Greek *sapros*	rotten, putrid, decay	LEADING ROOT COMPOUND: *sapr*: saprodontia (tooth decay) (*odontos* tooth) *sapro*: saprobe {saprobic} (*bios* life) saprogen {saprogenic, saprogenous} (*genere* to produce) sapronosis (*nosos* disease) saprophilous (*philein* to love—have an affinity for) saprophyte {saprophytic}, saprophytism (*phyton* plant: growth) saprozoic (also called *saprophytic*) (*zoon* animal) CROSS REFERENCE: caries, sep

Element	From	Meaning	Examples
sarc	Greek *sarx, sarkos*	flesh	SIMPLE ROOT: sarcous (pertaining to flesh or to muscular tissues)
			PREFIXED ROOT:
			anasarca (generalized massive edema) {anasarcous} (*ana* again)
			ectosarc (*ektos* outside)
			endosarc (also called *endoplasm*) (*endon* within)
			entosarc (or, endosarc) (*entos* inside)
			hyposarca (also called *anasarca*) (*hypo* under)
			polysarcia (corpulence or obesity) {polysarcous} (*polys* much)
			syssarcosis {syssarcotic} (*syn* with + *osis* condition)
			LEADING ROOT COMPOUND:
			sarc:
			sarcoid, sarcoidosis (*eidos* form + *osis* condition)
			sarcoma (pl., sarcomata) {sarcomatous}, sarcomatoid (*oma* tumor + *eidos* resemblance)
			sarcomatosis (*oma* tumor + *osis* condition)
			sarcosis (abnormal increase in flesh) {sarcotic} (*osis* condition)
			sarcostosis (ossification of the fleshy tissues) (*osteon* bone + *osis* condition)
			sarco:
			sarcoblast (also called *myoblast*) (*blastos* bud, shoot, germ)
			sarcocele (a fleshy tumor of the testicle) (*kele* tumor)
			sarcocystosis (*kystis* bladder + *osis* condition)
			sarcogenic (forming muscle) (*genere* to produce)
			sarcoglia (*glia* glue)
			sarcolemma {sarcolemmic, sarcolemmous} (*lemma* sheath)
			sarcology (also called *myology*) (*logos* study)
			sarcomere (*meros* part)
			sarconeme (also called *microneme*) (*nema* thread)
			sarcopenia (*penia* deficiency)
			sarcoplasm {sarcoplasmic}, sarcoplast (*plassein* to form)
			sarcopoietic (producing flesh or muscle) (*poiein* to produce)
			sarcosome (*soma* body)
			sarcoma: sarcomagenic (causing carcinoma; also called *cancerigenic*) (*oma* tumor + *genere* to produce)
			sarcomat fleshy tumor:
			sarcomatosis (*osis* condition)
			sarcomatoid (*eidos* form)
			TRAILING ROOT COMPOUND:
			sarcoma flesh tumor:
			adenomyosarcoma (*aden* gland + *myos* muscle)
			adenosarcoma (*aden* gland)
			angiosarcoma (*angeion* blood vessel)
			angiomysarcoma (*angeion* blood vessel + *myos* muscle)
			carcinosarcoma (*karkinos* crab, cancer)
			cholangiosarcoma (sarcoma of bile duct origin) (*chole* bile + *angeion* vessel)
			chondromyxosarcoma (*chondros* cartilage + *myxa* mucus)
			chondrosarcoma (*chondros* cartilage)
			chordosarcoma (also called *chordoma*) (*chorda* cord)
			cystosarcoma (*kystis* bladder, sac)
			fibrosarcoma (*fibra* fiber)
			fibroxanthosarcoma (also called *malignant fibrous histiocytoma*) (*fibra* fiber + *xanthos* yellow)
			gliosarcoma (*glia* glue)

A Thesaurus of Medical Word Roots

Element	From	Meaning	Examples
sarc (cont'd)		[flesh]	leiomyosarcoma (*leios* smooth + *myos* muscle)
			leukosarcoma (*leukos* white)
			liposarcoma (*lipos* fat)
			lymphosarcoma (*lympha* water, liquid)
			melanosarcoma (*melas* black, dark)
			myelosarcoma (also called *myeloma*) (*myelos* marrow)
			myosarcoma (*myos* muscle)
			myxosarcoma (*myxa* mucus)
			neurosarcoma (*neuron* nerve)
			osteosarcoma (*osteon* bone)
			pseudosarcoma (*pseudes* false)
			rhabdomyosarcoma (*rhabdos* rod + *myos* muscle)
			synoviosarcoma (synovial: *syn* with + *oon* egg)
			xanthosarcoma (*xanthos* yellow)
			CROSS REFERENCE: creat
scapul	Latin *scapula* shovel, spade	shoulder blade	SIMPLE ROOT: scapula (pl., scapulae) {scapular}, scapulary (a shoulder bandage)
			PREFIXED ROOT:
			infrascapular (also called *subscapular*) (*infra* below)
			interscapular (*inter* between)
			mesoscapular (*mesos* middle)
			parascapular (*para* alongside)
			postscapular (*post* posterior, behind)
			prescapular (*pre* before)
			subscapular (also called *infrascapular*) (*sub* below)
			suprascapular (*supra* above, over)
			LEADING ROOT COMPOUND:
			scapul:
			scapulalgia (also called *scapulodynia*) (*algos* pain)
			scapulectomy (*ektome* excision)
			scapulodynia (also called *scapulalgia*) (*odyne* pain)
			scapulo:
			scapuloanterior (*anterior* in front)
			scapuloclavicular (*clavicle* collarbone)
			scapulohumeral (*humerus*)
			scapuloperoneal (*perone* the fibula)
			scapulopexy (*pexis* fixation)
			TRAILING ROOT COMPOUND:
			acromioscapular (*acromion* tip of shoulder)
			cervicoscapular (*cervix* neck)
			costoscapular (*costa* rib)
			dorsoscapular (*dorsum* back — of the body)
			humeroscapular (*humerus*)
			sternoscapular (*sternon* chest, breast)
			CROSS REFERENCE: clavi, cleid
scel, skel	Greek *skelos*	leg	PREFIXED ROOT:
			scelia:
			macroscelia (abnormal size of legs) (*makros* large)
			polyscelia, polyscelus (an individual with polyscelia) (*polys* many)
			scelous:
			microscelous (short-legged) (*mikros* small)
			monoscelous (*monos* single)
			tetrascelus (*tetra* four)
			skel: brachyskelous (shortness of the legs) (*brachys* short)

Element	From	Meaning	Examples
scel (cont'd)		[leg]	LEADING ROOT COMPOUND: *scel*: scelalgia (or, skelalgia) (*algos* pain) *scelo*: scelotyrbe (*tyrbe* disorder) *skel*: skelalgia (or, scelalgia; pain in the leg) (*algos* pain) skelasthenia (*asthenia* weakness: *a* negative + *sthenos* strength) CROSS REFERENCE: crur
schesis	Greek *schesis*	holding, retention, suppression	TRAILING ROOT COMPOUND: galactoschesis (also called *galactischia*) (*galaktos* milk) hidroschesis (also called *anhidrosis*) (*hidros* sweat) lochioschesis (*lochia* vaginal discharge) menischesis (or, menoschesis) (*men* month: menstruation) menoschesis (or, menischesis) (*men* month: menstruation) sialoschesis (*sialon* saliva) spermatoschesis (*spermatos* seed: sperm) uroschesis (*ouron* urine) CROSS REFERENCE: isch

schis	Greek
	schistos
		split, divided;
		fissure
			SIMPLE ROOT: schistasis (a splitting, such as a cleft or fissure of
			  the body)
			PREFIXED ROOT:
			antischistosomal (*anti* against + *soma* body)
			diaschisis (*dia* across)
			LEADING ROOT COMPOUND:
			schistocelia (or, schistocoelia) (*koilia* belly)
			schistocephalus (*kephale* head)
			schistocoelia (also called *gastroschisis*) (*koilia* belly)
			schistocormia (also called *schistosomia*), schistocormus (a fetus ex-
			  hibiting schistocromia) (*kormos* trunk)
			schistocystis (also called *cystoschisis*) (*kystis* bladder)
			schistocyte, schistocytosis (schistocytes in the blood) (*kytos* cell +
			  osis condition)
			schistoglossia (*glossa* tongue)
			schistomelia (*melos* limb, member)
			schistoprosopia (also called *facial cleft*) (*prosopon* face)
			schistorrhachis (also called *rachischisis*) (*rhachis* spine)
			schistosomia (also called *schistocormia*) (*soma* body)
			schistosternia (also called *cleft sternum*) (*sternon* chest)
			schistothorax (also called *thoracoschisis*) (*thorax* chest)
			schistotrachelus (*trachelos* neck)
			TRAILING ROOT COMPOUND:
			abdominoschisis (a congenital fissure in the abdomen)
			alveoloschisis (*alveolus* trough—concave vessel)
			cardioschisis (*kardia* heart)
			celoschisis (or, celioschisis; also called *abdominal fissure*) (*koilia*
			  belly)
			cheilognathopalatoschisis (*cheilos* lip + *gnathos* jaw + palate)
			cheiloschisis (also called *cleft lip*) (*cheilos* lip)
			cranioschisis (also called *cranium bifidum*) (*kranion* skull)
			cystoschisis (also called *schistocystis*) (*kystis* bladder)
			encephaloschisis (*encephalon* brain)
			gastroschisis (also called *schistocoelia*) (*gaster* stomach, belly)
			gnathoschisis (also called *cleft jaw*) (*gnathos* jaw)
			iridoschisis (iris—of eye)
			meloschisis (also called *oblique facial cleft*) (*melon* cheek)

Element	From	Meaning	Examples
schis (cont'd)		[to split]	mitoschisis (also called *karyokinesis*) (*mitos* thread)
			myeloschisis (*myelos* spinal cord)
			palatoschisis (also called *cleft palate*) (*palatum* palate)
			penischisis (a fissured state of the penis, such as epispadias, hypospadias, or paraspadias)
			plasmoschisis (*plassein* to form)
			prosoposchisis (also called *facial cleft*) (*prosopon* face)
			rachischisis (*rhachis* spine)
			retinoschisis (cleft of the retina) (*rete* net: retina)
			somatoschisis (*somatos* body)
			spondyloschisis (also called *rachischisis*) (*spondylos* vertebra)
			staphyloschisis (also called *bifid uvula*) (*staphyle* bunch of grapes: uvula)
			sternoschisis (also called *cleft sternum*) (*sternon* chest)
			stomoschisis (also called *cleft lip*) (*stoma* mouth)
			thoracoschisis (also called *schistothorax*) (*thorax* chest)
			tracheloschisis (*trachelos* neck)
			tracheoschisis (*trachea* windpipe)
			trichoschisis (*trichos* hair)
			uranoschisis (also called *cleft palate*) (*ouranos* palate)
			uranostaphyloschisis (*ouranos* palate + *staphyle* uvula)
			schism: odontoschism (fissure of a tooth) (*odontos* tooth)
			PREFIXED TRAILING ROOT COMPOUND: hemirachischisis (rachischisis without prolapse of the spinal cord) (*hemi* half + *rhachis* spine)
			CROSS REFERENCE: schiz, sciss
schiz	Greek *schizein*	to divide	LEADING ROOT COMPOUND:
			schiz:
			schizamnion (an amnion developing, as in the human embryo, by the formation of a cavity over or within the inner cell mass) (*amnion* membrane)
			schizaxon (an axon that divides into two nearly equal branches) (*axon* axis)
			schizencephaly {schizencephalic} (*enkephalon* brain)
			schizoid, schizoidism (*eidos* form)
			schizont, schizonticide (*ontos* being + *caedere* to kill)
			schizonychia (splitting of the nails) (*onychos* nail)
			schizo:
			schizocephalia (*kephale* head)
			schizocyte (also called *schistocyte*), schizocytosis (also called *schistocytosis*) (*kytos* cell + *osis* condition)
			schizogenesis {schizogenous} (*genere* to produce)
			schizogony (*gone* seed)
			schizogyria (*gyros* circle: in this word, convolutions of brain)
			schizokinesis (*kinesis* movement)
			schizophasia (also called *word salad*) (*phanai* to speak)
			schizophrenia {schizophrenic} (*phren* mind)
			schizoprosopia (also called *facial cleft*) (*prosopon* face)
			schizothorax (also called *thoracoschisis*) (thorax)
			schizotonia (*tonos* tension, tone)
			schizotrichia (*trichia* hair condition)
			TRAILING ROOT COMPOUND: onychoschizia (*onychos* nail)
			CROSS REFERENCE: schis, sciss
sciat			See ischi- for *sciatic, sciatica*.

Element	From	Meaning	Examples
scirrh	Greek *skirrhos* hard	hard (hard tumor, scirrhus)	SIMPLE ROOT: scirrhus (a hard cancer with a marked predomi- nance of connective tissue) {scirrhous} LEADING ROOT COMPOUND: scirrhoid (resembling a scirrhous carcinoma) (*eidos* form) scirrhoma (a hard carcinoma or scirrhus) (*oma* tumor) scirrhophthalmia (*ophthalmia* eye condition) TRAILING ROOT COMPOUND: mastoscirrhus (*mastos* breast) parotidoscirrhus (parotid: *para* near + *otos* ear) CROSS REFERENCE: scler
sciss	Latin *scindere*	to split	SIMPLE ROOT: scission (fission), scissors (also called *shears*) scissura (cleft or fissure; a splitting; pl., scissurae) PREFIXED ROOT: abscission (removal by cutting or excision*) (*ab* away) discission (a cutting in two, or division, as of a soft cataract) (*dis* apart) LEADING ROOT COMPOUND: scissiparity (reproduction by fis- sion; also called *schizogenesis*) (*parere* to bear) *Excision itself comes from *ex* out + *caedere* to cut. CROSS REFERENCE: schis, schiz
scler	Greek *skleros*	hard, tough (sclera)	SIMPLE ROOT: sclera (the tough white supporting tunic of the eyeball; pl., scleras, sclerae) {scleral} sclerema (induration of subcutaneous fat) (<u>scler</u>a + ed<u>ema</u>) sclerosal (also called *scleroid*), sclerosant, sclerose (to harden; to undergo sclerosis), sclerosing, sclerous (indurated) sclerotium (in fungi, a hard mass of intertwined mycelia) PREFIXED ROOT: episclera {episcleral}, episcleritis (*epi* upon + *itis* inflammation) hyposcleral (*hypo* under) intrascleral (*intra* within) pansclerosis (*pan* all + *osis* condition) perisclerium (fibrous tissue encircling ossifying cartilage) (*peri* around) presclerotic (*pre* before) subscleral (or, subsclerotic; partly sclerosed) (*sub* slightly) suprascleral (*supra* above) LEADING ROOT COMPOUND: *scler*: scleradenitis (*adenos* gland + *itis* inflammation) sclerectasia (also called *scleral ectasia*) (*ektasis* dilatation) sclerectome, sclerectomy (*ektome* excision) scleredema (*edema* swelling) sclerencephalia (*enkephalon* brain) scleriasis (a hardened state of the eyelid) (*iasis* condition) scleriritomy (iris + *tomy* incision) scleritis (*itis* inflammation) scleroid (*eidos* form, resembling) scleroma (*oma* tumor) scleronychia (*onyx* nail) sclerophthalmia (*ophthalmia* eye condition) sclerosis (also called *induration*; pl., scleroses) {sclerotic} (*osis* con- dition)

A Thesaurus of Medical Word Roots

Element	From	Meaning	Examples
scler (cont'd)		[hard, tough]	*sclerato*: scleratogenous (or, sclerogenous) (*genere* to produce)

sclero:

scleroadipose (*adipose* fatty)

scleroblastema {scleroblastemic} (*blastos* bud, shoot, germ)

scleroconjunctival (conjunctiva: *con* with + *jungere* to join)

sclerocornea {sclerocorneal}

sclerodactylia (or, sclerodactyly) (*daktylos* finger, toe)

scleroderma {sclerodermatous} (*derma* skin)

sclerogenous (or, sclerogenic) (*genere* to produce)

scleroiritis (iris + *itis* inflammation)

sclerokeratitis (also called *sclerokeratosis*) (*keratos* horn: cornea + *itis* inflammation)

scleromalacia (*malakos* soft)

scleromere (*meros* part)

sclerometer (*metron* measure)

scleronyxis (*nyxis* puncture)

sclero-oophoritis (sclerosing inflammation of an ovary; also called *sclero-oothecitis*) (*oophor* ovary + *itis* inflammation)

sclero-oothecitis (also called *sclero-oophoritis*) (*ootheka* egg case + *itis* inflammation)

scleroplasty (*plassein* to form)

sclerostenosis (*stenosis* narrowing)

sclerostomy (*stoma* mouth, opening)

sclerotherapy (*therapy* treatment)

sclerothrix (or, sclerotrichia) (*thrix, trichos* hair)

sclerotome, sclerotomy (*tomy* incision)

sclerotrichia (or, sclerothrix) (*trichos* hair)

sclerotylosis (also called *scleroatrophy*) (*tylosis* callous)

sclerozone (*zona* zone)

TRAILING ROOT COMPOUND:

scleritis inflammation of the sclera:

keratoscleritis (*keratos* horn: cornea)

uveoscleritis (scleritis due to extension of uveitis) (uvea)

sclerosis a hardening condition:

adenosclerosis (*adenos* gland)

angiosclerosis (*angeion* blood vessel)

aortosclerosis (aorta)

arteriosclerosis (*arteria* artery)

arthrosclerosis (*arthron* joint)

atherosclerosis (*athere* gruel)

cardiosclerosis (*kardia* heart)

centrosclerosis (*kentron* center)

craniosclerosis (*kranion* upper skull)

cystosclerosis (*kystis* cyst)

dermatosclerosis (also called *scleroderma*) (*dermatos* skin)

encephalosclerosis (*enkephalon* brain)

inosclerosis (*inos* fiber)

myelosclerosis (also called *myelofibrosis*) (*myelos* spinal cord)

myosclerosis (*myos* muscle)

nephrosclerosis (*nephros* kidney)

osteosclerosis (*osteon* bone)

otosclerosis (*otos* ear)

phacosclerosis (*phakos* lens)

phlebosclerosis (also called *venosclerosis*) (*phlebos* vein)

Element	From	Meaning	Examples
scler (cont'd)		[hard, tough]	pneumosclerosis (*pneumon* lung) pseudosclerosis (*pseudes* false) pyosclerosis (*pyon* pus) splanchnosclerosis (*splanchnos* viscera) tympanosclerosis (*tympanon* eardrum) uterosclerosis (uterus) venosclerosis (also called *phlebosclerosis*) (*vena* vein) CROSS REFERENCE: scirrh
scol	Greek *skolex* grub, worm *skolios* twisted	worm, appendage; twisted, crooked	SIMPLE ROOT: scolex (the attachment end of a tapeworm, consisting of the head and neck; pl., scolices, or scoleces) LEADING ROOT COMPOUND: *scolec*: scoleciasis (the condition caused by the presence of larvae of moths or butterflies in the body) (*iasis* condition) scolecoid (resembling a worm; resembling a scolex) (*eidos* form) *scoleci*: scoleciform (*forma* shape) *scoleco*: scolecology (also called *helminthology*) (*logos* study) *scoli*: scoliosis (lateral curvature of the spine) {scoliotic} (*osis* condition) *scolio*: scoliokyphosis [combined lateral (scoliosis) and posterior (kyphosis) curvature of the spine] (*kyphosis* curvature, humpback) scoliometer (device for measuring curves, especially lateral ones of the spine), scoliometry (*metron* measure) scoliorachitic (affected with scoliosis and rickets) (*rhachis* spine) scoliotone (*tonos* tension) *scolioso*: scoliosometer (an apparatus for measuring curves, especially those of the vertical column) (*metron* measure) TRAILING ROOT COMPOUND: kyphoscoliosis (*kyphos* hump) lordoscoliosis (*lordos* bent back) rachioscoliosis (lateral curvature of the spine) (*rhachis* spine) CROSS REFERENCE: helminth, stroph, torq
scop	Greek *skopein* to view	to see, watch, examine, view	PREFIXED ROOT: *scopal*: abscopal (pertaining to the effect of irradiated tissue on remote tissue not exposed to radiation) (*ab* away) *scope*: diascope (a flat glass plate through which one can examine superficial skin lesions by means of pressure) (*dia* through) diploscope (*diploos* double) endoscope (an instrument for examining the inside of a hollow organ, as the bladder or rectum) (*endon* within) epidiascope (*epi* upon + diascope) euscope (a device for projecting the image from a compound microscope upon a barium screen in a dark chamber so that it may be easily viewed) (*eu* well) heteroscope (*heteros* other) isoscope (*isos* equal) mesoscope (*mesos* middle) microscope (*mikros* small) polyscope (*polys* many) *scopic*: amicroscopic (too small to be seen through a microscope; also called *submicroscopic*) (*a* negative + *mikros* small)

Element	From	Meaning	Examples
scop (cont'd)		[to examine, to see]	endoscopic (*endon* within)
			macroscopic (*makros* large)
			microscopic (*mikros* small)
			periscopic (viewing on all sides; providing a wide range of vision) (*peri* around)
			submicroscopic (also called *amicroscopic*) (*sub* under + microscopic)
			scopy:
			diascopy (*dia* through)
			ectoscopy (*ektos* outside)
			endoscopy (*endon* within)
			heteroscopy (*heteros* other)
			microscopy (*mikros* small)
			LEADING ROOT COMPOUND:
			scopolagnia (also called *scopophilia*) (*lagneia* lust)
			scopometer, scopometry (measurement of the optical density of a precipitate to determine the amount of a substance in suspension) (*metron* measure)
			scopophilia (sexual pleasure derived from visual sources such as nudity and obscene pictures; also called *voyeurism*) (*philein* to love)
			scopophobia (or, scoptophobia; a morbid fear of being seen or stared at) (*phobia* fear)
			TRAILING ROOT COMPOUNDS:
			abdominoscopy (also called *laparoscopy*) (abdomen)
			aeroscopy (the observation of the state and variations of the atomosphere) (*aer* air)
			amblyoscope (a stereoscope that can measure convergence and divergence of eyes) (*amblys* dull, blunted)
			amnioscope, amnioscopy (*amnion* membrane)
			angioscope, angioscopy (*angeion* vessel: blood vessel)
			anoscope, anoscopy (anus)
			antroscope, antroscopy (*antrum* cavity: sinus)
			arthroscope, arthroscopy (*arthron* joint)
			bioscopy (*bios* life)
			bronchoscope, bronchoscopy {bronchoscopic} (*bronchus* windpipe) [*bronchoscopic* applies to both]
			celioscope (also called *laparoscope*), celioscopy (also called *laparoscopy*) (*koilia* belly)
			cheiroscope (*cheiros* hand)
			chromatoscope, chromatoscopy (*chromatos* color)
			ciliariscope (*cilium* eyelash)
			colonoscope, colonoscopy (colon)
			colposcope, colposcopy {colposcopic} (*kolpos* vagina)
			cryoscope, cryoscopy {cryoscopical} (*kryos* cold)
			cystoscope, cystoscopy {cystoscopic} (*kystis* bladder)
			cryptoscope, cryptoscopy (examination by x-rays; also called *fluoroscopy*) (*kryptos* hidden)
			cytoscopy (*kytos* hollow vessel: cell)
			embryoscope (embryo)
			encephaloscope, encephaloscopy (*enkephalon* brain)
			enteroscope (*enteron* intestine)
			esophagoscope (esophagus)
			falloscopy (Fallopian tube)
			fetoscope, fetoscopy {fetoscopic} (fetus)

A Thesaurus of Medical Word Roots

Element	From	Meaning	Examples
scop (cont'd)		[to examine, see]	fibrinoscopy (also called *inoscopy*) (fiber)
			gastroscope, gastroscopy {gastroscopic} (*gaster* belly, stomach)
			glossoscopy (*glossa* tongue)
			gonioscope, gonioscopy (*gonia* angle—of the eye)
			hepatoscopy (*hepatos* liver)
			inoscopy (also called *fibrinoscopy*) (*inos* fiber)
			keratoscope, keratoscopy (*keratos* horn: cornea)
			kinetoscope, kinetoscopy (*kinein* to move)
			koroscopy (also called *retinoscopy*) (*kore* pupil—of eye)
			laparoscope, laparoscopy {laparoscopic} (*lapara* flank)
			laryngoscope, laryngoscopy {laryngoscopic} (larynx)
			leptoscope (used for measuring cell membranes) (*leptos* slender)
			myeloscope (*myelos* spinal cord)
			nasoscope (*nasus* nose)
			necroscopy (*nekros* dead)
			nephroscope, nephroscopy (*nephros* kidney)
			odontoscope, odontoscopy (*odontos* tooth)
			ophthalmoscope, ophthalmoscopy (*ophthalmos* eye)
			orthoscope, orthoscopy {orthoscopic} (*orthos* straight)
			otoscope, otoscopy (*otos* ear)
			pancreatoscopy (pancreas)
			peritoneoscope (also called *laparoscope*) (peritoneum)
			phacoscope, phacoscopy (*phakos* lens of eye)
			pharyngoscope, pharyngoscopy (pharynx)
			phonacoscope, phonacoscopy (*phone* sound + *akouein* to hear)
			phonoscope, phonoscopy (*phone* sound)
			photoscopy (*photos* light)
			pleuroscopy (also called *thoracoscopy*) (*pleura* rib, side)
			proctoscope, proctoscopy (*proktos* anus)
			pupilloscopy (also called *retinoscopy*) (pupil of eye)
			pyeloscopy (*pyelos* pelvis)
			pyloroscopy (*pyloros* gate guard—the distal portion of the stomach)
			radioscopy (radium; X-ray)
			rectoscope, rectoscopy (also called *proctoscopy*) (rectum)
			renoscopy (also called *nephroscopy*) (*ren* kidney)
			retinoscopy (also called *koroscopy, skiascopy*) (retina)
			rheoscope (*rheos* electric current)
			rhinoscope, rhinoscopy {rhinoscopic} (*rhinos* nose)
			scatoscopy (*skatos* dung, feces)
			scotoscopy (also called *retinoscopy*) (*skotos* darkness)
			sigmoidoscope, sigmoidoscopy (*sigma* the letter S + *eidos* form)
			skiascopy (also called *retinoscopy*) (*skieros* shady)
			somatoscopy (*somatos* body)
			spectroscope, spectroscopy {spectroscopic} (spectrum)
			spiroscope, spiroscopy (*spirare* to breathe)
			stereoscope {stereoscopic} (*stereos* solid)
			stethoscope, stethoscopy {stethoscopic} (*stethos* chest)
			stomatoscope (*stomatos* mouth)
			tachistoscope (*tachys* swift, fast)
			thoracoscopy (also called *pleuroscopy*) (thorax)
			tracheoscopy {tracheoscopic} (*trachea* windpipe)
			trichoscopy (*trichos* hair)
			ureteroscope, ureteroscopy (ureter)
			urethroscope, urethroscopy {urethroscopic} (urethra)

A Thesaurus of Medical Word Roots

Element	From	Meaning	Examples
scop (cont'd)		[to examine, see]	urinoscopy (also called *uroscopy*) (urine) uteroscope (also called *hysteroscope*) (uterus) vaginoscope (also called *colposcope*), vaginoscopy (also called *colposcopy*) (vagina) ventroscopy (also called *peritoneoscopy*) (*venter* belly) zymoscope (*zyme* leaven, yeast) CROSS REFERENCE: None
scoto	Greek *skotos*	darkness	SIMPLE ROOT: scotoma (an area of depressed vision within the visual field, surrounded by an area of less depressed or of normal vision; pl., scotomata) {scotomatous} PREFIXED ROOT: hemiscotosis (also called *hemianopia*) (*hemi* half + *osis* condition) LEADING ROOT COMPOUND: *scot*: scotopia (night vision) {scotopic} (*opia* vision condition) *scoto*: scotochromogen (*chroma* color + *genere* to produce) scotodinia (dizziness with blurring of vision and headache) (*dinos* whirl) scotograph (also called *noctograph*) (*graphein* to write) scotometer, scotometry (the measurement of isolated areas of depressed vision within the visual field) (*metron* measure) scotophilia (also called *nyctophilia*) (*philein* to love) scotophobia (*phobia* fear) scotoscopy (also called *retinoscopy*) (*skopein* to examine) *scotoma*: scotomagraph (an instrument for recording a scotoma) (*graphein* to write) TRAILING ROOT COMPOUND: phacoscotasmus (a clouding of the lens of the eye) (*phakos* lens) CROSS REFERENCE: melan, noct, nyct
scrot	Latin *scrotum* bag	testicle pouch	SIMPLE ROOT: scrotum (the double pouch of the male, which contains the testicles and part of the spermatic cord, found in most mammals; pl., scrotums, scrota) {scrotal} PREFIXED ROOT: intrascrotal (situated or occurring within the scrotum) (*intra* within) LEADING ROOT COMPOUND: *scrot*: scrotectomy (*ektome* excision) scrotitis (*itis* inflammation) *scroti*: scrotiform (having the shape or form of a scrotum) *scroto*: scrotocele (*kele* hernia) scrotoplasty (*plassein* to form) TRAILING ROOT COMPOUND: abdominoscrotal (relating to the abdomen and the scrotum) (abdomen) inguinoscrotal (*inguen* groin) labioscrotal (relating to or being a swelling or ridge on each side of the embryonic rudiment of the penis or clitoris which develops into one of the scrotal sacs in the male and one of the labia majora in the female) (*labium* lip) penoscrotal (penis) perineoscrotal (perineum) urethroscrotal (urethra) CROSS REFERENCE: didym, orchi, osche, test

Element	From	Meaning	Examples
sem	Greek *sema* sign	symptom, sign	SIMPLE ROOT: semantics (the study of the significance and development of the meaning of words) semeiosis (or, semiosis) {semeiotic or, semiotic; pertaining to the signs or symptoms of a disease} PREFIXED ROOT: asemia (loss of previous ability to comprehend any type of symbol; a form of aphasia; also called *asemasia, asymbolia*) (*a* privative) megaseme (denoting a large orbital aperture) (*megas* big) mesoseme (*mesos* middle) microseme (*mikros* small) LEADING ROOT COMPOUND: semeiography (a description of the signs of disease) (*graphein* to write) semeiology (the study of symptoms; also called *symptomatology*) (*logos* study) semeiopathic (or, semiopathic; the disordered use of symbols) (*pathos* disease) TRAILING ROOT COMPOUND: urosemiology (the study of urine as an aid to diagnosis) (*ouron* urine + *logos* study) CROSS REFERENCE: None
semen, semin	Latin *semen* seed *seminare* to sow	semen, sperm	SIMPLE ROOT: semen (pl., semina, semens) {seminal; also called *spermatic*} semination (the introduction of semen into the genital tract of the female; also called *insemination*) PREFIXED ROOT: insemination (the deposit of semen or seminal fluid within the vagina or cervix, as during sexual intercourse; also called *semination*) (*in* in) LEADING ROOT COMPOUND: *semen*: semenuria (or, seminuria) (*uria* urine condition) *semeno*: semenology (or, seminology) (*logos* study) *semin*: seminoma (a tumor of the testis) {seminomatous} (*oma* tumor) seminuria (also called *spermaturia*) (*uria* urine condition) *semini*: seminiferous (lit., seed-bearing; producing seed; pertaining to, or connected with the formation of semen; as seminiferous cells or vesicles) (*ferre* to bear) TRAILING ROOT COMPOUND: pyosemia (presence of pus in seminal fluid; also called *pyospermia*) (*pyon* pus) CROSS REFERENCE: gon[1], sperm, spers
semi-	Latin prefix	half	See Appendix B for examples of words with this prefix. Others are listed with the root to which it is attached. CROSS REFERENCE: demi-, hemi-
sens, sent	Latin *sentire*	to perceive, feel	SIMPLE ROOT: *sens*: sensate, sensation (an impression conveyed by an afferent nerve to the sensorium commune) sense (to perceive through a sense organ) sensibility, sensible, sensing, sensitive, sensitivity, sensitization, sensitize, sensitizer sensor, sensorium (any of the primary receptive areas; pl., sensoria, sensoriums) {sensorial}, sensory sensual (carnal; worldly), sensualism, sensuality, sensuous *sent*: sentient (capable of perceiving sensation), sentiment

Element	From	Meaning	Examples
sens (cont'd)		[to perceive]	PREFIXED ROOT: *sens*: consensual (excited by reflex stimulation) (*con* with) insensible (unconscious; not appreciable by the senses) (*in* not) *sensit*: desensitize (*de* reversal) hypersensitive, hypersensitivity (*hyper* over, beyond) hyposensitive, hyposensitivity, hyposensitization (*hypo* under) multisensitivity (*multus* many) polysensitivity (*polys* many) supersensitivity, supersensitization (*super* above) *sensory*: extrasensory—perception (ESP) (*extra* outside, beyond) hemisensory (*hemi* half) multisensory (*multus* many) polysensory (*polys* many) supersenory (*super* over, above) LEADING ROOT COMPOUND: *sensi*: sensiferous (*ferre* to bear) sensigenous (*genere* to produce) sensimeter (*metron* measure) *senso*: sensomobile, sensomobility, sensomotor (or, sensorimotor) (*movere* to move) *sensori*: sensoriglandular (gland) sensorimotor (or, sensomotor) (*movere* to move) sensorimuscular (producing reflex muscular action in response to a sensory impression) sensorineural (of or pertaining to a sensory nerve) sensorivascular (*vas* vessel: blood vessel) *senti*: sentisection (vivisection of an animal that is not anesthetized) (*sectare* to cut) TRAILING ROOT COMPOUND: chemosensory (relating to the perception of chemical substances) neurosensory (*neuron* nerve) psychosensory (*psyche* mind) somatosensory (*somatos* body) viscerosensory (*viscera* internal organs) visuosensory (*videre* to see) CROSS REFERENCE: esthes, path
sep	Greek *sepsis*	rotting, decaying, putrefaction	SIMPLE ROOT: sepsin, sepsis (also called *septicemia*; pl., sepses) septic (produced by or due to putrefaction) septicine (a ptomaine, or compound of hexylamine and amylamine, from putrid flesh) PREFIXED ROOT: *sepsis*: asepsis (sterile; a condition free from germs; also called *sterility*) {aseptic; also called *sterile*} (*a* negative) antisepsis {antiseptic} (*anti* against) endosepsis (*endon* within) *septic*: preantiseptic (*pre* before + antiseptic) *septicemia*: autosepticemia (*autos* self + septicemia)

Element	From	Meaning	Examples
sep (cont'd)		[rotting]	LEADING ROOT COMPOUND: *sept*: septemia (or, septicemia; presence in the blood of bacterial toxins) (*emia* blood condition) *septi*: septimetritis (*metra* uterus + *itis* inflammation) septineuritis (*neuron* nerve + *itis* inflammation) *septic*: septicemia (also called *blood poisoning*) {septicemic} (*emia* blood condition) *septico*: septicopyemia (*pyon* pus + *emia* blood condition) TRAILING ROOT COMPOUND: pyosepticemia (pyemia and septicemia combined) (*pyon* pus + *emia* blood condition) TERM: septic phlebitis (inflammation of the veins, due to septic poisoning) CROSS REFERENCE: caries, sapr
sept	Latin *septus*	wall, fence; septum	SIMPLE ROOT: septate (divided by a septum) septation (division into parts by a septum; a septum) septulum (a minute septum; pl., septula) septum (a partition dividing two cavities; pl., septa) {septal} PREFIXED ROOT: *sepiment*: dissepiment (a separating tissue, partition, or septum) (*dis* apart) *septal*: anteroseptal (*anterior* before) interseptal (between two septa) (*inter* between) preseptal (*pre* before) supraseptal (*supra* above) transseptal (*trans* across) *septate*: aseptate (*a* privative) biseptate (*bi* two) uniseptate (*uni* one) *septum*: hemiseptum (*hemi* half) interseptum (the diaphragm) (*inter* between) LEADING ROOT COMPOUND: *sept*: septectomy (*ektome* excision) *septo*: septodermoplasty (*derma* skin + *plassein* to form) septomarginal (margin) septonasal (*nasus* nose) septoplasty (*plassein* to form) septorhinoplasty (*rhinos* nose + *plassein* to form) septostomy (*stoma* mouth, opening) septotome, septotomy (*tomy* incision) TRAILING ROOT COMPOUND: myoseptum (also called *myocomma*) (*myos* muscle) nasoseptal, nasoseptitis (*nasus* nose + *itis* inflammation) CROSS REFERENCE: diaphragm, parie, phragm, phren[1]
ser	Latin *serum*	whey, watery substance	SIMPLE ROOT: serosa (a serous membrane) {serosal}, serosity, serous, serum (pl., serums, sera) {serumal} PREFIXED ROOT: antiserum (*anti* against) autoserum {autoserous} (*autos* self)

Element	From	Meaning	Examples
ser (cont'd)		[whey]	exoserosis (*exo* outside + *osis* condition)
			extraserous (*extra* outside)
			heteroantiserum (*heteros* other + antiserum)
			polyserositis (*polys* many + serositis)
			subserous (or, subserosal) (*sub* below)
			LEADING ROOT COMPOUND:
			ser:
			seralbumin (the albumin of the blood)
			seroma (*oma* tumor)
			seri: seriflux (a thin, watery discharge) (*fluere* to flow)
			serio: serioscopy (*skopein* to examine)
			sero:
			serocolitis (also called *pericolitis*) (colon + *itis* inflammation)
			seroculture (a bacterial culture on blood serum)
			serocystic (made up of serous cysts)
			serodiagnosis
			seroenteritis (inflammation of the serous coat of the intestine) (*enteron* intestine + *itis* inflammation)
			serofibrinous (also called *seroplastic*)
			serology {serologic} (*logos* study)
			serolysin (a lysin present in the blood stream)
			seromembranous (*membrum* a member: membrane)
			seromucus (a secretion which is part serum and part mucus) {seromucous}
			seromuscular (pertaining to the serous and muscular coats of the intestine)
			seromyotomy (*myos* muscle + *tomy* incision)
			serophilic (*philein* to love—have an affinity for)
			seroplastic (also called *serofibrinous*) (*plassein* to form)
			seroprognosis (the prognosis of a disease based on the results of serologic tests)
			seropurulent (containing both serum and pus)
			seropus (serum mingled with pus)
			serosanguineous (containing both serum and blood) (*sanguis* blood)
			seroserous (relating to two serous surfaces)
			serosynovial (both serous and synovial), serosynovitis (*itis* inflammation)
			serotaxis (*taxis* arrangement)
			serotherapy (*therapy* treatment)
			serothorax (also called *hydrothorax*) (*thorax* chest)
			serotoxin (*toxin* poison)
			seros: serositis (*itis* inflammation)
			serosa: serosamucin (mucoid material found in serous fluids, e.g., in ascitic or synovial fluid)
			CROSS REFERENCE: lymph
sex	Latin *secare* (possibly)	to cut	SIMPLE ROOT: sex, sexual, sexuality
			PREFIXED ROOT:
			asexual (having no sex; not sexual; not pertaining to sex), asexuality
			asexualization (sterilization of an individual, either by castration or by vasectomy) (*a* privative)
			ambisexual (bisexual; partial hermaphroditism) (*ambi* both)
			ambosexual (or, ambisexual) (*ambo* both)
			bisexual (pertaining to bisexuality: the condition of having gonads of both sexes or ovotestes) (*bi* two)

Element	From	Meaning	Examples
sex (cont'd)		[to cut]	contrasexual (pertaining to or characteristic of the opposite sex) (*contra* against) desexualize (to deprive of sexual characters) (*de* negative) heterosexual, heterosexuality (*heteros* other, different) homosexual, homosexuality (*homos* same) hypersexuality (*hyper* over) hyposexuality (*hypo* under) intersexual (also called *androgynous*) (*inter* between) isosexual (*isos* equal) monosexual (showing the traits of one sex only) (*monos* single) parasexual, parasexuality (*para* alongside) transsexual, transsexualism (*trans* across) unisexual (of only one sex; having the sexual organs of only one sex) (*uni* one) LEADING ROOT COMPOUND: sexology (*logos* study) sexopathy (also called *paraphilia*) (*pathos* disease) TRAILING ROOT COMPOUND: somatosexual (relating to the physical or physiological aspects of sexuality) (*somatos* body) urinosexual (pertaining to the genital and urinary organs; also called *genitourinary*) (*ouron* urine) CROSS REFERENCE: tom
sial	Greek *sialon*	saliva; saliva ducts	SIMPLE ROOT: sialic (also called *salivary*), sialidase, sialine (salivary) sialism (or, sialismus; an excessive secretion of saliva; also called *ptyalism*) PREFIXED ROOT: asialia (or, asialism; absence or deficiency of the secretion of saliva) (*a* privative) antisialic, antisialagogue (*anti* against + *agein* to lead) hyposialosis (also called *hypoptyalism*) (*hypo* under + *osis* condition) polysialia (*polys* much) LEADING ROOT COMPOUND: *sial*: sialaden (*adenos* gland) sialagogue (also called *ptyalagogue*) {sialagogic} (*agein* to lead) sialectasis (*ektasis* dilatation) sialemesis (or, sialemesia) (*emein* to vomit) sialendoscopy (*endon* within + *skopein* to examine) sialitis (*itis* inflammation) sialoma (*oma* tumor) sialosis (also called *ptyalism*) {sialotic} (*osis* condition) *sialo*: sialoaerophagy (*aer* air + *phagein* to swallow) sialoangiectasis (*angeion* vessel + *ektasis* dilatation) sialoangiitis (*angeion* vessel + *itis* inflammation) sialocele (cyst or tumor of a salivary gland) (*kele* tumor) sialodochitis (*dochos* receptacle + *itis* inflammation) sialodochoplast (*dochos* receptacle + *plassein* to form) sialogenous (producing saliva) (*genere* to produce) sialogram, sialography (*graphein* to write) sialolith (also called *salivary calculus*) (*lithos* stone)

A Thesaurus of Medical Word Roots

Element	From	Meaning	Examples
sial (cont'd)		[saliva]	sialolithotomy (*lithos* stone, calculus + *tomy* incision)
			sialometaplasia (squamous cell metaplasis in the salivary ducts)
			sialometry (*metron* measure)
			sialophagia (*phagein* to swallow)
			sialorrhea (also called *ptyalism*) (*rhein* to flow)
			sialoschesis (*schesis* suppression, retention)
			sialostenosis (*stenos* narrow + *osis* condition)
			TRAILING ROOT COMPOUND:
			glycosialia (also called *glycoptyalism*) (*glykys* sweet)
			oligosialia (also called *oligoptyalism*) (*oligos* scant, little)
			CROSS REFERENCE: ptyal
sider	Greek *sideros*	iron	SIMPLE ROOT: siderous (containing iron)
			PREFIXED ROOT:
			asiderosis (abnormal decrease of the iron reserve of the body) (*a* negative + *osis* condition)
			antisideric (counteracting the physiological action of iron, probably by chelating or precipitation) (*anti* against)
			LEADING ROOT COMPOUND:
			sider: siderosis (any disease of the lungs caused by the inhaling of particles of iron or other metal) {siderotic} (*osis* condition)
			siderin: siderinuria (excretion of iron in the urine) (*uria* urine condition)
			sidero:
			sideroblast (an erythroblast containing many iron granules in its cytoplasm) {sideroblastic} (*blastos* bud, shoot, germ)
			siderocyte (a red blood cell containing granules of iron that are not part of the cell's hemoglobin) (*kytos* cell)
			sideroderma (bronzed coloration of the skin from disorder of the metabolism of the iron from degenerated hemoglobin) (*derma* skin)
			siderofibrosis (fibrosis of the spleen with deposits of iron) (*fibra* fiber + *osis* condition)
			siderogenous (*genere* to produce)
			sideromycin (any of a class of antibiotics, synthesized by certain actinomycetes, that inhibit bacterial growth by interfering with iron uptake) (*mykes* fungus)
			sideropenia {sideropenic} (*penia* deficiency)
			siderophage (*phagein* to consume)
			siderophil (or, siderophile) {siderophilous} (*philein* to love)
			siderophore (a substance that binds iron) (*phorein* to bear)
			sideroscope (*skopein* to examine)
			TRAILING ROOT COMPOUND:
			hemosiderosis (*haima* blood + *osis* condition)
			silicosiderosis (*silex* silica + *osis* condition)
			CROSS REFERENCE: ferr
sigma	Greek *sigma* σ, Σ [18th letter of the Greek alphabet]	the letter σ, Σ; the sigmoid	SIMPLE ROOT: sigma, sigmatism (incorrect, difficult, or too frequent use of the *s* sound; also called *parasigmatism*)
			PREFIXED ROOT:
			sigma: parasigmatism (imperfect pronunciation of the letter "s"; also called *lisping, sigmatism*) (*para* abnormal)
			sigmoid similar to a sigma:
			macrosigmoid (also called *megasigmoid*) (*makros* large)
			megasigmoid (also called *macrosigmoid*) (*mega* large)
			mesosigmoid, mesosigmoiditis (*mesos* middle + *itis* inflammation)

Element	From	Meaning	Examples
sigma (cont'd)		[sigmoid]	mesosigmoidopexy (*mesos* middle + *pexis* fixation)
			perisigmoiditis (*peri* around + *itis* inflammation)
			retrosigmoidal (*retro* backward)
			LEADING ROOT COMPOUND:
			sigmoid similar to a sigma:
			sigmoid (shaped like the letter S, or like Greek *sigma*; the sigmoid flexure), sigmoidicity
			sigmoidectomy (*ektome* excision)
			sigmoiditis (*itis* inflammation)
			sigmoido:
			sigmoidopexy (*pexy* fixation)
			sigmoidoproctostomy (also called *sigmoidrectostomy*) (*proktos* anus + *stoma* mouth, opening)
			sigmoidoscope (or, sigmoscope) (*skopein* to examine)
			sigmoidostomy (*stoma* mouth, opening)
			sigmoidotomy (*tomy* incision)
			sigmoidovesical (*vesica* bladder)
			TRAILING ROOT COMPOUND:
			proctosigmoiditis (*proktos* anus + *itis* inflammation)
			vesicosigmoid (*vesica* bladder)
			CROSS REFERENCE: None
sin	Latin *sinus*	hollow, bend, fold: sinus	SIMPLE ROOT:
			sinuate (having wavy margins)
			sinuous (bending in and out; winding)
			sinus {sinal, sinusal}
			PREFIXED ROOT:
			sin: perisinuous (situated around a sinus) (*peri* around)
			sinus: retrosinus (the air cells posterior to the sigmoid sinus in the mastoid process of the temporal bone) (*retro* backward)
			sinusitis sinus inflammation:
			pansinusitis (inflammation involving all the paranasal sinuses) (*pan* all)
			perisinusitis (an inflammation of the structures around a sinus) (*peri* around)
			polysinusitis (*polys* many)
			sinusoidal similar to a sinus:
			parasinusoidal (also called *sinusoidal*) (*para* alongside)
			postsinusoidal (*post* after)
			presinusoidal (*pre* before)
			LEADING ROOT COMPOUND:
			sino:
			sinoatrial (or, sinuatrial; pertaining to the sinus venosus and the atrium of the heart)
			sinobronchitis (*bronchus* windpipe + *itis* inflammation)
			sinography (radiologic use of a contrast medium to opacify a sinus tract) (*graphein* to write)
			sinopulmonary (*pulmon* lung)
			sinospiral (pertaining to the sinus venosus and having a spiral course: said of certain muscle fibers of the heart)
			sinoventricular (pertaining to the sinus venosus and the ventricle of the heart)
			sinus:
			sinusitis (*itis* inflammation)
			sinusoid {sinusoidal} (*eidos* form)

Element	From	Meaning	Examples
sin (cont'd)		[sinus]	*sinuso*: sinusotomy (*tomy* incision) TRAILING ROOT COMPOUND: *sinusitis* sinus inflammation: aerosinusitis (inflammation of the paranasal sinuses caused by a difference between the pressure within the sinus cavities and the ambient pressure; also called *barosinusitis*) (*aer* air) barosinusitis (the painful symptoms related to the maxillary sinus resulting from a change in barometric pressure) (*baros* weight) bronchosinusitis (coexisting infection of the paranasal sinuses and the lower respiratory passages) (*bronchus* windpipe) dacryosinusitis (*dakyron* teardrop) nasosinusitis (also called *rhinosinusitis*) (*nasus* nose) rhinosinusitis (also called *nasosinusitis*) (*rhinos* nose) thrombosinusitis (also called *sinus thrombosis*) (*thrombos* clot) CROSS REFERENCE: cav, cel[1]
sinist	Latin *sinister*	left	SIMPLE ROOT: sinister (denotes the left hand of one of two similar structures), sinistrad (toward the left), sinistral, sinistrality, sinistrous (opposite of *dextral*) PREFIXED ROOT: ambisinister (the inability to perform acts requiring manual skill with either hand) {ambisinistrous; also called *ambilevous*} (*ambi* both) LEADING ROOT COMPOUND: *sinistr*: sinistraural (having better hearing in the left ear) (*auris* ear) sinistrocular (having stronger vision in the left eye) (*oculus* eye) *sinistro*: sinistrocardia (*kardia* heart) sinistrocerebral (*cerebrum* brain) sinistrogyration (a turning to the left) (*gyros* circle) sinistromanual (*manus* hand) sinistropedal (*pes* foot) sinistrorotation (also called *sinistrotorsion*) (*rotare* to turn) sinistrotorsion (also called *sinistrorotation*) (*torquere* to twist) DISGUISED ROOT: sinistrorse (turned or twisted to the left) (sinister + *vertere* to turn) CROSS REFERENCE: lev
sit	Greek *sitos*	food	PREFIXED ROOT: asitia (a loathing of food; also called *anorexia*) (*a* negative) autosite (the larger, more normally formed member of asymmetric conjoined twins, to which the other is attached) (*autos* self) eusitia (normal appetite) (*eu* well) parasite (*para* beside) [see separate entry: parasit-] LEADING ROOT COMPOUND: *sitio*: sitiology (or, sitology) (*logos* study) *sito*: sitology (science of food and nourishment) (*logos* study) sitomania (periodic abnormal craving for food) (*mania* craze) sitophobia (irrational fear of eating or of food) (*phobia* fear) sitotaxis (also called *sitotropism*) (*tassein* to arrange) sitotherapy (treatment by food; dietotherapy) sitotoxin, sitotoxism (*toxikon* poison) sitotropism (response of living cells to the presence of nutritive elements; also called *sitotaxis*) (*trepein* to turn) CROSS REFERENCE: None

Element	From	Meaning	Examples
som	Greek *soma*	body	SIMPLE ROOT: soma (the body as distinct from the mind; all of the body cells except the germ cells; also, the body exclusive of the extremities) {somal, somatic} somite (embryonic blocklike segment formed on either side of the neural tube and its underlying notochord; also called *mesoblastic, mesodermal segment*) PREFIXED ROOT: *soma*: asoma (a fetal monster with an imperfect head and the merest rudiments of a trunk) (*a* privative) megasoma (*mega* large) microsoma (a very short but not dwarfish stature) {microsomia) (*mikros* small) *somatia*: diplosomatia (or, diplosomia; a condition in which complete twins are joined at some part of their bodies), diplosome (*diploos* two-fold) macrosomatia (or, macrosomia) {macrosomatic} (*makros* large) *somatic*: ecsomatics (the study by laboratory methods of the materials removed from the body) (*ek* out) extrasomatic (*extra* outside) eurysomatic (having a thick-set body) (*eurys* broad) microsomatic (*mikros* small) *somatize*: exsomatize (to remove from the body) (*ex* out) *somato*: autosomatognosis (the sensation that an amputated portion of the body is still present) (*autos* self + *gnosis* knowledge) *some*: aposome (an inclusion within the cytoplasm which has been made by the activity of the cell itself) (*apo* from) autosome (*autos* self) centrosome (the cell center) (*kentron* point; center) diplosome (*diploos* two-fold) endosome (*endon* within) episome (*epi* upon) heterosome (a sex chromosome) (*heteros* other) mesosome (*mesos* middle) microsome {microsomal} (*mikros* small) monosome (an unpaired sex chromosome) (*monos* single) *somia*: diplosomia (*diploos* two-fold, double) hypersomia (gigantism) (*hyper* over, above) hyposomia (dwarfism) (*hypo* under) megasomia (also called *macrosomia*) (*megas* big) mesosomia (*mesos* middle) microsomia (*mikros* small) polysomia {polysomic} (*polys* much) *somic*: trisomic (*tri* three) tetrasomic (*tetra* four) *somus*: hemisomus (*hemi* half, imperfect) polysomus (*polys* much)

Element	From	Meaning	Examples
som (cont'd)		[body]	*somy*: disomy (a chromosome set having paired members) {disomic} (*di* two) monosomy (*monos* single) trisomy (*tri* three) LEADING ROOT COMPOUND: *som*: somasthenia (or, somatasthenia) (*asthenia* weakness) somesthesia (or, somatesthesia) {somesthetic} (*esthesia* feeling) *soma*: somaplasm (*plassein* to form) *somat*: somatagnosia (also called *somatotopagnosia*, where the *top* element is from *topos* place) (agnosia: *a* privative + *gnosis* knowledge) somatalgia (*algos* pain) somatasthenia (or, somasthenia) (*asthenia* weakness) somatesthesia (or, somesthesia; also called *somatognosis*) {somatesthetic} (*esthesia* feeling) *somatico*: somaticosplanchnic (relating to the body and the viscera; also called *somaticovisceral*) (*splanchnos* viscus) *somato*: somatochrome (*chroma* color) somatocrinin (also called *somatoliberin*) (*cernere* to separate) somatoderm (somatic layer) (*derma* skin) somatodidymus (*didymos* twin) somatoform (*forma* shape) somatogenesis {somatogenetic, somatogenic} (*genere* to produce) somatognosis (also called *cenesthesia, somatesthesia*) (*gnosis* knowledge) somatogram (*graphein* to write) somatoliberin (also called *somatocrinin*) (*liber* free) somatology (*logos* study) somatomegaly (also called *gigantism*) (*megalos* large) somatometry (*metron* measure) somatopagus (*pagos* thing fixed) somatopathy {somatopathic} (*pathos* disease) somatophrenia (*phrenia* mind condition) somatoplasm (*plassein* to form) somatopleure {somatopleural} (*pleura* rib, side) somatoprosthetics (prosthesis) somatopsychic (*psyche* mind) somatoschisis (*schisis* fissure) somatoscopy (*skopein* to examine) somatosensory (*sentire* to feel) somatosexual (pertaining to the physical manifestations of sexual development) somatostatin (*stasis* standing still) somatotherapy (*therapy* treatment) somatotonia (*tonos* tension) somatotopagnosia (or, somatagnosia) (*topos* place + *agnosia* lack of knowledge) somatotopic (*topos* place) somatotroph {somatotrophic} (*trephein* to nourish) somatotype (a particular category or type of body build, e.g., ectomorph, endomorph, mesomorph), somatotypy

A Thesaurus of Medical Word Roots

Element	From	Meaning	Examples
som (cont'd)		[body]	TRAILING ROOT COMPOUND:
			soma: pleurosoma (or, pleurosomus) (*pleura* side, rib)
			somatic:
			leptosomatic (having a light, thin body) (*leptos* slender)
			psychosomatic (also called *psychophysiologic*) (*psyche* mind)
			splanchnosomatic (also called *viscerosomatic*) (*splanchnos* viscus)
			viscerosomatic (also called *splanchnosomatic*) (*viscus* internal organ)
			some:
			acrosome (*akron* extremity)
			allosome (*allos* other)
			chromosome (*chroma* color)
			deuterosome (*deuteros* second)
			dictyosome (*diktyon* net)
			karyosome (irregular clumps of chromatin material seen in the nuclei of cells which are not dividing; also called *chromocenter, prochromosome*) (*karyon* nucleus)
			liposome (*lipos* fat)
			melanosome (*melanos* dark)
			pinosome (*pinein* to drink; liquid, fluid)
			sarcosome (*sarkos* flesh)
			trypanosome (*trypanon* a borer: an augur)
			somia:
			meromicrosomia (*meros* part + *mikros* small)
			pachysomia (*pachys* thick)
			somus:
			perosomus (also called *perocormus*) (*peros* maimed)
			schistosomus (also called *schistocormus*) (*schistos* split)
			CROSS REFERENCE: corp
son	Latin *sonus*	sound	SIMPLE ROOT:
			sone (a unit of loudness) {sonic}
			sonicate (to expose to sound waves; to disrupt bacteria by exposure to high-frequency sound waves), sonication
			sonitus (a sounding or tinkling in the ears; tinnitus aurium)
			sonorant (voiced), sonorous (resonant; sounding)
			PREFIXED ROOT:
			sonance:
			assonance (a morbid tendency to alliteration in speaking, that is, repetition of an initial sound in two or more words of a phrase) (*ad* to)
			dissonance, dissonant (*dis* apart)
			hyperresonance (*hyper* over + resonance)
			resonance, resonant, resonating, resonator (*re* back)
			transonance (*trans* across)
			sonic:
			hypersonic (*hyper* above)
			infrasonic (also called *subsonic*) (*infra* below)
			subsonic (also called *infrasonic*) (*sub* below)
			supersonic, supersonics (*super* more, greater)
			transonic (*trans* across)
			ultrasonic (*ultra* beyond)
			sonography writing of sound:
			endosonography (*endon* within)
			ultrasonography (*ultra* beyond)
			sound: ultrasound (*ultra* beyond)

Element	From	Meaning	Examples
son (cont'd)		[sound]	LEADING ROOT COMPOUND: *soni*: sonification, sonifier, sonify (*facere* to make) *sono*: sonochemistry sonogram (a record or display obtained by ultrasonic scanning), sonography {sonographic} (*graphein* to write) sonohysterography (*hystera* uterus + *graphein* to write) sonolucent {sonolucency} (*lucere* to shine) sonomicrometer (micrometer: *mikros* small + *metron* measure) sonomotor (*movere* to move) sonourethrography (urethra + *graphein* to write) FRENCH: sonde (sound) CROSS REFERENCE: phem, phon
spas	Greek *spasmos* from *span* to contract, draw, pull, wrench	convulsion; to pull, draw	SIMPLE ROOT: spasm (or, spasmus; a sudden, violent, involuntary contraction of a muscle or a group of muscles attended by pain and interference with function, producing involuntary movement and distortion) {spasmotic, spastic}, spasticity PREFIXED ROOT: *spasm*: antispasmodic (*anti* against) hemispasm (*hemi* half) monospasm (*monos* single) *spastic*: antispastic (*anti* against) epispastic (*epi* upon) LEADING ROOT COMPOUND: spasmogen {spasmogenic} (*genere* to produce) spasmolysis {spasmolytic} (*lysis* dissolution) spasmophemia (stuttering) (*pheme* speech) spasmophilia {spasmophilic} (*philein* to love) TRAILING ROOT COMPOUND: algospasm (*algos* pain) angiospasm (also called *vasospasm*) (*angeion* blood vessel) arteriospasm (*arteria* artery) blepharospasm (*blepharon* eyelid) bronchiospasm (or, bronchospasm) (*bronchus* windpipe) camptospasm (also called *camptocormia*) (*kamptos* bent) cardiospasm (*kardia* heart) cheirospasm (or, chirospasm) (*cheir* hand) clonospasm (also called *clonic spasm*) (*klonus* turmoil) colpospasm (also called *vaginal spasm*) (*kolpos* vagina) cystospasm (*kystis* bladder) dactylospasm (*daktylos* finger, toe) enterospasm (*enteron* intestine) esophagospasm (esophagus) gastrospasm (*gaster* stomach, belly) glossospasm (*glossa* tongue) graphospasm (also called *writer's cramp*) (*graphein* to write) gyrospasm (rotary spasm of the head) (*gyros* circle) hysterospasm (*hystera* uterus) idiospasm (a spasm of a limited area) (*idios* one's own) laryngospasm (also called *laryngismus, glottic spasm*) (larynx) logospasm (also called *logoclonia; stuttering*) (*logos* word) myospasm (*myos* muscle)

Element	From	Meaning	Examples
spas (cont'd)		[spasm]	neurospasm (*neuron* nerve) pharyngospasm (pharynx) phrenospasm (*phren* diaphragm) proctospasm (*proktos* anus) pylorospasm (*pyle* gate: the distal portion of the stomach) prosopospasm (facial tic) (*prosopon* face) stethospasm (*stethos* chest) urethrospasm (also called *urethrism*) (urethra) vasospasm (also called *angiospasm*) (*vas* vessel) CROSS REFERENCE: clon, stal, tetan
sperm	Greek *speirein* to sow *sperma,* *spermatos* seed	seed, sperm, semen (the male generative element)	SIMPLE ROOT: sperm (or, sperma; the semen or testicular ejaculate; pl., sperms) spermary, spermatic (also called *seminal*), spermatid spermium (mature male germ cell or sperm; pl., spermia) PREFIXED ROOT: *sperm:* endosperm (*endon* within) *spermia:* aspermia (lack of, or failure to ejaculate, semen) (*a* privative) dispermia (or, dispermy) (*di* two) dysspermia (an abnormality of the spermatozoa in the semen; diffi- cult or painful emission of sperm or semen) (*dys* abnormal) panspermia (or, panspermatism) (*pan* all) polyspermia (or, polyspermism) (*polys* much) *spermatitis:* perispermatitis (*peri* around + *itis* inflammation) *spermy:* dispermy (or, dispermia; the penetration of two spermatozoa into one ovum) (*di* two) monospermy (*monos* single) polyspermy (*polys* much) prespermatid (a secondary spermatocyte) (*pre* before) LEADING ROOT COMPOUND: *sperm:* spermacrasia (*akrasia* ill mixture) *spermat:* spermatemphraxis (*emphraxis* obstruction) spermatitis (inflammation of a vas deferens) (*itis* inflammation) spermatoid (*eidos* form) spermaturia (also called *seminuria*) (*uria* urine condition) *spermati:* spermaticide (or, spermicide) (*caedere* to kill) *spermato:* spermatoblast (*blastos* bud, shoot, germ) spermatocele (*kele* hernia) spermatocide {spermatocidal} (*caedere* to kill) spermatocyst (*kystis* sac) spermatocyte, spermatocytogenesis (*kytos* cell + *genere* to produce) spermatogenesis {spermatogenetic} (*genere* to produce) spermatogonium (pl., spermatogonia} (*gone* seed) spermatology (also called *seminology*) (*logos* study) spermatolysis {spermatolytic} (*lyein* to dissolve) spermatopathy (also called *dysspermia*) (*pathos* disease) spermatophobia (morbid fear of spermatorrhea or loss of semen) spermatophore (*pherein* to bear) spermatopoietic (also called *spermatogenic*) (*poiein* to produce) spermatorrhea (an involuntary discharge of semen, without orgasm) (*rhein* to flow)

A Thesaurus of Medical Word Roots

Element	From	Meaning	Examples
sperm (cont'd)		[seed, sperm]	spermatotoxin (or, spermatoxin, spermotoxin) (*toxin* poison)
			spermatozoan (*zoon* animal)
			spermi:
			spermicide (or, spermaticide) {spermicidal} (*caedere* to kill)
			spermiduct (also called *ductus deferens, ejaculatory duct*) (*ducere* to lead)
			spermio:
			spermiogenesis (*genere* to produce)
			spermiogram (*graphein* to write)
			spermo:
			spermoblast (spermatid) (*blastos* bud, shoot, germ)
			spermocytoma (also called *seminoma*) (*kytos* cell + *oma* tumor)
			spermolith (*lithos* stone)
			spermolysis (or, spermatolysis) (*lyein* to dissolve)
			spermoplasm (*plassein* to form)
			spermotoxic (also called *spermicidal*) (*toxikon* poison)
			TRAILING ROOT COMPOUND:
			sperm:
			oosperm (*oon* egg, ovum)
			zygosperm (also called *zygospore*) (*zygon* yoke)
			spermia sperm condition:
			asthenospermia (also called *asthenozoospermia*) (*asthenia* weakness: *a* negative + *sthenos* strength)
			bacteriospermia (the presence of bacteria in semen or ejaculate)
			hematospermia (or, hemospermia) (*hematos* blood)
			leukospermia (also called *leukocytospermia*) (*leukos* white)
			necrospermia (*nekros* dead)
			nematospermia (*nematos* thread)
			normospermia {normospermic} (*norma* rule: normal, usual)
			oligospermia (also called *oligozoospermia*) (*oligos* little, few)
			pyospermia (*pyon* pus)
			spherospermia (*sphaira* sphere: ball, globe)
			teratospermia (*teratos* monster)
			spermatism: bradyspermatism (*bradys* slow)
			PREFIXED TRAILING ROOT COMPOUND:
			azoospermia (lack of live spermatozoa in the semen; failure to form live spermatozoa) (*a* privative + *zoa* animal)
			dyszoospermia (*dys* abnormal + *zoa* animal)
			CROSS REFERENCE: blast, gon[1], semen, spor
sphen	Greek *sphen, sphenos* wedge	wedge (the sphenoid bone)	SIMPLE ROOT: sphenion (point at apex of the sphenoidal angle of the parietal bone)
			PREFIXED ROOT:
			esosphenoiditis (osteomyelitis of the sphenoid bone) (*eso* within + *eidos* form + *itis* inflammation)
			parasphenoid (*para* alongside, near + sphenoid)
			postsphenoid (*post* after + sphenoid)
			presphenoid (anterior region of the body of the sphenoid bone) (*pre* before + sphenoid)
			supersphenoid (*super* above + sphenoid)
			transsphenoidal (*trans* across + sphenoid)
			LEADING ROOT COMPOUND:
			sphen:
			sphenoid {sphenoidal} (*eidos* form) [sphenoid bone: an irregular wedge-shaped bone at the base of the skull]

Element	From	Meaning	Examples
sphen (cont'd)		[wedge]	sphenorbital (*orbit* eye socket) sphenosis (a wedging of the fetus in the pelvis) (*osis* condition) *spheno*: sphenobasilar (relating to the sphenoid bone and the basilar process of the occipital bone; also called *sphenooccipital*) sphenocephaly (*kephale* head) sphenoethmoid, sphenoethmoidectomy (the ethmoid process: *ethmos* sieve + *ektome* excision) sphenofrontal (pertaining to the sphenoid and frontal bones) sphenomaxillary (*maxilla* upper jaw) sphenometer (*metron* measure) sphenooccipital (also called *sphenobasilar*) (*occiput* back of head) sphenopagus (*pagos* fixed) sphenopalatine (*palatum* roof of mouth) sphenoparietal (*paries* wall) sphenotemporal (temporal region) *sphenoid*: sphenoiditis (*itis* inflammation) *sphenoido*: sphenoidostomy (*stoma* mouth, opening) sphenoidotomy (*tomy* incision) TRAILING ROOT COMPOUND: *sphenoid* wedge-shaped: basisphenoid (also called *postsphenoid*) (basion) ethmosphenoid (*ethmos* sieve) orbitosphenoid (*orbit* eye socket) parietosphenoid (*paries* wall) petrosphenoid (*petra* stone) squamosphenoid (*squama* thin plate—of bone) temporosphenoid (temporal process) zygomaticosphenoid (*zygon* yoke: zygomatic process) CROSS REFERENCE: cune
spher	Greek *sphaira*	ball, sphere	SIMPLE ROOT: sphere {spherical}, spherule (a small sphere) PREFIXED ROOT: ectosphere (*ektos* outer) hemisphere, hemispherectomy (*hemi* half + *ektome* excision) microsphere (also called *centrosome*) (*mikros* small) microspherocyte (also called *spherocyte*), microspherocytosis (*mikros* small + *kytos* cell + *osis* condition) microspherolith (*mikros* small + *lithos* stone) LEADING ROOT COMPOUND: *spher*: spheresthesia (the disturbing subjective sensation of a lump in the throat: seen in hysteria) (*esthesia* feeling) spheroid {spheroidal} (*eidos* form) spheroma (*oma* tumor) *sphero*: spherocylinder (a combined spherical and cylindrical lens) spherocyte (also called *microspherocyte*) {spherocytic}, spherocytosis (*kytos* cell + *osis* condition) spherolith (any one of the minute spherical deposits found in the kidney tissue of the newborn) (*lithos* stone) spherometer (*metron* measure) spherophakia (*phakos* lens) spheroplast (*plassein* to form)

A Thesaurus of Medical Word Roots

Element	From	Meaning	Examples
spher (cont'd)		[ball, globe]	spherospermia (*sperm* seed) TRAILING ROOT COMPOUND: centrosphere (also called *statosphere*) (*kentrum* point) myospherulosis (*myos* muscle + *osis* condition) oosphere (*oon* egg, ovum) zygosphere (also called *zygosperm*) (*zygon* yoke) CROSS REFERENCE: glob
sphinct	Greek *sphingein* to draw tight *sphinkter* a band	to draw tight	SIMPLE ROOT: sphincter (circular muscle constricting an orifice, especially the anus) {sphincterial, sphincteric} sphincterismus (spasmodic contraction of the sphincter) PREFIXED ROOT: intersphincteric (between the internal and external anal sphincters) (*inter* between) LEADING ROOT COMPOUND: *sphincter*: sphincteralgia (*algos* pain) sphincterectomy (*ektome* excision) sphincteritis (*itis* inflammation) sphincteroid (*eidos* form, resemblance) *sphinctero*: sphincterolysis (*lyein* to loosen) sphincterometry (also called *cystosphincterometry*) (*metron* measure) sphincteroplasty (*plassein* to form) sphincteroscope, sphincteroscopy (*skopein* to examine) sphincterotome, sphincterotomy (*tomy* incision) TRAILING ROOT COMPOUND: lissosphincter (*lissos* smooth) CROSS REFERENCE: systol
sphygmo, sphyx	Greek *sphygmos, sphyzein* to throb	pulse, throb	SIMPLE ROOT: sphygmic (pertaining to the pulse) PREFIXED ROOT: *sphygia*: asphygmia (temporary disappearance of the pulse) (*a* privative) anisosphygmia (*aniso* unequal: *an* negative + *iso* equal) hemisphygmia (*hemi* half) hyposphygmia (*hypo* under) microsphygmia (or, microsphyxia) (*mikros* small) *sphygmic*: postsphygmic (*post* after) presphygmic (*pre* before) *sphyxia*: asphyxia (condition caused by insufficient intake of oxygen) {asphyxial}, asphyxiate (to suffocate, smother) (*a* privative) hypersphyxia (*hyper* over, beyond) microsphyxia (or, microsphygmy) (*mikros* small) LEADING ROOT COMPOUND: *sphygm*: sphygmoid (*eidos* form, resemblance) *sphygmo*: sphygmocardiograph (also called *sphygmocardioscope*) (*kardia* heart + *graphein* to write) sphygmochronograph (*chronos* time + *graphein* to write) sphygmogram, sphygmograph (*graphein* to write) sphygmomanometer (*manos* thin, scanty + *metron* measure) sphygmometer, sphygmometroscope (*metron* measure + *skopein* to view)

Element	From	Meaning	Examples
sphygm (cont'd)		[pulse, throb]	sphygmooscillometer (*oscillare* to swing + *metron* measure) sphygmopalpation (*palpare* to touch) sphygmophone (*phone* sound) sphygmoscope, sphygmoscopy (*skopein* to examine) sphygmosystole (*systole* a contracting) sphygmotonograph (*tonos* tension + *graphein* to write) sphygmotonometer (*tonos* tension + *metron* measure) TRAILING ROOT COMPOUND: *sphygm*: bradysphygmia (*bradys* slow) *sphyxia*: acroasphyxia (cold, pale condition of hands and feet; also called *acrocyanosis*) (*akron* extremity + *a* privative) CROSS REFERENCE: crot, ict, puls
spin	Latin *spina* spine	spine, back	SIMPLE ROOT: spina (or, spine; a thornlike process or projection: used in anatomical nomenclature as a general term to denote such a process; pl., spinae) {spinal, spinalis, spinate, spinous, spinose} PREFIXED ROOT: *spinal*: epispinal (*epi* upon) infraspinal (below the vertebral column; below the spine; also called *subvertebral, infraspinate, infraspinous*) (*infra* below) interspinal (or, interspinous) (*inter* between) intraspinal (also called *intrarachidian*) (*intra* within) juxtaspinal (also called *paravertebral*) (*juxta* close, nearby) paraspinal (*para* alongside, near) prespinal (*pre* anterior) semispinal (*semi* half) supraspinal (or, supraspinous) (*supra* above) *spinous*: infraspinous (inferior to the spine of the scapula) (*infra* below) interspinous (or, interspinal) (*inter* between) subspinous (*sub* below) supraspinous (or, supraspinal) (*supra* above) LEADING ROOT COMPOUND: *spini*: spinifugal (*fugere* to flee) spinipetal (*petere* to seek) *spino*: spinobulbar (relating to the medulla oblongata and spinal cord; also called *bulbospinal*) spinocellular (*cella* cell) spinocerebellum (also called *paleocerebellum*) (*cerebrum* brain) spinocollicular (also called *spinotectal*) (*collis* hill) spinocostalis (*costa* rib) spinoglenoid (*glene* socket of a joint + *eidos* appearance) spinogram (*graphein* to write) spinomuscular (muscle) spinoneural (*neuron* nerve) spinopetal (*petere* to seek) spinotectal (also called *spinocollicular*) (*tectum* roof) spinothalamic (thalamus) TRAILING ROOT COMPOUND: anospinal (anus) cerebrospinal (*cerebrum* brain) ciliospinal (*cilium* eyelash: ciliary structure or body)

Element	From	Meaning	Examples
spin (cont'd)		[spine, back]	corticospinal (*cortex* rind: outer layer of the brain) craniospinal (*kranion* skull) dorsispinal (*dorsum* back — of body) iliospinal (*ilium*) oculospinal (*oculus* eye) propriospinal (pertaining wholly to the spinal cord) (*propios* one's own) rubrospinal (relating to the nerve fibers passing from the red nucleus to the spinal cord) (*rubrum* red) sacrospinal (or, sacrospinous) (*sacrum*) tectospinal (extending from the tectum of the midbrain to the spinal cord) (*tectum* rooflike structure) vesicospinal (pertaining to the urinary bladder and the spinal cord) (*vesica* bladder) vestibulospinal (vestibule) CROSS REFERENCE: noto, rachi, spondyl, vertebr
spir	Greek *speira* Latin *spira* coil	turn, wrap, coil, spiral	SIMPLE ROOT: spiral, spirem (or, spireme; the threadlike, continuous or segmented figure formed by the chromosome material during the prophase of mitosis or meiosis; also called *skein*) spirillum (a relatively rigid, spiral-shaped bacterium; pl., spirilla) PREFIXED ROOT: dispireme (the stage of cell division which follows the diaster; so called because the protoplasm is divided into two parts) (*di* two) LEADING ROOT COMPOUND: *spir*: spiradenoma (*adenos* gland + *oma* tumor) spiroid (*eidos* form) *spirill*: spirillosis (*osis* condition) *spirilli*: spirillicide (*caedere* to kill) *spirillo*: spirillotropic (having an affinity for spirilla), spirillotropism (*tropein* to turn) *spiro*: spirochete, spirochetemia (presence of spirochetes in the blood) (*chaite* hair + *emia* blood condition) TRAILING ROOT COMPOUND: fusospirillary (*fusus* spindle) sinospiral (sinus) CROSS REFERENCE: cochl, cycl, helix, rhomb, trop
splanchn	Greek *splanchnos*	viscus (any of the internal organs of the body)	SIMPLE ROOT: splanchnic (pertaining to the viscera) PREFIXED ROOT: eusplanchnia (a normal condition of the internal organs) (*eu* well) macrosplanchnic (also called *megalosplanchnic*) (*makros* large) microsplanchnic (*mikros* small) perisplanchnic, perisplanchnitis (also called *perivisceritis*) (*peri* around + *itis* inflammation) trisplanchnic (relating to the three visceral cavities: skull, thorax, and abdomen) (*tri* three) LEADING ROOT COMPOUND: *splanchn*: splanchnapophysis (*apophysis* offshoot) splanchnectopia (also called *splanchnodiastasis*) (*ektopia* displaced) splanchnesthesia {splanchnesthetic} (*esthesia* feeling) *splanchnic*: splanchnicectomy (*ektome* excision) *splanchnico*: splanchnicotomy (*tomy* incision)

A Thesaurus of Medical Word Roots

Element	From	Meaning	Examples
splanchn (cont'd)		[viscus]	*splanchno*: splanchnocele (*kele* hernia; *koilos* hollow) [two meanings] splanchnocoele (*koilia* cavity) splanchnocranium (also called *viscerocranium*) (*kranion* skull) splanchnoderm (also called *splanchnopleure*) (*derma* skin) splanchnodiastasis (also called *splanchnectopia*) (*diastasis* separation, displacement) splanchnography (*graphein* to write) splanchnolith (*lithos* stone) splanchnology (*logos* study) splanchnomegaly (also called *visceromegaly*) (*megalos* large) splanchnomicria (*mikros* small) splanchnopathy (*pathos* disease) splanchnopleure {splanchnopleural, splanchnopleuric} (*pleura* side) splanchnoptosis (or, splanchnoptosia; also called *visceroptosis*) (*ptosis* prolapse: a falling) splanchnosclerosis (*sklerosis* hardening, induration) splanchnoscopy (*skopein* to examine) splanchnoskeletal (also called *visceroskeletal*) splanchnosomatic (also called *viscerosomatic*) (*somatos* body) splanchnotomy (*tomy* incision) splanchnotribe (*tribein* to crush) TRAILING ROOT COMPOUND: *splanchnia*: perosplanchnia (*pero* maimed) *splanchnic*: neurosplanchnic (pertaining to the cerebrospinal and sympathetic nervous systems) (*neuron* nerve) parietosplanchnic (also called *parietovisceral*) (*paries* wall) somaticosplanchnic (also called *somaticovisceral*) (*soma* the body) CROSS REFERENCE: enter, ventr, visc
splen, spleen	Greek *splen, splenos*	spleen	SIMPLE ROOT: *spleen*: spleen (a large, ductless organ situated in the upper part of the abdominal cavity) *splen*: splen {splenic, splenetic; also called *lienal*}, spleneolus, splenial, splenulus (or, splenunculus; also called *lienculus*; an accessory or rudimentary spleen; splenic exclave; pl., splenuli) PREFIXED ROOT: *splen*: autosplenectomy (almost complete disappearance of the spleen due to progressive fibrosis and shrinkage) (*autos* self + *ektome* excision) *splenia*: asplenia (*a* privative) eusplenia (*eu* good, well) hypersplenia (*hyper* over, above) megalosplenia (also called *splenomegaly*) (*megalos* large) microsplenia {microsplenic} (*mikros* small) polysplenia (*polys* many) *splenic*: asplenic (*a* privative) infrasplenic (*infra* below) intrasplenic (*intra* within) parasplenic (*para* beside) perisplenic (*peri* around) postsplenic (*post* posterior)

A Thesaurus of Medical Word Roots

Element	From	Meaning	Examples
splen (cont'd)		[spleen]	*splenism*:

hypersplenism (*hyper* above)
hyposplenism (*hypo* under)
splenitis inflammation of the spleen:
episplenitis (inflammation of the capsule of the spleen) (*epi* upon)
perisplenitis (*peri* around, near)
LEADING ROOT COMPOUND:
splen:
splenalgia (also called *splenodynia*) (*algos* pain)
splenatrophy (atrophy: *a* negative + *trephein* to nourish)
splenauxe (also called *splenomegaly*) (*auxein* to increase)
splenceratosis (induration of the spleen) (*keras* horn + *osis* condi-
    tion)
splenectasis (also called *splenomegaly*) (*ektasis* dilatation)
splenectomy (*ektome* excision)
splenectopia, splenectopy (*ektopia* displaced)
splenelcosis (*helkos* ulcer + *osis* condition) [h of helkos elided]
splenemia (*emia* blood condition)
splenemphraxis (*emphraxis* obstruction)
splenicterus (*ikteros* jaundice)
splenitis (*itis* inflammation)
splenodynia (also called *splenalgia*) (*odyne* pain)
splenoid (also called *spleniform*) (*eidos* form)
splenoma (also called *splenoncus*) (*oma* tumor)
splenoncus (also called *splenoma*) (*onkos* mass, tumor)
splenosis (*osis* condition)
spleni:
spleniserrate (pertaining to the splenius and the serratus muscles)
spleniform (also called *splenoid*) (*forma* shape)
spleno:
splenoblast (*blastos* bud, shoot, germ)
splenocele (*kele* hernia)
splenoceratosis (or, splenokeratosis) (*keratosis* hardening)
splenocleisis (inducing the formation of new fibrous tissue on the
    surface of the spleen by friction or wrapping with gauze) (*kleisis*
    closure)
splenocolic (*kolon* colon)
splenogenous (*genere* to produce)
splenogram, splenography (*graphein* to write)
splenohepatomegalia (*hepatos* liver + *megalos* large)
splenokeratosis (or, splenoceratosis) (*keratosis* horny condition)
splenolaparotomy (also called *laparosplenotomy*) (*lapara* flank +
    tomy incision)
splenolymphatic (pertaining to the spleen and lymph nodes)
splenolysin, splenolysis (*lysis* destruction)
splenomalacia (*malakos* soft)
splenomedullary (*medulla* marrow)
splenomegaly (also called *splenauxe*) (*megas* large)
splenometry (*metron* measure)
splenomyelogenous (*myelos* marrow + *genere* to produce)
splenomyelomalacia (*myelos* marrow + *malakos* soft)
splenonephric (also called *splenorenal*) (*nephros* kidney)
splenonephroptosis (downward displacement of the spleen and kid-
    ney on the same side) (*nephros* kidney + *ptosis* a falling)

Element	From	Meaning	Examples
splen (cont'd)		[spleen]	splenopancreatic (pancreas)
			splenopathy (*pathos* disease)
			splenopexy (or, splenopexia) (*pexy* fixation)
			splenophrenic (*phren* diaphragm)
			splenoptosia (or, splenoptosis) (*ptosis* a falling)
			splenorenal (also called *splenoneprhic*) (*ren* kidney)
			splenorrhagia (*rhagia* bursting forth)
			splenorrhaphy (*rhaphe* suture)
			splenotomy (*tomy* incision)
			splenotoxin (*toxin* poison)
			TRAILING ROOT COMPOUND:
			gastrosplenic (*gaster* stomach, belly)
			hepatosplenitis (*hepatos* liver + *itis* inflammation)
			phrenosplenic (*phren* diaphragm)
			NB: *Splenium*, from Greek *splenion*, bandage, is not related to this family. It is not otherwise listed.
			CROSS REFERENCE: lien
spondyl	Greek *spondylos*	vertebra (spinal column)	SIMPLE ROOT: spondylous (pertaining to a vertebra; vertebral)
			PREFIXED ROOT:
			dysspondylism (abnormal development of the spine) (*dys* abnormal)
			perispondylic, perispondylitis (*peri* around + *itis* inflammation)
			polydysspondylism (*polys* many + dysspondylism)
			prespondylolisthesis (*pre* before + *olisthesis* slipping)
			retrospondylolisthesis (*retro* backward + *olisthesis* slipping)
			LEADING ROOT COMPOUND:
			spondyl:
			spondylalgia (also called *spondylodynia*) (*algos* pain)
			spondylarthritis (*arthron* joint + *itis* inflammation)
			spondylarthrocace (tuberculosis of the vertebrae) (*arthron* joint + *kakos* bad)
			spondylarthropathy (*arthron* joint + *pathos* disease)
			spondylexarthrosis (*exarthrosis* joint dislocation)
			spondylitis (also called *rachitis*) {spondylitic} (*itis* inflammation)
			spondylizema (*izemia* depression)
			spondylodynia (also called *spondylalgia*) (*odyne* pain)
			spondylolisthesis {spondylolisthetic} (*olisthanein* to slip)
			spondylosis {spondylotic} (*osis* condition)
			spondylo:
			spondyloarthropathy (*arthron* joint + *pathos* disease)
			spondylocace (tuberculosis of the vertebrae) (*kakos* bad)
			spondylodidymia (*didymos* twin)
			spondylolysis (*lysis* loosening)
			spondylomalacia (*malakos* soft)
			spondylopathy (also called *rachiopathy*) (*pathos* disease)
			spondyloptosis (also called *spondylolithesis*) (*ptosis* a falling)
			spondylopyosis (*pyosis* suppuration)
			spondyloschisis (embryologic failure of fusion of the vertebral arch) also called *rachischisis*) (*schisis* fissure)
			spondylosyndesis (spinal fusion) (*syn* together + *desis* binding)
			spondylothoracic (thorax)
			spondylotomy (*tomy* incision)
			TRAILING ROOT COMPOUND: platyspondylia (or, platyspondylisis; flatness of the vertebral bodies) (*platys* broad, flat)
			CROSS REFERENCE: atlanto, rachi, spin, vertebr

Element	From	Meaning	Examples
spor	Greek *speirein* to sow, strew *sporos* seed	seed, spore	SIMPLE ROOT: sporadic (occurring occasionally or in scattered instances, as a disease) sporation (also called *sporulation*), spore sporidium (pl., sporidia), sporulation (also called *sporation*, *sporogenesis*, *sporogeny*, *sporogony*), sporule (a small spore) sporulate (to produce or release spores) PREFIXED ROOT: *sporangium* seed vessel: microsporangium (*mikros* small) megasporangium (*mega* large) *spore*: adiaspore (*a* negative + *dia* through) anisospore (*aniso* unequal; *an* negative + *isos* equal) archespore (or, archesporium) (*archein* to begin) bispore (also called *dispore*) (Latin *bi* two; Greek *di* two) endospore (*endon* within) exospore (*exo* outside) heterospore {heterosporous} (*heteros* different, other) hemispore (*hemi* half) homospore {homosporous} (*homos* same) isospore {isosporous} (*isos* equal) macrospore (also called *megaspore*) (*makros* large, long) megalospore (also called *macrospore*) (*megalos* large) megaspore (also called *macrospore*) (*mega* large) microspore (*mikros* small) protospore (*protos* first) *sporium*: endosporium (*endon* within) exosporium (*exo* outside) *sporoblast*: pansporoblast (*pan* all + *blastos* germ, sprout) *sporogenic*: asporogenic (*a* negative + *genere* to produce) *sporous*: asporous (*a* privative) disporous (*di* two) *sporulate*: asporulate (*a* privative) LEADING ROOT COMPOUND: *spor*: sporangium (pl., sporangia) {sporangial}, sporangiophore (*angeion* vessel + *phorein* to bear) sporangiospore (a spore contained in a sporangium) sporont (*ontos* being) *spori*: sporicide {sporicidal} (*caedere* to cut, kill) sporiferous (also called *sporiparous*) (*ferre* to bear) sporiparous (also called *sporiferous*) (*parere* to bear, produce) *sporo*: sporoblast (*blastos* bud, shoot, germ) sporocyst (*kystis* cyst, sac) sporoduct (*ducere* to lead) sporogenesis {sporogenic, sporogenous} (*genere* to produce) sporogony (also called *sporogenesis*, *sporogeny*) (*gone* seed) sporophore (*phorein* to carry) sporophyte (*phyton* plant: growth)

Element	From	Meaning	Examples
spor (cont'd)		[seed]	sporoplasm {sporoplasmic} (*plassein* to form) sporotheca (*theke* case) sporotrichosis {sporotrichotic} (*trichos* hair + *osis* condition) sporozoan, sporozoite (*zoon* animal) TRAILING ROOT COMPOUND: *sporangium*: merosporangium (*meros* part + *angeion* vessel) *spore*: arthrospore (*arthron* joint) ascospore (*askos* bag) basidiospore (*basidium* base) blastospore (also called *blastoconidium*) (*blastos* shoot, bud) chlamydospore (*chlamys* cloak) gymnospore (*gymnos* naked) oospore (*oon* egg, ovum) zygospore (*zygon* yoke) CROSS REFERENCE: blast, gon[1], semin, sperm
squam	Latin *squama* scale	scale, plate	SIMPLE ROOT: squama (a scale or platelike structure; pl., squamae) {squamate, squamous} squamatization, squame squamosa (scaly, or platelike; pl., squamosae) {squamosal} PREFIXED ROOT: desquamate, desquamation (shedding of the epidermis) {desquamative, desquamatory} (*de* off) LEADING ROOT COMPOUND: squamocellular (*cella* cell) squamocolumnar (column) squamofrontal (pertaining to the squamous part of the frontal bone, or *squama frontalis*) squamomastoid (pertaining to the squamous and mastoid portions of the temporal bone) squamo-occipital (pertaining to the *squama occipitalis*) squamoparietal (also called *parietosquamosal*) (*paries* wall) squamopetrosal (pertaining to the squamous and petrous portions of the temporal bone; also called *petrosquamosal*) squamozygomatic (zygomatic process) TRAILING ROOT COMPOUND: parietosquamosal (also called *squamoparietal*) (parietal bone) petrosquamosal (also called *squamopetrosal*) (*petra* stone) sphenosquamosal (*sphenos* wedge) tympanosquamosal (*tympanon* drum: eardrum) CROSS REFERENCE: cort, lam, lep[1], plak
stal, **stol**	Greek *stellein* to send *stalsis* contraction	to set, place, send	PREFIXED ROOT: *stalsis*: antiperistalsis (*anti* against + peristalsis) catastalsis {catastaltic} (*kata* down) diastalsis (a wave of inhibition before a downward contraction in the intestine) {diastaltic} (*dia* apart) hypoperistalsis (abnormally sluggish peristalsis) (*hypo* under) peristalsis (the movement by which the alimentary canal and other tubular organs propel their contents) {peristaltic} (*peri* around) retrostalsis (*retro* backward) *staltic*: anastaltic (highly astringent; styptic) (*ana* again) systaltic (lit., drawing together; alternating contracting and expanding, as the action of the heart; pulsating) (*syn* with)

Element	From	Meaning	Examples
stal (cont'd)		[to set, place]	*stole*:
			diastole (*dia* across) [see separate entry: diastol-]
			peristole {peristolic} (*peri* around)
			systole {systolic} (*syn* with) [see separate entry: systol-]
			stolic: pansystolic (lasting throughout systole, extending from first to second heart sound; also called *holosystolic*) (*pan* all)
			CROSS REFERENCE: spas, stas, stat, thes
staphyl	Greek *staphyle* bunch of grapes	uvula; staphylococci	SIMPLE ROOT:
			staphyline (also called *botryoid*, *uvular*), staphylinus (uvular)
			staphylion (an encephalometric landmark on the posterior edge of the hard palate at the median line)
			PREFIXED ROOT: peristaphyline (*peri* around)
			LEADING ROOT COMPOUND:
			staphyl:
			staphylectomy (also called *uvulectomy*) (*ektome* excision)
			staphyledema (or, staphyloedema) (*edema* swelling)
			staphylitis (also called *uvulitis*) (*itis* inflammation)
			staphyloma {staphylomatous} (*oma* tumor)
			staphyloncus (a tumor or swelling of the uvula) (*onkos* mass, tumor)
			staphylo:
			staphyloangina (a mild form of sore throat) (*anchein* to squeeze)
			staphylococcemia (septicemia caused by staphylococci) (*kokkos* berry: a berry-shaped bacterium + *emia* blood condition)
			staphylococcosis (infection caused by staphylococci) (*kokkos* berry: a berry-shaped bacterium + *osis* condition)
			staphylococcus (pl., staphylococci) {staphylococcal} (*kokkos* berry: a berry-shaped bacterium)
			staphyloderma (pyoderma due to staphylococci) (*derma* skin)
			staphylodialysis (also called *uvuloptosis*) (*dialysis* loosening)
			staphyloedema (or, staphyledema) (*edema* swelling)
			staphylopharyngorrhaphy (pharynx + *rhaphe* suture)
			staphyloplasty (plastic surgery of the uvula and the soft palate) (*plassein* to form)
			staphyloptosia (also called *uvuloptosis*) (*ptein* to fall)
			staphylorrhaphy (also called *palatorrhaphy*) (*rhaphe* suture)
			staphyloschisis (also called *bifid uvula*) (*schisis* fissure)
			staphylotomy (also called *uvulotomy*) (*tomy* incision)
			staphylotoxin (*toxin* poison)
			TRAILING ROOT COMPOUND:
			brachystaphyline (having a short, wide palate) (*brachys* short)
			leptostaphyline (*leptos* narrow)
			mesostaphyline (*mesos* middle, moderate)
			platystaphyline (*platys* flat, broad)
			stylostaphyline (*stilus* stake, pole; styloid process)
			uranostaphyloschisis (*ouraniskos* palate + *schisis* fissure)
			CROSS REFERENCE: uvul
stas, stat, stem	Greek *histanai* to cause to stand	to stand, place; a standing still	SIMPLE ROOT:
			stas: stasis (stagnation of normal flow of fluids, as of the blood, urine, or of the intestinal mechanisms; pl., stases)
			static (at rest; in equilibrium; not in motion), statics
			PREFIXED ROOT:
			stase: diastase (a white, amorphous, soluble enzyme produced during germination of seeds, and contained in malt; converts starch into simple sugars), diastasis (separation) (*dia* apart)

Element	From	Meaning	Examples
stas (cont'd)		[to stand]	*stasia*:

astasia (difficulty in standing because of muscular incoordination) {astatic} (*a* privative)

dysstasia (or, dystasia; difficulty in standing) {dysstatic} (*dys* abnormal)

stasis:

apostasis (the end or crisis of an attack of disease) (*apo* from)

catastasis (a condition or state; restoration to a normal condition or a normal place) (*kata* down)

epistasis (or, epistasy; suppression of a secretion, as of blood, menses, or lochia; scum on the surface of urine) {epistatic} (*epi* upon)

homeostasis {homeostatic} (*homoios* like, resembling)

hypostasis {hypostatic} (*hypo* under)

metastasis {metastatic} (*meta* after)

parastasis (*para* alongside)

peristasis (also called *peristatic hyperemia*) (*peri* around)

state: prostate (*pro* before) [see separate entry: prostat-]

stem:

diastema (an interval; pl., diastemata) (*dia* apart)

epistemology (the science of the methods and validity of knowledge) (*epi* upon + *logos* study)

system (or, systema; a complex or organized whole) {systemic}

systematic, systemoid (*syn* with + *eidos* resemblance)

LEADING ROOT COMPOUND:

stasi: stasimorphy (deformity or abnormality of shape in any organ, due to arrest of development; a type of dysmorphogenesis) (*morphe* form)

stato:

statoacoustic (pertaining to balance and hearing)

statoconium (also called *otoconium, statolith*; pl., statoconia) (*konis* dust)

statocyst (*kystis* bladder)

statoliths (also called *otoliths*) (*lithos* stone)

statometer (also called *exophthalometer*) (*metron* measure)

statosphere (also called *centrosphere*) (*sphaira* ball)

TRAILING ROOT COMPOUND:

stasis:

bacteriostasis (*bakterion* rod-shaped organism)

brachystasis (*brachys* short)

cholestasis (*chole* bile)

coprostasis (impaction of the feces in the intestine) (*kopros* feces)

cytostasis (*kytos* cell)

fungistasis (also called *mycostasis*) (fungus)

galactostasis (cessation of *lactation*) (*galaktos* milk)

hemostasis (or, hemostasia) (*haima* blood)

karyostasis (*karyon* nut, kernel: nucleus)

laryngostasis (commonly known as *croup*) (larynx)

leukostasis (*leukos* white: white blood cells)

lochiostasis (*lochia* vaginal discharge)

lymphostasis (*lymph* water, liquid)

menostasis (suppression of the menses; cessation of menstruation; also called *menopause*) (*mene* month: menstruation)

metrostasis (*metra* uterus)

mycostasis (also called *fungistasis*) (*mykes* fungus)

Element	From	Meaning	Examples
stas (cont'd)		[to stand]	orthostasis (also called *postural hypotension*) (*orthos* straight)
			phlebostasis (also called *venous stasis*) (*phlebos* vein)
			poikilostasis (*poikilos* varied, mottled)
			presbyastasis (*presbys* old age + *a* privation)
			proctostasis (*proktos* anus, rectum)
			thrombostasis (*thrombos* clot)
			stat:
			blepharostat (*blepharos* eyelid)
			cephalostat (*kephale* head)
			cryostat (*kryos* cold)
			fungistat (also called *mycostat*) (fungus)
			gnathostat (*gnathos* jaw)
			hemostat (*haima* blood)
			melanostatin (inhibits synthesis and release of melanotropin; also called *melanotropin release-inhibiting hormone*) (*melanos* dark)
			mycostat (also called *fungistat*) (*mykes* fungus)
			rheostat (an appliance for regulating the resistance and thus controlling the amount of current entering an electric circuit) (*rheos* flow)
			thermostat (*therme* heat)
			static:
			cytostatic (*kytos* cell)
			glycostatic (*glykys* sugar)
			hemostatic (*haima* blood)
			orthostatic (*orthos* straight)
			pyostatic (*pyon* pus)
			virostatic (*virus* poison)
			CROSS REFERENCE: stal, thes
stear, **steat**	Greek *stear,* *steatos* tallow	fat, tallow	SIMPLE ROOT: stearate, stearin (also called *tristearin*)
			PREFIXED ROOT:
			asteatosis (scantiness or absence of the sebaceous secretion) (*a* privative + *osis* condition)
			hypersteatosis (*hyper* above + *osis* condition)
			hyposteatolysis (*hypo* under + *lysis* loosening)
			LEADING ROOT COMPOUND:
			steari: steariform (fatlike) (*forma* shape)
			stearo: stearopten (*ptenos* volatile)
			steat:
			steatitis (inflammation of adipose tissue) (*itis* inflammation)
			steatoma, steatomatosis (*oma* tumor + *osis* condition)
			steatosis (also called *adiposis, fatty degeneration*) (*osis* condition)
			steato:
			steatocele (a fatty mass formed within the scrotum) (*kele* tumor)
			steatocystoma (*kystis* sac + *oma* tumor)
			steatogenesis {steatogenous} (*genere* to produce)
			steatohepatitis (*hepatos* liver + *itis* inflammation)
			steatolysis (lipolysis) {steatolytic} (*lyein* to loosen)
			steatomery (*meros* thigh)
			steatonecrosis (also called *fat necrosis*) (*nekrosis* deadness)
			steatopyga (or, steatopygia) {steatopygous} (*pyge* buttocks)
			steatorrhea (also called *stearrhea*) (*rhein* to run)
			steatocystoma (*kystis* sac + *oma* tumor)
			TRAILING ROOT COMPOUND: cholesteatosis (fatty deposits of cholesterol esters in a tissue) (*chole* bile + *osis* condition)
			CROSS REFERENCE: adip, ather, lip, pimel

Element	From	Meaning	Examples
sten(o)	Greek *stenos* narrow	narrow, compressed, close, little	PREFIXED ROOT: poststenotic (located or occurring distal to or beyond a stenosed segment) (*post* after) restenosis (recurrent stenosis) (*re* back) LEADING ROOT COMPOUND: *sten*: stenopeic (or, stenopaic; provided with a narrow opening or slit, as in stenopeic spectacles) (*ope* opening) stenosis (a narrowing) {stenosal, stenosed} (*osis* condition) *steno*: stenobregmatic (*bregma* forehead) stenocardia (severe constricting chest pain) (*kardia* heart) stenocephalia (or, stenocephaly) (*kephale* head) stenochoria (abnormal contraction of any canal or orifice) (*chora* place, room) stenocoriasis (*kore* pupil + *iasis* condition) stenocrotaphy (narrowness of the skull in the temporal region; the condition of a stenobregmate skull) (*krotaphos* temple) stenostenosis (stricture of the parotid duct; also called *Steno's duct* or *Stensen's duct*) [fr. Nicolas Steno (1638-86), Danish physician, anatomist in Italy] stenostomia (*stoma* mouth) stenothermal (or, stenothermic) (*therme* heat) stenothorax (*thorax* chest) TRAILING ROOT COMPOUND: *stenosis* a narrowing condition: angiostenosis (*angeion* blood vessel) aortostenosis (also called *aortarctia*) (aorta) arteriostenosis (artery) blepharostenosis (or *blepharophimosis*) (*blepharon* eyelid) bronchiostenosis (or, bronchostenosis) (*bronchos* windpipe) colpostenosis (*kolpos* vagina) craniostenosis (*kranion* skull) dacryostenosis (*dakryon* teardrop: lacrimal duct) enterostenosis (*enteron* intestine) episiostenosis (*epision* pubic region: vulvar orifice) esophagostenosis (esophagus) faciostenosis (*facies* face) gastrostenosis (*gaster* stomach, belly) hemadostenosis (contraction of the arteries) (*haima* blood) laryngostenosis (larynx) metrostenosis (*metra* uterus) pharyngostenosis (pharynx) phlebostenosis (*phlebos* vein) proctostenosis (also called *rectostenosis*) (*proktos* anus, rectum) pyloristenosis (also called *pyloric stenosis*) (pylorus) rectostenosis (also called *proctostenosis*) (rectum) rhinostenosis (also called *rhinocleisis*) (*rhis* nose: nasal passage) sclerostenosis (induration and contraction of the tissues) (*skleros* hard) sialostenosis (*sialon* saliva: salivary duct) tracheostenosis (*trachea* windpipe) ureterostenosis (ureter) urethrostenosis (urethra) CROSS REFERENCE: angin, arct

Element	From	Meaning	Examples
stere	Greek *stereos*	solid	SIMPLE ROOT: stere (a measure of capacity equivalent to a cubic meter or a kilometer)

PREFIXED ROOT:

isostere (*isos* equal)

macrostereognosis (*makros* large + stereognosis)

retrosteroid (*retro* reversed + steroid)

LEADING ROOT COMPOUND:

ster: steroid, steroidal (*eidos* form)

stere: stereopsis (*opsis* vision)

stereo:

stereoagnosis (loss of power to recognize objects or to appreciate their form by touching or feeling them; also called *astereognosis, tactile agnosia*) (*a* negative + *gnosis* knowledge)

stereoanesthesia (also called *astereognosis, tactile agnosia*) (*an* privative + *esthesia* feeling)

stereoarthrolysis (operative formation of a movable new joint in cases of bony ankylosis) (*arthron* joint + *lyein* to loosen)

stereoausculation (*ausculare* to listen)

stereoblastula (a solid blastula, all of whose cells reach the external surface) (*blastos* bud, shoot, germ)

stereocampimeter (an instrument for studying unilateral central scotoma and defects in the central retinal area) (*campus* field + *metron* measure)

stereochemistry {stereochemical}

stereocilium (a non-motile protoplasmic filament on the free surface of a cell) (*cilium* hairlike process)

stereocognosy (also called *stereognosis*) (*gnosis* knowledge)

stereocolpogram, stereocolpography (*kolpos* vagina + *graphein* to write)

stereoencephalometry (*enkephalos* brain + *metron* measure)

stereoencephalotomy (stereotaxic surgery) (*enkephalon* brain + *tomy* incision)

stereognosis (the faculty of perceiving and understanding the form and nature of objects by the sense of touch; perception by the senses of the solidity of objects; also called *stereocognosy*) {stereognostic} (*gnosis* knowledge)

stereogram, stereograph (*graphein* to write)

stereoisomer, stereoisomerism (*isos* equal + *meros* part)

stereology (*logos* study)

stereometer, stereometry (*metron* measure)

stereo-orthopter (*orthos* straight + *optikos* optical)

stereopathy (persistent stereotypical thinking) (*pathos* disorder)

stereophoroscope (*phorein* to bear + *skopein* to examine)

stereoplasm (*plassein* to form)

stereoradiography (radio + *graphein* to write)

stereoradiometry (radio + *metron* measure)

stereosalpingography (*salpingos* tube + *graphein* to write)

stereoscope {stereoscopic}, stereoscopy (*skopein* to examine)

stereoskiagraphy (also called *stereoradiography*) (*skia* shadow + *graphein* to write)

stereotactic (*tactus* touch)

stereotaxis {stereotactic, stereotaxic} (*tassein* to arrange)

stereotropism (also called *thigmotropism*) (*tropism* a turning)

stereotypy (type)

Element	From	Meaning	Examples
stere (cont'd)		[solid]	TRAILING ROOT COMPOUND: androsterone (a steroid hormone reinforcing masculine characteristics) (*andros* man) cholesterol (solid fat which was first isolated in the gall bladder) (*chole* gall + *ol* oil) testosterone (the principal androgenic hormone) (testis) CROSS REFERENCE: None
steres	Greek *sterein* to deprive	privation, loss	TRAILING ROOT COMPOUND: glossosteresis (also called *glossectomy*) (*glossa* tongue) halisteresis [or, halosteresis; a loss or lack of lime salts (calcium) of bone; also called *osteomalacia*] {halisteretic} (*hals* salt) iridosteresis (iris, of eye) ophthalmosteresis (*ophthalmos* eye) osteohalisteresis (*osteon* bone + *halos* salt) ovariosteresis (also called *ovariectomy*) (*ovum* egg) thermosteresis (*therme* heat) NB: *Hysteresis*, a time lag in the occurrence of two associated phenomena, is not related to this element, and is not otherwise listed. CROSS REFERENCE: apheres, priv
stern	Greek *sternon*	chest (sternum)	SIMPLE ROOT: sternad (toward the sternum) sternen (pertaining to the sternum alone) sternum (a longitudinal unpaired plate of bone forming the middle of the anterior wall of the thorax; pl., sterna) {sternal} PREFIXED ROOT: *sternal*: adsternal (near or toward the sternum) (*ad* to) infrasternal (also called *substernal*) (*infra* below) intersternal (*inter* between) intrasternal (*intra* within) parasternal (*para* alongside) quartisternal (*quartus* fourth) quintisternal (*quintus* fifth) retrosternal (*retro* behind) substernal (also called *infrasternal*) (*sub* below) suprasternal (*supra* above) transsternal (*trans* through) ultimisternal (pertaining to the xiphoid process) (*ultima* last) *sternation*: prosternation (also called *camptocormia*) (*pro* before) *sternia*: asternia {asternal} (*a* privative) *sternum*: episternum {episternal} (*epi* upon) mesosternum (the corpus sterni; also called *midsternum, body of sternum*) (*mesos* middle) metasternum (also called *xiphoid process*) (*meta* after) midsternum (the body of the breast bone; also called *mesosternum*) presternum (the manubrium; the cranial part of the sternum) (*pre* before) LEADING ROOT COMPOUND: *stern*: sternalgia (also called *sternodynia*) (*algos* pain) sternebra (any one of the segments of the sternum in the embryo) (sternum + vertebrae) sternodynia (also called *sternalgia*) (*odyne* pain)

Element	From	Meaning	Examples
stern (cont'd)		[chest]	sternoid (resembling the breastbone) (*eidos* form) *sterno*: sternoclavicular (also called *sternocleidal*) (*clavicle* collarbone) sternocostal (*costa* rib, side) sternoglossal (*glossa* tongue) sternomastoid [mastoid (breast-shaped) process] sternopagus (also called *thoracopagus*) (*pagos* thing fixed) sternopericardial (pericardium — around the heart) sternoscapular (*scapula* shoulder blade) sternoschisis (also called *cleft sternum*) (*schisis* fissure) sternotomy (*tomy* incision) sternotracheal (*trachea* windpipe) sternotrypesis (*trypesis* trephination — a boring) sternovertebral (*vertebra*) TRAILING ROOT COMPOUND: *sternal*: chondrosternal (*chondros* cartilage) costosternal (*costa* rib) vertebrosternal (*vertebra*) *sternia*: schistosternia (also called *schistothrorax*) (*schistos* split) *sternum*: ensisternum (also called *xiphoid process*) (*ensis* sword) omosternum (*omos* shoulder) pelvisternum (pelvis) xiphisternum {xiphisternal} (*xiphos* sword) CROSS REFERENCE: pect, steth, thora
steth	Greek *stethos*	chest	PREFIXED ROOT: endostethoscope (*endon* within + *skopein* to examine) LEADING ROOT COMPOUND: *steth*: stethacoustic (heard with the stethoscope) (*akouein* to hear) stethalgia (also called *pectoralgia, thoracalgia*) (*algos* pain) stetharteritis (*arteria* artery + *itis* inflammation) *stetho*: stethogoniometer (an apparatus for measuring the curvature of the chest) (*gonia* angle + *metron* measure) stethograph, stethography (*graphein* to write) stethometer (an instrument for measuring the circular dimension or expansion of the chest) (*metron* measure) stethomyitis (or, stethomyositis) (*myos* muscle + *itis* inflammation) stethoparalysis (paralysis of the chest muscles) stethophonometer (*phone* sound + *metron* measure) stethoscope {stethoscopic} (*skopein* to examine) stethospasm (*spasmos* contraction) CROSS REFERENCE: pect, stern, thora
sthen	Greek *sthenos*	strength	SIMPLE ROOT: sthenia (a condition of strength and activity) {sthenic} PREFIXED ROOT: *sthenia*: asthenia (lack of or loss of strength) {asthenic} (*a* privative) [see separate entry: asthen-] eusthenia (*eu* well; normal) hypersthenia {hypersthenic} (*hyper* above) hyposthenia (weakness) {hyposthenic} (*hypo* under)

Element	From	Meaning	Examples
sthen (cont'd)		[strength]	*sthenic*: anisosthenic (of unequal strength: said of paired muscles) (*aniso* unequal: *an* negative + *isos* equal)
			sthenuria urine strength condition:
			hypersthenuria (*hyper* over)
			hyposthenuria (*hypo* under)
			isosthenuria (*isos* equal)
			LEADING ROOT COMPOUND: sthenometer, sthenometry (*metron* measure)
			TRAILING ROOT COMPOUND:
			myosthenometer (*myos* muscle + *metron* measure)
			normosthenuria (*norma* rule + *uria* urine condition)
			zymosthenic (*zyme* yeast)
			CROSS REFERENCE: asthen
stol			See stal- for *diastole*.
stom	Greek *stoma* mouth	mouth, opening, orifice	SIMPLE ROOT: stoma (a mouth, small opening, or a pore; pl., stomas, stomata) {stomal, stomatal}, stomatic, stomion
			PREFIXED ROOT:
			stome:
			peristome (or, peristoma; a groove running from the cytosome in certain protozoa; also called *buccal cavity*) {peristomial} (*peri* around)
			protostome (or, protostoma; also called *blastopore*) (*protos* first)
			stomia:
			astomia (without a mouth or oral aperture) (*a* privative)
			cacostomia (a diseased or gangrenous state of the mouth) (*kakos* bad)
			hypostomia (*hypo* under)
			macrostomia (*makros* large)
			microstomia (*mikros* small)
			stomosis:
			anastomosis (communication between vessels by collateral channels) {anastomotic} (*ana* up + *osis* condition)
			microanastomosis (*mikros* small + anastomosis)
			stomous: astomous (*a* privative)
			LEADING ROOT COMPOUND:
			stom: stomodeum (the oral cavity in the digestive track of an embryo) (*hodos* way) [h of hodos elided]
			stoma:
			stomacace (also called *ulcerative stomatitis*) (*kakos* bad)
			stomatomy (the surgical incision of the ostium uteri) (*tomy* incision) [ostium uteri: the vaginal opening of the uterus]
			stomat:
			stomatalgia (also called *stomatodynia*) (*algos* pain)
			stomatitis (pl., stomatitides) (*itis* inflammation)
			stomatodynia (also called *stomatalgia*) (*odyne* pain)
			stomatosis (also called *stomatopathy*) (*osis* condition)
			stomato:
			stomatocace (also called *ulcerative stomatitis*) (*kakos* bad)
			stomatocyte, stomatocytosis (*kytos* cell + *osis* condition)
			stomatodysodia (also called *halitosis*) (*dysodia* bad odor)
			stomatogenesis (*genesis* beginning)
			stomatoglossitis (*glossa* tongue + *itis* inflammation)
			stomatognathic (*gnathos* jaw)
			stomatography (*graphein* to write)

Element	From	Meaning	Examples
stom (cont'd)		[mouth]	stomatolalia (also called *hyponasality*) (*lalein* to speak)
			stomatology {stomatologic} (*logos* study)
			stomatomalacia (*malakos* soft)
			stomatomenia (*mene* menses)
			stomatomycosis (*mykes* fungus + *osis* condition)
			stomatonecrosis (also called *noma*, a spreading sore) (*nekrosis* death)
			stomatopathy (also called *stomatosis*) (*pathos* disease)
			stomatoplasty {stomatoplastic} (*plassein* to form)
			stomatorrhagia (*rhagia* bursting forth)
			stomatoschisis (or, stomoschisis; also called *cleft lip*) (*schisis* fissure)
			stomatoscope (*skopein* to examine)
			stomo:
			stomocephalus (a fetus with rudimentary head and jaws so that the skin hangs in folds about the mouth) (*kephale* head)
			stomoschisis (also called *cleft lip*) (*schisis* fissure)
			TRAILING ROOT COMPOUND:
			stoma: pseudostoma (*pseudes* false)
			stomatitis: pyostomatitis (*pyon* pus + *itis* inflammation)
			stome: archistome (blastopore) (*archein* to be first)
			stomia:
			ozostomia (bad breath; halitosis) (*oze* stench)
			stenostomia (*stenos* narrow)
			xerostomia (*xeros* dry)
			stomy:
			angiostomy (*angeion* blood vessel)
			antrostomy (*antrum* cavity)
			arthrostomy (*arthron* joint)
			bronchostomy (*bronchos* windpipe)
			cecostomy (*cecum* blind gut)
			cerebrostomy (*cerebrum* brain)
			colostomy (*kolon* colon)
			cystostomy (also called *vesicostomy*) (*kystis* bladder)
			enterostomy (*enteron* intestine)
			esophagogastrostomy (esophagus + *gaster* stomach, belly)
			ganglionostomy (*ganglion* knot)
			gastroenterostomy (*gaster* stomach, belly + *enteron* intestine)
			hepatostomy (*hepatos* liver)
			jejunostomy (*jejunus* empty: a part of the small intestine)
			lipostomy (*leipein* to fail) [The first element is *not* from *lipos* fat.]
			myringotomy (also called *tympanostomy*) (*myringos* membrane)
			neocystostomy, neostomy (*neos* new + *kystis* bladder)
			nephrostomy (*nephros* kidney)
			oophorostomy (*oophoros* egg-bearer)
			pericardiostomy (pericardium)
			pharyngostomy (pharynx)
			proctostomy (*proktos* anus, rectum)
			pyelostomy (*pyelos* pelvis)
			pylorostomy (pylorus)
			rectostomy (rectum)
			sclerostomy (surgical perforation of the sclera, as for the relief of glaucoma) (*skleros* hard)
			septostomy (*septum* partition)
			tracheostomy (*trachea* windpipe)
			tympanostomy (also called *myringotomy*) (*tympanon* eardrum)

A Thesaurus of Medical Word Roots

Element	From	Meaning	Examples
stom (cont'd)		[mouth]	ureterostomy (ureter) urethrostomy (urethra) vasostomy (also called *vasotomy*) (*vas* vessel) vesicostomy (also called *cystostomy*) (*vesica* bladder) PREFIXED TRAILING ROOT COMPOUND: aglossostomia (congenital absence of the tongue and mouth opening) (*a* privative + *glossa* tongue) CROSS REFERENCE: for, or, pyl
stomach	Greek *stomachos* gullet, stomach from *stoma* mouth	stomach	SIMPLE ROOT: stomach (the musculomembranous expansion of the alimentary canal; also called *gaster*) {stomachal; also called *gastric*) stomachic (pertaining to the stomach; a medicine which promotes the functional activity of the stomach; also called *gastric*) LEADING ROOT COMPOUND: stomachalgia (also called *stomachodynia, gastrodynia*) (*algos* pain) stomachodynia (also called *stomachalgia, gastrodynia*) (*odyne* pain) CROSS REFERENCE: gast(r), ventr
streph			See stroph-.
strob			See stroph- for *strobila*.
stroph, streph, strept, strob	Greek *strephein*	to twist	SIMPLE ROOT: strobila (pl., strobilae) PREFIXED ROOT: diastrophic (bent or curved), diastrophism (*dia* across, through) enstrophe (inversion; a turning inward, especially of the eyelids; also called *entropion, blepharelosis, trichoma*) (*en* in) epistropheus (the pivot; the second cervical vertebra) (*epi* upon) exstrophy (or, extrophe; the turning inside out of an organ) (*ex* out) LEADING ROOT COMPOUND: *streph*: strephenopodia (talipes varus) (*en* in + *pous* foot) strephexopodia (talipes valgus) (*exo* outside + *pous* foot) *strepho*: strephopodia (talipes equinus) (*pous* foot) strephosymbolia (a disorder of perception in which objects—symbols—seem reversed, as in a mirror) *strepsi*: strepsinema (the threads of chromatin in the strepsitene stage) (*nema* thread) *streptic*: strepticemia (streptococci present in the blood, causing infection; also called *streptococcemia*) (*emia* blood condition) *strepto*: streptobacillus (pl., streptobacilli) (*bacillus* rod) streptococcemia (*kokko* berry + *emia* blood condition) streptomycin (*mykes* fungus) *strobil*: strobiloid (*eidos* form, resemblance) *strobilo*: strobilocercus (*kerkos* tail) *strobo*: stroboscopy {stroboscopic} (*skopein* to examine) *stropho*: strophocephaly (*kephale* head) strophosomia, strophosomus (*soma* body) CROSS REFERENCE: torq
styl	Greek *stylos* pillar	pillar the styloid process of the temporal bone	SIMPLE ROOT: stylet (or, stylette; a wire run through a catheter to render it stiff or to remove debris from its lumen) See Appendix B for examples of words with this initial combining form. Others are placed with the roots to which it is attached. CROSS REFERENCE: None

Element	From	Meaning	Examples
sub-	Latin prefix	under, below	See Appendix B for examples of words with this prefix. Others are listed with the root to which it is attached. CROSS REFERENCE: hypo-, infra-
sud	Latin *sudare*	to perspire, sweat	SIMPLE ROOT: sudamen (pl., sudamina) {sudaminal}, sudation (perspiration) sudor (perspiration), sudoresis (also called *diaphoresis*) PREFIXED ROOT: antisudoral (or, antisudorific) (*anti* against + *facere* to make) exudate {exudative}, exude (*ex* out) [s is elided because of x sound] insudate (*in* in) transudate {transudation}, transude (*trans* across) LEADING ROOT COMPOUND: *sudo*: sudogram (*graphein* to write) sudomotor (*motor* mover) sudorrhea (also called *hyperhidrosis*) (*rhein* to flow) *sudor*: sudoresis (profuse sweating) (*esis* condition) *sudori*: sudoriferous (carrying or producing sweat) (*ferre* to bear) sudorific (causing sweat) (*facere* to make) sudoriparous (*parere* to bear) *sudoro*: sudorometer (*metron* measure) CROSS REFERENCE: hidr
super-, supra-	Latin prefix	above, beyond, extreme	See Appendix B for examples of words with these prefixes. Others are listed with the root to which they are attached. CROSS REFERENCE: extra-, ultra-
surgery			See chir-.
sympath	Greek *sym* with + *pathos* feeling, disease	sympathy	SIMPLE ROOT: sympathism (suggestibility), sympathy {sympathetic, sympathic}, sympathizer PREFIXED ROOT: antisympathetic (also called *sympatholytic*) (*anti* against) parasympathetic (*para* alongside) LEADING ROOT COMPOUND: *sympath*: sympathectomy (or, sympath<u>e</u>tectomy, sympath<u>i</u>cectomy), sympathectomize (*ektome* excision) *sympathetico*: sympatheticomimetic (*mimetic* simulation, mimicking) sympatheticotonia {sympathicotonic} (*tonos* tone) *sympatheto*: sympathetoblast (*blastos* bud, shoot, germ) *sympathico*: sympathicoblast (or, sympathoblast) (*blastos* bud, shoot, germ) sympathiconeuritis (*neuron* nerve + *itis* inflammation) sympathicopathy (*pathos* suffering) sympathicotonia {sympathicotonic} (*tonos* tone) sympathicotripsy (*tribein* to crush) sympathicotropic (*tropein* to turn) *sympatho*: sympathoadrenal (adrenal glands) sympathoblast (or, sympathicoblast) (*blastos* bud, shoot, germ) sympathogonia (*gone* seed) sympatholysis {sympatholytic} (*lyein* to dissolve) sympathomimetic (producing physiological effects mimicking those caused by the action of the sympathetic nervous system) CROSS REFERENCE: esthes, path

Element	From	Meaning	Examples
syn-	Greek prefix	together, with	See Appendix B for examples of words with this prefix. Others are listed with the root to which it is attached. CROSS REFERENCE: com-
syndes	Greek *syn* with + *dein* to bind	a binding together; ligament	SIMPLE ROOT: syndesis (condition of being bound together; also called *arthrodesis, synapsis*) PREFIXED ROOT: asyndesis (a pattern of language in which words and phrases are juxtaposed without grammatical linkage; seen in schizophrenic and other mental disorders) (*a* negative) metasyndesis (also called *metasynapsis*) (*meta* after) parasyndesis (also called *parasynapsis*) (*para* alongside) LEADING ROOT COMPOUND: *syndesm*: syndesmectomy (*ektome* excision) syndesmectopia (*ektopos* out of place) syndesmitis (*itis* inflammation) syndesmo-odontoid (*odontos* tooth + *eidos* form) syndesmosis {syndesmotic} (*osis* condition) *syndesmo*: syndesmochorial (*chorion* membrane) syndesmography (*graphein* to write) syndesmology (also called *arthrology*) (*logos* study) syndesmo-odontoid (*odontos* tooth + *eidos* form) syndesmopexy (*pexis* fixation) syndesmophyte (*phyton* plant: excrescence, growth) syndesmoplasty (*plassein* to form) syndesmorrhaphy (*rhaphe* suture) syndesmotomy (the dissection or cutting of a ligament) (*tomy* incision) TRAILING ROOT COMPOUND: spondylosyndesis (also called *spinal fusion*) (*spondylos* vertebra) CROSS REFERENCE: desm, lig
synov	Greek *syn* with + *oon* egg	synovia; synovial membrane	SIMPLE ROOT: synovia (a transparent, colorless, viscid, lubricating fluid resembling the white of an egg, secreted by the synovial membrane, and contained in joint cavities, bursae, and tendon sheaths; also called *synovial fluid*) {synovial, synovialis}, synovin, synovium PREFIXED ROOT: asynovia (deficiency of the synovial secretion) (*a* privative) intrasynovial (*intra* within) parasynovitis (*para* alongside + *itis* inflammation) perisynovial (*peri* around) polysynovitis (*polys* many + *itis* inflammation) LEADING ROOT COMPOUND: *synov*: synovectomy (*ektome* excision) synovitis (*itis* inflammation) *synovi*: synovianalysis (the laboratory examination of joint fluid, or synovia) synovioma (or, synovialoma; a tumor arising from synovial membranes) (*oma* tumor) synoviorthesis (irradiation of the synovium to destroy inflamed synovial tissue) (*orthos* straight)

A Thesaurus of Medical Word Roots

Element	From	Meaning	Examples
synov (cont'd)		[synovia]	synoviparous (*parere* to produce) *synovio*: synovioblast (a fibroblast of synovial membrane origin) (*blastos* bud, germ, shoot) synoviocyte (*kytos* cell) synoviosarcoma (*sarkos* flesh + *oma* tumor) TRAILING ROOT COMPOUND: *synovial*: meniscosynovial (pertaining to a meniscus and the synovial membrane) serosynovial (both serous and synovial) *synovitis*: tendosynovitis (also called *tenosynovitis*) (tendon + *itis* inflammation) CROSS REFERENCE: None
syphil	Greek *Syphilis* a shepherd having the disease in a Latin poem	infectious venereal disease	SIMPLE ROOT: syphilid (or, syphilide; a general term for the skin lesions of secondary syphilis, appearing in a series of lesions lasting a few days to a few months; also called *syphiloderm, syphiloderma*) syphilis (a subacute to chronic infectious disease usually transmitted by sexual contact) {syphilitic; also called *luetic*} PREFIXED ROOT: mesosyphilis (the second stage of syphilis) (*mesos* middle) metasyphilis (also called *parasyphilis*) (*meta* after) parasyphilis (also called *metasyphilis*) (*para* alongside) LEADING ROOT COMPOUND: *syphil*: syphilemia (*emia* blood condition) syphiloid (resembling syphilis) (*eidos* form) syphiloma (also called *gumma*) (*oma* tumor) *syphili*: syphilimetry (*metron* measure) *syphilo*: syphiloderm (or, syphiloderma) (*derma* skin) syphilology (*logos* study) syphilomania (also called *syphilophobia*) (*mania* madness) syphilophobia (also called *syphilomania*) (*phobia* fear) syphilophyma (any growth or excrescence due to syphilis) (*phyma* growth) TRAILING ROOT COMPOUND: neurosyphilis (*neuron* nerve) CROSS REFERENCE: None
syring, **syrinx**	Greek *syrinx,* *syringos* pipe	pipe, duct, tube, fistula	SIMPLE ROOT: syringe (an instrument for injecting or withdrawing fluids) syrinx (an abnormal cavity in the spinal cord in syringomyelia) {syringeal} PREFIXED ROOT: microsyringe (*mikros* small) perisyringitis (inflammation of tissues around ducts of the sweat glands) (*peri* around + *itis* inflammation) LEADING ROOT COMPOUND *syring*: syringadenoma (or, syringoadenoma; also called *syringocystadenoma*) (*aden* gland + *oma* tumor) syringadenosus (relating to the sweat glands) (*aden* gland) syringectomy (the excision of the walls of a fistula) (*ektome* excision)

Element	From	Meaning	Examples
syring (cont'd)		[pipe, duct]	syringitis (inflammation of the auditory or eustachian tube) (*itis* inflammation) syringoid (*eidos* form, resemblance) syringoma (adenoma of the sweat glands) (*oma* tumor) *syringo*: syringoacanthoma (*akantha* spine, thorn + *oma* tumor) syringoadenoma (*aden* gland + *oma* tumor) syringobulbia (*bulbus* bulb) syringocarcinoma (carcinoma of a sweat gland) CROSS REFERENCE: fistul, salping, tub[1]
systol	Greek *sys* together + *stellein* to set up, order	to draw together; contraction	SIMPLE ROOT: systole (that part of the heart cycle in which the heart is in contraction) {systolic} PREFIXED ROOT: *systole*: asystole (absence of the heartbeat) (*a* privative) eusystole (a normal state of the systole of the heart) (*eu* well) hyposystole (*hypo* under) parasystole (*para* alongside) perisystole (the period preceding the systole in the cardiac rhythm; also called *presystole*) (*peri* around) presystole (also called *perisystole*) (*pre* before) tachysystole (*tachys* rapid) *systolic*: eusystolic (*eu* well) extrasystolic (*extra* outside) holosystolic (also called *pansystolic*) (*holos* entire) pansystolic (lasting throughout systole, extending from first to second heart sound; also called *holosystolic*) (*pan* all) mesosystolic (*mesos* middle) perisystolic (*peri* around) presystolic (*pre* before) CROSS REFERENCE: distol, peristol, sphinct

$\mathcal{T}$

Element	From	Meaning	Examples
tach	Greek *tachys* swift	speed; swift, rapid	See Appendix B for examples of words with this initial combining form. Others are listed with the roots to which it is attached. CROSS REFERENCE: None
tact			See tax- for *atactic*.
tal	Latin *talus*	ankle	SIMPLE ROOT: talus (the ankle bone; pl., tali) PREFIXED ROOT: subtalar (*sub* under) LEADING ROOT COMPOUND: *tal*: talalgia (*algos* pain) *tali*: taliped (clubfooted; a clubfooted person) {talipedic} (*pes* foot) talipes (also called *clubfoot*) (*pes* foot) [There are many types of talipes.] *talipo*: talipomanus (clubhand) (*manus* hand) *talo*: talocalcaneal (or, talocalcanean; pertaining to the talus and cal-caneus) (*calcaneum* heel) talocrural (pertaining to the talus and the bones of the leg; the ankle joint) (*crus* leg; genitive: *cruris*) talofibular (fibula) talonavicular (also called *astragaloscaphoid, taloscaphoid*; pertain-ing to the talus and the navicular bone) talotibial (tibia) CROSS REFERENCE: astrag, tars[1]
tars[1]	Greek *tarsos* a broad, flat surface	root of foot; also, ankle	SIMPLE ROOT: tarsen, tarsus (the region of articulation between the foot and the leg) {tarsal, tarsalis; also listed under tars[2]} PREFIXED ROOT: *tarsal*: extratarsal (*extra* outside) intertarsal (also called *tarsotarsal*) (*inter* between) intermetarsal (*inter* between + metatarsal) intratarsal (*intra* within, inner) mediotarsal (also called *mesotarsal, midtarsal*) (*medius* middle) mesotarsal (also called *mediotarsal, midtarsal*) (*mesos* middle) posttarsal (*post* posterior) pretarsal (*pre* anterior, or inferior) subtarsal (*sub* under) *tarsalgia*: metatarsalgia (*meta* after + *algos* pain) *tarsalia*: polymetatarsalia (congenital anomaly characterized by supernumerary metatarsal bones) (*polys* many + *meta* after) *tarsectomy*: metatarsectomy (*meta* after + *ektome* excision) *tarsia*: polymetatarsia (*polys* many + metatarsus) *tarso*: metatarsophalangeal (pertaining to the metatarsus and the phalanges of the toes) (*meta* after + phalanges) *tarsus*: metatarsus (pl., metatarsi) {metatarsal} (*meta* after) LEADING ROOT COMPOUND: *tars*: tarsalgia (pain in the ankle or foot) (*algos* pain) tarsectomy (*ektome* excision) [also listed under tars[2]] tarsectopia (dislocation of the tarsus of the foot) (*ektopia* displaced)

Element	From	Meaning	Examples
tars[1] (cont'd)		[ankle]	tarsitis (*itis* inflammation) [also listed under tars[2]] *tarso*: tarsoclasis (or, tarsoclasia) (*klaein* to break) tarsomegaly (also called *Trevor disease*) (*megalos* large) tarsometatarsal (pertaining to the tarsus and the metatarsal) tarsophalangeal (pertaining to the tarsus and the phalanges of the toes) tarsoptosis (falling of the tarsus; flatfoot) (*ptein* to fall) tarsotarsal (also called *intertarsal, tarsotibial, tibiotarsal*) TRAILING ROOT COMPOUND: tibiotarsal (tibia) CROSS REFERENCE: astrag, tal
tars[2]	Greek *tarsos* a broad, flat surface	edge of the eyelid	SIMPLE ROOT: tarsus {tarsal, tarsalis; also listed under tars[1]) PREFIXED ROOT: epitarsus (a congenital anomaly of the eye) (*epi* upon) retrotarsal (*retro* behind) LEADING ROOT COMPOUND: *tars*: tarsectomy (*ektome* excision) [also listed under tars[1]] tarsitis (*itis* inflammation) [also listed under tars[1]] *tarso*: tarsocheiloplasty (*cheilos* lip + *plassein* to form) tarsomalacia (*malakos* soft) tarsophyma (a growth or tumor of the eyelid) (*phyma* growth) tarsoplasia (or, tarsoplasty; plastic surgery of the tarsus of an eyelid; also called *blepharoplasty*) (*plassein* to form) tarsorrhaphy (also called *blepharorrhaphy*) (*rhaphein* to suture) tarsotomy (also called *blepharotomy*) (*tomy* incision) CROSS REFERENCE: blephar, cili, palpebr
tas			See ten[1] for *ectasis*.
tax, **tact**	Greek *tassein* to arrange *taxis* arrange- ment	order, arrangement	SIMPLE ROOT: taxis (manual replacement or reduction of a hernia or dislocation), taxon (pl., taxa) PREFIXED ROOT: *tact*: atactiform (resembling ataxia) (*a* privative + *forma* shape) syntactics (*syn* with, together) *taxia*: ataxia (total or partial inability to coordinate voluntary bodily movements, especially muscular movements) {ataxic, atactic} (*a* privative) [see separate entry: atax-] dystaxia (difficulty in controlling voluntary movements) (*dys* abnormal) hypotaxia (*hypo* under) parataxia (or, parataxis) (*para* abnormal) *taxis*: allelotaxis (*allos* other) heterotaxis (or, heterotaxia) {heterotaxic} (*heteros* other) parataxis (or, parataxia) {parataxic} (*para* alongside) syntaxis {syntactic} (*syn* with) *taxy*: epitaxy (*epi* upon) LEADING ROOT COMPOUND: taxology (also called *taxonomy*) (*logos* study) taxonomy (also called *taxology*) {taxonomic} (*nomos* law) TRAILING ROOT COMPOUND: *taxia*: acroataxia (*akros* extremities + *a* privative)

Element	From	Meaning	Examples
tax (cont'd)		[arrangement]	*taxis:* aerotaxis (*aer* air) barotaxis (*baros* weight) biotaxis (the ability of cells to develop into certain forms and arrangements) (*bios* life) chemotaxis (*chein* to pour: chemical) chromatotaxis (*chromatos* color) cytobiotaxis (also called *cytoclesis*) (*kytos* cell + *bios* life) cytotaxis (the attraction or repulsion of cells for one another) {cytotactic} (*kytos* cell) ecotaxis (the migration of lymphocytes from the thymus and bone marrow into tissues possessing an appropriate microenvironment) (*oikos* environment) eosinotaxis (movement of eosinophils with reference to stimulus which attracts or repels them) (*eosin* fr. *eos* dawn) galvanotaxis (also called *electrotaxis*) geotaxis (also called *geotropism*) (*geo* earth) glycotaxis (*glykys* sweet) hydrotaxis (*hydor* water, fluid) leukotaxis (also called *leukocytotaxis*) (*leukos* white) lymphotaxis (*lympha* water, fluid) neutrotaxis (neutrophil) osmotaxis (*osmos* impulse) phototaxis (also called *heliotaxis*) (*photos* light) rheotaxis (also called *rheotropism*) (*rhein* to flow) serotaxis (*serum* whey) sitotaxis (also called *sitotropism*) (*sitos* food) stereotaxis (also called *thigmotaxis*) (*stereos* solid) thermotaxis (*therme* heat) thigmotaxis (also called *stereotaxis*) (*thigma* touch) trophotaxis (*trophein* to nourish) CROSS REFERENCE: None
tect, **teg**	Greek *tekton* builder Latin *tectus* roof; *tegere* to cover	builder, cover (skin)	SIMPLE ROOT: *tect:* tectonic (pertaining to plastic surgery or to surgery for the restoration of parts) tectorium (an overlaying structure) {tectorial} tectum (any rooflike covering or structure; pl., tecta) {tectal} *teg:* tegmen (any covering, shelter, or roof; pl., tegmina) {tegmental}, tegmentum (pl., tegmenta), tegument (the integument or skin) {tegumental, tegumentary} PREFIXED ROOT: *tect:* detection (discovery of the presence or existence of something), detector (*de* from) dystectia (defective closure of the neural tube) (*dys* abnormal) pretecta (orad to the hidden part of the duodenum) (*pre* before) protectant (or, protective; covering, preventing infection, providing immunity), protectin, protector (*pro* for) *teg:* integument (a covering or investment; the covering of the body, or skin), integumentary (serving as a covering, like the skin), integumentum (*in* in, on) subtegumental (also called *subcutaneous*) (*sub* below)

Element	From	Meaning	Examples
tect (cont'd)		[cover, skin]	LEADING ROOT COMPOUND: *tecti*: tectiform (roof-shaped) (*forma* shape) *tecto*: tectocephaly (also called *scaphocephaly*) {tectocephalic; also called *scaphocephalic*} (*kephale* head) tectology (the science which treats of the building up of organisms from organic elements; structural morphology) (*logos* study) tectospinal (pertaining to the tectum mesencephali and the spinal cord) (*spina* spine) *tegmento*: tegmentotomy (production of lesions in the reticular formation of the midbrain tegmentum) (*tomy* incision) TRAILING ROOT COMPOUND: *tect*: immunodetection (also called *immunoscintigraphy*) (immunity) *tegm*: thalamotegmental (thalamus) CROSS REFERENCE: cut, derm
tele[1]	Greek *telos*	the end; complete	SIMPLE ROOT: telesis (a goal to be attained by planned actions), telotism (the perfect performance of a function) PREFIXED ROOT: atelia (imperfect or incomplete development) {ateliotic} (*a* privative) [see separate entry: atel-] autotelic (denoting those traits closely associated with the central purposes of an individual) (*autos* self) dysteleology (the doctrine of purposelessness in nature) (*dys* abnormal + *logos* study) entelechy (full development or realization) (*en* intensive) subtelocentric (*sub* under + telocentric) LEADING ROOT COMPOUND: *tel*: telangion (*angeion* vessel—blood vessel) telencephalon {telencephalic} (*enkephale* brain) *tele*: telediastolic (pertaining to or occurring toward the end of ventricular diastole) (*diastole* dilation) teleneurite, teleneuron (a nerve ending) (*neuron* nerve) teleorganic (manifesting life; necessary to life) *teleo*: teleology {teleological} (*logos* study) teleomitosis (*mitos* thread + *osis* condition) teleomorph (*morphe* form) teleonomy (the doctrine that life is endowed with a project or purpose) {teleonomic} (*nomos* law) *telo*: telocentric (*kentron* point, center) telodendrion, telodendron (pl., telodendra) (*dendron* tree: growth) telogen (resting phase of hair cycle) (*genere* to produce) teloglia (*glia* glue) telomere (the distal end of a chromosome) (*meros* part) telepeptide telophase (*phasis* appearance) telosynapsis (*synapsis* conjunction) CROSS REFERENCE: atel
tele[2]	Greek *tele*	distant, far off	See Appendix B for examples of words with this element. Others are listed with the roots to which it is attached. CROSS REFERENCE: dist

Element	From	Meaning	Examples
temp	Latin *temperare* to observe proper measure *temporis*	time, timely, or fatal spot; temple of the body	SIMPLE ROOT: temper, temperament (the peculiar physical character and mental cast of an individual), temperance, temperate, temperature temple (also called *tempora*), tempora (the regions on either side of the head; the temples), temporal, temporalis tempus (the temple; also time; pl., tempora) PREFIXED ROOT: bitemporal (*bi* two) inferotemporal (*inferus* low) infratemporal (*infra* below) posterotemporal (*posterior* behind) pretemporal (*pre* before, in front of) subtemporal (*sub* below) supratemporal (*supra* above) transtemporal (crossing the cerebrum) (*trans* across) LEADING ROOT COMPOUND: *tempo*: tempolabile (*labilis* perishable) tempostabile (not subject to change with the passage of time) (*stabilis* stable, abiding) *temporo*: temporoauricular (*auris* ear) temporofacial (*facies* face) temporofrontal (*frontis* front) temporohyoid (hyoid bones) temporomalar (also called *temporozygomatic*) (*mala* cheek) temporomandibular (*mandible* lower jaw) temporomaxillary (*maxilla* upper jaw) temporo-occipital (*occipitus* back of head: *ob* against + *caput* head) temporoparietal (parietal bones) temporopontile (*pontis* bridge) temporospatial (space) temporosphenoid (*sphen* wedge + *eidos* form) TRAILING ROOT COMPOUND: auriculotemporal (*auris* ear) basitemporal (*basis* basion) frontotemporal (*frontis* front) occipitotemporal (or, temporo-occipital) (*occiput* back of head) orbitotemporal (*orbita* the cavity that contains the eyeball) parietotemporal (*paries* wall) sphenotemporal (*sphen* wedge) tympanotemporal (*tympanon* drum—eardrum) zygomaticotemporal (zygomatic process) CROSS REFERENCE: chron
ten			See ten³ for *tenalgia*.
ten¹, tas, tet	Greek *teinein* to stretch, strain	to stretch, intensify; tension; dilatation	SIMPLE ROOT: *ten*: tenesmus (straining, especially ineffectual and paining at stool or in urination) *tet*: tetanus [see separate listing: tetan-] PREFIXED ROOT: anectasis (congenital atelectasis due to developmental immaturity) (*an* privative + ectasis) ectasia (or, ectasis; dilatation, expansion, or distention) (*ek* out) entasia (a constrictive spasm; spasmodic muscular action) (*en* in)

Element	From	Meaning	Examples
ten[1] (cont'd)		[to stretch}	parectasis (excessive stretching or distention of a part or organ) (*para* alongside + ectasis) [term is now obsolete]
			LEADING ROOT COMPOUND: tenonometer (an instrument for measuring intraocular pressure; also called *tonometer*) (*metron* measure)
			TRAILING ROOT COMPOUND:
			ectasia a stretching out:
			angiectasia (or, angiectasis) {angioectatic} (*angeion* vessel)
			aortectasia (aorta)
			arteriectasia (artery)
			chylectasia (*chylus* juice)
			colpectasia (or, colpectasis) (*kolpos* vagina)
			cystectasia (or, cystectasy) (*kystis* sac, bladder)
			keratoectasia (or, kerectasis) (*keratos* cornea)
			nephrectasia (or, nephrectasis) (*nephros* kidney)
			neurectasia (or, neurectasis, neurectasy) (*neuron* nerve)
			osteoectasia (bowing of the bones) (*osteon* bone)
			pharyngectasia (pharynx)
			proctectasia (*proktos* anus)
			prosopectasia (oversize of the face) (*prosopon* face)
			ureterectasia (also called *megaloureter*) (ureter)
			ectasis a stretching out:
			angiectasis (or, angiectasia; also called *hemangiectasia*) (*angeion* vessel; blood vessel)
			appendicectasis (appendix)
			arteriectasis (artery)
			atelectasis (*ateles* incomplete)
			bronchiectasis (*bronchus* windpipe)
			caliectasis (or, calicectasis) (calyx; the renal calyx)
			cardiectasis (*kardia* heart)
			cholangiectasis (*chole* bile + *angeion* blood vessel)
			colpectasis (or, colpectasia) (*kolpos* vagina)
			corectasis (morbid dilatation of the pupil of the eye) (*kore* pupil)
			desmectasis (*desmos* band, ligament)
			enterectasis (*enteron* intestine)
			esophagectasis (esophagus)
			gastrectasis (*gaster* stomach, belly)
			hemangiectasis (*haima* blood + *angeion* blood vessel)
			nephrectasis (or, nephrectasia) (*nephros* kidney)
			neurectasis (also called *neurotension*) (*neuron* nerve)
			phlebectasis (also called *varicosity*) (*phlebos* vein)
			pneumonectasis (*pneumon* lung)
			pseudobronchiectasis (*pseudes* false + *bronchos* windpipe)
			ptyalectasis (*ptyalon* saliva)
			pyelectasis (*pyelos* pelvis)
			pyopyelectasis (*pyon* pus + *pyelos* pelvis)
			sclerectasis (or, sclerectasia) (*sklera* hard; the outer coat of the eyeball)
			sialectasis (*sialon* saliva: saliva glands)
			splenectasis (also called *splenomegaly*) (*splen* spleen)
			typhlectasis (*typhlon* cecum)
			ureterectasis (or, ureterectasia) (ureter)
			tasis: myotasis {myotatic} (*myos* muscle)
			CROSS REFERENCE: ten[3], ton

Element	From	Meaning	Examples
ten², **tend**, **tens**, **tent**	Latin *tendere*, *tensus*, *tentus*	to stretch; tension	SIMPLE ROOT: *ten*: tenuity (the state or condition of being thin, as blood) *tens*: tense (drawn tight), tension (the act of stretching; mental, emotional, or nervous strain) tensor (any muscle that stretches or makes tense; pl., tensores) *tent*: tent, tentorium (an anatomical part resembling a tent or a covering) PREFIXED ROOT: *ten*: attenuant, attenuate (to make thin), attenuation (*ad* to) *tend*: ambitendency (the existence of conflicting tendencies in the same individual) (*ambi* both) distend (to expand, as by pressure from within; to make or become swollen or bloated) (*dis* apart, away) extend (to straighten a limb; unbend) (*ex* out) superextended (*super* beyond + extend) *tens*: distensibility (the capability of being distended or stretched) (*dis* apart) extension, extensor (*ex* out) hyperextension (*hyper* + extension) hypertension (high arterial blood pressure) {hypertensive} (*hyper* above) hypotension {hypotensive} (*hypo* below) intensity, intensive, intensivist (*in* in, at, on) intensification (intensity + *facere* to make) isointense (*isos* equal + intense) protensity (the time attribute of mental process) (*pro* forward) superextension (*super* beyond + extension) *tention*: attention (directing or concentrating one's consciousness on only one object or an internal or external stimulus) (*ad* to) distention (or, distension; the state of being distended) (*dis* apart) hyperdistention (*hyper* above + distention) inattention (*in* negative + attention) superdistention (*super* above + distention) *tentorial*: subtentorial (situated beneath the tentorium of the cerebellum) (*sub* below) supratentorial (*supra* above) transtentorial (*trans* across) LEADING ROOT COMPOUND: tensiometer (*metron* measure) TRAILING ROOT COMPOUND: normotensive (also called *normotonic*) (normal) CROSS REFERENCE: ten², ton
ten³	Greek *teinein* to stretch [influenced by Latin *tendere* to stretch]	tendon	SIMPLE ROOT: tendinous (pertaining to, resembling, or of the nature of a tendon) tendo (or, tendon; pl., tendines) tendon (a fibrous cord by which muscle is attached) PREFIXED ROOT: *tendinitis*: polytendinitis (*polys* many + *itis* inflammation) *tendinous*: intratendinous (*intra* within)

Element	From	Meaning	Examples
ten³ (cont'd)		[tendon]	semitendinous (or, semitendinosus) (*semi* partly)
			subtendinous (deep to a tendon; typically used in relationship to bursae) (*sub* below)
			tendineum:
			endotendineum (*endon* within)
			epitendineum (also called *epitenon*) (*epi* upon)
			mesotendineum (also called *mesotendon*) (*mesos* middle)
			peritendineum (pl., peritendinea) {peritendinous}, peritendinitis (also called *peritenonitis*) (*peri* around + *itis* inflammation)
			tendino: polytendinobursitis (*polys* many + *bursitis*)
			tendon: mesotendon (*mesos* middle)
			teno: polytenosynovitis (*polys* many + *synovitis*)
			tenon:
			endotenon (also called *endotendineum*) (*endon* within)
			epitenon (the connective tissue holding a tendon within the sheaths; also called *epitendineum*) (*epi* upon)
			mesotenon (also called *mesotendineum*) (*mesos* middle)
			paratenon (*para* alongside)
			peritenon, peritenoneum, peritenonitis (*peri* around + *itis* inflammation)
			LEADING ROOT COMPOUND:
			ten:
			tenalgia (also called *tenodynia, tenontodynia*) (*algos* pain)
			tenectomy (*ektome* excision)
			tenodynia (also called *tenalgia, tenontodynia*) (*odyne* pain)
			tenostosis (or, tenonostosis) (*osteon* bone + *osis* condition)
			tendin: tendinitis (or, tendonitis) (*itis* inflammation)
			tendino:
			tendinoplasty (or, tenoplasty) (*plassein* to form)
			tendinosuture (the suturing of a tendon) (*suere* to sew)
			tendo:
			tendolysis (or, tenolysis) (*lyein* to loosen)
			tendomucin (a mucin derivable from tendons and closely related to submaxillary mucin and to the colloid of cancers)
			tendomucoid (also called *tendomucin*) (mucus + *eidos* form)
			tendoplasty (reparative surgery of an injured tendon) (*plassein* to form)
			tendosynovitis (or, tenosynovitis)
			tendotome (or, tenotome), tendotomy (or, tenotomy) (*tomy* incision)
			tendovaginitis (or, tenosynovitis) (*vagina* sheath + *itis* inflammation)
			tendon: tendonitis (or, tendinitis) (*itis* inflammation)
			teno:
			tenodesis (tendon fixation) (*dein* to bind)
			tenofibril (also called *tonofibril*) (fiber)
			tenolysis (or, tendolysis; release of a tendon from adhesions) (*lyein* to loosen)
			tenomyoplasty (*myos* muscle + *plassein* to form)
			tenomyotomy (also called *myotenotomy*) (*myos* muscle + *tomy* incision)
			tenophony (or, tendophony) (*phone* sound)
			tenophyte (*phyte* plant: growth)
			tenoplasty (or, tendinoplasty) {tenoplastic} (*plassein* form)
			tenoreceptor (receptor) (*re* again + *capere* to hold)
			tenorrhaphy (also called *tenosuture*) (*rhaphe* suture)

Element	From	Meaning	Examples
ten³ (cont'd)		[tendon]	tenosuture (also called *tenorrhaphy*) (*suere* to sew) tenosynitis (or, tenosynovitis) (synovia + *itis* inflammation) tenosynovectomy (synovia + *ektome* excision) tenosynovitis (also called *tenosynitis*) (synovia + *itis* inflammation) tenotome, tenotomy (*tomy* incision) tendovaginal, tenovaginitis (*vagina* sheath + *itis* inflammation) *tenon*: tenonectomy (*ektome* excision) tenonitis (*itis* inflammation) tenonostosis (or, tenostosis; ossification of a tendon) (*osteon* bone + *osis* condition) *tenono*: tenonometer (also called *tonometer*; an apparatus for measuring intraocular pressure) (*metron* measure) *tenont*: tenontagra (*agra* seizure) tenontitis (*itis* inflammation) tenontodynia (also called *tenalgia*) (*odyne* pain) *tenonto*: tenontography (*graphein* to write) tenontolemmitis (also called *tenosynovitis*) (*lemma* sheath—egg membrane + *itis* inflammation) tenontology (*logos* study) tenontomyoplasty (or, tenomyoplasty; also called *myotenotomy*) (*myos* muscle + *plassein* to form) tenontomyotomy (or, tenomyotomy) (*myos* muscle + *tomy* incision) tenontophyma (*phyma* tumor, growth) tenontoplasty (or, tenoplasty) (*plassein* to form) tenontothecitis (also called *tenosynovitis*) (*theka* sheath + *itis* inflammation) tenontotomy (or, tenotomy) (*tomy* incision) *tenos*: tenositis (or, tendinitis) (*itis* inflammation) TRAILING ROOT COMPOUND: myotenositis (*myos* muscle + tenositis) myotenotomy (*myos* muscle + tenotomy) CROSS REFERENCE: ten²
terat	Greek *teras* monster	fetal monster	SIMPLE ROOT: teras (a malformed fetus with deficient, redundant, misplaced, or misshapen parts; pl., terata) {teratic} teratism (an anomaly of formation or development; the condition of a fetal monster; also called *teratosis*) PREFIXED ROOT: hemiterata (a grouping of congenitally deformed individuals whose deformities are less severe than teratism) {hemiteratic} (*hemi* half: partly) LEADING ROOT COMPOUND: *terat*: teratoid (resembling a monster, or teras) (*eidos* form) teratoma (also called *teratoblastoma*) {teratomatous} (*oma* tumor) teratosis (also called *teratism*) (*osis* condition) *terato*: teratoblastoma (also called *tertoma*) (*blastos* germ + *oma* tumor) teratocarcinogenesis (*karkinos* cancer + *genere* to produce) teratocarcinoma (*karkinos* cancer + *oma* tumor) teratogenesis {teratogenic, teratogenetic} (*genere* to produce) teratology {teratologic} (*logos* study)

Element	From	Meaning	Examples
terat (cont'd)		[fetal monster]	teratophobia (morbid fear of carrying and giving birth to a malformed infant) (*phobia* fear) teratospermia (the presence of malformed spermatozoa in the semen; also called *teratozoospermia*) (*sperma* seed) CROSS REFERENCE: None
tess			See tetra- for *tessellated*.
test	Latin *testis*	male gonad, testis	SIMPLE ROOT: testicle (or, testis), testis (the male gonad; an egg-shaped gland normally situated in the scrotum, which produces spermatozoa; pl., testes) {testicular; pertaining to testes; also called *orchidic*}, testiculus (testis; pl., testiculi) PREFIXED ROOT: hypertestoidism (*hyper* above + *eidos* form) intratesticular (*intra* within) LEADING ROOT COMPOUND: *test*: testalgia (also called *orchialgia, orchiodynia*) (*algos* pain) testectomy (also called *orchiectomy*) (*ektome* excision) testitis (also called *orchitis*) (*itis* inflammation) testoid (also called *androgenic, androgen*) (*eidos* form) *testi*: testicond (*condere* to hide, conceal) *testo*: testosterone (*stereos* solid) testotoxicosis (*toxikon* poison + *osis* condition) *testicul*: testiculoma (also called *testicular tumor*) (*oma* tumor) *testo*: testopathy (also called *orchiopathy*) (*pathos* disease) CROSS REFERENCE: orchi, osche
tetan	Greek *teinein* to stretch	spasm, tetanus	SIMPLE ROOT: tetanism (also called *neonatal tetany*), tetanize {tetanization} tetanus (an acute infectious disease caused by a toxin in the body) {titanic}, tetany PREFIXED ROOT: antitetanic (*anti* against) hemitetany (*hemi* half) subtetanic (mildly tetanic) (*sub* under) LEADING ROOT COMPOUND: *tetan*: tetanoid (also called *tetaniform*) (*eidos* form) *tetani*: tetaniform (also called *tetanoid*) (*forma* form) tetanigenous (*genere* to produce) *tetano*: tetanolysin (*lyein* to loosen) tetanometer (*metron* measure) tetanomotor (*movere* to move) tetanospasmin (spasm) tetanotoxin (*toxikon* poison) TRAILING ROOT COMPOUND: gutturotetany (laryngeal spasm causing a temporary stutter) (*guttur* throat) CROSS REFERENCE: clon, spas
tetra, **tess**	Greek *tetras* four; *tessara* square	four, square	SIMPLE ROOT: *tess*: tessellated (divided into squares, like a checkerboard) *tetra*: tetrad (a group of four things with something in common) See Appendix C for examples of words beginning with this element. Others are listed with the root to which it is attached. CROSS REFERENCE: quadr

A Thesaurus of Medical Word Roots

Element	From	Meaning	Examples
thalam	Greek *thalamus* inner chamber	thalamus	SIMPLE ROOT: thalamus (pl., thalami) {thalamic} PREFIXED ROOT: *thalamic*: interthalamic (*inter* between) transthalamic (*trans* across) *thalamus*: epithalamus {epithalamic} (*epi* upon) hypothalamus {hypothalamic} (*hypo* under) metathalamus (the most caudal part of the thalamus) (*meta* after) subthalamus {subthalamic} (*sub* under) LEADING ROOT COMPOUND: *thalam*: thalamectomy (also called *thalamotomy*) (*ektome* excision) thalamencephalon (the part of the diencephalon comprising the thalamus) {thalamencephalic} (*enkephalon* brain) *thalamo*: thalamocortical (*cortex* rind: outer covering) thalamolenticular (lens) thalamotegmental (*tegmen* covering) thalamotomy (also called *thalamectomy*) (*tomy* incision) TRAILING ROOT COMPOUND: neothalamus (the phylogenetically newer part of the thalamus) (*neos* new) rubrothalamic (pertaining to the red nucleus and the thalamus) (*rubeus* red) CROSS REFERENCE: atri, cell
theca	Greek *thekion* case, cover	case, sheath, repository	SIMPLE ROOT: theca (any sac enclosing an organ or a whole organism, as the covering of an ovarian follicle or tendon; pl., thecae) {thecal} PREFIXED ROOT: apothecary (lit., put away; orig., a storehouse; a druggist or pharmacist) (*apo* from) hyperthecosis (hyperplasia and excessive luteinization of the cells of the inner stromal layer of the ovary) (*hyper* over + *osis* condition) intrathecal (pertaining to a structure, process, or substance within a sheath, such as within the spinal cord) (*intra* within) perithecium (pl., perithecia) (*peri* around) LEADING ROOT COMPOUND: *thec*: thecitis (inflammation of the sheath of a tendon; also called *tenosynovitis*) (*itis* inflammation thecodont (having teeth inserted in sockets) (*odontos* tooth) thecoma (a theca cell tumor), thecomatosis (*oma* tumor + *osis* condition) *theco*: thecostegnosis (constriction, or contraction, of a tendon sheath) (*stegnosis* a narrowing) TRAILING ROOT COMPOUND: karyotheca (nuclear membrane) (*karyon* nucleus) odontotheca (the dental sac) (*odontos* tooth) ootheca (an egg case, such as is found in certain animals; ovarium) (*oon* egg, ovum) sporotheca (the envelope enclosing the minute needle-like spores of certain Sporozoea) (*sporos* seed) CROSS REFERENCE: lemma, vagin

Element	From	Meaning	Examples
thel	Greek *thele*	nipple, teat	SIMPLE ROOT: thelium (a small nipple-shaped projection or elevation; nipple; pl., thelia), thelotism (also called *thelerethism*)
			PREFIXED ROOT:
			thelia:
			athelia (congenital absence of the nipples) (*a* privative)
			hyperthelia (also called *polythelia*) (*hyper* above)
			microthelia (*mikros* small)
			polythelia (or, polythelism; also called *hyperthelia*) (*polys* many)
			thelium:
			endothelium (*endon* within) [see separate entry: endothel-]
			epithelium (*epi* upon) [see separate entry: epithel-]
			mesothelium (pl., mesothelia) (*mesos* middle)
			perithelium (pl., perithelia) {perithelial} (*peri* around)
			LEADING ROOT COMPOUND:
			thel:
			thelalgia (*algos* pain)
			thelarche (the beginning of development of the breasts at puberty) (*archein* to begin)
			thelerethism (erection or protrusion of the nipple) (*erethisma* a stirring up)
			thelitis (also called *mammillitis*) (*itis* stimulation)
			theloncus (a tumor of a nipple) (*onkos* mass)
			thele: theleplasty (*plassein* to form)
			thelio: theliolymphocyte (*lympha* water, liquid + *kytos* cell)
			thelo: thelorrhagia (*rhagia* bursting forth)
			TRAILING ROOT COMPOUND:
			meningothelioma (*meningos* membrane + *oma* tumor)
			retothelium (*rete* net)
			CROSS REFERENCE: mamm, papill
therap	Greek *therapeia*	medical treatment	SIMPLE ROOT:
			therapeusis (or, therapeutics), therapeutics (the branch of medicine concerned with the remedial treatment of disease)
			therapia (or, therapy, therapeutics}, therapist
			PREFIXED ROOT:
			therapeutic: eutherapeutic (*eu* well)
			therapy:
			autotherapy (*autos* self)
			heterotherapy (*heteros* other)
			isotherapy (also called *isopathy*) (*isos* equal)
			monotherapy (*monos* single)
			teletherapy (*tele* afar)
			TRAILING ROOT COMPOUND:
			therapy:
			actinotherapy (also called *phototherapy*) (*aktinos* a ray)
			aerohydrotherapy (*aer* air + *hydor* water)
			acutherapy (*acus* needle)
			alkalitherapy (alkali)
			ammotherapy (treatment with warm dry sand or of damp sand)
			apitherapy (*apis* bee)
			aromatherapy (aroma)
			aurotherapy (also called *chrysotherapy*) (*aurum* gold)
			balneotherapy (*balneum* bath)
			biotherapy (also called *biological therapy*) (*bios* life)
			brachytherapy (*brachys* short)

Element	From	Meaning	Examples
therap (cont'd)		[treatment]	bromatotherapy (also called *diet therapy*) (*broma* food)
			cardiotherapy (*kardia* heart)
			chemotherapy {chemotherapeutic} (chemical)
			choletherapy (*chole* bile)
			chromotherapy (*chroma* light)
			chronotherapy (*chronos* time)
			chrysotherapy (also called *aurotheraphy*) (*chrysos* gold)
			climatotherapy (climate)
			crymotherapy (also called *cryotherapy*) (*krymos* frost, cold)
			cryotherapy (also called *crymotherapy, frigotherapy*) (*kryos* cold)
			curietherapy (radioactive source) (from Marie Curie, discoverer of radium)
			dermatotherapy (*dermatos* skin)
			dipsotherapy (*dipsa* thirst)
			electrotherapy (electricity)
			eleotherapy (also called *oleotherapy*) (*elaion* oil)
			ergotherapy (*ergon* work)
			ferrotherapy (*ferrum* iron)
			heliotherapy (*helios* sun)
			hemotherapy (or, hematherapy, hematotherapy) (*haima* blood)
			hepatotherapy (*hepatos* liver)
			histotherapy (*histos* web, tissue)
			homeotherapy (*homoios* like, resembling)
			hormonotherapy (also called *endocrine therapy*) (*hormaein* to set in motion: hormone)
			hydrotherapy (*hydor* water)
			hypnotherapy (*hypnos* sleep)
			hypsotherapy (*hypso* high)
			immunotherapy (immunization)
			iodotherapy (*iode* iodine)
			kinesitherapy (movement, exercise) (*kinein* to move)
			lucotherapy (also called *phototherapy*) (*lucis* light)
			massotherapy (massage) (*massein* to knead)
			mechanotherapy (mechanical)
			myelotherapy (*myelos* spinal cord)
			myotherapy (*myos* muscle)
			odontotherapy (*odontos* tooth)
			oncotherapy (*onkos* tumor)
			osmotherapy (*osmos* impulse)
			pharmacotherapy (*pharmakon* medicine, drug)
			phototherapy (also called *lucotherapy*) (*photos* light)
			physiotherapy (also called *physical therapy*)
			phytotherapy (herbal therapy) (*phyton* plant)
			pneumotherapy (*pneuma* lung)
			psychotherapy (*psyche* mind)
			pyretotherapy (*pyretos* fever)
			radiotherapy (also called *irradiation, radiation therapy*)
			reflexotherapy (also called *reflex therapy*)
			serotherapy (serum, antitoxin)
			sitotherapy (also called *bromatotherapy, dietotherapy*) (*sitos* food)
			somatotherapy (*somatos* body)
			thermotherapy (*therme* heat)
			traumatherapy (*trauma* wound, injury)
			CROSS REFERENCE: iat

Element	From	Meaning	Examples
therm	Greek *therme*	heat	SIMPLE ROOT: therm {thermal, thermic}, thermion thermotics (the science of heat) PREFIXED ROOT: *therm*: allotherm (also called *poikilotherm, heterotherm*) (*allos* other) ectotherm {ectothermic}, ectothermy (*ektos* outside) endotherm (also called *homeotherm*) {endothermal, endothermic} (*endon* within) heterotherm (also called *allotherm*) {heterothermic} (*heteros* other) homotherm {homothermal, homothermic} (*homos* same) ultratherm (a shortwave diathermy machine) (*ultra* beyond) *thermal*: diathermal (or, diathermic) (*dia* through) endothermal (*endon* within) eurythermal (or, eurythermic) (*eurys* wide, broad) exothermal (or, exothermic) (*exo* outside) hyperthermal (*hyper* above) hypothermal {hypothermic} (*hypo* under) isothermal (*isos* equal) synthermal (*syn* with) *thermancy*: athermancy (*a* negative) adiathermancy (state of being impervious to heat waves) (*a* negative + *dia* across) *thermanous*: athermanous (not transmitting heat) (*a* negative) diathermanous (permeable by heat waves) (*dia* through) *thermia*: hyperthermia (*hyper* above) hypothermia (or, hypothermy; lower than normal body temperature) {hypothermic} (*hypo* under) monothermia (*monos* single) normothermia {normothermic} (*norma* normal) transthermia (also called *diathermy*) (*trans* across) *thermic*: athermic (afebrile) (*a* negative) antithermic (also called *antipyretic*; that which reduces fever) (*anti* against) diathermic (*dia* through) ectothermic (*ektos* outside) endothermic (*endon* within) euthermic (characterized by the proper temperature) (*eu* well) eurythermic (*eurys* wide, broad) exothermic (*exo* outside) *thermo*: hemithermoanesthesia (*hemi* half + *an* negative + *esthesia* feeling) hyperthermoesthesia (*hyper* above + *esthesia* feeling) isothermognosis (a dysesthesia in which pain, cold, and heat stimuli are all perceived as heat) (*isos* equal + *gnosis* knowledge) *thermous*: athermous (without fever or rise of temperature) (*a* negative) *thermy*: diathermy {diathermal, diathermic} (*dia* across)

Element	From	Meaning	Examples
therm (cont'd)		[heat]	ectothermy (*ektos* outside)
			endothermy (*endon* within)
			heterothermy {heterothermic} (*heteros* other)
			LEADING ROOT COMPOUND:
			therm:
			ther<u>mac</u>ogenesis (the elevation of body temperature by drug action) (phar<u>makon</u> drug + *genere* to produce)
			thermalgia (also called *causalgia*) (*algos* pain)
			thermanalgesia (also called *thermoanesthesia*) (analgesia: *an* negative + *algesia* sense of pain)
			thermelometer (*electric* + *metron* measure)
			thermesthesia (or, thermoesthesia), thermesthesiometer (*esthesia* feeling + *metron* measure)
			thermato: thermatology (*logos* study)
			thermo:
			thermoacoustics (also called *optoacoustic imaging*) (*akouein* to hear)
			thermoalgesia (or, thermalgesia) (*algos* pain)
			thermoanesthesia (also called *thermoanalgesia*) (anesthesia: *an* negative + *esthesia* feeling)
			thermocautery, thermocauterectomy (cauterization by means of a hot wire) (*ektome* excision)
			thermochroic, thermochroism (or, thermochrosis) (*chrosis* color)
			thermoduric (*durus* enduring, lasting)
			thermodynamics (*dynamis* force)
			thermoesthesia, thermoesthesiometer (*esthesia* feeling + *metron* measure)
			thermogenesis {thermogenetic, thermogenic} (*genere* to produce)
			thermogram, thermograph, thermography (*graphein* to write)
			thermoinhibitory (inhibiting or arresting thermogenesis)
			thermolabile (*labilis* perishable)
			thermology (also called *thermotics*) (*logos* study)
			thermolysis {thermolytic} (*lyein* to loosen)
			thermomassage (combination of heat and massage in physical therapy)
			thermometer {thermometric}, thermometry (*metron* measure)
			thermoneurosis (*neuron* nerve + *osis* condition)
			thermonuclear (pertaining to nuclear reactions brought about by nuclear fusion)
			thermopalpation (*palpare* to touch)
			thermophile {thermophilic} (*philein* to love)
			thermophore (*phorein* to bear)
			thermopile (*pila* pillar)
			thermoplacentography (placenta + *graphein* to write)
			thermoplegia (heat stroke or sunstroke) (*plessein* to strike)
			thermoscope (a differential thermometer) (*skopein* to examine)
			thermostabile (or, thermostable; not affected by heat) (*stabilis* stable)
			thermostasis (*stasis* a setting)
			thermostat (*histanai* to halt)
			thermosteresis (*steresis* loss, privation)
			thermosystaltism {thermosystaltic} (*systaltikos* contractile)
			thermotaxis {thermotaxic, thermotactic} (*taxis* arrangement)
			thermotherapy (*therapy* treatment)
			thermotonometer (*tonos* tone + *metron* measure)

Element	From	Meaning	Examples
therm (cont'd)		[heat]	thermotropic, thermotropism (*tropein* to turn) TRAILING ROOT COMPOUND: *therm*: electrotherm (*electrum* shining, amber: electricity) *thermal*: hemathermal (*haima* blood) hydrothermal (pertaining to the temperature effects of water, as in hot baths) (*hydor* water) stenothermal {stenothermic} (*stenos* narrow) *thermic*: homeothermic (*homoios* like, similar) myothermic (*myos* muscle) normothermic (pertaining to or characterized by normal temperature, neither hyperthermic nor hypothermic) *thermo*: aerothermotherapy (*aer* air + *therapy* treatment) *thermy*: acrohypothermy (*akros* extremities + hypothermy) phototherapy (*photos* light) poikilothermy (also called *ectothermy*) (*poikilos* mottled, varied) CROSS REFERENCE: caum, phleg, pyr
thes	Greek *tithenai*	to place, do	SIMPLE ROOT: thesis (any theory or hypothesis advanced as a basis for discussion; pl., theses) PREFIXED ROOT: *thesis*: diathesis (constitutional predisposition to a certain disease, condition, or group of diseases) {diathetic} (*dia* across) enthesis (the use of metallic or other inert substances to substitute for or to replace lost tissue) (*en* in) epithesis (*epi* upon) hypothesis (*hypo* under) metathesis {metathetic} (*meta* after) prosthesis (*pros* to, at) synthesis (the artificial building up of a chemical compound by the union of the elements; pl., syntheses) (*syn* with) *thesitis*: enthesitis (inflammation of the muscular or tendinous attachment to bone) (*en* in + *itis* inflammation) *theso*: enthesopathy (a disease process occurring at the site of insertion of muscle tendons and ligaments into bones or joint capsules) {enthesopathic} (*en* in + *pathos* suffering) *thetic*: polythetic (*polys* many) prosthetic, prosthetics (*pros* to, at) synthetic (*syn* with, together) *thetosis*: athetosis (a form of dyskinesia; also called *mobile spasm*) {athetosic, athetotic} (*a* negative + *osis* condition) hemiathetosis (*hemi* half + athetosis) monathetosis (athetosis affecting a single part of the body) (*monos* single + athetosis) *thesize*: synthesize (to make something by synthesis) (*syn* with) TRAILING ROOT COMPOUND: *thesis*: biosynthesis (*bios* life + synthesis) cytothesis (*kytos* cell) CROSS REFERENCE: stal, stas

Element	From	Meaning	Examples
thora	Greek *thorax,* *thorakos*	chest, breastplate	SIMPLE ROOT: thorax (the part of the body between the base of the neck superiorly and the diaphragm inferiorly; pl., thoraces) {thoracal, thoracic; also called *pectoral*}

PREFIXED ROOT:

thoracic:

endothoracic (also called *intrathoracic*) (*endon* within)

infrathoracic (*infra* below)

intrathoracic (also called *endothoracic*) (*intra* within)

perithoracic (*peri* around)

suprathoracic (*supra* above)

transthoracic (*trans* across)

thoraco: transthoracotomy (*trans* across + *tomy* incision)

thorax:

hemithorax (*hemi* half)

synthorax (also called *thoracopagus*) (*syn* together)

LEADING ROOT COMPOUND:

thor: thoradelphus (duplicitas posterior in which the individual is duplicated from the umbilicus downward) (*adelphos* brother)

thora: thoracentesis (also called *pleuracentesis, pleurocentesis*) (*kentesis* puncture)

thorac:

thoracalgia (also called *pectoralgia, stethalgia*) (*algos* pain)

thoracectomy (*ektome* excision)

thoracodynia (pain in the chest; also called *thoracalgia, pectoralgia*) (*odyne* pain)

thoraci: thoracispinal (spine)

thoracico:

thoracicoabdominal (or, thoracoabdominal)

thoracicohumeral (humerus)

thoraco:

thoracoabdominal (or, thoracicoabdominal)

thoracoacromial (*acromion* highest point of the shoulder)

thoracoceloschisis (also called *thoracogastroschisis*) (*koilia* belly + *schisis* fissure)

thoracocentesis (or, thoracentesis; also called *pleuracentesis*) (*kentein* to puncture)

thoracocyllosis (*kyllosis* crippling, deformed)

thoracocyrtosis (*kyrtosis* curvature, crooked)

thoracodelphus (or, thoradelphus) (*adelphos* brother, twin)

thoracodorsal (*dorsum* back)

thoracogastroschisis (also called *thoracoceloschisis*) (*gaster* belly, stomach + *schisis* fissure)

thoracolaparotomy (*lapara* flank, loins + *tomy* incision)

thoracolumbar (*lumbar* loin)

thoracolysis (breaking up of pleural adhesions) (*lysis* dissolution)

thoracomeleus (unequaled conjoined twins) (*melos* limb)

thoracometer (also called *stethometer*) (*metron* measure)

thoracomyodynia (also called *pectoralgia*) (*myos* muscle + *odyne* pain)

thoracopagus (also called *synthorax, thoracodidymus*) (*pagus* thing fixed)

thoracopathy (*pathos* disease)

thoracoplasty (*plassein* to form)

thoracopneumoplasty (*pneumon* lung + *plassein* to form)

Element	From	Meaning	Examples
thora (cont'd)		[chest]	thoracoschisis (*schisis* fissure)
			thoracoscope, thoracoscopy (also called *pleuroscopy*) (*skopein* to examine)
			thoracostenosis (*stenosis* narrowing)
			thoracosternotomy (*sternon* chest + *tomy* incision)
			thoracostomy (*stoma* mouth, opening)
			thoracotomy (*tomy* incision)
			TRAILING ROOT COMPOUND:
			thoracic:
			abdominothoracic (abdomen)
			acromiothoracic (*acromion* tip of shoulder)
			cardiothoracic (*kardia* heart)
			cephalothoracic (*kephale* head)
			cervicothoracic (*cervix* neck)
			scapulothoracic (*scapula* shoulder blade)
			thorax:
			chylothorax (also called *chylopleura*) (*chylus* juice)
			fibrothorax (*fibra* fiber)
			hemothorax (or, hemathorax, hematothorax) (*haima* blood)
			hydrothorax (also called *serothorax*) (*hydor* water)
			oleothorax (*oleum* oil)
			planithorax (*planus* plane)
			pyothorax (also called *empyema*) (*pyon* pus)
			schistothorax (also called *thoracoschisis*) (*schistos* split)
			serothorax (also called *hydrothorax*) (*serum* whey)
			stenothorax (*stenos* narrow)
			urinothorax (*ouron* urine)
			CROSS REFERENCE: pect, stern, steth
thrix			See trich-.
thromb	Greek *thrombos* a clot	blood clot	SIMPLE ROOT:
			thrombin (an enzyme, formed in shed blood)
			thrombus (a plug or clot in a blood vessel or in one of the cavities of the heart; pl., thrombi)
			PREFIXED ROOT:
			athrombia (defective blood clotting) (*a* negative)
			antithrombin, antithrombotic (*anti* against)
			hypoprothrombinemia (also called *prothrombinopenia*) (*hypo* below + *pro* for + *emia* blood condition)
			hypothrombinemia (*hypo* under + *emia* blood condition)
			metathrombin (*meta* change)
			microthrombus, microthrombosis (*mikros* small + *osis* condition)
			prothrombin (also called *serozyme, thrombinogen*) (*pro* for)
			LEADING ROOT COMPOUND:
			throm: thrombolus (an embolus composed mainly of agglutinated platelets) {thrombolic} (embolus)
			thromb:
			thrombapheresis (also called *thrombocytapheresis*; the selective separation and removal of platelets from withdrawn blood, the remainder being retransfused to the donor) (*apheresis* removal)
			thrombasthenia (or, thromboasthenia) (*asthenia* weakness)
			thrombectomy (*ektome* excision)
			thromboid (*eidos* form)
			thrombosis (the formation, development, or presence of a thrombus) {thrombosed, thrombotic} (*osis* condition)

Element	From	Meaning	Examples
thromb (cont'd)		[clot]	*thrombo*: thromboangiitis (*angeion* blood vessel + *itis* inflammation) thromboarteritis (artery + *itis* inflammation) thromboblast (also called *megakaryocyte*) (*blastos* germ, cell) thrombocytapheresis (also called *thrombapheresis*) (*kytos* cell + *apheresis* removal) thromboclasis (also called *thrombolysis*) {thromboclastic; also called *thrombolytic*} (*klaein* to break) thrombocyst (or, thrombocystis), thrombocystasthenia (*kystis* sac + *asthenia* weakness: *a* negative + *sthenos* strength) thrombocyte (*kytos* cell) thromboelastogram, thromboelastograph (*elastreo* to push + *graphein* to write) thromboembolism, thromboembolectomy (*embolism* obstruction + *ektome* excision) thromboendarterectomy (*endon* within + artery + *ektome* excision) thrombogenesis {thrombogenic} (*genere* to produce) thrombokinesis (blood coagulation) (*kinein* to move) thrombolymphangitis (*lympha* fluid + *angeion* vessel + *itis* inflammation) thrombolysis (also called *thromboclasis*) (*lysis* dissolving) thrombonecrosis (*nekrosis* death) thrombopathy (also called *thrombocytopathy*) (*pathos* disease) thrombopenia (also called *thrombocytopenia*) (*penia* deficiency) thrombophilia (*philein* to love—have an affinity for) thrombophlebitis (*phlebos* vein + *itis* inflammation) thromboplastic (*plassein* to form) thrombopoiesis (also called *thrombogenesis, thrombocytopoiesis*) {thrombopoietic} (*poiein* to produce) thrombosinusitis (sinus + *itis* inflammation) thrombostasis (*stasis* standing still) TRAILING ROOT COMPOUND: *thrombo*: poikilothrombocyte (*poikilos* varied + *kytos* cell) *thrombosis* clotting condition: atherothrombosis (*athere* gruel) osteothrombosis (thrombosis of the veins of a bone) (*osteon* bone) phlebothrombosis (*phlebos* vein) pylethrombosis (*pyle* gate: portal vein) CROSS REFERENCE: coagul
thym[1]	Greek *thymus* a gland	thymus	SIMPLE ROOT: thymus (a ductless glandlike body situated in the anterior mediastinal cavity which reaches its maximum development during the early years of childhood; pl., thymi, thymuses) {thymic} PREFIXED ROOT: athymia (congenital absence of the thymus) (*a* privative) [also listed under thym[2]] euthymism (normal condition of thymus activity) (*eu* well) hyperthymism {hyperthymic} (*hyper* over, above) hypothymism {hyperthymic} (*hypo* under) megalothymus (*megalos* large) LEADING ROOT COMPOUND: *thym*: thymectomy {thymectomize} (*ektome* excision) thymitis (*itis* inflammation)

Element	From	Meaning	Examples
thym[1] (cont'd)		[thymus]	thymoma (*oma* tumor) *thymo*: thymocyte (lymphocyte within the thymus, usually applied to an immature lymphocyte) (*kytos* cell) thymokesis (enlargement of the remnant of the thymus that is found in the adult) thymokinetic (activating the thymus) (*kinein* to move) thymolysis {thymolytic} (*lyein* to loosen) thymopathy {thymopathic} (*pathos* disease) thymoprivous (or, thymoprival, thymoprivic) (*privus* without) thymotoxin, thymotoxic (poisonous to the thymus tissue) (*toxikon* poison) thymotrophic (*trophein* to nourish) CROSS REFERENCE: acin, aden, gland
thym[2]	Greek *thymos*	soul, spirit, mind	PREFIXED ROOT: athymia (without feeling or emotion) (*a* privative) [also listed under thym[1]] catathymia (the existence of unconscious material so emotionally charged or affect-laden that conscious effects are produced) (*kata* down) dysthymia (also called *dysthymic disorder*) {dysthymic} (*dys* abnormal) euthymia {euthymic} (*eu* well) hyperthymia {hyperthymic} (*hyper* above, beyond) hypothymia (depression of spirits; the "blues") {hypothymic} (*hypo* below) parathymia (a perverted, contrary, or inappropriate mood) (*para* alongside; abnormal) LEADING ROOT COMPOUND: thymogenic (of effective origin) (*genere* to produce) thymoleptic (any drug that favorably modifies mood in serious affective disorders) (*leptein* to hold) TRAILING ROOT COMPOUND: alexithymia (inability to verbalize one's emotions) (*a* privative + *lexos* word) cyclothymia (also called *cyclothymic disorder*) (*kyklos* circle) lipothymia (a condition or feeling of faintness; also called *syncope*) {lipothymic} (*leipein* to fail, leave) poikilothymia (a mental state marked by abnormal variations in mood) (*poikilos* varied) CROSS REFERENCE: phren[2], psych
thyr	Greek *thyreos* large shield from *thyra* door	a ductless gland (thyroid)	SIMPLE ROOT: thyroidea (also called *thyroid gland*) PREFIXED ROOT: *thyroid*: antithyroid (*anti* against) dysthyroid (*dys* abnormal) euthyroid (*eu* well) hypoparathyroid (*hypo* under + parathyroid) hypothyroid (*hypo* under) parathyroid (pl., parathyroid glands) {parathyroidal} (*para* alongside) prethyroid {prethyroideal} (*pre* before) *thyroidectomy* excision of the thyroid: hemithyroidectomy (*hemi* half) parathyroidectomy (*para* alongside)

A Thesaurus of Medical Word Roots

Element	From	Meaning	Examples
thyr (cont'd)		[thyroid]	*thyroidism*:

athyroidism {athyrotic} (*a* privative)

dysthyroidism (*dys* abnormal)

euthyroidism {euthyroid} (*eu* well)

hyperthyroidism (excessive functional activity of the thyroid gland; also called *thyrointoxication*) {hyperthyroid} (*hyper* above)

hypothyroidism (deficiency of thyroid activity or the condition resulting therefrom; also called *thyroprival*) (*hypo* under)

thyroiditis: perithyroiditis (or, perithyreoiditis) (*peri* around + *itis* inflammation)

thyrotropic: parathyrotropic (*para* alongside + *tropein* to turn)

LEADING ROOT COMPOUND:

thyr: thyroid (lit., resembling a shield; as a noun, the thyroid gland) (*eidos* form)

thyro:

thyroactive (stimulating activity of the thyroid gland)

thyroadenitis (or, thyroiditis) (*adenos* gland + *itis* inflammation)

thyroaplasia (*a* privative + *plassein* to form)

thyrocardiac (*kardia* heart)

thyrocele (goiter) (*kele* tumor, swelling)

thyrocervical (*cervix* neck)

thyrogenous (or, thyrogenic) (*genere* to produce)

thyroglossal (also called *thyrolingual*) (*glossa* tongue)

thyrohyal, thyrohyoid (hyoid bone)

thyrointoxication (also called *hyperthyroidism*)

thyrolaryngeal (larynx)

thyrolingual (also called *thyroglossal*) (*lingua* tongue)

thyrolytic (destructive to thyroid tissue) (*lyein* to loosen, dissolve)

thyromegaly (enlargement of the thyroid gland) (*megalos* large)

thyromimetic (producing effects similar to those of thyroid hormones or the thyroid gland) (*mimetic* simulation)

thyropalatine (denoting the palatopharyngeus muscle) (palate)

thyropathy (*pathos* disease)

thyropharyngeal (pharynx)

thyroplasty (*plassein* to form)

thyroprivia (also called *hypothyroidism*) {thyroprivic, thyroprivous, thyroprival} (*privare* to deprive, remove)

thyroprotein (also called *thyroglobulin*)

thyroptosis (*ptosis* a falling: downward displacement)

thyrotomy (*tomy* incision)

thyrotoxicosis (*toxikon* poison + *osis* condition)

thyrotrophic (also called *thyrotropic*) (*trophein* to nourish)

thyrotropic (also called *thyrotrophic*) (*tropein* to turn)

thyroid:

thyroidectomy {thyroidectomize} (*ektome* excision)

thyroiditis (also called *thyroadenitis*) (*itis* inflammation)

thyroido:

thyroidology (the study of the thyroid gland, both normal and pathologic) (*logos* study)

thyroidotherapy (*therapy* treatment)

thyroidotomy (also called *laryngofissure*) (*tomy* incision)

thyroidotoxin (*toxin* poison)

TRAILING ROOT COMPOUND: sternothyroid (sternum)

CROSS REFERENCE: None

Element	From	Meaning	Examples
tib	Latin *tibia* a pipe, flute	shinbone	SIMPLE ROOT: tibia {tibial, tibialis}, tibiad, tibiale PREFIXED ROOT: posttibial (*post* posterior) pretibial (in front of the tibia) (*pre* before) LEADING ROOT COMPOUND: *tibi*: tibialgia (*algos* pain) *tibio*: tibiocalcanean (pertaining to the tibia and the calcaneus) tibiofemoral (pertaining to the tibia and the femur) tibiofibular (pertaining to the tibia and the fibula) tibioperoneal (also called *tibiofibular*) (*perone* fibula) tibiotarsal (pertaining to the tibia and the tarsus) TRAILING ROOT COMPOUND: peroneotibial (pertaining to the fibula and the tibia; also called *tibiofibular, tibioperoneal*) (*perone* fibula) pubotibial (pubic bone) CROSS REFERENCE: None
toc, **tok**	Greek *tiktein* to give birth; *tokos* birth	childbirth, labor	PREFIXED ROOT: atocia (also called *nulliparity*) (*a* privative) dystocia (*dys* abnormal) eutocia (normal labor, or childbirth) (*eu* well) monotocous (*monos* single) polytocous (*polys* many) LEADING ROOT COMPOUND: *toco*: tocodynagraph (also called *tocograph*) (*dynamis* force + *graphein* to write) tocograph (also called *tocodynagraph*) (*graphein* to write) tocology (science of parturition and obstetrics) (*logos* study) tocolysis (inhibition of uterine contractions) {tocolytic} (*lysis* loosening) tocometer (also called *tokodynamometer*) (*metron* measure) tocophobia (*phobia* fear) *toko*: tokodynagraph (*dynamis* power + *graphein* to write) tokodynamometer (*dynamis* power + *metron* measure) TRAILING ROOT COMPOUND: bradytocia (slow, tedious childbirth) (*bradys* slow) deuterotocia (asexual reproduction in which the female produces offspring of both sexes) (*deuteros* second) oxytocia (rapid labor) {oxytocic} (*oxys* sharp, keen) CROSS REFERENCE: nat, par
tom, **tme**	Greek *temnein*	to cut	NOTE: The root is often joined with *ec-* to form *ectomy*, excision, or to surgically remove (see below). There is one word that doesn't fit the format: peritectomy (*peri* around, with an inserted *t* for easier pronunciation). The word means the same as *peritomy* as well as *circumcision*, literally, to cut around. PREFIXED ROOT: *tom*: atom (lit., that which cannot be cut further) (*a* negative) diatom {diatomaceous} (*dia* across, through) *tome*: macrotome (*makros* large) microtome (*mikros* small)

Element	From	Meaning	Examples
tom (cont'd)		[to cut]	*tomic*:

tomic:

[1]diatomic (made up of two atoms; also called *dibasic*)

[2]diatomic (diatomaceous; composed of diatoms)

hexatomic (*hex* six + atom)

tomist: peritomist (one who performs circumcision) (*peri* around)

tomo:

pantomography (*pan* all + *graphein* to write)

polytomography (*polys* many + *graphein* to write)

tomy:

anatomy (*ana* thorough, complete)

microtomy (also called *histotomy*) (*mikros* small)

peritomy (lit., a cutting around; circumcision; also called *peritectomy*) (*peri* around)

trichotomy (a division into three parts) (*trichia* threefold)

LEADING ROOT COMPOUND:

tomogram, tomograph (any x-ray machine which makes roentgeno-grams at any depth), tomography (also called *body section radiography*) (*graphein* to write)

tomomania (tendency of a surgeon to resort to unnecessary surgical operations; also, abnormal desire to be operated upon) (*mania* madness)

TRAILING ROOT COMPOUND:

tmesis:

axonotmesis (damage to nerve fibers of such severity that complete peripheral degeneration follows) (*axon* axle)

neurotmesis (*neuron* nerve)

tome an instrument for cutting; a segment:

adenotome (*adenos* gland; adenoids)

angiotome (*angeion* blood vessel)

arthrotome (*arthron* joint)

bioptome (a cutting instrument for taking biopsy specimens) (*bios* life + *opsis* vision)

bronchotome (*bronchos* windpipe)

chondrotome (*chondros* cartilage)

encephalotome (*encephalon* brain)

enterotome (*enteron* intestine)

gastrotome (*gaster* belly, stomach)

herniotome (*hernia* a protrusion)

lithotome (*lithos* stone)

myotome (*myos* muscle)

myringotome (*myringa* membrane)

periostotome (periosteum)

polymicrotome (*polys* many + *mikros* small)

rachitome (*rhachis* spine)

tenotome (*tenon* sinew: tendon)

tomy the operation of cutting, or incision:

adenotomy (*adenos* gland)

androtomy (dissection of the human body, as distinguished from *zootomy*; also called *anthropotomy*) (*andros* man)

angiotomy (the cutting or severing of a blood or lymphatic vessel) (*angeion* vessel)

antrotomy (also called *antrostomy*) (*antrum* cavity: sinus)

aortotomy (aorta)

arteriotomy (artery)

Element	From	Meaning	Examples
tom (cont'd)		[to cut]	arthrotomy (*arthron* joint)
			blastotomy (also called *blastomerotomy*) (*blastos* germ, bud)
			bronchotomy (*bronchos* windpipe)
			chondrotomy (*chondros* cartilage)
			desmotomy (*desmos* a band: ligament)
			dichotomy (the process or result of division into two parts) (*dicha* twofold)
			encephalotomy (also called *cerebrotomy*) (*enkephalon* brain)
			enterotomy (*enteron* intestine)
			episiotomy (an incision of the perineum, often performed during childbirth to prevent injury to the vagina) (*episeion* pubic region)
			esophagotomy (esophagus)
			gastrotomy (*gaster* belly, stomach)
			herniotomy (also called *celotomy, kelotomy*) (hernia)
			histotomy (also called *microtomy*) (*histos* web, tissue)
			hymenotomy (*hymen* membrane)
			lithotomy (*lithos* stone)
			meatotomy (also called *porotomy*) (*meatus* passage)
			myelotomy (*myelos* spinal cord)
			myotomy (*myos* muscle)
			myringotomy (*myringa* membrane)
			necrotomy (also called *dissection*) (*nekros* death)
			nephrotomy (*nephros* kidney)
			odontotomy (*odontos* tooth)
			omentotomy (*omentum* fat skin)
			omphalotomy (*omphalos* navel, umbilicus)
			onychotomy (*onyx* nail)
			oncotomy (the incision of a tumor, abscess, or swelling) (*onkos* mass)
			ophthalmotomy (*ophthalmos* eye)
			orbitotomy (*orbit* eye socket)
			orchiotomy (or, orchidotomy) (*orchis* testicle)
			osteotomy (*osteon* bone)
			ototomy (*otos* ear)
			ovariotomy (ovary)
			pelviotomy (pelvis)
			pericardiotomy (pericardium)
			perineotomy (perineum)
			periosteotomy (periosteum)
			peritoneotomy (peritoneum)
			phallotomy (*phallos* penis)
			pharyngotomy (pharynx)
			phlebotomy (*phlebos* vein)
			pneumonotomy (*pneumon* lung)
			porotomy also called *meatotomy*) (*poros* pore)
			proctotomy (also called *rectotomy*) (*proktos* anus, rectum)
			pubiotomy (severance of the pubic bone a few centimeters lateral to the symphysis to facilitate childbirth) (pubis bone)
			pyelotomy (*pyelos* pelvis)
			pylorotomy (pyloros)
			radicotomy (also called *rhizotomy*) (*radix* root)
			rectotomy (also called *proctotomy*) (rectum)
			rhinotomy (*rhinos* nose)
			rhizotomy (also called *radicotomy*) (*rhizos* root)
			sacrotomy (sacrum)

Element	From	Meaning	Examples
tom (cont'd)		[to cut]	sclerotomy (*skleros* hard—sclera of the eye)
			septotomy (*septum* wall, partition)
			splanchnicotomy (*splanchnos* viscus)
			splenotomy (spleen)
			spondylotomy (*spondylos* vertebra)
			staphylotomy (*staphyle* uvula)
			sternotomy (*sternon* chest)
			syndesmotomy (*syndesis* bound together—ligament)
			tarsotomy (also called *blepharotomy*) (*tarsus* eyelid)
			tenotomy (*tenon* sinew, tendon)
			thalamotomy (also called *thalamectomy*) (thalamus)
			thoracotomy (*thorax* chest)
			thyrotomy (thyroid gland)
			tonsillotomy (tonsil)
			trachelotomy (also called *cervicotomy*) (*trachelos* neck)
			tympanotomy (also called *tympanocentesis, myringotomy*) (*tympanon* eardrum)
			typhlotomy (also called *cecotomy*) (*typhlon* cecum: blind gut)
			[1]ulotomy (*oulon* gums)
			[2]ulotomy (*oule* scar, cicatrix)
			ureterotomy (ureter)
			uterotomy (uterus)
			vaginotomy (vagina)
			vagotomy (*vagus* wandering nerve)
			varicotomy (*varix* varicose vein)
			vasotomy (also called *vasopuncture, vasostomy*) (*vas* vessel)
			venotomy (*vena* vein)
			ventrotomy (*venter* abdomen, belly)
			vesicotomy (also called *cystotomy*) (*vesica* bladder)
			vestibulotomy (vestibule)
			viscerotomy (*viscera* internal organs)
			zonulotomy (*zona* zone: encircling region)
			ectomy excision—to surgically remove:
			abdominohysterectomy (also called *abdominal hysterectomy*)
			adenectomy (*adenos* gland)
			adipectomy (excision of fat or adipose tissue, usually a large quantity; also called *lipectomy*) (*adeps* fat)
			adrenalectomy (also called *suprarenalectomy*) (adrenal gland)
			alveolectomy (*alveus* hollow: saclike structure)
			aneurysmectomy (aneurysm)
			angiectomy (*angeion* blood vessel)
			antrectomy (Greek *antron* cave; Latin *antrum* cavity, chamber)
			appendectomy (appendix) [from *appendere* to hang to]
			arteriectomy (artery)
			arthrectomy (*arthron* joint)
			atherectomy (*athere* gruel)
			blepharectomy (*blepharon* eyelid)
			bursectomy (*bursa* sac)
			carpectomy (*karpos* wrist)
			cecectomy (*cecum* blind gut)
			celiectomy (*koilia* belly)
			ceratectomy (also called *keratectomy*) (*keratos* horn: cornea)
			cervicectomy (also called *trachelectomy*) (*cervix* neck—of uterus)
			cheilectomy (*cheilos* lip)

Element	From	Meaning	Examples
tom (cont'd)		[to cut]	chondrectomy (*chondros* cartilage)
			cicatrectomy (*cicatrix* scar)
			ciliectomy (*cilium* eyelash)
			clitoridectomy (clitoris)
			colectomy (colon)
			colpectomy (also called *vaginectomy*) (*kolpos* vagina)
			cordectomy (or, chordectomy) (*chorda* cord, usually vocal cord)
			corectomy (also called *iridectomy*) (*kore* pupil—of eye)
			corticectomy (also called *topectomy*) (*cortex* rind: external layer)
			costectomy (*costa* rib)
			craniectomy (*kranion* skull)
			cryptectomy (*kryptos* hidden: crypt)
			cyclectomy (*kyklos* circle: ciliary body)
			dacryoadenectomy (*dakryon* tear + *adenos* gland)
			diskectomy (or, discectomy) (disk of vertebra)
			duodenectomy (duodenum: part of the small intestine)
			embolectomy (*embolus* plug)
			embryectomy (embryo)
			enterectomy (*enteron* intestine)
			esophagectomy (esophagus)
			facetectomy (facet of a vertebra)
			fasciectomy (*fascia* band)
			frenectomy (*frenum* bridle: restraining structure)
			gangliectomy (*ganglion* knot)
			gastrectomy (also called *gastric resection*) (*gaster* stomach)
			gingivectomy (*gingivae* gums of the mouth)
			glomectomy (*glomus* ball)
			glossectomy (*glossa* tongue)
			gonadectomy (*gonad* ovary, testis)
			gyrectomy (*gyros* circle; cerebral gyrus, cerebral cortex)
			hepatectomy (*hepatos* liver)
			hysterectomy (*hystera* uterus)
			ileectomy (*ileum* distal portion of the small intestine)
			iridectomy (also called *corectomy*) (iris of eye)
			ischiectomy (*ischion* hip)
			keratectomy (or, kerectomy) (*keras* horn: cornea)
			laminectomy (*lamina* layer)
			laryngectomy (larynx)
			lipectomy (*lipos* fat)
			lithectomy (also called *lithotomy*) (*lithos* stone)
			lobectomy (lobe—of the thyroid, liver, brain, or lung)
			lumpectomy (*lump* mass)
			mammectomy (also called *mastectomy*) (*mamma* breast)
			maxillectomy (*maxilla* upper jaw)
			medullectomy (*medulla* marrow: interior portion of an organ)
			membranectomy (membrane)
			meniscectomy (*meniskos* crescent, as in the knee joint)
			myringectomy (also called *tympanectomy*) (*myringa* membrane)
			necrectomy (*nekros* death: corpse)
			nephrectomy (*nephros* kidney)
			neurectomy (*neuron* nerve)
			odontectomy (tooth extraction) (*odontos* tooth)
			omentectomy (*omentum* fat skin)
			omphalectomy (*omphalos* umbilicus)

A Thesaurus of Medical Word Roots

Element	From	Meaning	Examples
tom (cont'd)		[to cut]	onychectomy (*onychos* nail)
			oophorectomy (also called *ovariectomy*) (*oophoros* ovary)
			ophthalmectomy (*ophthalmos* eye)
			orchiectomy (or, orchidectomy) (*orchis* testicle, testis)
			ostectomy (or, osteoectomy) (*osteon* bone)
			oulectomy[1] (*oulon* gingivae—gums of the mouth)
			oulectomy[2] (*oule* scar)
			ovariectomy (also called *oophorectomy*) (ovary)
			pancreatectomy (also called *pancreectomy*) (pancreas)
			penectomy (also called *phallectomy*) (penis)
			pericardiectomy (pericardium)
			phallectomy (also called *penectomy*) (*phallos* penis)
			pharyngectomy (pharynx)
			phlebectomy (*phlebos* vein)
			phrenectomy (*phrenos* diaphragm)
			pituitectomy (also called *hypophysectomy*) (*pituita* phlegm)
			pleurectomy (*pleura* rib, side)
			pneumonectomy (*pneumon* lung)
			polypectomy (polyp)
			proctectomy (*proktos* anus)
			prostatectomy (prostate)
			pulmonectomy (also called *pneumonectomy*) (*pulmon* lung)
			pulpectomy (also called *root canal therapy*) (pulp—of tooth)
			pylorectomy (*pyle* gate: *pylorus* distal portion of the stomach)
			radectomy (also called *root amputation*) (*radix* root)
			rectectomy (also called *proctectomy*) (rectum)
			sacrectomy (sacrum)
			salpingectomy (also called *tubectomy*) (*salpingos* tube)
			saphenectomy (*saphenes* manifest: a type of vein)
			scalenectomy (*scalenus* uneven: scalenus muscle)
			scapulectomy (*scapula* shoulder blade)
			sclerectomy (*skleros* hard; sclera, the tough coat of the eyeball)
			scrotectomy (*scrotum* bag: testicle pouch)
			septectomy (*septum* wall, partition)
			sigmoidectomy (sigmoid flexure)
			sphincterectomy (*sphingein* to draw tight: sphincter)
			splanchnicectomy (*splanchnos* viscus)
			splenectomy (*splen* spleen)
			staphylectomy (also called *uvulectomy*) (*staphyle* uvula)
			syndesmectomy (*syndesis* bound together: ligament)
			[1]tarsectomy (excision of the tarsus of the foot)
			[2]tarsectomy (excision of all or part of an eyelid)
			tenectomy, tenonectomy (tendon)
			testectomy (also called *orchiectomy*) (testis, testicle)
			thalamectomy (also called *thalamotomy*) (*thalamus* inner chamber)
			thoracectomy (*thorax* chest)
			thrombectomy (*thrombos* clot)
			thymectomy (thymus)
			tonsillectomy (tonsils)
			topectomy (also called *corticectomy*) (*topos* place)
			uterectomy (also called *hysterectomy*) (uterus)
			vasectomy (also called *vasoresection*) (*vas* vas deferens)
			vertebrectomy (vertebra)
			CROSS REFERENCE: sex

Element	From	Meaning	Examples
ton	Greek *tonos;* Latin *tonus* from Greek *teinein* to stretch; yields *tetatnus*	tone, tension	SIMPLE ROOT: tone (the normal degree of vigor and tension) {tonic}, tonicity, tonus (body or muscular tone) PREFIXED ROOT: *toneum*: peritoneum (*peri* around) [see separate entry: periton-] *tonia*: atonia (or, atony) {atonic} (*a* privative) catatonia (a phase of schizophrenia in which the patient is unresponsive) {catatonic} (*kata* down) dystonia {dystonic} (*dys* abnormal) hemidystonia (*hemi* half + dystonia) hemihypertonia (also called *hemitonia*) (*hemi* half + hypertonia) hemihypotonia (*hemi* half + hypotonia) hemitonia (also called *hemihypertonia*) (*hemi* half) heterotonia (a state of abnormality or variation in tension or tone) {heterotonic} (*heteros* other) hypertonia (a condition of excessive tone, tension, or activity; compare *hypertension*) {hypertonic} (*hyper* above) hypotonia {hypotonic}, hypotonicity (*hypo* under) isotonia (a condition of equal tone, tension, or activity) {isotonic}, isotonicity (*isos* equal) paratonia (counterpressure; also called German *gegenhalten*) semihypertonia (*semi* half + hypertonia) *tonic*: anisotonic (*aniso* unequal: *an* negative + *isos* equal) antitonic (diminishing tone or tonicity) (*anti* against) entonic (having great tension, or exaggerated action) (*en* in) epitonic (*epi* upon) eutonic (also called *normotonic*) (*eu* well) homotonic (*homos* same) hyperisotonic (also called *hypertonic*) (*hyper* beyond + isotonic) hypoisotonic (less than isotonic) (*hypo* under + isotonic) syntonic (describing the stable type of personality which responds normally to the environment, as contrasted with the schizoid type) (*syn* with, together) *tono*: microtonometer (*mikros* small + *metron* measure) *tonos*: emprosthotonos (*emprosthen* forward) *tony*: atony (or, atonia, atonicity) {atonic} (*a* privative) amphotony (hyperexcitability of both the sympathetic and parasympathetic nervous systems) (*ampho* both) LEADING ROOT COMPOUND: *ton*: tonaphasia (inability to recall a familiar tune; musical aphasia; also called *amusia*) (aphasia: *a* privative + *phanein* to appear) tonoscillograph (*oscillein* to swing + *graphein* to write) *tonico*: tonicoclonic (or, tonoclonic) (*klonos* tumult) *tono*: tonoclonic (or, tonicoclonic; both tonic and clonic, said of muscular spasms) (*klonos* tumult) tonofilament (*filum* thread) tonogram, tonograph, tonography (*graphein* to write) tonometer, tonometry (*metron* measure) tonophant (an instrument for visualizing sound waves) (*phanein* to appear)

Element	From	Meaning	Examples
ton (cont'd)		[tension]	tonoplast (*plassein* to form)
			tonotopic {tonotopicity} (*topikos* place)
			tonotropic (*tropein* to turn)
			TRAILING ROOT COMPOUND:
			tonia:
			acromyotonia (contracture of the hand or foot resulting in spastic deformity) (*akros* extremities + *myos* muscle)
			angiotonia (also called *vasotonia*) {angiotonic; also called *vasotonic*} (*angeion* blood vessel)
			antrotonia (tonus of the muscular walls of an antrum, such as that of the stomach) (*antrum* chamber)
			cerebrotonia (*cerebrum* brain)
			myotonia {myotonic}, myotonus, myotony (*myos* muscle)
			pupillotonia (pupil of eye)
			somatotonia (*somatos* body)
			vagotonia {vagotonic} (*vagus* wandering nerve)
			vasotonia (also called *angiotonia*) {vasotonic} (*vas* vessel)
			viscerotonia (*viscera* internal organs)
			tonic:
			auxotonic (contracting against increasing resistance) (*auxein* to increase)
			cardiotonic (relating to or having a favorable effect upon the action of the heart) (*kardia* heart)
			normotonic (also called *normotensive, eutonic*) (*norma* normal)
			uterotonic (increasing the tone of the uterine muscle; an agent that so acts) (*uterus*)
			tonin: serotonin (a chemical produced by the brain that functions as a neurotransmitter) (*serum* whey)
			tono: aerotonometer (an instrument for estimating the tension or pressure of a gas) (*aer* air + *metron* measure)
			tonos:
			opisthotonos (a tetanic spasm in which the head and feet are drawn backward and the spine arches forward) (*episthen* behind)
			orthotonos (a form of tetanic spasm in which the neck, limbs, and body are held fixed in a straight line, resulting from strychnine poisoning or tetanus infection) (*orthos* straight)
			tonus: electrotonus (the modified condition of a nerve, when a constant current of electricity passes through any part of it)
			tony:
			arteriotony (blood pressure) (artery)
			myodystony (a condition of slow relaxation interrupted by a succession of slight contractions following electrical stimulation of a muscle) (*myos* muscle + *dys* abnormal)
			orthoarteriotony (normal arterial pressure) (*orthos* right + artery)
			PREFIXED TRAILING ROOT COMPOUND:
			myotonia muscle tone condition:
			amyotonia (also called *myatonia*) (*a* privative)
			dysmyotonia (also called *dystonia*) (*dys* abnormal)
			hypermyotonia (*hyper* above)
			paramyotonia (*para* alongside)
			tonus: anelectrotonus (*ana* up + *electro* shining)
			tony: dysarteriotony (abnormal blood pressure) (*dys* abnormal + artery)
			CROSS REFERENCE: ten[1], ten[2]

Element	From	Meaning	Examples
tonsil	Latin *tonsilla*	tonsil	SIMPLE ROOT: tonsil (either of a pair of oval masses of lymphoid tissue, one on each side of the throat at the back of the mouth) tonsilla (also called *palatine tonsil*; pl., tonsillae) {tonsillar} PREFIXED ROOT: infratonsillar (*infra* below) intratonsillar (*intra* within) peritonsillar, peritonsillitis (*peri* around + *itis* inflammation) supratonsillar (*supra* above) LEADING ROOT COMPOUND: *tonsil*: tonsillith (or, tonsillolith, tonsolith) (*lithos* stone) *tonsill*: tonsillectomy (*ektome* excision) tonsillitis {tonsillitic} (*itis* inflammation) *tonsillo*: tonsillolith (or, tonsolith) (*lithos* stone) tonsillomycosis (also called *mycotic tonsillitis*) (*mykes* fungus + *osis* condition) tonsillopathy (*pathos* disease) tonsillopharyngitis (*pharynx* throat + *itis* inflammation) tonsillotome (also called *guillotine*), tonsillotomy (*tomy* incision) TRAILING ROOT COMPOUND: pharyngotonsillitis (pharynx + *itis* inflammation) CROSS REFERENCE: amygdal
top	Greek *topos*	place	SIMPLE ROOT: topica (remedies for local external use) topic {topical}, topistic PREFIXED ROOT: *top*: autotopagnosia (*autos* self + *a* privative + *gnosis* knowledge) *tope*: epitope (*epi* upon) isotope (*isos* equal) paratope (*para* alongside) *topia*: allotopia (also called *dystopia*) (*allos* other) dystopia (abnormal or anomalous position of an organ or part; also called *allotopia*, *malposition*) {dystopic} (*dys* abnormal) ectopia (*ek* out) [see separate entry: ectop-] heterotopia (or, heterotopy; also called *malposition, ectopia, choristoma*) {heterotopic} (*heteros* other) *topic*: atopic (displaced; also called *ectopic*) (*a* negative) entopic (occurring in the proper place; opposed to *ectopic*) (*en* in) eutopic (situated normally) (*eu* well) heterotopic (*heteros* different) homotopic (relating to or occurring in the same or corresponding place or part of the body) (*homos* same) isotopic (*isos* equal) *topism*: anatopism (a mental condition in which patients fail to conform to the customs of the social group to which they belong; also called *ectopism*) (*ana* again) *topo*: atopognosia (or, atopognosis; loss of power of correctly locating a sensation) (agnosia: *a* privative + *gnosis* knowledge) *topous*: heterotopous (*heteros* different)

Element	From	Meaning	Examples
top (cont'd)		[place]	*topy*: atopy (an allergy for which there was a genetic disposition; also called *atopic allergy*) (*a* uncertain meaning) holotopy (*holos* whole) syntopy (the position of an organ relative to other organs) (*syn* together) LEADING ROOT COMPOUND: *top*: topagnosia (or, topagnosis; also called *atopognosia*) (agnosia: *a* privative + *gnosis* knowledge) topalgia (localized pain: seen in neurasthenia) (*algos* pain) topanesthesia (also called *topagnosis*) (anesthesia: *an* privative + *esthesia* feeling) topectomy (*ektome* excision) topesthesia (also called *topognosis*) (*esthesia* feeling) toponym (the name of a region as distinguished from an organ), toponymy (terminology pertaining to the position and direction of organs and parts) (*onyma* name) *topo*: topoanesthesia (also called *atopognosia*) (anesthesia: *an* privative + *esthesia* feeling) topognosis (or, topognosia; recognition of the location of tactile sensation; also called *topesthesia*) (*gnosis* knowledge) topogometer (*gonia* angle + *metron* measure) topographic, topography {topographical} (*graphein* to write) topology (the relation between the presenting part of the fetus and the birth canal) {topological} (*logos* study) toponarcosis (localized cutaneous anesthesia) (*narkoun* to benumb + *osis* condition) topophylaxis (*phylaxis* protection) TRAILING ROOT COMPOUND: biotope (*bios* life) idiotope (*idios* one's own) nomotopic (occurring normally) (*nomos* custom, law) normotopia {normotopic} (*norma* rule: normal) orthotopic (*orthos* straight) planotopokinesia (*planan* to wander + *kinein* to move) somatotopic (*somatos* body) tonotopic (*tonos* tension) CROSS REFERENCE: loc
torq, **tors,** **tort**	Latin *torquere*	to twist	SIMPLE ROOT: *torq*: torque (a rotary force; the rotation of a tooth on its long axis), torquing (the twisting of a tooth into position) *tors*: torsion, torsive, torso (a twisted column; the main part of the body, to which the head and limbs are attached) *tort*: tortua (agony), tortuous (twisted; full of turns and twists) PREFIXED ROOT: *tors*: abtorsion (also called *extorsion*) (*ab* away) adtorsion (conclination: inward rotation of the pole of the vertical meridian of each eye; also called *intorsion*) (*ad* to) detorsion (the correction of a curvature or deformity) (*de* reversal) extorsion (rotation of an organ or limb; also called *abtorsion, disclination*) (*ex* out)

Element	From	Meaning	Examples
torq (cont'd)		[to twist]	intorsion (also called *adtorsion, conclination*) (*in* toward)
			retrotorsion (*retro* backward)
			tort:
			distortion, distortor (*dis* apart)
			extortor (*ex* outward)
			intortor (also called *medial rotator*) (*in* in)
			LEADING ROOT COMPOUND:
			torsi: torsiversion (*vertere* to turn)
			torsiono: torsionometer (*metron* measure)
			torti:
			torticollis (also called *wry neck*) {torticollar} (*collum* neck)
			tortipelvis (*pelvis* basin)
			TRAILING ROOT COMPOUND:
			acutorsion (the twisting of an artery with a needle to arrest a hemor-rhage) (*acus* needle)
			dextrotorsion (also called *dextroclination*) (*dexter* right)
			laterotorsion (*lateris* side)
			levotorsion (also called *levoclination*) (*laevus* left)
			sinistrotorsion (a twisting toward the left; said mainly of the eye) (*sinister* left)
			tubatorsion (torsion or twisting of the uterine tube) (*tubus* tube)
			tubotorsion (a twisting of a tube, especially of the auditory tube) (*tubus* tube)
			CROSS REFERENCE: scol, stroph
tox	Greek *toxikon*	poison	SIMPLE ROOT: toxicant, toxication (poisoning), toxicity, toxin {toxinic; also called *poisonous, venomous*}, toxon (or, toxone)
			PREFIXED ROOT:
			tox: intoxation (poisoning), intoxicant, intoxication (*in* in)
			toxemia toxic blood condition
			autotoxemia (*autos* self)
			endotoxemia (*endon* within)
			toxic:
			atoxic (not poisonous; not due to poison) (*a* negative)
			autotoxic (*autos* self)
			endotoxic (*endon* within)
			exotoxic (*exo* outside)
			hypertoxic (*hyper* over, above)
			toxicity:
			hypertoxicity (*hyper* over, above)
			hypotoxicity (*hypo* under)
			toxicate: detoxicate (or, detoxify) (*de* negative)
			toxicosis toxic condition:
			autotoxicosis (*autos* self)
			endotoxicosis (*endon* within)
			toxify: detoxify (or, detoxicate) (*de* negative + *facere* to make)
			toxin:
			allotoxin (any substance formed by tissue change within the body which serves as a defense against toxins by neutralizing their poi-sonous properties) (*allos* other)
			anatoxin (also called *toxoid*) {anatoxic} (*ana* again)
			antitoxin (antibody to the toxin of a microorganism, usually the bac-terial exotoxins, that combines specifically with the toxin, in vivo and in vitro, with neutralization of toxicity) {antitoxic} (*anti* against)

Element	From	Meaning	Examples
tox (cont'd)		[poison]	autotoxin (also called *autointoxicant*) (*autos* self)
			endotoxin (a heat-stable toxin present in the bacterial cell but not in cell-free filtrates of cultures of intact bacteria) (*endon* within)
			exotoxin (or, ectotoxin) (*exo* outside)
			hemiantitoxin (*hemi* half + antitoxin)
			hemitoxin (*hemi* half)
			isotoxin {isotoxic} (*isos* equal)
			toxoid: epitoxoid (*epi* upon + *eidos* form)
			LEADING ROOT COMPOUND:
			tox:
			toxanemia (also called *toxic hemolytic anemia*) (anemia: *an* privative + *emia* blood condition)
			toxemia (or, toxicemia) {toxemic} (*emia* blood condition)
			toxoid (*eidos* form)
			toxi:
			toxicide (*caedere* to kill)
			toxidrome (the constellation of symptoms and signs resulting from any given poison) (*dromos* a course)
			toxiferous (also called *toxicogenic*) (*ferre* to bear)
			toxigenic (also called *toxiferous*), toxigenicity (*genere* to produce)
			toxignomic (*gnome* a means of knowing)
			toxipathy (also called *toxicosis*) (*pathos* disease)
			toxiphobia (or, toxicophobia) (*phobia* fear)
			toxic:
			toxicoid (*eidos* form)
			toxicyst (*kystis* sac)
			toxicophidia (venomous snakes) (*ophis* snake)
			toxicosis (any disease of toxic origin; also called *toxipathy, system poisoning*) (*osis* condition)
			toxico:
			toxicodermatitis (*derma* skin + *itis* inflammation)
			toxicodermatosis (or, toxicoderma) (*derma* skin + *osis* condition)
			toxicogenic (*genere* to produce)
			toxicohemia (also called *toxemia*) (*hemia* blood condition)
			toxicokinetics (*kinein* to move)
			toxicology {toxicologic} (*logos* study)
			toxicomania (the addiction to a drug) (*mania* craze, madness)
			toxicopathy {toxicopathic} (*pathos* disease)
			toxicopexis (or, toxicopexy) {toxicopectic, toxicopexic} (*pexis* fixation)
			toxicophobia (or, toxiphobia) (*phobia* fear)
			toxin:
			toxinemia (*emia* blood condition)
			toxinosis (or, toxonosis; any disease condition due to the presence of a toxin) (*osis* condition)
			toxino:
			toxinogenic, toxinogenicity (*genere* to produce)
			toxinology (*logos* study)
			toxo:
			toxogen (*genere* to produce)
			toxoglobulin (*globus* ball, sphere)
			toxophil {toxophilic, toxophilous} (*philein* to love)
			toxophore {toxophorous} (*pherein* to bear)
			toxoplasma, toxoplasmosis (*plassein* to form + *osis* condition)

Element	From	Meaning	Examples
tox (cont'd)		[poison]	TRAILING ROOT COMPOUND: *toxemia* condition of toxins in the blood: actinotoxemia (*aktinos* ray) enterotoxemia (*enteron* intestines) gonotoxemia (*gone* seed) hepatotoxemia (*hepatos* liver) radiotoxemia (radium) *toxic*: bacteriotoxic (bacteria) cardiotoxic (*kardia* heart) fungitoxic, fungitoxicity (fungus) genotoxic (*genere* to produce: genes) hemotoxic (or, hematotoxic) (*haima* blood) hepatotoxic, hepatotoxicity (*hepatos* liver) histotoxic (*histos* web, tissue) ichthyotoxic (*ichthys* fish) leukotoxic (*leukos* white: white blood cells) myelotoxic (*myelos* marrow) nephrotoxic {nephrotoxicity} (*nephros* kidney) neurotoxic {neurotoxicity} (*neuron* nerve) ototoxic {ototoxicity} (*otos* ear) phacotoxic (*phakos* lens of eye) phototoxic {phototoxicity} (*photos* light) phytotoxic (*phyton* plant) vasculotoxic (*vascule* small vessel) *toxin*: apitoxin (*apis* bee) biotoxin (*bios* life) ichthyotoxin (*ichthys* fish) mycotoxin {mycotoxinization} (*mykes* fungus) immunotoxin (immune system) serotoxin (*serum* whey) sitotoxin (*sitos* food) spermatotoxin (or, spermatoxin, spermotoxin) (*spermatos* seed) splenotoxin (spleen) thymotoxin (thymus) trichotoxin (*trichos* hair) CROSS REFERENCE: vir
trache	Greek orig., *tracheia arteria* rough windpipe	trachea, windpipe	SIMPLE ROOT: trachea (pl., tracheae) {tracheal}, tracheole PREFIXED ROOT: endotracheal (*endon* within) extratracheal (*extra* outside) infratracheal (*infra* below) intratracheal (*intra* within) paratracheal (*para* alongside) peritracheal (*peri* around) pretracheal (*pre* before) transtracheal (*trans* across, through) LEADING ROOT COMPOUND: *trache*: trachealgia (*algos* pain) tracheitis (or, trachitis) (*itis* inflammation) *tracheo*: tracheoaerocele (*aer* air + *kele* hernia)

Element	From	Meaning	Examples
trache (cont'd)		[trachea, windpipe]	tracheobiliary (relating to the trachea or bronchi and the biliary duct system) tracheobroncheal, tracheobronchitis (*bronchos* windpipe + *itis* inflammation) tracheobronchomegaly (*bronchos* windpipe + *megalos* large) tracheobronchoscopy (*bronchos* windpipe + *skopein* to examine) tracheocele (*kele* hernia) tracheoesophageal (also called *esophagotracheal*) (esophagus) tracheofistulization (*fistula* pipe, passage) tracheogenic (*genere* to produce) tracheolaryngeal (also called *laryngotracheal*) (larynx) tracheomalacia (*malakos* soft) tracheomegaly (*megalos* large) tracheopathia (or, tracheopathy) (*pathos* disease) tracheopharyngeal (pharynx) tracheophonesis, tracheophony (*phone* sound: voice) tracheoplasty (*plassein* to form) tracheopyosis (*pyon* pus + *osis* condition) tracheorrhagia (*rhagia* hemorrhage) tracheorrhaphy (*rhaphe* suture) tracheoschisis (*schisis* fissure) tracheoscopy {tracheoscopic} (*skopein* to examine) tracheostenosis (*stenosis* narrowing) tracheostoma, tracheostomy (*stoma* mouth, opening) tracheotome, tracheotomy (*tomy* incision) TRAILING ROOT COMPOUND: bronchotracheal (*bronchos* windpipe) esophagotracheal (also called *tracheoesophageal*) (esophagus) laryngotracheal (larynx) nasotracheal (*nasus* nose) orotracheal (*oris* mouth) sternotracheal (*sternon* chest) CROSS REFERENCE: bronch, laryn
trachel	Greek *trachelos*	neck; neck of an organ	SIMPLE ROOT: trachelism (or, trachelismus) PREFIXED ROOT: endotrachelitis (also called *endocervicitis*) (*endon* within + *itis* inflammation) LEADING ROOT COMPOUND: *trachel*: trachelagra (*agra* seizure) trachelectomy (also called *cervicectomy*) (*ektome* excision) trachelematoma (*hematos* blood + *oma* tumor) [h of hematos elided] trachelitis (also called *cervicitis*) (*itis* inflammation) trachelodynia (called *cervicodynia*) (*odyne* pain) *trachelo*: trachelocyllosis (also called *torticollis*) (*kyllosis* crooking) trachelocyrtosis (also called *trachelokyphosis*) (*kyrtos* curved) trachelocystitis (also called *cystitis colli*) (*kystis* sac, bladder + *itis* inflammation) trachelology (*logos* study) trachelopanus (swelling of the lymphatic vessels of the neck) (*panus* tumor, swelling) trachelopexy (or, trachelopexia; also called *cervicopexy*) (*pexis* fixation) trachelophyma (*phyma* tumor, growth)

Element	From	Meaning	Examples
trachel (cont'd)		[neck]	tracheloplasty (*plassein* to form) trachelorrhaphy (*rhaphe* suture) tracheloschisis (*schisis* fissure) trachelotomy (also called *cervicotomy*) (*tomy* incision) TRAILING ROOT COMPOUND: hematotrachelos (*hematos* blood) rhinotracheitis (*rhinos* nose + *itis* inflammation) schistotrachelus (*schistos* split) CROSS REFERENCE: cervi
trans-	Latin prefix	through, across	See Appendix B for examples of words with this prefix. Others are listed with the root to which it is attached. CROSS REFERENCE: dia-

trauma	Greek
	trauma
		wound, hurt	SIMPLE ROOT: trauma (injury; psychological or emotional dam-
			   age; pl., traumas, traumata) {traumatic}, traumatism, traumatize
			PREFIXED ROOT:
			atraumatic (not producing injury or damage) (*a* negative)
			microtrauma (a very slight injury or lesion; a microscopic lesion or
			   injury) (*mikros* small)
			polytrauma (*polys* many)
			posttraumatic (*post* after)
			LEADING ROOT COMPOUND:
			trauma:
			traumatherapy (or, traumatotherapy) (*therapy* treatment)
			traumatropism (*trepein* to turn)
			traumat: traumatosis (or, traumatism) (*osis* condition)
			traumato:
			traumatogenic (*genere* to produce)
			traumatology (*logos* study)
			traumatonesis (*neis* spinning)
			traumatopathy (*pathos* disease)
			traumatophilia (*philein* to love)
			traumatopnea (*pnein* to breathe)
			traumatosepsis (*sepsis* putrefaction)
			traumatotherapy (*therapy* treatment)
			TRAILING ROOT COMPOUND:
			barotrauma (*baros* weight, pressure)
			neurotrauma (*neuron* nerve)
			volutrauma (volume)
			CROSS REFERENCE: None

treph			See troph- for *trephocyte*.

tres	Greek
	tresis
		hole,
		perforation
			SIMPLE ROOT: tresis (also called *perforation*)
			PREFIXED ROOT: atresia (congenital absence or closure of a
			   normal body opening or tubular structure; also called *clausura*)
			   (*a* privative) [see separate entry: atres-]
			CROSS REFERENCE: ethm, for

tri-
tripl-
	Greek
	and Latin
	tri three +
	Latin
	plicare
	to fold
		three;
		threefold
			SIMPLE ROOT:
			tri: triad (any three things having something in common)
			tripl: triplet, triplex (threefold)
			See Appendix B for examples of words with these prefixes. Others
			   are listed with the root to which they are attached.
			FRENCH: trocar (a sharply pointed surgical instrument contained in
			   a metal cannula and used for aspiration or removal of fluids from
			   cavities) [*trois carre* three sides]

A Thesaurus of Medical Word Roots

Element	From	Meaning	Examples
tri- (cont'd)		[three]	NB: *Triage*, from French *trier*, and from which *try* and *trial* are derived, is not in this family; pronounced tree AHZH, *triage* originally designated a system of assigning priorities of medical treatment to battlefield casualties on the basis of urgency, chance for survival, etc. It is now a general term. CROSS REFERENCE: None
trib, **trig**, **trip**, **trit**	Greek *tribein* to rub	to rub, crush; friction	SIMPLE ROOT: *trib*: tribadism (lesbianism; a relationship in which women attempt to imitate heterosexual intercourse with each other) *trip*: tripsis (also called *trituration*; *massage*) *trit*: triturate (to rub into a powder) {triturable}, trituration PREFIXED ROOT: *trigo*: intertrigo (irritant dermatitis) {intertriginous} (*inter* between) *tripsis*: anatripsis (therapeutic rubbing or friction) {anatriptic} (*ana* again) paratripsis (chafing) (*para* beside) syntripsis (also called *comminuted fracture*) (*syn* with) *trition*: attrition (the physiologic wearing away of a substance or structure in the course of normal use) (*ad* to) detrition (a wearing away, as of the teeth, by friction) (*de* away) LEADING ROOT COMPOUND: tribology (the study of the lubrication, friction, and wear of the joints) (*logos* study) triboluminescence (luminosity produced by friction) TRAILING ROOT COMPOUND: *trib*: angiotribe (*angeion* blood vessel) osteotribe (or, osteotrite; an instrument for crushing off bits of necrosed or carious bone) (*osteon* bone) splanchnotribe (an instrument used for occluding the intestine temporarily prior to resection) (*splanchnos* viscus) *tripsis*: odontotripsis (wearing away the teeth) (*odontos* tooth) ulotripsis (*oulon* gums) xerotripsis (dry friction) (*xeros* dry) *tripsy*: cholelithotripsy (or, cholelithotrity; the crushing of gallstones) (*chole* bile + *lithos* stone) cysticolithotripsy (*kystis* bladder + *lithos* stone) lithotripsy (crushing of a calculus in the bladder or urethra) (*lithos* stone) neurotripsy (*neuron* nerve) omphalotripsy (crushing, instead of cutting, the umbilical cord after childbirth) (*omphalos* navel) phrenicotripsy (also called *phreniclasia*) (phrenic nerve) *trite*: osteotrite (or, osteotribe; an instrument for grinding away carious bone) (*osteon* bone) CROSS REFERENCE: None
trich, **thrix**, **trix**	Greek *thrix*, *trichos*	hair, cilia	SIMPLE ROOT: trichion (an anthropometric landmark, the point at which the midsagittal plane of the head intersects the hairline) trichite (also called *trichocyst*) trichoma (also called *entropion, blepharelosis, enstrophe*)

Element	From	Meaning	Examples
trich (cont'd)		[hair]	PREFIXED ROOT: *trich*: atrichia (absence of hair; also called *alopecia*) (*a* privative) amphitrichate (or, amphitrichous; having a single flagellum at each end: applied to a bacterial cell) (*amphi* around, both) districhiasis (a condition in which two hairs grow from a single follicle) (*dis* twice + *iasis* condition) epitrichium (superficial layers of the epidermis of the fetus; also called *periderm*) (*epi* upon) eutrichosis (*eu* well + *osis* condition) heterotrichosis (growth of hair of different colors on the body) (*heteros* other + *osis* condition) holotrichous (covered uniformly with cilia) (*holos* whole) hypertrichosis (or, hypertrichiasis; also called *polytrichia, polytrichosis, trichauxis*) (*hyper* over + *osis* condition) hypotrichosis (*hypo* under + *osis* condition) Isotricha (a genus of ciliate protozoa) (*isos* equal) monotrichous (having a single polar flagellum: applied to a bacterial cell) (*monos* single) paratrichosis (*para* abnormal + *osis* condition) peritrichous (or, peritrichate, peritrichic; having flagella over the entire surface: said of a bacterial cell) (*peri* around) polytrichia (or, polytrichosis; also called *hypertrichosis*) (*polys* much) *thrix*: ectothrix (a sheath of spores on the outside of a hair) (*ektos* outside) endothrix (*endon* within) *trix*: distrix (splitting of the hairs at their ends) (*dis* double, twice) LEADING ROOT COMPOUND: *trich*: trichalgia (also called *trichodynia*) (*algos* pain) trichatrophia (atrophy: *a* privative + *trephein* to nourish) trichauxis (excessive growth of the hair, in respect to both quantity and length; also called *hypertrichosis*) (*auxein* to increase) trichiasis (inversion of eyelashes so that they rub against the cornea, causing a continual irritation of the eyeball) (*iasis* condition) trichitis (inflammation of the hair bulbs) (*itis* inflammation) trichodynia (also called *trichalgia*) (*odyne* pain) trichoid (*eidos* form) trichoma, trichomatosis (both also called *trichiasis*) (*oma* tumor) trichosis (also called *trichopathy*) (*osis* condition) *trichi*: trichilemmoma (*lemma* husk + *oma* tumor) *tricho*: trichobacteria (bacteria possessing flagella) (*bakterion* rod) trichobezoar (a hair ball or concretion of hairs in the intestine or stomach) (Persian *pad-zahr* concretion) trichocardia (a hairy appearance upon the heart, due to exudative pericarditis) (*kardia* heart) trichochrome (*chroma* color) trichoclasia (or, trichoclasis: brittleness of the hair) (*klaein* to break) trichocryptosis (any disease of the hair follicles) (*kryptein* to hide + *osis* condition) trichocyst (a cell structure derived from the protoplasm) (*kystis* sac) trichodystrophy (*dys* abnormal + *trophein* to nourish)

Element	From	Meaning	Examples
trich (cont'd)		[hair]	trichoepithelioma (epithelioma)
			trichoesthesia (*esthesia* feeling)
			trichofolliculoma (follicle + *oma* tumor)
			trichogen (an agent stimulating hair growth) (*genere* to produce)
			trichoglossia (also called *hairy tongue*) (*glossa* tongue)
			tricholeukocyte (hairy cell) (*leukos* white + *kytos* cell)
			tricholith (a hairy concretion) (*lithos* stone)
			trichology (*logos* study)
			trichomegaly (congenital condition characterized by abnormally long eyelashes, associated with dwarfism) (*megalos* large)
			trichomycosis (also called *trichomycetosis*) (*mykes* fungus + *osis* condition)
			trichonodosis (a condition characterized by apparent or actual knotting of the hair) (*nodus* knot + *osis* condition)
			trichonosis (any diseased condition of the hair; also called *trichopathy*) (*nosos* disease)
			trichopathy (also called *trichonosis, trichosis*) (*pathos* disease)
			trichophagia (or, trichophagy; the habit of eating hair or wool) (*phagein* to devour, consume)
			trichophobia (morbid disgust caused by the sight of loose hairs on clothing or elsewhere) (*phobia* fear)
			trichophytosis (a fungal infection) (*phyton* growth + *osis* condition)
			trichopoliosis (also called *poliosis*) (*polios* gray + *osis* condition)
			trichoptilosis (a splitting of the shaft of the hair, giving it a feathery appearance) (*ptilon* feather + *osis* condition)
			trichorrhexis (*rhexis* fracture, break)
			trichoschisis (*schisis* fissure, split)
			trichoscopy (*skopein* to examine)
			trichosomatous (*soma* body)
			trichotillomania (a compulsion to pull one's own hair) (*tillein* to pull out + *mania* frenzy)
			trichotoxin (*toxin* poison)
			trichotrophy (nutrition of the hair) (*trophein* to nourish)
			TRAILING ROOT COMPOUND:
			trich:
			lissotrichous (*lissos* smooth)
			lophotrichous (having a tuft of flagella at one end: applied to a bacterial cell) (*lophos* ridge, tuft)
			melanotrichous (*melanos* dark)
			oligotrichia (congenital thinness of the growth of hair; also called *hypotrichosis*) (*oligos* little, scanty)
			schizotrichia (*schizein* to split)
			sporotrichosis (also called *Schenck's disease*) (*sporos* seed + *osis* condition)
			ulotrichous (*ulos* woolly)
			thrix:
			clastothrix (splitting of the hair) (*klaein* to break)
			monilethrix (a genetic defect of the hair shaft in which the hair becomes beaded and brittle) (*monile* necklace)
			sclerothrix (abnormal hardness and dryness of the hair) (*skleros* hard)
			CROSS REFERENCE: capill
tripsis			See trib-.
trit			See trib- for *attrition*.

Element	From	Meaning	Examples
trop	Greek *trepein* to turn	to turn, react	SIMPLE ROOT: tropia (a manifest deviation of an eye from the normal position), tropism

PREFIXED ROOT:

trope: antitrope (any organ which forms a symmetrical pair with another; antibody) {antitropic} (*anti* against)

tropia:

anatropia {anatropic} (*ana* again)

anotropia (*ano* upward)

esotropia (a condition in which only one eye fixes on an object while the other turns inward, producing the appearance of a cross-eye) {esotropic} (*eso* within, inward)

exotropia {exotropic} (*exo* outside)

heterotropia (or, heterotropy; strabismus; also called *manifest deviation, squint*) {heterotropic} (*heteros* other)

hypertropia (upward deviation of the visual axis of the eye) *hyper* above)

hypotropia (*hypo* under)

tropic:

allotropic (*allos* other)

anisotropic (*aniso* unequal: *an* negative + *isos* equal)

bitropic (having affinity for two issues or two organisms) (*bi* two)

homotropic (*homos* same)

isotropic (*isos* equal)

mesotropic (*mesos* middle)

monotropic (*monos* one, single)

pantropic (or, pantotropic; having an affinity for many tissues) (*pan* all)

pleiotropic (*pleon* more)

polytropic (*polys* many)

syntropic (*syn* with)

tropism:

allotropism (*allos* other)

homotropism (*homos* same)

pleiotropism (*pleon* more)

tropous: isotropous (or, isotropic) (*isos* equal)

tropy:

allotropy (*allos* other)

entropy (*en* in, inward)

isotropy (*isos* equal)

pleiotropy (or, pleiotropism) {pleiotropic} (*pleon* more)

syntropy (*syn* with, together)

LEADING ROOT COMPOUND: tropometer (*metron* measure)

TRAILING ROOT COMPOUND:

tropic:

adrenotropic (adrenal gland)

aerotropic (*aer* air)

arthrotropic (*arthron* joint)

bathmotropic (*bathmos* threshold)

chemotropic (*cheein* to pour—chemistry)

chromotropic (*chroma* color)

chronotropic (*chronos* time)

corticotropic (also called *adrenocorticotropic*) (*cortex* covering)

cytotropic (*kytos* cell)

dentotropic (*dens* tooth)

Element	From	Meaning	Examples
trop (cont'd)		[to turn]	dermotropic (having a selective affinity for the skin and mucous membranes) (*derma* skin)
			dextrotropic (opposed to *leotropic*) (*dexter* right)
			dromotropic (*dramein* to run: course)
			ecotropic (*oikos* house: environment)
			egotropic (*ego* I, self)
			enterotropic (*enteron* intestine)
			ergotropic (*ergon* work)
			glycotropic (*glykys* sweet)
			gonadotropic (*gone* seed: procreation)
			hematotropic (*hematos* blood)
			idiotropic (also called *introspective*; *egocentric*) (*idios* one's own)
			inotropic (*inos* fiber)
			leotropic (opposed to *dextrotropic*) (*laios* left)
			lipotropic (*lipos* fat)
			lyotropic (also called *lyophilic*) (*lyein* to dissolve)
			mammotropic (*mamma* breast, nipple)
			melanotropic (*melanos* black)
			myotropic (*myos* muscle)
			nephrotropic (also called *renotropic*) (*nephros* kidney)
			neurotropic (*neuron* nerve)
			nootropic (denotes an agent having an effect on memory) (*noos, nous* mind)
			nosotropic (*nosos* disease)
			oncotropic (*onkos* mass, tumor)
			organotropic (*organon* organ)
			orthotropic (*orthos* straight)
			phototropic (*photos* light)
			phrenotropic (*phrenos* mind)
			renotropic (also called *renotrophic, nephrotropic*) (*ren* kidney)
			stereotropic (*stereos* solid)
			thermotropic (also called *caloritropic*) (*therme* heat)
			thigmotropic (also called *stereotropic*) (*thigma* touch)
			thyrotropic (also called *thyrotrophic*) (thyroid gland)
			uterotropic (uterus)
			vagotropic (*vagus* wandering nerve)
			vasotropic (*vas* vessel: blood vessel)
			viscerotropic (*viscera* internal organs)
			xenotropic (*xenos* strange, foreign)
			tropism:
			cytotropism (*kytos* cell)
			hydrotropism (*hydor* water)
			lipotropism (*lipos* fat)
			pathotropism (*pathos* disease)
			phototropism (*photos* light)
			plasmotropism (plasma)
			rheotropism (also called *rheotaxis*) (*rhein* to flow)
			sitotropism (also called *sitotaxis*) (*sitos* food)
			stereotropism (also called *thigmotropism*) (*stereos* solid)
			thermotropism (*therme* heat)
			thigmotropism (also called *stereotropism*) (*thigma* touch)
			trophotropism (*trophein* to nourish)
			tropy: rhizodontropy (*rhiza* root + *odontos* tooth)
			CROSS REFERENCE: rhomb, spir

Element	From	Meaning	Examples
troph, **treph**, **trep**	Greek *trephein* to nourish *threpsis* nutrition	to nourish, nutrition	SIMPLE ROOT: trophic (nutritional), trophicity, trophism PREFIXED ROOT: *trep*: atrepsy (infantile atrophy; progressive wasting and emaciation; also called *marasmus*, *athrepsia*) (*a* privative) *troph*: autotroph (*autos* self) heterotroph (*heteros* different) metatroph (*meta* different, change) prototroph (*protos* first) *trophia*: atrophia (or, atrophy) {atrophic} (*a* privative) [see separate entry: atroph-] dystrophia (or, dystrophy) {dystrophic} (*dys* abnormal) [see separate entry: dystroph-] eutrophia (or, eutrophy) {eutrophic} (*eu* well, good) heterotrophia (or, heterotrophy) {heterotrophic} (*heteros* different) macrodystrophia (*makros* large + dystrophia) metatrophia (a change in diet) {metatrophic} (*meta* change) polytrophia (or, polytrophy; excessive nutrition) {polytrophic} (*polys* many, much) *trophic*: allotrophic (*allos* other) antatrophic (correcting or preventing atrophy) (*anti* against) autotrophic (*autos* self) ectotrophic (*ektos* outside) metatrophic (*meta* change) paratrophic (requiring living material or complex matter for food) (*para* alongside) *trophism*: syntrophism (also called *crossfeeding*) (*syn* with) *tropho*: dystrophoneurosis (*dys* abnormal + *neurosis* nerve condition) syntrophoblast (*syn* with + *blastos* bud, shoot, germ) *trophy*: cacotrophy (malnutrition; impaired or disordered nourishment) (*kakos* bad) hemidystrophy (*hemi* half + dystrophy) hemihypertrophy (*hemi* half + hypertrophy) hypertrophy (or, hypertrophia) {hypertrophic} (*hyper* above) hypotrophy (also called *abiotrophy*) (*hypo* under) panatrophy (or, pantatrophia) (*pan* all + atrophy) paratrophy (also called *dystrophy*) (*para* abnormal) polydystrophy {polydystrophic} (*polys* many + dystrophy) hemihypertrophy (*hemi* half + hypertrophy) LEADING ROOT COMPOUND: *treph*: trephocyte (or, trophocyte; a cell that furnishes nutrition to other cells) (*kytos* cell) *troph*: trophedema (or, trophoedema; permanent edema of the lower limbs or feet; also called *hereditary lymphedema*) (*edema* swelling) *tropho*: trophoblast {trophoblastic} (*blastos* bud, shoot, germ) trophocyte (or, trephocyte) (*kytos* cell) trophoderm (*derma* skin) trophodermatoneurosis (*dermatos* skin + neurosis)

Element	From	Meaning	Examples
troph (cont'd)		[to nourish]	trophodynamics (*dynamis* power)
			trophology (also called *nutriology*) (*logos* study)
			trophoneurosis {trophoneurotic} (*neuron* nerve + *osis* condition)
			trophonucleus (also called *macronucleus*) (*nucleus* kernel: core)
			trophopathy (or, trophopathia) (*pathos* disease)
			trophoplast (an elementary constructive unit, as a cell; also called *plastid*) (*plassein* to form)
			trophospongium (pl., trophospongia) (sponge)
			trophotaxis (also called *trophotropism*) (*taxis* arrangement)
			trophotherapy (diet therapy) (*therapy* treatment)
			trophotropism (also called *trophotaxis*) {trophotropic} (*trepein* to turn)
			TRAILING ROOT COMPOUND:
			troph:
			hemotroph (or, hemotrophe) {hemotrophic} (*haima* blood)
			histotroph {histotrophic} (*histos* web, tissue)
			lactotroph (*lactis* milk)
			phagotroph (a holozoic organism) {phagotrophic; also called *holozoic*} (*phagein* to devour, consume)
			somatotroph (*somatos* body)
			trophia:
			bradytrophia (*bradys* slow)
			oligotrophia (also called *malnutrition*) (*oligos* little, scant)
			osteodystrophia (*osteon* bone + dystrophia)
			trophic:
			angiotrophic (also called *vasotrophic*) (*angeion* blood vessel)
			bradytrophic (*bradys* slow)
			brephotrophic (*brephos* embryo, newborn infant)
			chondrotrophic (*chondros* cartilage)
			glycotrophic (*glykys* sweet)
			idiotrophic (*idios* one's own)
			mammotrophic (also called *mammotropic*) (*mamma* breast)
			phagotrophic (also called *holozoic*) (*phagein* to devour, consume)
			phototrophic (*photos* light)
			prototrophic (*protos* first)
			renotrophic (also called *renotropic*) (*ren* kidney)
			thymotrophic (thymus)
			thyrotrophic (also called *thyrotropic*) (thyroid gland)
			vasotrophic (*vas* vessel)
			viscerotrophic (*viscera* internal organs)
			trophism: tachytrophism (rapid metabolism) (*tachys* swift, rapid)
			tropho: cytotrophoblast (*kytos* cell, vessel + *blastos* bud, germ)
			trophy:
			lipotrophy (increase in bodily fat) {lipotrophic} (*lipos* fat)
			myotrophy {myotrophic} (*myos* muscle)
			neurotrophy {neurotrophic} (*neuron* nerve)
			oligotrophy (also called *malnutrition*) (*oligos* few, little, scant)
			ophthalmatrophy (atrophy of the eye) (*ophthalmos* eye + atrophy)
			PREFIXED TRAILING ROOT COMPOUND:
			abiotrophy (trophic failure; degeneration or failure of vitality; compare *abiatrophy*) (*a* privative + *bios* life)
			amyotrophy (muscular wasting) (*a* negative + *myos* muscle)
			hypermyotrophy (*hyper* beyond + myotrophy)
			CROSS REFERENCE: al, nur

Element	From	Meaning	Examples
tub[1]	Latin *tubus*	tube	SIMPLE ROOT: tuba (or, tube; an elongated hollow cylindrical organ; pl., tubae) tubal (relating to a tube, especially the uterine tube) tubule {tubular; also called *tubuliform*} tubulose (or, tubulous), tubulus (pl., tubuli), tubus (pl., tubi) PREFIXED ROOT: *tubal*: extratubal (*extra* outside) infratubal (*infra* below) intratubal (*intra* within) *tubate*: extubate (to remove a tube) (*ex* out) intubate (to insert a tube into a hollow organ or body passage) (*in* in) *tubation*: detubation (also called *extubation*) (*de* negative) extubation (also called *detubation*) (*ex* out) intubation (*in* in) *tubular*: intertubular (*inter* between) intratubular (*intra* within) *tubule*: microtubule (*mikros* small) LEADING ROOT COMPOUND: *tub*: tubectomy (also called *salpingectomy*) (*ektome* excision) *tuba*: tubatorsion (or, tubotorsion) (*torquere* to twist) *tubo*: tuboabdominal (abdomen) tuboligamentous (ligament) tubo-ovarian, tubo-ovaritis (ovary + *itis* inflammation) tuboperitoneal (peritoneum) tuboplasty [plastic repair of a tube, such as the uterine tube (salpingoplasty) or auditory tube (eustachian tuboplasty)] (*plassein* to form) tuborrhea (discharge from the auditory tube) (*rhein* to flow) tubotorsion (or, tubatorsion; twisting of the uterine tube, or oviduct) (*torquere* to twist) tubotympanum (the auditory tube and tympanic cavity considered together) {tubotympanal} (*tympanon* a drum; eardrum) tubouterine (relating to the oviduct and the uterus) (*uterus* womb) tubovaginal (vagina) *tubul*: tubulitis (inflammation of a renal tubule) (*itis* inflammation) *tubulo*: tubulocyst (*kystis* sac) tubulodermoid (*derma* skin + *eidos* form) tubuloglomerular (also called *glomerulotubular*) (*glomus* ball) tubulointerstitial (*inter* between + *stare* to stand) tubuloneogenesis (*neos* new + *genesis* formation) tubuloracemose (denoting a gland of combined tubular and racemose structure) tubulopathy (*pathos* disease) tubulorrhexis (*rhexis* rupture) tubulovesicle (*vesica* bladder) TRAILING ROOT COMPOUND: vesiculotubular (*vesicula* small bladder) CROSS REFERENCE: fistul, salping, syring

Element	From	Meaning	Examples
tub²	Latin *tuber* lump, swelling	swelling, node, bulge	SIMPLE ROOT:
			tuber (pl., tubers, or tubera)
			tubercle (a little swelling)
			tubercular, tuberculate (or, tuberculated), tuberculation
			tuberculid (recurrent eruptions of the skin)
			tuberculin, tuberculum (pl., tubercula)
			tuberose (tuberous; covered with tubers; knobby, lumpy or nodular; presenting many tubers or tuberosities; also called *tubiferous*)
			tuberositas (or, tuberosity; an elevation or protuberance)
			PREFIXED ROOT:
			tuberal: subtuberal (*sub* below)
			tuberance: protuberance (or, protuberantia) (*pro* forth)
			tubercular:
			antitubercular (*anti* against)
			intertubercular (*inter* between)
			quadritubercular (*quattuor* four)
			tritubercular (*tri* three)
			tuberculate: multituberculate (*multus* many)
			tuberculosis:
			epituberculosis (*epi* upon)
			paratuberculosis (*para* alongside)
			tuberculotic: antituberculotic (*anti* against + *osis* condition)
			LEADING ROOT COMPOUND:
			tuber: tuberosis {tuberosity} (*osis* condition)
			tubercul:
			tuberculitis (*itis* inflammation)
			tuberculoid (*eidos* form)
			tuberculoma (*oma* tumor)
			tuberculosis (an infectious disease caused by the formation of tubercules and caseous necrosis in the tissues) (*osis* condition)
			tubi: tubiferous (also called *tuberose*, *tuberous*) (*ferre* to bear)
			CROSS REFERENCE: bulb, cel², gangli, onc, tum
tum	Latin *tumere* to swell	swelling, node, bulge, tumor	SIMPLE ROOT:
			tumescence, tumentia (a swelling; also called *tumefaction*)
			tumid (swollen, as by congestion, edema, hyperemia; also called *turgid*) {tumidity}
			tumor (swelling, one of the cardinal signs of inflammation; morbid enlargement; a neoplasm; a mass of new tissue which persists and grows independently of its surrounding structures, and which has no physiologic use) {tumoral, tumorous}, tumorlet
			PREFIXED ROOT:
			antitumorigenic (*anti* against + *genere* to produce)
			detumescence (the subsidence of swelling, or turgor) (*de* down)
			intumesce (to swell up), intumescence, intumescent (*in* intensive)
			LEADING ROOT COMPOUND:
			tume: tumefacient, tumefaction (also called *tumescence*) {tumefactive, or tumefacient}, tumefy (*facere* to make)
			tumor:
			tumoraffin (also called *oncotropic*) (*affinis* related)
			tumorectomy (*ektome* excision)
			tumori:
			tumoricidal (also called *oncolytic*) (*caedere* to cut, kill)
			tumorigenesis (also called *oncogenesis*) (*genere* to produce)
			CROSS REFERENCE: cel², gangli, onc, tub²

Element	From	Meaning	Examples
tympan	Greek *tympanon* drum	the eardrum; hollow, like a drum	NOTE: This root usually refers to the middle ear cavity (the eardrum), but also means "distention," as though stretched like a drum, e.g., tympanites (distention of the abdomen or intestines by gas), and tympany.

SIMPLE ROOT:

tympanism (abdominal inflation from gas; also called *tympanites*) {tympanitic, tympanous}

tympanum (the eardrum; pl., tympana, tympanums) {tympanal, tympanic}

tympanites, tympany, tympanous (distended with gas)

PREFIXED ROOT:

tympanic:

entotympanic (*enton* within)

extratympanic (*extra* outside)

infratympanic (also called *subtympanic*) (*infra* below)

intratympanic (*intra* within)

mesotympanum (*mesos* middle)

pretympanic (*pre* anterior)

subtympanic (below the tympanum; having a somewhat tympanic quality; also called *infratympanic*) (*sub* below)

supratympanic (*supra* over, above)

transtympanic (*trans* across, through)

tympanotomy: hypotympanotomy (*hypo* under + *tomy* incision)

tympanum:

epitympanum {epitympanic} (*epi* upon, over)

hypotympanum (a space in the middle ear) (*hypo* below)

mesotympanum (*mesos* middle)

LEADING ROOT COMPOUND:

tympan:

tympanectomy (*ektome* excision)

tympanitis (also called *myringitis*) (*itis* inflammation)

tympano:

tympanocentesis (also called *tympanotomy*, *myringotomy*) (*kentein* to puncture)

tympanochord (also called *chorda tympani*) {tympanichordal}

tympanoeustachian (eustachian tube)

tympanogenic (*genere* to produce)

tympanogram (*graphein* to write)

tympanohyal (hyoid arch)

tympanomalleal (*malleus* hammer: part of the ear)

tympanomandibular (*mandible* lower jaw)

tympanomastoidectomy (mastoid process + *ektome* excision)

tympanomastoiditis (mastoid process + *itis* inflammation)

tympanometry {tympanometric} (*metron* measure)

tympanophonia (or, tympanophony) (*phone* sound)

tympanoplasty {tympanoplastic} (*plassein* to form)

tympanosclerosis {tympanosclerotic} (*sklerosis* a hardening)

tympanosquamosal (also called *squamotympanic*) (*squama* scale)

tympanostapedial (*stapes* stirrup—of ear)

tympanostomy (also called *myringotomy*) (*stoma* mouth, opening)

tympanotomy (also called *tympanocentesis*) (*tomy* incision)

TRAILING ROOT COMPOUND:

tympanic:

antrotympanic (*antrum* sinus, cavity)

Element	From	Meaning	Examples
tympan (cont'd)		[the eardrum]	craniotympanic (*kranion* skull) osteotympanic (also called *otocranial*) (*osteon* bone) petrotympanic (*petra* stone) vesiculotympanic (or, vesiculotympanitic) (*vesica* bladder) *tympanum*: hemotympanum (or, hematotympanum) (*haima* blood) tubotympanum {tubotympanic} (*tubus* pipe, tube) CROSS REFERENCE: myring
typh	Greek *typhos* fever	fog, stupor, delirium	SIMPLE ROOT: typhinia (stupor arising from fever; also called *relapsing fever*) typhus {typhous} PREFIXED ROOT: antityphoid (*anti* against + typhoid) paratyphoid (also called *paratyphoid fever*) (*para* alongside, similar to + typhoid) posttyphoid (*post* after + typhoid) LEADING ROOT COMPOUND: *typh*: typhoid (typhuslike; stuporous from fever) (*eidos* form) *typho*: typhobacterin (typhoid vaccine) typhogenic (causing typhus or typhoid fever) (*genere* to produce) typhomania (*mania* madness) TRAILING ROOT COMPOUND: pyretotyphosis (*pyr* fire, fever + *osis* condition) pseudotyphus (*pseudes* false) CROSS REFERENCE: None
typhl	Greek *typhlon* cecum from *typhlos* blind (next entry)	cecum, the first part of the large intestine; blind gut	SIMPLE ROOT: typhlon (cecum) PREFIXED ROOT: epityphlitis (also called *appendicitis, paratyphlitis*) (*epi* upon + *itis* inflammation) paratyphlitis (*para* alongside + *itis* inflammation) perityphlic (also called *pericecal*), perityphlitis (inflamed condition of tissues around the cecum and appendix; also called *appendicitis*) (*peri* around + *itis* inflammation) LEADING ROOT COMPOUND: *typhl*: typhlectasis (cecal distention) (*ektasis* dilatation) typhlectomy (also called *cecectomy*) (*ektome* excision) typhlenteritis (or, typhloenteritis; also called *cecitis*) (*enteron* intestine + *itis* inflammation) typhlitis (also called *cecitis*) (*itis* inflammation) *typhlo*: typhlocele (also called *cecocele*) (*kele* hernia) typhlodicliditis (*diklis* door + *itis* inflammation) typhloempyema (*empyema* abscess) typhloenteritis (also called *cecitis*) (*enteron* intestine + *itis* inflammation) typhlolithiasis (*lithos* stone + *iasis* condition) typhlopexy (or, typhlopexia) (*pexy* fixed) typhlorrhaphy (also called *cecorrhaphy*) (*rhaphe* suture) typhlostomy (also called *cecostomy*) (*stoma* mouth, opening) typhlotomy (also called *cecotomy*) (*tomy* incision) CROSS REFERENCE: cec

$\mathcal{U}$

Element	From	Meaning	Examples
ud			See sud- for *exudate*.
ul			See oulo- for *ulalgia*.
ul	Greek *oule*	scar, cicatrix	SIMPLE ROOT: ulosis (formation of a scar) PREFIXED ROOT: epulosis (cicatrization) {epulotic} (*epi* upon) synulosis (complete cicatrization) {synulotic} (*sym* intensive) LEADING ROOT COMPOUND: *ul*: ulectomy (or, oulectomy) (*ektome* excision) ulerythema (an erythematous disease of the skin characterized by the formation of cicatrices and by atrophy) (*erythema* redness) *ule*: ulegyria (a defect of the cerebral cortex characterized by narrow and distorted gyri; may be congenital or the result of scars) (*gyrus* circle) *ulo*: ulodermatitis (inflammation of the skin resulting in destruction of tissue and formation of scars) (*derma* skin + *itis* inflammation) ulotomy (the cutting or division of scar tissue) (*tomy* incision) [another *ulotomy* is listed under oulo-] CROSS REFERENCE: None
ulc	Latin *ulcus*	abscess, ulcer	SIMPLE ROOT: ulcer {ulcerous}, ulcerate, ulceration (the formation or development of an ulcer; an ulcer) {ulcerated, ulcerative}, ulcus (ulcer; pl., ulcera) PREFIXED ROOT: antiulcerative (*anti* against) LEADING ROOT COMPOUND: ulcerogangrenous (characterized by both ulceration and gangrene; pertaining to a gangrenous ulcer) ulcerogenic (*genere* to produce) ulceroglandular ulceromembranous (*membrane* a thin skin) CROSS REFERENCE: aphtha, helc[1]
ultra-	Latin prefix	beyond	See Appendix B for examples of words with this prefix. Others are listed with the root to which it is attached. CROSS REFERENCE: extra-, meta-
umbilic	Latin *umbilicus*	navel	SIMPLE ROOT: umbilicus {umbilicate, umbilical, umbilicated} PREFIXED ROOT: exumbilication (protrusion of the navel) (*ex* out) infraumbilical (also called *subumbilical*) (*infra* below) paraumbilical (also called *paraomphalic*) (*para* alongside) periumbilical (also called *periomphalic*) (*peri* around, near) subumbilical (also called *infraumbilical*) (*sub* below) supraumbilical (*supra* above) LEADING ROOT COMPOUND: umbilectomy (also called *omphalectomy*) (*ektome* excision) TRAILING ROOT COMPOUND: pyoumbilicus (infection of the umbilicus) (*pyon* pus) vesicoumbilical (pertaining to the urinary bladder and the umbilicus) (*vesica* bladder) CROSS REFERENCE: omphal

A Thesaurus of Medical Word Roots

Element	From	Meaning	Examples
uni-	Latin prefix	one	See Appendix B for examples of words with this prefix. Others are listed with the root to which it is attached. CROSS REFERENCE: mono-
ur	Latin *urina* Greek *ouron* urine	urine	SIMPLE ROOT: urate (any salt or anion of uric acid; see *uratemia, uraturia* below) {uratic} urea {ureal, ureic}, urease (an enzyme that catalyzes the hydrolysis of urea to form ammonium carbonate) uresis (the passage of urine; urination) ureter [see separate entry]; urethra [see separate entry] urinal, urinary (also called *ureteric, uretic, urinous*) urinate, urination, urine {urinous} PREFIXED ROOT: *uremia*: hypouremia (an abnormally low level of urea in the blood) (*hypo* under + *emia* blood condition) *uresis* the passage of urine: anuresis (retention of urine in the bladder; anuria) (*an* negative) diuresis (discharge of urine, especially in large amounts) (*dia* through) ecuresis (absolute dehydration of the body) (*ek* out) emuresis (absolute hydration of the body) (*em* in) enuresis (bedwetting) {enuretic} (*en* in) hyperuresis (also called *polyuria*) (*hyper* over, above) hypouresis (also called *oliguria*) (*hypo* under) paruresis (also called *shy bladder syndrome*) (*para* abnormal) *uria urine* condition: anisuria (*aniso* unequal, dissimilar: *an* negative + *isos* equal) anuria (absence of urine formation; also called *anuresis*) {anuric} (*an* privative) dysuria (painful or difficult urination) {dysuric} (*dys* abnormal) paruria (any disorder of the urine or abnormal state of the urine or its discharge) (*para* abnormal) polyuria (the passage of a large volume of urine in a given period, as in diabetes mellitus; also called *hyperuresis*) (*polys* much) *uric*: antidysuric (*anti* against + dysuric) *uricemia* condition of uric acid in the blood: hyperuricemia {hyperuricemic} (*hyper* above) hypouricemia (*hypo* under) *uricuria* condition of uric acid in the urine: hyperuricuria (*hyper* above) hypouricuria (*hypo* under) *urolith*: antiurolithic (*anti* against + *lithos* stone) *urology*: endourology (*endon* within + *logos* study) LEADING ROOT COMPOUND: *ur*: uracrasia (a disordered state or composition of the urine) (*a* negative + *krasis* a mixing) uracratia (urinary incontinence) (*akrateia* lack of self control) uragogue (*agein* to lead) urapostema (pus which contains urine) (*apostema* pus, abscess) uredema (or, uroedema) (*edema* swelling) uremia {uremic} (*emia* blood condition) uridrosis (*hidrosis* sweat condition) [h of hidrosis elided] urodynia (*odyne* pain) uroncus (also called *urinoma*) (*onkos* mass)

Element	From	Meaning	Examples
ur (cont'd)		[urine]	*urat*: uratemia (the presence of urates in the blood) (*emia* blood condition) uratoma (also called *gouty tophus*) (*oma* tumor) uratosis (*osis* condition) uraturia (the presence of an excess of urates in the urine; lithuria; also called *hyperuricosuria*) (*uria* urine condition) *urato*: uratolysis {uratolytic} (*lysis* solution) *urea*: ureagenesis (also called *ureapoiesis*) {ureagenetic} (*genere* to produce) ureapoiesis (also called *ureagenesis*) (*poiesis* a producing) *ureo*: ureolysis {ureolytic} (*lysis* a loosening) ureotelia {ureotelic} (*telos* end) *uresi*: uresiesthesia (or, uriesthesia; the desire to urinate) (*esthesia* feeling) *uri*: uriposia (urine-drinking) (*posis* drinking) *uric*: uricacidemia (the accumulation of uric acid in the blood; also called *hyperuricemia*) (acid + *emia* blood condition) *urico*: uricocholia (*cholia* bile condition) uricolysis (decomposition of uric acid) {uricolytic} (*lysis* a loosening) uricometer (*metron* measure) uricopoiesis (*poiein* to produce) uricotelia {uricotelic} (*telos* end, outcome) *uricos*: uricosuria {uricosuric} (*uria* urine condition) *urin*: urinalysis (urine + analysis) urinoma (*oma* tumor) *urini*: uriniferous (*ferre* to bear) urinific (*facere* to make) uriniparous (*parere* to produce) *urino*: urinocryoscopy (*kryos* cold + *skopein* to examine) urinogenital (also called *genitourinary*) urinometer, urinometry (*metron* measure) urinoscopy (also called *uroscopy*) (*skopein* to examine) urinosexual (also called *genitourinary*) *uro*: urobiline, urobilinemia (*bilis* bile + *emia* blood condition) urobilinuria (*bilis* bile + *uria* urine condition) urocele (*kele* hernia) urocheras (also called *uropsammus*) (*cherados* gravel) urochesia (*chezein* to defecate) urochrome (also called *urian*), urochromogen (*chroma* color + *genere* to produce) uroclepsis (the unconscious escape of urine) (*kleptein* to steal) urocyanosis (*kyanos* the color blue + *osis* condition) urocystis (the urinary bladder) {urocystic}, urocystitis (*kystis* bladder + *itis* inflammation) uroedema (or, uredema) (*edema* swelling) urogenital (also called *genitourinary*, *urinosexual*) urogenous (or, urinogenous) (*genere* to produce)

A Thesaurus of Medical Word Roots

Element	From	Meaning	Examples
ur (cont'd)		[urine]	urogram, urography (*graphein* to write)
			urolagnia (*lagneia* lust)
			urolith {urolithic}, urolithiasis (*lithos* stone + *iasis* condition)
			urolithology (*lithos* stone + *logos* study)
			urology {urologic, urological} (*logos* study)
			urometer (or, urinometer) (*metron* measure)
			uronephrosis (also called *hydronephrosis*) (*nephrosis* kidney condition)
			uropathogen (*pathos* disease + *genere* to produce)
			uropathy (*pathos* disease)
			uropenia (also called *oliguria*) (*penia* deficiency)
			urophanic (appearing in the urine) (*phainein* to show)
			uroplania (extravasation of urine) (*planan* to wander)
			uropoiesis (also called *urogenesis*) {uropoietic} (*poiesis* production)
			uropsammus (also called *urocheras*) (*psammous* gravel)
			urorectal (rectum)
			uroschesis (*schesis* retention)
			uroscopy (also called *urinoscopy*) {uroscopic} (*skopein* to examine)
			urosemiology (*semeion* sign + *logos* study)
			urosepsis {uroseptic} (*sepsis* putrefaction)
			urostealith (*stear* fat + *lithos* stone)
			urothelium (the epithelial lining of the urinary tract)
			urothorax (the presence of urine in the thoracic cavity, usually following complex multiple organ injuries)
			urotoxin {urotoxic} (*toxin* poison)
			TRAILING ROOT COMPOUND:
			uresis passage of urine:
			chloruresis (chlorides)
			hydrodiuresis (*hydor* water + diuresis)
			kaliuresis (*kalium* potassium)
			lithuresis (*lithos* stone)
			melanuresis (also called *melanuria*) (*melanos* dark)
			natriuresis (*natrium* sodium)
			saluresis (*sal* salt)
			strontiuresis (strontium: fr. Strontian, a town in Scotland)
			uria urine condition:
			acetonuria (also called *ketonuria*) (acetone)
			aciduria (*acidus* sharp: acid)
			adiposuria (also called *lipiduria*) (*adipos* fat)
			albiduria (also called *albinuria*) (*albus* white)
			alkalinuria (alkaline)
			ameburia (ameba)
			aminuria (amines)
			amylasuria (*amylase* a starch compound)
			bacteriuria (bacteria)
			biliuria (bile)
			blennuria (*blenna* mucus)
			bradyuria (*bradys* slow)
			chloriduria (chlorides)
			cholesteroluria (cholesterol)
			diuria (frequency of urination during the day) (*dies* day)
			erythruria (*erythros* red)
			fecaluria (feces)
			fructosuria (fructose)

Element	From	Meaning	Examples
ur (cont'd)		[urine]	glycosuria (also called *glucosuria*) (*glykys* sweet)
			heptosuria (presence of heptose in the urine) (*hepta* seven)
			inosuria (*inos* fiber)
			ketonuria (also called *acetonuria*) (ketone)
			melanuria (also called *melanuresis*) {melanuric} (*melanos* dark)
			meninguria (*meningos* membrane)
			nocturia (or, nycturia; excessive urination at night, or more during the night than in the day) (Latin *nox*; Greek *nyx* night)
			oliguria (or, oliguresis) {oliguric} (*oligos* little, scant)
			pepsinuria (pepsin)
			pimeluria (*pimele* fat)
			pollakiuria (or, pollakisuria; abnormally frequent passage of urine) (*pollakis* often)
			pneumaturia (*pneumatos* gas)
			proteinuria (protein)
			pyuria (*pyon* pus)
			semenuria (or, seminuria; also called *spermaturia*) (*semen* sperm)
			spermaturia (also called *seminuria*) (*sperma* seed, sperm)
			sucrosuria (sucrose)
			xanthiuria (*xanthos* yellow)
			CROSS REFERENCE: None
uran	Greek *ouraniskos* from *Ouranos* god of heaven; thus, over-arching	roof of mouth; palate	SIMPLE ROOT: uraniscus (the palate)
			LEADING ROOT COMPOUND:
			uranisco:
			uraniscochasm (fissure of the palate; also called *uranischisis*) (*chasma* a cleft)
			uraniscolalia (a speech defect due to cleft palate) (*lalein* to speak)
			uraniscoplasty (also called *palatoplasty*) (*plassein* to form)
			uraniscorrhaphy (also called *staphylorrhaphy*) (*rhaphe* suture)
			uraniscon: uranisconitis (also called *palatitis*) (*itis* inflammation)
			urano:
			uranoplasty (also called *palatoplasty*) (*plassein* to form)
			uranoplegia (also called *palatoplegia*) (*plessein* to strike)
			uranorrhaphy (also called *palatorrhaphy*) (*rhaphe* suture)
			uranoschisis (cleft palate; also called *uraniscochasm*) (*schisis* fissure)
			uranostaphyloschisis (*staphle* uvula + *schisis* fissure)
			CROSS REFERENCE: palat
ureter	Greek *oureter* fr. *ouron* urine	urinary canal	SIMPLE ROOT: ureter (a duct or tube that carries urine from a kidney to the bladder or cloaca) {ureteral, ureteric, uretic} [cloaca: a passage]
			PREFIXED ROOT:
			ureter: megaloureter (also called *megaureter, ureterectasia*) (*megalos* large)
			ureteral:
			endoureteral (also called *intraureteral*) (*endon* within)
			interureteral (or, interureteric) (*inter* between)
			intraureteral (also called *endoureteral*) (*intra* within)
			periureteral (or, periureteric), periureteritis (*peri* around + *itis* inflammation)
			LEADING ROOT COMPOUND:
			ureter:
			ureteralgia (*algos* pain)
			uretercystoscope (*kystis* bladder + *skopein* to view, examine)
			ureterectasia (or, ureterectasis) (*ectasia* dilatation)

Element	From	Meaning	Examples
ureter (cont'd)		[urinary canal]	ureterectomy (*ektome* excision)
			ureteritis (*itis* inflammation)
			ureteric:
			endoureteric (also called *intraureteral*) (*endon* within)
			periureteric (*peri* around)
			uretero:
			uretercolostomy (colon + *stoma* mouth, opening)
			ureterocalicostomy (*kalyx* cup + *stoma* mouth, opening)
			ureterocele, ureterocelectomy (*kele* hernia + *ektome* excision)
			ureterocelorraphy (*kele* hernia + *raphe* suture)
			ureterocervical (*cervix* neck—of uterus)
			ureterocolic (colon)
			ureterocystoscope (*kystis* bladder + *skopein* to examine)
			ureterocystostomy (also called *ureterocystoneostomy*) (*kystis* bladder + *stoma* mouth, opening)
			ureteroduodenal (duodenum)
			ureteroenteric (also called *ureterointestinal*) (*enteron* intestine)
			ureteroenterostomy (*enteron* intestine + *stoma* mouth, opening)
			ureterogram, ureterography (*graphein* to write)
			ureterohydronephrosis (*hydor* water + *nephrosis* kidney condition)
			ureteroileostomy (ileum + *stoma* mouth, opening)
			ureterolith, ureterolithiasis (*lithos* stone + *iasis* condition)
			ureterolithotomy (*lithos* stone + *tomy* incision)
			ureterolysis (*lysis* a loosening)
			ureteroneocystostomy (*neos* new + *kystis* bladder + *stoma* mouth, opening)
			ureteronephrectomy (also called *nephroureterectomy*) (*nephros* kidney + *ektome* excision)
			ureteropathy (*pathos* disease)
			ureteropelvic (also called *pelviureteral*), ureteropelvioplasty (also called *ureteropyelostomy*) (pelvis + *plassein* to form)
			ureteroplasty (*plassein* to form)
			ureteroproctostomy (also called *ureterorectostomy*) (*proktos* anus + *stoma* mouth, opening)
			ureteropyelitis (*pyelos* pelvis + *itis* inflammation)
			ureteropyeloneostomy (also called *ureteropyelostomy*) (*pyelos* pelvis + *neo* new + *stoma* mouth, opening)
			ureteropyosis (also called *pyoureter*) (*pyon* pus + *osis* condition)
			ureterorectal, ureterorectoneostomy (rectum + *neos* new + *stoma* mouth, opening)
			ureterorrhagia (*rhagia* bursting forth)
			ureterorrhaphy (*rhaphe* suture)
			ureteroscope, ureteroscopy (*skopein* to examine)
			ureterosigmoid, ureterosigmoidostomy (sigmoid colon + *stoma* mouth, opening)
			ureterostenosis (*stenosis* a narrowing)
			ureterostomy (*stoma* mouth, opening)
			ureterotomy (*tomy* incision)
			ureteroureteral (relating to two segments of the same ureter or to both ureters)
			ureterouterine (uterus)
			ureterovaginal (vagina)
			ureterpyeloplasty (*pyelos* pelvis + *plassein* to form)
			ureterpyelostomy (*pyelos* pelvis + *stoma* mouth, opening)

A Thesaurus of Medical Word Roots

Element	From	Meaning	Examples
ureter (cont'd)		[urinary canal]	ureterovesical (also called *vesicoureteral*), ureterovesicotomy (*vesica* bladder + *tomy* incision) TRAILING ROOT COMPOUND: *ureter*: pyoureter (*pyon* pus) *ureteral*: pelviureteral (also called *ureteropelvic*) (pelvis) vesicoureteral (also called *ureterovesical*) {vesicourerteric} (*vesica* bladder) CROSS REFERENCE: None
urethr	Greek *ourethra* fr. *ouron* urine	urethra	SIMPLE ROOT: urethra (the canal through which urine is discharged from the bladder) {urethral}, urethrism (or, urethrismus; also called *urethrospasm*) PREFIXED ROOT: endourethral (also called *intraurethral*) (*endon* within) intraurethral (also called *endourethral*) (*intra* within) megalourethra (*megalos* large) paraurethral, paraurethritis (also called *periurethritis*) (*para* alongside + *itis* inflammation) periurethral, periurethritis (*peri* around + *itis* inflammation) preurethritis (*pre* before + *itis* inflammation) suburethral (*sub* under) transurethral (*trans* across) LEADING ROOT COMPOUND: *urethr*: urethralgia (also called *urethrodynia*) (*algos* pain) urethratresia (also called *urethral atresia*) (*atresia* imperforation) urethrectomy (*ektome* excision) urethremorrhagia (*haima* blood + *rhagia* bursting forth) [h of haima (hemo) elided] urethremphraxis (*emphraxis* obstruction) urethritis (*itis* inflammation) urethrodynia (also called *urethralgia*) (*odyne* pain) *urethro*: urethroanal (also called *anourethral*) (anus) urethrobulbar (also called *bulbourethral*) (bulb) urethrocele (*kele* tumor, hernia) urethrocystitis (*kystis* bladder + *itis* inflammation) urethrography (*graphein* to write) urethrometer (*metron* measure) urethropenile (penis) urethroperineal, urethroperineoscrotal (perineum + scrotum) urethropexy (also called *bladder neck suspension*) (*pexy* fixation) urethrophyma (*phyma* tumor, growth) urethroplasty (*plassein* to form) urethroprostatic (prostate gland) urethrorectal (also called *rectourethral*) (rectum) urethrorrhagia (*rhagia* bursting forth) urethrorrhaphy (*raphe* suture) urethrorrhea (*rhein* to flow) urethroscope {urethroscopic}, urethroscopy (*skopein* to examine) urethroscrotal (*scrotum* bag: testicle pouch) urethrospasm (also called *urethrism*) (*spasmos* contraction) urethrostaxis (*staxis* dripping) urethrostenosis (*stenosis* a narrowing)

Element	From	Meaning	Examples
urethr (cont'd)		[urethra]	urethrostomy (*stoma* mouth, opening)
			urethrotome, urethrotomy (*tomy* incision)
			urethrovaginal (vagina)
			urethrovesical (also called *vesicourethral*), urethrovesicopexy (*vesica* bladder + *pexis* fixation)
			TRAILING ROOT COMPOUND:
			urethral:
			bulbourethral (bulb—of the penis)
			rectourethral (rectum)
			vestibulourethral (vestibule)
			vesicourethral (*vesica* bladder)
			urethria: ankylurethria (*ankylos* stiff)
			CROSS REFERENCE: None
urg			See erg- for *micrurgical*.
uter	Latin *uterus*	womb, uterus	SIMPLE ROOT: uterus (pl., uteri) {uterine}
			PREFIXED ROOT:
			endouterine (also called *intrauterine*) (*endon* within)
			extrauterine (*extra* outside)
			intrauterine (also called *endouterine*) (*intra* within)
			parauterine (*para* alongside)
			periuterine (also called *perimetric*) (*peri* around)
			postuterine (posterior to the uterus) (*post* behind)
			retrouterine (behind the uterus) (*retro* back)
			LEADING ROOT COMPOUND:
			uter:
			uteralgia (also called *hysteralgia*) (*algos* pain)
			uterectomy (also called *hysterectomy*) (*ektome* excision)
			uteritis (also called *metritis*) (*itis* inflammation)
			uterodynia (also called *hysteralgia, metralgia, metrodynia*) (*odyne* pain)
			utero:
			uteroabdominal (abdomen)
			uterocervical (*cervix* neck—of uterus)
			uterocystostomy (*kystis* bladder + *stoma* mouth, opening)
			uterofixation (also called *hysteropexy*) (*fixere* to fasten)
			uterogenic (formed in the uterus) (*genere* to produce)
			uterogestation (*gerare* to bear)
			uteroglobin (globulin)
			uterography (also called *hysterography*) (*graphein* to write)
			uterolith (also called *hysterolith, uterine calculus*) (*lithos* stone)
			uterometer, uterometry (*metron* measure)
			utero-ovarian (ovary)
			uteroparietal (relating to the uterus and the abdominal wall) (*paries* wall—of an organ)
			uteropelvic (pelvis)
			uteropexy (also called *hysteropexy*) (*pexis* fixation)
			uteroplacental (placenta)
			uteroplasty (*plassein* to form)
			uterorectal (also called *rectouterine*) (rectum)
			uterosacral (sacrum)
			uterosalpingography (*salpingos* tube + *graphein* to write)
			uterosclerosis (*sklerosis* hardness)
			uteroscope (also called *hysteroscope*), uteroscopy (also called *hysteroscopy*) (*skopein* to examine)

Element	From	Meaning	Examples
uter (cont'd)		[womb]	uterotomy (also called *hysterotomy*) (*tomy* incision)
			uterotonic (*tonus* tone)
			uterotropic (*tropein* to turn; have an affinity for)
			uterotubal (also called *tubouterine*), uterotubography (tube + *graphein* to write)
			uterovaginal (vagina)
			uteroventral (*venter* belly, stomach)
			uterovesical (*vesica* bladder)
			TRAILING ROOT COMPOUND:
			cervicouterine (*cervix* neck—of uterus)
			rectouterine (also called *uterorectal*) (rectum)
			sacrouterine (sacrum)
			tubouterine (Fallopian tube)
			ureterouterine (ureter)
			vesicouterine (*vesica* bladder)
			vulvouterine (vulva)
			CROSS REFERENCE: colp, hyster[1], metr
uv	Latin *uva* grape	uvea (part of the eye)	SIMPLE ROOT: uvea (the iris, ciliary body, and choroid considered together; also referred to as *vascular layer of the eyeball*) {uveal, uveitic}
			PREFIXED ROOT: panuveitis (*pan* all + *itis* inflammation)
			LEADING ROOT COMPOUND:
			uve: uveitis (pl., uvetides) {uveitic} (*itis* inflammation)
			uveo:
			uveoencephalitis (*enkephalon* brain + *itis* inflammation)
			uveomeningitis (*meningos* membrane + *itis* inflammation)
			uveoparotid (affecting the parotid gland and the uvea)
			uveoscleritis (*scleritis* inflammation of the sclera)
			CROSS REFERENCE: None
uvul	Latin *uvula* little grape	uvula	SIMPLE ROOT: uvula (small soft structure hanging from the free edge of soft palate in midline above the root of the tongue) {uvular}, uvularis (also called *muscle of uvula*)
			PREFIXED ROOT: periuvular (*peri* around)
			LEADING ROOT COMPOUND:
			uvi: uviform (having the form of a grape; also called *botryoid*) (*forma* shape)
			uvul:
			uvulectomy (*ektome* excision)
			uvulitis (inflammation of the uvula; also called *staphylitis*) (*itis* inflammation)
			uvulo:
			uvulopalatopharyngoplasty (also called *palatopharyngoplasty*) (palate + pharynx + larynx + *plassein* to form)
			uvuloptosis (relaxed and pendulous condition of the palate) (*ptein* to fall)
			uvulotome (also called *staphylotome*), uvulotomy (also called *staphylotomy*) (*tomy* incision)
			CROSS REFERENCE: staphyl

A Thesaurus of Medical Word Roots

Element	From	Meaning	Examples
vag	Latin *vagari* to wander	to wander; wandering nerve [vagus]	SIMPLE ROOT: vagus (designating the tenth cranial nerve; often called *the wandering nerve*; pl., vagi) {vagal} PREFIXED ROOT: divagation (incoherent speech and thought) (*dis* away) hemivagotony (vagotonia on one side) (*hemi* half) LEADING ROOT COMPOUND: vagoglossopharyngeal (*glossa* tongue + pharynx) vagogram (also called *electrovagogram*) (*graphein* to write) vagolysis {vagolytic} (*lyein* to loosen) vagomimetic (*mimesis* imitation) vagosympathetic (sympathetic nervous system) vagotomy (*tomy* incision) vagotony (or, vagotonia) {vagotonic} (*tonos* tension) vagotropic, vagotropism (*trepein* to turn) vagovagal (pertaining to both afferent and efferent impulses) CROSS REFERENCE: noma, plan[2]
vagin	Latin *vagina*	sheath, vagina	SIMPLE ROOT: vagina (pl., vaginae) {vaginal} vaginate (to enclose in a sheath; provided with a sheath) vaginismus (or, vaginism; a painful spasm of the vagina making coital penetration difficult or impossible) vagitus (the cry of an infant in the uterus or vagina) PREFIXED ROOT: *vaginal*: extravaginal (*extra* outside) intervaginal (*inter* between) intravaginal (*intra* within) paravaginal (*para* alongside) perivaginal (*peri* around) subvaginal (*sub* below) supravaginal (*supra* superior) transvaginal (*trans* across, through) *vaginat*: disinvagination (*dis* negative + invagination) evagination (an outpouching of a layer or part) (*ex* out) invaginate, invagination (*in* in) *vaginator*: invaginator (an instrument for pushing inward any tissue) (*in* in) *vaginitis* vagina inflammation: paravaginitis (also called *paracolpitis*) (*para* alongside) perivaginitis (also called *pericolpitis*) (*peri* around) LEADING ROOT COMPOUND: *vagin*: vaginectomy (excision of the vagina or a portion of it; also called *colpectomy*) (*ektome* excision) vaginitis (pl., vaginitides) (*itis* inflammation) vaginodynia (also called *colpodynia*) (*odyne* pain) vaginosis (*osis* condition, disease) *vagina*: vaginapexy (also called *vaginofixation*) (*pexis* fixation)

Element	From	Meaning	Examples
vagin (cont'd)		[sheath, vagina]	*vagino*: vaginoabdominal (abdomen) vaginocele (also called *colpocele*) (*kele* hernia) vaginocutaneous (*cutis* skin) vaginofixation (also called *vaginapexy*) (*fixare* to fix) vaginogram, vaginography (*graphein* to write) vaginohysterectomy (also called *vaginal hysterectomy*) (*hyster* uterus + *ektome* excision) vaginolabial (*labium* lip—of the vagina) vaginometer (*metron* measure) vaginomycosis (also called *colpomycosis*) (*mycosis* fungal condition) vaginopathy (*pathos* disease) vaginoperineoplasty (perineum + *plassein* to form) vaginoperineorrhaphy (perineum + *rhaphe* suture) vaginoperitoneal (peritoneum) vaginopexy (also called *colpopexy, vaginofixation*) (*pexy* fixation) vaginoplasty (also called *colpoplasty*) (*plassein* to form) vaginoscopy (also called *colposcopy*) (*skopein* to examine) vaginotomy (also called *colpotomy*) (*tomy* incision) vaginovesical (also called *vesicovaginal*) (*vesica* bladder) vaginovulvar (also called *vulvovaginal*) (vulva) TRAILING ROOT COMPOUND: *vaginal*: anovaginal (anus) colovaginal (colon) enterovaginal (*enteron* intestine) ischiovaginal (*ischium* hip) perineovaginal (perineum) rectovaginal (rectum) tendovaginal (tendon) tubovaginal (tube) ureterovaginal (ureter) urethrovaginal (urethra) uterovaginal (uterus) vesicovaginal (also called *vaginovesical*) (*vesica* bladder) vulvovaginal (*vulvae* external female genitalia) *vaginitis* vaginal inflammation: cervicovaginitis (*cervix* neck—of uterus) pachyvaginitis (*pachys* thick) tendovaginitis (also called *tenosynovitis*) (tendon) vulvovaginitis (*vulvae* external female genitalia) TERM: per vaginam (through the vagina) CROSS REFERENCE: colp, lemma, theca
vari	Latin *variare* to change	vein (enlarged)	SIMPLE ROOT: varication (the formation of a varix; a varicose condition) varicosity (a varix, or the quality or state of being varicose) varicula (also called *conjunctival varix*) varicule (a small varicose vein) varix (a permanent and irregularly swollen or dilated blood or lymph vessel, especially a vein; pl., varices) {variceal} LEADING ROOT COMPOUND: *varic*: varicoid (also called *variciform*) (*eidos* form) varicomphalus (*omphalos* navel)

Element	From	Meaning	Examples
vari (cont'd)		[enlarged vein]	varicose, varicosis (pl. varicoses) (*osis* condition)
			varici: variciform (also called *varicoid, varicose*) (*forma* shape)
			varico:
			varicoblepharon (*blepharon* eyelid)
			varicocele, varicocelectomy (*kele* hernia + *ektome* excision)
			varicography (*graphein* to write)
			varicophlebitis (*phlebos* vein + *itis* inflammation)
			varicotomy (*tomy* incision)
			CROSS REFERENCE: cirs, phleb, ven
vas	Latin *vas*	vessel, duct	SIMPLE ROOT:
			vas (any canal for carrying fluid, such as blood, lymph, spermatozoa; pl., vasa) {vasal}
			vascular, vascularization (also called *vasculogenesis*)
			vasculature (the circulatory system), vasculum (pl., vascula)
			PREFIXED ROOT:
			vasate: extravasate (*extra* beyond, outside)
			vasation:
			devasation (destruction of blood vessels) (*de* negative)
			extravasation (*extra* beyond)
			intravasation (*intra* within)
			vascular:
			avascular (lacking in blood vessels or having a poor blood supply) (*a* privative)
			circumvascular (also called *perivascular*) (*circum* around)
			dysvascular (*dys* abnormal)
			endovascular (also called *intravascular*) (*endon* within)
			extravascular (*extra* outside)
			hypervascular (*hyper* beyond)
			intervascular (*inter* between)
			intravascular (also called *endovascular*) (*intra* within)
			microvascular (*mikros* small)
			perivascular (also called *circumvascular*) (*peri* around)
			vascularization:
			avascularization (diversion of blood from tissues, as by ligation or bandaging) (*a* privative)
			devascularization (*de* negative)
			neovascularization (*neos* new)
			revascularization (*re* again)
			supervascularization (*super* over, above)
			vasculitis vessel inflammation:
			endovasculitis (also called *endangiitis*) (*endon* within)
			perivasculitis (*peri* around)
			LEADING ROOT COMPOUND:
			vas:
			vasectomy {vasectomized} (*ektome* excision)
			vasitis (also called *deferentitis*) (*itis* inflammation)
			vastomy (*tomy* incision)
			vascul: vasculitis {vasculitic} (*itis* inflammation)
			vasculo:
			vasculocardiac (*kardia* heart)
			vasculogenesis (also called *angiogenesis*)} (*genere* to produce)
			vasculolymphatic (lymphatic vessels) (*lympha* fluid, liquid)
			vasculomotor (also called *vasomotor*) (*movere* to move)
			vasculomyelinopathy (*myelos* marrow + *pathos* disease)

Element	From	Meaning	Examples
vas (cont'd)		[vessel, duct]	vasculopathy (*pathos* disease)
			vasculotoxic (*toxikon* poison)
			vasi:
			vasifaction (formation of blood or lymphatic vessels; also called *angiopoiesis*) {vasifactive} (*facere* to make)
			vasiform (*forma* shape)
			vaso:
			vasoactive (exerting an effect upon the caliber of blood vessels)
			vasoconstriction, vasoconstrictor (*con* with + *stringere* to bind)
			vasodilatation (or, vasodilation) (*dilatation* widening)
			vasoepididymostomy (epididymis + *stoma* mouth, opening)
			vasofactive (also called *angiogenic, angiopoietic*) (*facere* to make)
			vasoformative (also called *angiogenic, angiopoietic*) (*forma* shape)
			vasoganglion (a mass of blood cells) (*ganglion* swelling, knot)
			vasohypertonic (also called *vasodilator*) (*hyper* above + *tonos* tone)
			vasoinert (exerting no effect on the caliber of blood vessels)
			vasolabile (*labilis* liable to slip; unstable)
			vasoligation (*ligare* to bind)
			vasomotion, vasomotor, vasomotoricity (*movere* to move)
			vasoneuropathy (*neuron* nerve + *pathos* disease)
			vasoneurosis (also called *vasoneuropathy*) (*neurosis* nerve condition)
			vaso-orchidostomy (*orchis* testicle + *stoma* mouth, opening)
			vasoparesis (also called *angioparesis*) (*paresis* paralysis)
			vasopermeability (the extent to which a blood vessel is permeable)
			vasopressor (*premere* to press: contraction)
			vasopuncture (also called *vasotomy*) (*pungere* to pierce)
			vasosection (also called *vasotomy*) (*secare* to cut)
			vasosensory (supplying sensory filaments to the vessels)
			vasospasmolytic (arresting spasm of the vessels) (*spasmos* contraction + *lytic* loosening)
			vasostimulant (also called *vasotonic*) (*stimulus* goad, incentive)
			vasostomy (also called *vasopuncture, vasotomy*) (*stoma* opening)
			vasotomy (also called *vasopuncture, vasostomy*) (*tomy* incision)
			vasotonia (also called *angiotonia*) {vasotonic} (*tonos* tension)
			vasotrophic (*trophein* to nourish: nutrition)
			vasotropic (*tropein* to turn)
			vasovagal (*vagal* wandering)
			vasovasostomy (reversal of a vasectomy) (*stoma* mouth, opening)
			vasovesiculectomy (excision of the vas deferens and seminal vesicles) (*vesica* bladder + *ektome* excision)
			vasovesiculitis (*vesica* bladder + *itis* inflammation)
			TRAILING ROOT COMPOUND:
			algiovascular (or, algovascular) (*algos* pain)
			cardiovascular (*kardia* heart)
			cerebrovascular (*cerebrum* brain)
			dermovascular (*derma* skin)
			emotiovascular (emotions)
			fibrovascular (*fibra* fiber)
			meningovascular (*meningos* membrane)
			myovascular (*myos* muscle)
			neurovascular (*neuron* nerve)
			ophthalmovascular (*ophthalmos* eye)
			renovascular (*ren* kidney)
			CROSS REFERENCE: angi, syring

Element	From	Meaning	Examples
ven	Latin *vena*	vein	SIMPLE ROOT: vena (in English, vein; pl., venae) venation (the manner of distribution of the veins of a part) venose, venosity, venous venula (or, venule; pl., venulae) {venular, venulous} venule (or, venula; a tiny vein continuous with a capillary) PREFIXED ROOT: *venation*: intravenation (*intra* within) *venitis*: endovenitis (also called *endophlebitis*) (*endon* within + *itis* inflammation) *venosity*: hypovenosity (*hypo* under) supervenosity (*super* over, above) *venous*: endovenous (also called *intravenous*) (*endon* within) intravenous (also called *endovenous*) (*intra* within) paravenous (*para* beside) perivenous (*peri* around, near) transvenous (*trans* across) LEADING ROOT COMPOUND: *ven*: venectasia (a varicosity of a vein; also called *phlebectasia*) (*ektasis* dilatation) venectomy (also called *phlebectomy*) (*ektome* excision) *vena*: venacaval (pertaining to a vena cava; also called *caval*) *vene*: venepuncture (or, venipuncture) (*pungere* to prick) venesection (also called *phlebotomy*) (*sectare* to cut) venesuture (also called *phleborrhaphy*) (*suere* to sew) *veni*: venipuncture (also called *phlebotomy*) (*pungere* to prick) venisection (also called *phlebotomy*) (*sectare* to cut) venisuture (also called *phleborrhaphy*) (*suere* to sew) *veno*: venoatrial (pertaining to the vena cava and the right atrium) venoclysis (also called *phleboclysis*) (*klysis* a drenching) venofibrosis (also called *phlebosclerosis*) (*fibrosis* fibrous condition) venography (also called *phlebography*) (*graphein* to write) venomotor (*movere* to move) venoperitoneostomy (peritoneum + *stoma* mouth, opening) venopressor (relating to the venous blood pressure) venosclerosis (also called *phlebosclerosis*) (*sklerosis* hardening) venosinal (pertaining to the vena cava and the atrial sinus of the heart) venostasis (also called *venous stasis*) (*stasis* standing) venostat (an instrument for stopping bleeding) (*statikos* standing) venotomy (also called *phlebotomy*) (*tomy* incision) venovenostomy (*stoma* mouth, opening) TRAILING ROOT COMPOUND: arteriovenous (both arterial and venous, pertaining to or affecting an artery and a vein) enterovenous (communicating between the intestinal lumen and the lumen of the vein) (*enteron* intestine)

Element	From	Meaning	Examples
ven (cont'd)		[vein]	peritoneovenous (communicating with the peritoneal cavity and the venous system) (peritoneum)
			pyelovenous (*pyelos* pelvis)
			venovenous (beginning and ending at a vein)
			CROSS REFERENCE: phleb, vari
ventr, **venter**	Latin *venter,* *ventris*	belly, abdomen, stomach, cavity	SIMPLE ROOT:
			venter (the abdomen, or belly; the uterus; the wide swelling portion, as though a belly, of the muscle) {ventral, or ventralis}
			ventrad (toward the belly; also called *ventralward*; opposed to *dorsad*, toward the back)
			ventricle (a small cavity, either of the heart or brain) [see separate entry: ventricul-]
			ventrose (having a bellylike expansion)
			PREFIXED ROOT:
			anteroventral (*anterior* before)
			biventer (two-bellied, as two-bellied muscles) (*bi* two)
			biventral (also called *digastric*) (*bi* two)
			eventration (also called *evisceration*) (*e* out)
			LEADING ROOT COMPOUND:
			ventri:
			ventricumbent (lying upon the belly) (*cumbere* to lie down)
			ventriduct, ventriduction (*ducere* to lead)
			ventriflexion (*flectere* to bend)
			ventrimeson {ventrimesal} (*meson* middle)
			ventro:
			ventrocystorrhaphy (*kystis* bladder + *rhaphe* suture)
			ventrodorsad, ventrodorsal (*dorsum* back)
			ventrofixation (also called *ventrosuspension*) (*fixare* to fix)
			ventrohysteropexy (*hystera* uterus + *pexis* fixation)
			ventroinguinal (also called *inguinoabdominal*) (*inguen* groin)
			ventrolateral (both ventral and lateral) (*laterus* side)
			ventromedian (both ventral and median) {ventromedial}
			ventroposterior (both ventral and posterior)
			ventroptosis (also called *gastroptosis*) (*ptosis* a falling)
			ventroscopy (also called *peritoneoscopy*) (*skopein* to examine)
			ventrosuspension (also called *ventrofixation*)
			ventrotomy (also called *celiotomy, laparotomy*) (*tomy* incision)
			TRAILING ROOT COMPOUND:
			dorsoventrad (in a direction from the dorsal to the ventral aspect)
			dorsoventral (passing from the back to the belly surface) (*dorsum* back)
			uteroventral (uterus)
			CROSS REFERENCE: cel[1], gast(r), lapar, stomach
ventricul	Latin diminutive of *venter* belly (cavity)	ventricle	SIMPLE ROOT: ventriculus (or, ventricle; a small, normal cavity in an organ such as the heart or brain; pl., ventriculi) {ventricular}
			PREFIXED ROOT:
			ventricular:
			biventricular (*bi* two)
			circumventricular (*circum* around)
			extraventricular (*extra* outside)
			interventricular (*inter* between)
			intraventricular (*intra* within)
			periventricular (*peri* around)
			supraventricular (*supra* over)

Element	From	Meaning	Examples
ventricul (cont'd)		[ventricle]	transventricular (*trans* across) *ventriculus*: preventriculus (*pre* before) LEADING ROOT COMPOUND: *ventricul*: ventriculectomy (*ektome* excision) ventriculitis (inflammation of a ventricle, especially one of the brain) (*itis* inflammation) ventriculostium (*ostium* mouth, opening) *ventriculo*: ventriculoatriostomy (also called *ventriculocisternostomy, ventriculoatrial shunt*) (atrium + *stoma* opening) ventriculoencephalitis (*enkephalon* brain + *itis* inflammation) ventriculogram, ventriculography (*graphein* to write) ventriculomegaly (*megalos* large) ventriculomastoidostomy (mastoid + *stoma* mouth, opening) ventriculometry (*metron* measure) ventriculomyotomy (*myos* muscle + *tomy* incision) ventriculonector (*nectere* to join) ventriculoplasty (*plassein* to form) ventriculopuncture (also called *ventricular puncture*) ventriculoscope, ventriculoscopy (*skopein* to examine) ventriculostomy (*stoma* mouth, opening) ventriculotomy (*tomy* incision) ventriculovenostomy (also called *ventriculovenous shunt*) (*vena* vein + *stoma* mouth, opening) TRAILING ROOT COMPOUND: atrioventricular (atrium) idioventricular (*idios* one's own, particular) sinoventricular (sinus) CROSS REFERENCE: None
vertebr	Latin *vertere* to turn	a bone of the spinal column (vertebra)	SIMPLE ROOT: vertebra (pl., vertebrae) {vertebral}, vertebrarium (the vertebral column), vertebrate {vertebrated} PREFIXED ROOT: *vertebra*: hemivertebra (*hemi* half) protovertebra {provertebral} (*protos* first) *vertebral*: intervertebral (*inter* between) intravertebral (also called *intraspinal*) (*intra* within) paravertebral (*para* alongside) perivertebral (also called *perispondylic*) (*peri* around) postvertebral (*post* behind, after) prevertebral (*pre* before) subvertebral (*sub* below) LEADING ROOT COMPOUND: *vertebr*: vertebrarterial (or, vertebroarterial) (artery) vertebrectomy (*ektome* excision) *vertebro*: vertebrochondral (*chondros* cartilage) vertebrocostal (*costa* rib, side) vertebrodidymus (*didymos* twin, double) vertebrogenic (*genere* to produce) vertebroplasty (*plassein* to form)

Element	From	Meaning	Examples
vertebr (cont'd)		[vertebra]	vertebrosacral (sacrum) vertebrosternal (sternum) TRAILING ROOT COMPOUND: basivertebral (basion) costovertebral (*costa* rib) ischiovertebral (*ischion* hip) oculovertebral (*oculus* eye) sacrovertebral (sacrum) sternovertebral (sternum) uncovertebral (*uncus* hook) CROSS REFERENCE: rachi, spondyl
vesic	Latin *vesica*	bladder, blister, sac	SIMPLE ROOT: vesica (bladder; pl., vesicae) {vesical} vesicant (or, vesicatory; causing blisters) vesicate (to blister; to form a vesicle), vesication vesicle (a small cavity or sac filled with fluid, especially a small, round elevation of the skin containing a serous fluid; blister) vesicula (pl., vesiculae) {vesicular}, vesiculated, vesiculation PREFIXED ROOT: *vesical*: extravesical (*extra* outside) infravesical (*infra* below) intravesical (*intra* within) juxtavesical (also called *perivesical*) (*juxta* near, close by) microvesicle (*mikros* small) paravesical (also called *perivesical*) (*para* beside) perivesical (also called *paravesical, pericystic*) (*peri* around) prevesical (*pre* before) retrovesical (*retro* behind, posterior) supravesical (*supra* above) transvesical (*trans* through) *vesiculitis*: perivesiculitis (*peri* around + *itis* inflammation) LEADING ROOT COMPOUND: *vesico*: vesicoabdominal (also called *abdominovesical*) vesicocavernous (both vesicular and cavernous) vesicocele (also called *cystocele*) (*kele* hernia) vesicocervical (*cervix* neck—of uterus) vesicoclysis (*klysis* a drenching) vesicocolonic (or, vesicocolic) (colon) vesicoenteric (also called *enterovesical*) (*enteron* intestine) vesicofixation (*fixare* to fix) vesicointestinal (also called *enterovesical*) vesicolithiasis (also called *cystolithiasis*) (*lithos* stone + *iasis* condi- tion) vesicoperineal (perineum) vesicoprostatic (prostate) vesicopubic (also called *pubovesical*) (pubes) vesicopustule (pustule) vesicorectal (also called *rectovesical*) (rectum) vesicorenal (*ren* kidney) vesicosigmoid (also called *sigmoidovesical*) vesicospinal (spine; spinal cord) vesicostomy (*stoma* mouth, opening)

Element	From	Meaning	Examples
vesic (cont'd)		[bladder, sac, blister]	vesicotomy (also called *cystotomy*) (*tomy* incision) vesicoumbilical (*umbilicus* navel) vesicourachal (also called *urachovesical*) (*urachus* fetal canal) vesicoureteral (also called *ureterovesical*) (ureter) vesicovaginal, vesicovaginorectal (vagina + rectum) vesicovisceral (*viscera* internal organs) *vesicul*: vesiculectomy (*ektome* excision) vesiculitis (*itis* inflammation) vesiculose (*osis* condition) *vesiculi*: vesiculiform (*forma* shape) *vesiculo*: vesiculobronchial (*bronchos* windpipe) vesiculography (*graphein* to write) vesiculopapular (*papula* papule, pimple) vesiculoprostatitis (prostate + *itis* inflammation) vesiculopustular (pustule) vesiculotomy (*tomy* incision) vesiculotubular (tube) vesiculotympanic (having both a vesicular and tympanic quality: said of percussion sounds) (*tympanon* drum) vesiculovisceral (*viscera* internal organs) TRAILING ROOT COMPOUND: *vesical*: anovesical (anus) cervicovesical (also called *vesicocervical*) (*cervix* neck—of uterus) colovesical (also called *vesicocolonic*) (colon) enterovesical (also called *vesicoenteric, vesicointestinal*) (*enteron* intestine) ileovesical (also called *vesicoileal*) (ileum) omphalovesical (also called *vesicoumbilical*) (*omphalos* navel) prostaticovesical (also called *vesicoprostatic*) (prostate) pubovesical (also called *vesicopubic*) (pubic bone) sigmoidovesical (also called *vesicosigmoid*) urachovesical (also called *vesicourachal*) (*urachus* fetal canal) ureterovesical (also called *vesicoureteral*) (ureter) uterovesical (also called *vesicouterine*) (uterus) vaginovesical (also called *vesicovaginal*) (vagina) *vesicle*: tubulovesicle {tubulovesicular} (*tubus* tube) *vesiculosis*: pyovesiculosis (*pyon* pus + *osis* condition) CROSS REFERENCE: bursa, cyst
vestibul	Latin *vestibulum* entrance hall, ante-chamber	cavity or space [serving as an entrance]	SIMPLE ROOT: vestibulum (or, vestibule; pl., vestibula) {vestibular} LEADING ROOT COMPOUND: *vestibul*: vestibulitis (*itis* inflammation) *vestibulo*: vestibulocerebellum (*cerebrum* brain) vestibulocochlear (cochlea) vestibulogenic (*genere* to produce) vestibulo-ocular (*oculus* eye) vestibulopathy (*pathos* disease) vestibuloplasty (*plassein* to form) vestibulospinal (spine) vestibulotomy (*tomy* incision)

Element	From	Meaning	Examples
vestibul (cont'd)		[vestibule]	TRAILING ROOT COMPOUND: cochleovestibular (pertaining to the cochlea and vestibule of the ear) rectovestibular (rectum) stapediovestibular (pertaining to the stapes and vestibule of the ear) CROSS REFERENCE: alveol, antr, cell
vir	Latin *virus*	poison	SIMPLE ROOT: virion (the complete virus particle that is structurally intact) virulent (exceedingly pathogenic), virus (pl., viruses) {viral} PREFIXED ROOT: avirulence, avirulent (*a* negative) antiviral (or, antivirotic) (*anti* against) provirus (*pro* before) subvirion (an incomplete viral particle) (*sub* under: incomplete) LEADING ROOT COMPOUND: *vir*: viremia (*emia* blood condition) viroid (*eidos* form) virosis (*osis* condition) viruria (*uria* urine condition) *viri*: viricide {viricidal} (*caedere* to kill) *viro*: virogene, virogenetic (caused by a virus) (*genere* to produce) viropexis (*pexis* fixation) viroplasm (*plassein* to form) virostatic (*statikos* causing to stand: inhibition) virotherapy (*therapy* treatment) *viru*: virucide {virucidal} (*caedere* to kill) virucopria (*kopros* feces) *viruli*: virulicidal (*caedere* to kill) viruliferous (*ferre* to bear, carry) *virus*: virusoid (*eidos* form, resembling) TRAILING ROOT COMPOUND: enterovirus (*enteron* intestine) herpesvirus (*herpein* to creep) poliovirus (*polios* gray) CROSS REFERENCE: tox
visc	Latin *viscus*	inner part of the body	SIMPLE ROOT: viscera (the internal organs of the body, especially of the thorax and abdomen, as the heart, lungs, liver, kidneys, intestines, etc; specifically, in popular usage, the intestines; also called *vitals*) {visceral}, viscerad (toward the viscera) viscus (any large interior organ in one of the three great cavities of the body, especially of the abdomen; pl., viscera) PREFIXED ROOT: *visceral*: paravisceral (*para* alongside, beside) perivisceral (*peri* around) *visceration*: devisceration (also called *evisceration*) (*de* away) evisceration (also called *devisceration, eventration*) (*ex* out) plurivisceral (pertaining to or affecting several viscera, or organs) (*pluris* more)

Element	From	Meaning	Examples
visc (cont'd)		[intestines]	*visceritis*: perivisceritis (inflammation around a viscus or the viscera) (*peri* around + *itis* inflammation)
			viscero: evisceroneurotomy (*eviscero* to disembowel + *neuron* nerve + *tomy* incision)
			LEADING ROOT COMPOUND:
			viscer: visceralgia (*algos* pain)
			viscero:
			viscerocranium (*kranion* skull)
			viscerogenic (*genere* to produce)
			viscerography (radiography of the viscera) (*graphein* to write)
			visceromegaly (also called *splanchnomegaly*) (*megalos* large)
			visceromotor (or, viscerimotor) (*movere* to move)
			visceroparietal (*paries* abdominal wall)
			visceroperitoneal (peritoneum)
			visceropleural (*pleura* side, rib)
			visceroptosis (or, visceroptosia) (*ptosis* a falling)
			viscerosomatic (relating to the viscera and the body; also called *splanchnosomatic*) (*soma* body)
			viscerotome, viscerotomy (*tomy* incision)
			viscerotonia (personality traits of love of food, sociability, general relaxation, friendliness, and affection) (*tonos* tension)
			viscerotrophic (*trephein* to nourish)
			viscerotropic (affecting the viscera) (*trepein* to turn)
			TRAILING ROOT COMPOUND:
			neurovisceral (also called *neurosplanchnic*) (*neuron* nerve)
			parietovisceral (*paries* wall)
			pleurovisceral (*pleura* rib, side)
			somaticovisceral (*somatos* body)
			vesicovisceral (*vesica* bladder)
			CROSS REFERENCE: cel[1], enter, lapar, ventr, splanchn
vitell	Latin *vitellus*	egg yolk	SIMPLE ROOT:
			vitellarium (an accessory genital gland found in tapeworms which secretes the yolk or albumin for the fertilized egg; also called *vitelline gland*)
			vitellary (also called *vitelline*)
			vitellicle (the yolk sac), vitellin (also called *ovovitellin*)
			vitellin (also called *lipovitellin, ovovitellin*)
			vitelline (resembling or pertaining to the yolk of an egg or ovum)
			vitellose (a form of proteose derived from vitellin)
			vitellus (the yolk of an egg or ovum) {vitelline}
			PREFIXED ROOT:
			bivitelline (*bi* two)
			intravitelline (*intra* within)
			perivitelline (*peri* around)
			univitelline (*unus* one, single)
			LEADING ROOT COMPOUND:
			vitelli: vitelliform (relating to or resembling the yolk of an egg)
			vitello:
			vitellogenesis, vitellogenin (*genere* to produce)
			vitellolutein (lutein from the yolk of egg) (*luteus* saffron-yellow)
			vitellorubin (*rubin* red)
			TRAILING ROOT COMPOUND:
			lecithovitellin (a saline extract of egg yolks used in an egg-yolk agar to test for bacterial lecithinase) (*lekithos* yolk)

Element	From	Meaning	Examples
vitell (cont'd)		[egg yolk]	lipovitellin (most abundant protein in egg yolk) (*lipos* fat) ovovitellin (also called *vitellin*) (*ovum* egg) phytovitellin (vitelline of vegetable origin) (*phyton* plant) CROSS REFERENCE: lecith
vulv	Latin *vulva, volva* wrapper, covering, womb	external genital organs of the female	SIMPLE ROOT: vulva (pl., vulvae) {vulval, vulvar), vulvismus (also called *vaginismus*) LEADING ROOT COMPOUND: *vulv*: vulvectomy (*ektome* excision) vulvitis (*itis* inflammation) vulvodynia (*odyne* pain) *vulvo*: vulvocrural (relating to the vulva and the thigh) (*crus*; pl., *crura* leg, thigh) vulvopathy (*pathos* disease) vulvorectal (pertaining to the vulva and to the rectum) vulvouterine (*uterus* womb) vulvovaginal (also called *vaginovulvar*), vulvovaginitis (vagina + *itis* inflammation) TRAILING ROOT COMPOUND: rectovulvar (rectum) vaginovulvar (also called *vulvovaginal*) (vagina) CROSS REFERENCE: episio, labi[1]

Element	From	Meaning	Examples
xanth	Greek *xanthos*	yellow, blond	SIMPLE ROOT: xanthate (any salt of xanthic acid) xanthene, xanthic (yellow; pertaining to xanthine) xanthine (a yellow pigment obtained from flowers), xanthism xanthous (yellowish; yellow-colored) PREFIXED ROOT: heteroxanthine (*heteros* other) hypoxanthine (*hypo* under) paraxanthine (*para* alongside, similar to) LEADING ROOT COMPOUND: *xanth*: xanthelasma (*elasma* plate) xanthodontous (having yellowish teeth) (*odontos* tooth) xanthoma, xanthomatosis (*oma* tumor + *osis* condition) xanthopsia (also called *yellow vision*) (*opsia* vision condition) xanthosis (*osis* condition) *xanthi*: xanthiuria (or, xanthinuria) (*uria* urine condition) *xantho*: xanthochromia {xanthochromatic, xanthochromic} (*chroma* color) xanthocyanopsia (*kyanos* blue + *opsia* vision condition) xanthoderma (*derma* skin) xanthoerythrodermia (*erythros* red + *dermia* skin condition) xanthogranuloma {xanthogranulomatous} (granule + *oma* tumor) xanthophore (*pherein* to bear) xanthophyll (*phyllon* leaf) xanthosarcoma (*sarkos* flesh + *oma* tumor) TRAILING ROOT COMPOUND: lipoxanthine (*lipos* fat) CROSS REFERENCE: cirrh, lut
xen	Greek *xenos* stranger	strange or foreign material	SIMPLE ROOT: xenia, xenon (Xe) PREFIXED ROOT: *xenic*: axenic (not contaminated by or associated with any other living organisms; sterile) (*a* negative) antixenic (pertaining to the reaction of living tissue to any foreign substance) (*anti* against) monoxenic (*monos* single) synxenic (*syn* together) *xenitis*: perixenitis (inflammation occurring around a foreign body in a tissue or organ; also called *perialienitis*) (*peri* around + *itis* inflammation) *xenous*: heteroxenous (requiring more than one host in order to complete the life cycle: said of parasitic organisms; also called *metoxenous*; compare *monoxenous*) (*heteros* other) homoxenous (requiring only one host in the life cycle; said of certain parasites; also called *monoxenous*) (*homos* same) metoxenous (also called *heteroxenous, heterecious*) (*meta* beyond) monoxenous (requiring only one host in order to complete the life cycle; also called *homoxenous*) (*monos* single, one)

Element	From	Meaning	Examples
xen (cont'd)		[stranger]	metoxenous (requiring a change of host by a parasite; also called *heteroxenous*) (*meta* change)
			polyxenous (capable of infecting more than one species) (*polys* many)
			LEADING ROOT COMPOUND:
			xen:
			xenophthalmia (ophthalmia caused by a foreign body in the eye) (*ophthalmia* eye condition)
			xenorexia (an appetite disorder leading to the repeated swallowing of nonnutritive substances, such as ice, dirt, gravel, laundry starch; also called *pica*) (*orexia* appetite)
			xeno:
			xenoantigen (*anti* against + *genere* to produce)
			xenobiotic (*bios* life + *osis* condition)
			xenocytophilic (*kytos* cell + *philein* to love)
			xenogeneic (also called *heterogenic, heterologous*), xenogenesis {xenogenous} (*genere* to produce)
			xenograft (also called *heterograft*)
			xenology (the science of the relations of parasites to their hosts) (*logos* study)
			xenomenia (menstruation from a part of the body other than the normal one) (*mene* month: menstruation)
			xenoparasite (parasite: *para* alongside + *sitos* food)
			xenophobia (*phobia* fear)
			xenophonia (*phone* sound)
			xenotropic (*tropic* a turning)
			TRAILING ROOT COMPOUND: lipoxeny (the desertion of the host by a parasite) (*leipein* to leave)
			CROSS REFERENCE: allotrio
xer	Greek *xeros*	dry	SIMPLE ROOT:
			xeransis (a gradual loss of moisture in the tissues)
			xerantic (causing dryness; also called *siccant, siccative*)
			xerasia (a condition of the hair characterized by dryness)
			xeroma (a dryness of the conjunctiva and cornea due to vitamin A deficiency; also called *xerophthalmia*)
			PREFIXED ROOT: antixerotic (*anti* against)
			LEADING ROOT COMPOUND:
			xer:
			xerophthalmia (or, xerophthalmus) (*opthalmia* eye condition)
			xerosis (also called *xeronosus*) {xerotic} (*osis* condition)
			xero:
			xerochilia (dryness of the lips; a type of cheilitis) (*cheilos* lip)
			xerocyte, xerocytosis (presence of xerocytes in the blood) (*kytos* cell + *osis* condition)
			xeroderma (excessive or abnormal dryness of the skin, as in ichthyosis; also called *ichythyosis*) (*derma* skin)
			xerogel (a gel containing little fluid)
			xerography (also called *xeroradiography*) (*graphein* to write)
			xeromammography (*mamma* breast + *graphein* to write)
			xeromenia (the occurrence of the usual manifestations at the menstrual period but without the show of blood) (*mene* menstruation)
			xeromycteria (dryness of the nasal mucous membrane) (*mykter* nose)
			xeronosus (dryness of the skin; also called *xerosis*) (*nosos* disease)
			xerophagia (the eating of dry food only) (*phagein* to devour)

A Thesaurus of Medical Word Roots

Element	From	Meaning	Examples
xer (cont'd)		[dry]	xerostomia (dryness of the mouth resulting from diminished or arrested salivary secretion) (*stoma* mouth)
			xerotripsis (dry friction) (*tripsis* rubbing)
			TRAILING ROOT COMPOUND:
			xerosis dry condition:
			colpoxerosis (*kolpos* vagina)
			laryngoxerosis (larynx)
			mycteroxerosis (also called *xeromycteria*) (*mykter* nose)
			ophthalmoxerosis (*ophthalmos* eye)
			pharyngoxerosis (pharynx)
			CROSS REFERENCE: None
xiph	Greek *xiphos* sword	xiphoid process	PREFIXED ROOT: supraxiphoid (*supra* over)
			LEADING ROOT COMPOUND:
			xiph:
			xiphodynia (pain in the xiphoid process) (*odyne* pain)
			xiphoid (also called *ensiform*; see Term) (*eidos* form)
			xiphi: xiphisternum {xiphosternal} (*sternon* chest)
			xipho:
			xiphocostal (*costa* rib)
			xiphodidymus (also called *xiphopagus*) (*didymos* twin)
			xiphopagus (symmetrical conjoined twins fused in the region of the xiphoid process) (*pagos* thing fixed)
			xiphoid:
			xiphoidalgia (*algos* pain)
			xiphoiditis (*itis* inflammation)
			TRAILING ROOT COMPOUND: ilioxiphopagus (ilium + *pagus* fixed)
			TERM: xiphoid process (the pointed process of cartilage, supported by a core of bone, connected with the lower end of the body of the sternum)
			CROSS REFERENCE: None

Z

Element	From	Meaning	Examples
zein, **zem**, **zeo**	Greek *zein*	to boil, seethe	PREFIXED ROOT: antieczematic (*anti* against + eczema) apozema (a medicinal or medicated decoction) (*apo* from) eczema (acute or chronic cutaneous inflammatory condition) (*ek* out) LEADING ROOT COMPOUND: *zei*: zeiosis (bubbling or blebbing activity, giving the appearance of boiling in slow motion, observed at the periphery of cells cultured in artificial media) (*osis* condition) [bleb: a large flaccid vesicle] *zeo*: zeoscope (a device for determining the alcoholic content of a liquid by ascertaining its exact boiling point) (*skopein* to examine) CROSS REFERENCE: zym
zo	Greek *zoion*	life; animal	SIMPLE ROOT: zoic (pertaining to animal life) PREFIXED ROOT: *zoan*: protozoan (also called *microzoon*) (*protos* first) *zoiasis*: protozoiasis (infection with protozoa; any disease caused by protozoa) (*protos* first + *iasis* condition) *zoic*: azoic (containing no living organisms) (*a* privative) heterozoic (*heteros* different) holozoic (also called *phagotrophic*) (*holos* entire, whole) homozoic (*homos* same) *zoo*: dyszoospermia (*dys* abnormal + *spermia* sperm condition) protozoology (*protos* first + *logos* study) protozoophage (*protos* first + *phagein* to consume) *zoon*: ectozoon (also called *ectoparasite*; pl., ectozoa) (*ektos* outside) entozoon (pl., entozoa) {*entozoal*} (*entos* within) epizoon (pl., epizoa) {*epizoic*}, epizootic (*epi* upon) microzoon (a protozoan) (*mikros* small) protozoon (pl., protozoa) {*protozoal*} (*protos* first) *zot*: azote (nitrogen, because the gas does not support life) [see separate entry: azo-] LEADING ROOT COMPOUND: *zo*: zoanthropy (a delusion that one is an animal) (*anthropos* man) zooid (resembling an animal) (*eidos* resembling) *zoo*: zooblast (*blastos* germ, cell) zoochrome (*chroma* color) zooerastia (also called *bestiality, zoophilia*) (*eros* love) zoogenesis (*genere* to produce) zoograft (a graft of tissue from an animal to a human) zoolagnia (sexual attraction toward animals) (*lagneia* lust) zoology (*logy* study) zoomania (an excessive, abnormal love of animals) (*mania* craze) zoophilia (also called *bestiality, zooerastia*) (*philein* to love) zoophobia (*phobia* fear) zoophyte (any plantlike animal, as a sponge) (*phyton* plant) zooplasty (grafting of tissue from an animal to a human; also called *zoograft*) (*plassein* to form)

Element	From	Meaning	Examples
zo (cont'd)		[life; animal]	zoospermia (the presence of live spermatozoa in the ejaculated semen) (*sperma* seed) TRAILING ROOT COMPOUND: *zoan*: sporozoan (*sporos* seed) *zoic*: cytozoic (living within or attached to cells) (*kytos* cell) enterozoic (*enteron* intestine) hemozoic (also called *hematozoan*) (*haima* blood) histozoic (*histos* web, tissue) karyozoic (*karyon* nucleus) saprozoic (also called *saprophytic*) (*sapros* rotten) CROSS REFERENCE: azo, bio
zon	Latin *zona* girdle	encircling region	SIMPLE ROOT: zona (or, zone; pl., zonae), zone {zonal, zonary), zoning zonula (pl., zonulae), zonule (or, zonula) {zonular} PREFIXED ROOT: metazonal (situated after or below a sclerozone) (*meta* after, below) prezonular (pertaining to the posterior chamber of the eye, between the iris and ciliary zonule) (*pre* before) subzonal (*sub* under) trizonal (having, or arranged in, three zones or layers) LEADING ROOT COMPOUND: *zon*: zonesthesia (also called *cincture sensation; girdle sensation, stranglesthesia*) (*esthesia* feeling) *zoni*: zonifugal (passing outward from a zone or region) (*fugere* to flee) zonipetal (*petere* to seek) *zono*: zonography (*graphein* to write) *zonul*: zonulitis (inflammation of the ciliary zonule) *zonulo*: zonulolysis (or, zonulysis) (*lyein* to loosen) zonulotomy (*tomy* incision) TRAILING ROOT COMPOUND: sclerozone (any surface on a bone giving attachment to the muscles from a given myotome) (*skleros* hard) CROSS REFERENCE: None
zyg	Greek *zygon*	yoke, pair	SIMPLE ROOT: zygal (shaped like a yoke) zygoma (also called *zygomatic bone*), zygomatic zygon, zygosis (conjugation) {zygosity} zygote {zygotic} PREFIXED ROOT: *zygium*: syzygium (or, syzygy; fusion of two parts or structures without loss of identity of the parts) {syzygial} (*syn* together) *zygomatic*: bizygomatic (*bi* two) subzygomatic (*sub* under) suprazygomatic (*supra* above) *zygosis*: prozygosis (also called *syncephaly*) (*pro* before) *zygote*: heterozygote (*heteros* different) hemizygote (*hemi* half) *zygotic*: enzygotic (*en* in)

Element	From	Meaning	Examples
zyg (cont'd)		[yoke, pair]	monozygotic (or, monozygous) (*monos* single)
			polyzygotic (*polys* many)
			postzygotic (*post* after)
			prezygotic (*pre* before)
			zygous:
			azygous (unmatched; not one of a pair; having no mate; odd; as an azygous muscle) (*a* negative)
			autozygous (*autos* self)
			heterozygous (*heteros* different)
			hemizygous (*hemi* half)
			homozygous (*homos* same)
			LEADING ROOT COMPOUND:
			zygo:
			zygoapophysis (*apophysis* offshoot)
			zygodactyly (*dactylos* finger, toe)
			zygomaxillary (*maxilla* upper jaw)
			zygomycosis (*mykes* fungus + *osis* condition)
			zygonema (also called *zygotene*) (*nema* thread)
			zygopodium (*podos* foot)
			zygosperm (also called *zygospore*) (*sperma* seed)
			zygosphere (*sphere* ball, globe)
			zygospore (also called *zygosperm*) (*sporos* seed)
			zygotene (also called *zygonema*) (*tainia* band)
			zygomatico:
			zygomaticofacial
			zygomaticofrontal
			zygomaticomaxillary (*maxilla* jaw)
			zygomaticoorbital
			zygomaticosphenoid (*sphenos* wedge)
			zygomaticotemporal (temporal process)
			zygoto:
			zygotoblast (*blastos* germ)
			zygotomere (also called *sporoblast*) (*meros* part)
			TRAILING ROOT COMPOUND: oculozygomatic (*oculus* eye)
			CROSS REFERENCE: jug
zym	Greek *zyme*	ferment, leaven	SIMPLE ROOT: zyme (a ferment)
			PREFIXED ROOT:
			abzyme (a catalytic antibody) (*ab* away)
			allozyme (*allos* other)
			enzyme (*en* in) [see separate entry]
			microzyme (*mikros* small)
			synzyme (*syn* with)
			LEADING ROOT COMPOUND:
			zymogenesis {zymogenic, zymogenous} (*genere* to produce)
			zymogram (*graphein* to write)
			zymoscope (*skopein* to examine)
			zymosthenic (*sthenos* strength)
			TRAILING ROOT COMPOUND:
			angiozyme (*angeion* vessel)
			lysozyme (*lyein* to loosen)
			CROSS REFERENCE: zein

Appendix A
English to Roots Index

Roots are listed in alphabetical order in the thesaurus proper

A

abdomen: *abdom, cel¹, ile, lapar, stomach, ventr*
aberration (mental): *mania*
abnormal: *caco*
abortion: *ectro*
above: *hyper-, super-*
abscess: *ulc*
absent (congenitally): *ectro*
acorn: *gland*
adrenal gland: *adren*
adult: *pub*
afar: *dist, tele²*
affinity for: *phil*
against: *anti-, contra-, ob-*
age (old): *ger², presby*
agnosia: *agnos*
air: *aer, phys², pneumat, pneumo*
alimentary canal: *esophag*
all: *omni, pan*
almond: *amygdal*
alone: *mono-*
alongside: *para-*
amber: *electr*
angle: *canth, gon²*
animal: *zo*
ankle: *astrag, tal, tars¹*
another: *all*
antrum: *antr*
anus: *an, proct*
aorta: *aort*
apex: *apic*
appearance: *eid, ide, form, morph, phan, plas*
appendage: *scol*
appetite: *orex*
arm (upper): *brachi*
around: *peri-*
arrangement: *tax*
artery: *arter*
atrium: *atri*
attach: *fix, pact, pex*
away: *ab-, apo-, de-*
axis: *ax*

B

back (of body): *dors, noto, rachi, spin, spondyl*
back (of head): *ini, occip*

back of: *dors, opist*
backbone: *rachi, spin, spondyl, vertebr*
backward: *opist, palin*
bad: *cac-, dys-, mal-*
bag: *cyst, scrot, vesic*
ball: *glob, spher*
band: *desm, fasci*
bark (noun): *cort*
base: *bas*
bear (verb): *fer, ger¹, phor*
bearing ova: *gon¹, oo, oophor, ov*
beat: *crot, ict, sphygm*
becoming an adult: *pub*
before: *ante, antero, pro*
beginning: *arch, prot*
behind: *dors, opist, palin*
below: *hypo-, sub-*
bend: *ankyl, camp*
berry: *cocc*
beyond: *extra-, meta-, ultra-*
bile: *bil, chol*
bile duct: *choledoch*
bind: *desm, lig, syndes*
birth: *nat, par, toc*
black: *melan*
bladder: *cyst, vesic*
blade (shoulder): *scapul*
blemish: *macul*
blind gut: *cec, typhl*
blinking: *blephar, cili, palpebr*
blister: *vesic*
blond: *xanth*
blood: *hem, sangui*
blood condition: *emia*
blood vessel: *angi*
blow (verb): *phys²*
bodily tissue: *hist*
body (inner part): *visc*
body: *corp, som*
boil: *zein*
bone: *oss, ost(e)*
bone (of the spinal column): *coccy, spondyl, vertebr*
bone protuberance: *condyl, epiphys*
born (to be): *grav*
both: *ambi-, amphi-*
brain: *cerebr, encephal, phren*
break: *clas, rupt*
breaking forth: *rhex*

breast: *mamm, mast, pect, stern, steth, thora*
breathe: *phys², pnea, pneumat, spir¹*
bride: *nymph*
bring forth: *phyt*
broad: *eury, later, platy*
bud: *blast, graft*
builder: *tect*
bulb: *bulb, tub²*
bulk: *gangl, onc, phyma*
burn: *caum, phleg, pyr*
bursting: *rhex*
buttocks: *glut¹, pyg*

C

calculus: *calc, lith*
cancer: *cancr, carcin*
capillary: *capill*
capsule: *caps*
care for: *med(ic)*
carry: *fer, ger¹, phor*
cartilage: *cartilag, chondr*
case: *theca*
caudal portion of of the body: *pelvi, pyel*
caul: *hymen*
cause: *fac*
cavity: *alveol, antr, cell, vestibul*
cecum (blind gut): *typhl¹*
cell: *alveol, cell*
cell layer: *epithel*
center: *centr*
cervix: *cervi, trachel*
chamber: *atri, thalam*
change: *muta*
check (verb): *isch, schesis*
cheek: *bucc, mel²*
chest: *pect, stern, steth, thora*
chief: *arch*
child: *ped¹, puer*
childbirth: *nat, par, toc*
childish: *puer*
chin: *geni¹, ment*
cicatrix: *ul*
circle: *cycl, gyr, orb*
circle (colored): *irid*
clavicle: *clavi, cleid*
claws: *onych, ungu*
cleft: *schis*

close (adj.): *angin, arct, steno*
clot: *coagul, thromb*
coil: *helic, spir*
cold: *cry*
collarbone: *clavi, cleid*
colon: *col*
color: *chrom*
column: *styl*
comb-like: *pecten*
common: *cen, hom*
complete: *tele¹*
complete (not): *atel*
compressed: *arct, steno*
conceal: *crypt*
condition: *osis*
cone: *con, pine*
congenitally absent: *ectro*
connection: *arthr*
contracture: *diastol, peristol, systol*
cook (verb): *pept*
cord: *chord, funi*
cornea: *kerat*
corner: *canth*
corpse: *mort, necr*
cortex: *cort*
covering: *tect*
covering (fat skin): *epiplo, oment*
crescent: *men, menisc*
crooked: *ankyl, scol*
crush: *trib*
cure: *iat(r), therap*
curved: *camp*
cut (verb): *cide, sex, tom*

𝒟

dark: *melan, scoto*
death: *mort, necr, than*
decay: *caries, sapr, sep*
deep: *bath*
defecate: *chez*
deficiency: *penia*
delicate: *lept*
depression: *foll*
deprive: *priv*
depth: *bath*
destroy: *clas*
diaphragm: *phragm, phren¹*
die (verb): *mort*
different: *all-, heter-*
digest: *pept*
dilatation: *ectas, ten¹*
disease: *noso, path*

disease (blood): *-emia*
displaced: *ectop*
dissimilar: *all-, aniso-, heter-*
dissolve: *lys*
distant: *dist*
distinguish: *crin*
diverse: *multi-, poly-*
divide: *clas, schis, schiz, sciss*
do: *fac, prax, thes*
door: *pyl*
double: *didym, diplo*
down (adverb): *de-, cata-*
doze: *nystagm*
draw tight: *sphinct, systol*
dream: *oneir*
drenching: *clys*
drive: *puls*
drum membrane: *chori, myring, tympan*
dry: *xero*
duct: *vas*
duct (bile): *choledoch*
dull: *ambly*
duodenum: *duoden*
dust: *coni*
dwarf: *nan*

𝑬

ear: *aur, ot*
eardrum: *myring, tympan*
eat: *phag*
edge: *cheil, labi¹*
edge of eyelid: *tars²*
egg: *oo, ov*
egg yolk: *lecith, vitell*
eight: *oct*
elbow: *ancon, olecran*
empty: *jejun*
encircling region: *zon*
enclosure: *phragm, phren¹, sept*
end: *tele¹*
enlarged vein: *vari*
entire: *hol-*
environment: *eco*
epididymis: *epididym*
equal: *iso*
every: *pan-, omni-*
examine: *scop*
exempt: *immun*
exercise: *prax*
extension: *ectas*
external female genitals: *episio, labi¹, vulv*

external layer: *cort*
extremity: *acro-*
eye: *ocul, op, ophthalm*
eye corner: *canth*
eyelash: *cili*
eyelid: *blephar, palpebr*
eyelid (edge of): *tars²*

ℱ

face: *faci, opo, prosop*
fall: *pto*
false: *pseud*
far off: *dist, tele²*
fast (make): *fix, pact, pex*
fat: *adip, ather, lip, pimel, stear*
fat skin covering: *oment*
fear: *phob*
feed: *al, nur, troph*
feeling: *alg, esthes, path, sens*
female: *gyn*
female external general organs: *vulv*
ferment: *zym*
fever: *caum, phleg, pyr*
few: *olig, penia*
fiber: *fibr, in*
finger: *dactly*
fire: *pyr*
first: *arch, prot*
fistula: *syring*
fix: *fix, pact, pex*
flagellum: *mastig*
flank: *lapar*
flat: *plan¹, platy*
flesh: *creat, sarc*
flow: *rhe*
flow (excessive): *rrhag*
fluid (of body): *lymph*
flux: *rheum*
fold (noun): *sin*
fold (verb): *ploid*
food: *sit*
foot: *ped², pod*
forehead: *fron*
foreign: *all, allotrio, xen*
foremost: *arch*
foreskin: *posth*
form: *eid, form, ide, morph, plas*
foundation: *bas*
four: *quadr, tetra*
fracture: *clas*
free: *immun, lys*

fruit stone: *kary, nuc(le), pyren*
fungus: *myc*
fused: *ankyl*

G

gall: *bil, chol*
gas: *aer, phys², pneumat*
gastric juice: *chyl*
germ: *blast*
give birth to: *nat, par, toc*
gland: *acin, aden, gland, thym¹*
glans penis: *balano*
globe: *glob, spher*
glucose: *glyc*
glue: *colla, gli, glut²*
go: *meat*
gonad (male): *orchi, test*
gout: *agra*
grain: *chondr, gran*
grapes (bunch of): *staphyl, uv*
gray: *polio*
great: *mega-*
green: *chlor*
gristle: *cartilag*
groin: *ili, inguen*
grow: *aug, embryo, phys¹*
gruel: *ather*
guard (against): *phylax*
gums: *gingiv, oulo*
gut (blind): *cec*

H

hair: *capill, trich*
hand: *chir*
hand (right): *dextr*
hanging: *append*
hard: *scirrh, scler*
hatred of: *phob*
haunch: *cox, ischi*
head: *capit, cephal*
head (back of): *ini, occip*
heal: *iat(r), therap*
hear: *acou, aur*
heart: *card*
heat: *caum, phleg, therm*
heavy: *bar, grav*
heel bone: *calcan*
hernia: *cel², hern*
hide (verb): *crypt*
high: *acro-*
hip: *cox, ischi*
hold (verb): *lep², syndes*
hold fast: *hapt*

holding: *isch, schesis*
hole: *for, or, stoma, tres*
hollow: *cav, cel¹, sin*
hollow (like a drum): *tympan*
horn: *cerat, corn*
humped: *kyph*
hunger, hungry: *jejun*

I

ileum: *ileo*
ilium: *ilio*
ill: *caco-*
image: *eid*
imitate: *mim*
implement: *organ*
incomplete: *atel*
increase: *aug*
infectious venereal disease:
   syphil
inflammation: *itis, phleg*
inflation: *aer, phys², pneumat*
injury: *trauma*
inner chamber: *thalam*
inner part (of the body): *visc*
insanity: *mania*
instrument: *organ*
intestines: *enter, intestin, visc*
intestines (lower): *ile*
iodine: *iod*
iris: *irid*
iris (opening): *pupil*
iron: *ferr, sider*
irregular: *anomal, poikilo*
island: *insul, nesi*
itch: *psor*

J

jaw: *geni¹, gnath*
jaw bone (lower): *mandib*
jaw (upper): *maxill*
joined: *gam, jug, zyg*
joint: *arthr, articul*
juice: *chyl, chym*

K

kernel: *karyo, nuc(le), pyren*
ketone: *keto*
kidney: *nephr, ren*
kidney (above the): *supraren*
knee: *geni², gon³*
knee cap: *patell*

knot: *cel², gangli, nod, onc*

L

labia minora: *nymph*
labor: *nat, par, toc*
lack of: *penia*
language: *gloss, lingu*
large: *macr-, mega-*
layer (external): *cort. lam*
leading: *agog*
leaven: *zym*
left: *lev, sinist*
leg: *crur, scel*
lens: *lens, phac*
leprosy: *lep¹*
lesion: *les, trauma*
less: *mio*
life: *bio, zo*
ligament: *desm, lig, syndes*
light: *lum, phos*
like: *eid*
limb: *brachi, mel¹*
limestone: *calc*
lip: *cheil, labi¹*
liquid: *hydr, liqu, lymph*
listen: *acou, aur, auscul*
little: *olig, penia*
liver: *hepa*
living: *bio, zo*
lobe: *lob*
loin: *lapar, lumb*
long: *dolicho-, macr-*
loosen: *lys*
loss: *apheres, priv, steres*
lost: *clas*
loving: *phil*
lower abdomen: *ile*
lower jawbone: *mandib*
lungs: *pneumo, pulmo(n)*

M

madness: *mania*
maimed: *pero*
make: *fac, gen, poie*
make fast: *fix, pact, pex*
male gonad: *orchi, test*
mammary gland: *mast*
man: *andr, anthrop*
mandible: *gnath*
many: *multi-, poly-*
mark: *sem*
marriage: *gam*
marrow: *medull, myel*

mass: *cel²*, *gangli*, *onc*, *phyma*
maze: *labyrinth*
measles: *rub(r)*
measure (proper): *temp*
measure (verb): *mens*, *meter*
meat: *creat*
member (of body): *mel¹*
membrane: *ependym*, *hymen*,
  membran, *mening*, *myring*,
  pia
membrane (drum): *myring*
membranes (inner fetal):
  amnio
memory: *mne(m)*
menses, menstruation: *men*
mental aberration: *mania*
middle: *medi-*, *meso-*
milk: *galact*, *lact*
mimic: *mim*
mind: *psych*, *thym²*
mingling: *misc*
mix (verb): *cras*, *misc*
mold (verb): *plas*
moldy: *muc*, *myx*
month: *men*, *mens*
more: *plei-*, *pluri-*
mottled: *poikilo*
mouth: *or*, *stom*
move: *cin*, *mot*
much: *multi-*, *poly-*
mucus: *blenn*, *muc*, *myx*
muscle: *musc*, *my*
mutually: *all-*, *muta*

N

nail: *onych*, *ungu*
name: *onom*, *onym*
narrow: *angin*, *arct*, *steno*
natural opening: *for*, *por*, *stom*
navel: *omphal*, *umbilic*
near: *juxta-*
neck: *cervi*, *trachel*
neck of an organ: *trachel*
negative: *a-*, *ab-*, *de-*, *dis-*
neither: *neutr*
nematode worm: *nema*
nerve: *neur*
net: *ret*
new: *neo-*
night: *noct*, *nyct*
nipple: *mamm*, *papill*, *thel*
nitrogen: *azo*
nod: *nystagm*
node: *tub²*

normal: *norm*, *ortho*
nose: *nari*, *nas*, *rhin*
not complete: *atel*
not perforated: *atres*
nucleus: *karyo*, *nuc(le)*, *pyren*
nurture: *al*, *nur*, *troph*
nut: *karyo*, *nuc(le)*
nutrition: *al*, *nur*, *troph*

O

obstruction: *angin*, *arct*,
  emphrax, *steno*
occiput: *ini*, *occip*
oily: *lip*
old age: *ger²*, *presby*
omentum: *epiplo*
one: *hapl-*, *mono-*
one's own: *auto*, *idi*, *noe*
opening: *or*, *stom*
opening (natural): *for*, *por*,
  stom
opposite: *anti-*, *contra-*, *de-*,
  ob-
opsonin: *opson*
orange-yellow: *cirrh*
order: *tax*
organ (neck of): *cervi*, *trachel*
orifice: *pyl*, *stom*
origin: *arch*
originate: *gen*
other: *all-*, *heter-*
out of place: *ectop*
outside: *ecto-*, *ex-*, *exo-*
ova (bearing of): *oophora*
over: *hyper-*, *meta-*
ovum: *oo*, *ov*

P

pain: *alg*, *odyn*
pair: *jug*, *zyg*
palate: *palat*, *uran*
pancreas: *pancrea*
papule: *papu*
paralysis: *paraly*, *pares*, *pleg*
parasite: *mensa*, *parasit*
part: *mer*
particle: *gran*
partition: *diaphragm*, *phragm*,
  phren¹, *sept*
passage: *for*, *meat*, *por*, *tub¹*
passage (tubelike): *fistul*
patella: *patell*
pea-shaped: *lens*

pelvis: *pelvi*, *pyel*
penis: *balano*, *peni*, *phall*
people: *anthrop*
perception: *esthes*, *sens*
perforation: *for*, *tres*
perforated (not): *atres*
perineum: *perine*
periosteum: *periost*
peritoneum: *periton*
perspire: *hidr*, *sud*
phalanx: *phalang*
phallus: *balano*, *peni*, *phall*
pharynx: *pharyn*
phlegm: *pituit*
phosphorus: *phosphor*
pierce: *cente*, *nyx*, *punct*
pillar: *styl*
pimple: *papul*
pineal body: *pine*
pipe: *syring*
pit: *alveol*
pituitary gland: *hypophys*
place (noun): *loc*, *place*, *top*
place (out of): *ectop*
place (verb): *stal*, *stas*, *thes*
placenta: *placent*
plane: *plac*, *plan¹*
plant (noun): *phyt*
plate: *lam*, *plak*, *squam*
plug: *embol*
pneumonia: *pneumo*
point: *centr*, *punct*
poison: *tox*, *vir*
pore: *por*
pouch: *burs*, *cyst*, *sac*
pouch (testicle): *scrot*
pour: *chem*, *chys*, *fund*
powder: *coni*
power: *dynam*, *sthen*
prattle: *lal*
pregnant: *cyes*, *grav*
prepuce: *posth*
pressure: *bar*, *pies*
prevention: *phylax*
prick: *nyx*, *punct*
produce (verb): *fac*, *fer*, *gen*,
  par, *poie*
projecting: *geni¹*, *ment²*
prostate gland: *prostat*
protein (whitish): *album*
protrusion: *hern*, *rhex*
protuberance: *gangli*, *nod*
protuberance (bone): *condyl*
puberty: *ped¹*, *pub*, *puer*
pudenda: *episio*, *labi¹*, *vulv*
pulse: *crot*, *puls*, *sphygm*

puncture: *cente, nyx, punct*
pus: *pur, py*
pushing: *osm², puls*
pylorus: *pylor*

ℛ

rapid: *tach*
ray: *actin, rad¹*
reading: *lex*
recent: *neo*
rectum: *an, proct, rect*
red: *erythr, rub(r)*
region (encircling): *zon*
relaxation: *chalas, pares*
remedy: *iat(r), therap*
remember: *mne(m)*
remote: *dist*
remove: *apheres, ectom, priv, steres*
repository: *theca*
reproduction (sexual): *gam*
respiration: *pneumat, pneumo*
retention: *isch, schesis*
retina: *ret*
rheum: *pituit*
rhythm: *rhythm*
rib: *cost, later, pleur*
rickets: *rachi*
ridge: *rhaph*
right: *dextr, orth, rect*
rind: *cort*
ring: *an, gyr*
rock: *lith, petr*
rod: *bac, bacteri, rhabd*
roof of mouth: *palat, uran*
room: *cell*
root: *rad², rhiz*
rope: *chord, funi*
rose-colored: *erythr, rub(r)*
rotten: *caries, sapr, sep*
round: *cycl, gyr, orb*
rub: *trib*
rule: *arch, norm*
rump: *glut¹, pyg*
run: *drom, rhe*
rupture: *hern, rhex*

S

sac (excretory): *foll*
sac(k): *burs, cyst, vesic*
sacrum: *sacr*
saliva: *ptyal, sial*
salt: *hal*

saltpeter: *nitr*
same: *hom, iso*
scale [scaly]: *lep¹, squam*
scanty: *olig, penia*
scar: *ul*
scion: *blast, graft, sperm, spor*
scrotum: *scrot*
seam: *rhaph*
second: *deuter*
seed: *blast, gon¹, sperm, spor*
seethe: *zein*
seizure: *agra, epilep, hapt, lep²*
self: *auto, propri*
semen: *gon¹, semen, sperm, spor*
sense of touch: *hapt, palp*
septum: *diaphragm, parie, phragm, phren¹, sept*
serum: *lymph, ser*
sew: *rhaph*
sexual reproduction: *gam*
shake: *cuss*
shape: *eid, form, morph, plas*
shared: *cen, mer*
sharp: *ox*
sheath: *lemma, theca, vagin*
shield (noun): *thyr*
shin: *crur, scel*
shinbone: *tib*
shoot (noun): *blast, graft*
short: *brachy*
shoulder: *omo*
shoulder blade: *clavi, cleid, scapul*
side: *canth, cost, later, pleur*
sieve: *ethm, for, tres*
sight: *ocul, op, ophthalm, optic*
sigmoid: *sigma*
sign: *sem*
simple: *hapl*
single: *hapl, mono*
sinus: *antr, sin*
skin (thin): *chori, membr*
skin: *chori, cut, derm*
skull: *cephal, cran*
slender: *lept*
slime: *blenn, muc, myx*
slip (verb): *olist*
slow: *brady*
small: *lept, micro, mio, nan*
smell: *olfact, osm¹, osphr*
soft: *malac, pia*
sole [alone]: *hapl-, mono-*
solid: *ster*
soul: *psych, thym²*
sound: *phem, phon, son*

spasm: *clon, spas, tetan*
speak: *lal, lingua, logo, loqui, or, phas, phras*
speed: *tach*
sperm: *semen, sperm*
sphere: *glob*
spider: *arachn*
spinal cord: *medull, myel*
spine: *noto, rachi, spin, spondyl*
spiny: *acanth*
spiral: *cochl, helix, spir*
spirit: *psych, thym²*
spittle: *ptyal, sial*
spleen: *lien, splen*
split: *schis, schiz, sciss*
spoon: *cochl*
spore: *coni, spor*
spot: *macul, punct*
spread (verb): *rad¹, noma, ulc*
sprout: *blast, graft*
square: *quadr, tetra*
staff: *bac, bacteri*
stain: *macul*
stand (verb): *stas, thes*
starch: *amyl*
steal: *klept*
stench: *brom, oz*
stick: *bac, bacteri, rhabd*
sticky: *muc, visci*
stiffness: *ankyl*
stitch: *rhaph, sut*
stomach: *abdomen, cel¹, gast(r), stomach, ventr*
stone: *calc, lith, petr*
stone (fruit): *pyren*
stoppage: *emphrax*
stopper: *embol*
straight: *orth, rect*
strain (verb): *ethm, tres*
strange: *allotrio*
stranger: *xen*
strength: *sthen*
stretch: *ten¹, ten²*
strike: *cuss, pact*
string: *chord, funi*
stroke (medical): *apople, pleg*
stroke (noun): *crot, ict, palp, pleg, puls, sphyg*
strong: *sthen*
stupor: *typh*
sucrose: *glyc, sacchar*
suffer: *path*
sugar: *glyc, sacchar*
summit: *acro, apex*
suppress: *isch, schesis*

A Thesaurus of Medical Word Roots

surface (of a body structure): *faci*
surroundings: *eco*
suture: *rhaph*
swallow: *phag*
sweat: *hidr, sud*
sweet: *glyc, sacchar*
swell (verb): *edema*
swellng: *cel², edema, gangli, onc, tub², tum*
swift: *tach*
symptom: *sem*
synovia: *synovi*

T

table: *mensa*
tail: *peni*
take: *heres, lep²*
tallow: *adip, ather, lip, pimel, stear*
taste: *geus*
tear (as in teardrop): *dacry, lachry*
teat: *mamm, papill, thel*
temple: *temp*
temporal bone (part of): *petr*
tender: *pia*
tendon: *ten³*
tension: *ten¹, ten², ton*
testicle: *orchi, osche, test*
testicle pouch: *scrot*
thalamus: *thalam*
thick: *pachy, pykn*
thigh: *femor*
thin: *lept, mano*
thin skin: *membr*
thorax: *pect, stern, steth, thor*
thorny: *acanth*
thoughts: *idi, noe*
thread: *fil, mit, nema*
three: *tri*
throat: *pharyn*
throb: *crot, puls, sphygm*
through: *dia-, per-, trans-*
throw: *ball*
thymus: *thym¹*
tight: *angin*
time: *chron, temp*
tip: *apex*
tissue: *hist*
toe: *dactyl*
together: *com-, jug, syn-, zyg-*
tone: *ton*
tongue: *gloss, lingu*

tonsil: *amygdal, tonsil*
tooth: *dent, odont*
torso: *corm, som*
touch: *hapt, palp, tact*
tough: *scirrh, scler*
treatment: *iat(r), therap*
trumpet: *salping, tub¹*
trunk (of body): *corm*
tube: *fistul, salping, syring, tub¹*
tumor: *cel², gangli, onc, phyma, tum*
turmoil: *clon, spas, tetan*
turn: *cycl, rhomb, spir, trop*
twelve: *duoden*
twin: *diplo*
twist: *scol, helminth, stroph, torq*
two: *bi-, di-, dicho-*
two-fold: *diplo-*

U

ulcer: *helc, noma, ulc*
umbilical cord: *funi*
under: *hypo-, infra-, sub-*
unequal: *aniso*
uneven: *anomal, poikilo*
united: *gam, syn-*
unstable: *labi²*
upper arm: *brachi, humer*
upper jaw: *maxill*
urine deficiency: *diabet*
urine: *ur*
uterus: *colp, hyster, metr*
uvea [part of the eye]: *uv*
uvula: *staphyl, uvul*

V

vagina: *colp, vagin*
vaginal discharge: *lochi*
varied: *poikilo*
varix: *cirs, vari*
vein: *phleb, ven*
vein (enlarged): *vari*
venereal (infectious disease): *syphil*
ventricle: *ventricul*
vertebra: *spondyl, vertebr*
vessel: *angi, vas*
violet: *iod*
viscus: *splanchn, visc*
vision: *op*
voice: *phem, phon*

vomit (verb): *emes*
vulva: *episio, labi¹, vulv*

W

walk: *bas*
wall: *diaphragm, parie, phragm, phren¹, sept*
wander: *plan², noma, vag*
ward off: *phylax*
warmth: *caum, phleg, pyr, therm*
waste away: *atroph, phthis*
watch: *scop*
water: *hydr, lymph*
watery substance: *lymph, ser*
weak: *asthen, lept, lys, pares*
web: *hist*
wedge: *cune, sphen*
weight: *bar, grav*
well: *eu-*
wheel: *cycl*
whey: *lymph, ser*
whip: *mastig*
white: *leuk*
whitish protein: *album*
whole: *hol-*
wide: *eury, later*
widening: *aneurys*
windpipe: *bronch, laryn, trache*
woman: *gyn*
womb: *colp, hyster, metr, uter*
word: *lex, logo*
work: *erg*
worm: *helminth, scol*
wound: *trauma*
wrap (verb): *spir*
wrist: *carp*
write: *graph*

X

xiphoid process (sword-shaped): *xiph*

Y

yeast: *zym*
yellow: *cirrh, lut, xanth*
yoke: *zyg*
yolk: *lecith, vitell*
young: *neo*

Appendix B
Prefixes and Initial Combining Forms

Prefix	Other Forms	Meaning	Examples
a- 	 an-	negative	ablepsia, ametria, atrophy anomaly [second form: (h)omo]
ab- 	 abs-	away from	abducent abscess
abdomino- 	 abdomin-	abdomen, belly	abdominocentesis, abdominopelvic abdominalgia
acantho- 	 acanthro- acanth-	thorny, spiny	acanthocyte acanthrocyte acanthesthesia
aceto-		vinegar	acetometer
acido- 	 acidi- acid-	acid, sharp, sour	acidocyte acidify acidemia
acousto- 	 acou	hearing	acoustogram acouesthesia
acro- 	 acr-	high, height	acrocephalic, acrophobia acrodynia
actino- 	 actin-	rays; of a radiated nature	actinology, actinolyte actinoid
acu-		needle, sharp	acupressure, acupuncture
ad-	Assimilated forms: ac- af- ag- ap- as- at-	to, at, toward	adaptation, addiction, adduction accelerant, acclimation, accretion affection, afferent, affinity agglutinant, aggregate appendage, appendix assessment, assimilation attenuate, attrition
adeno- 	 aden-	gland	adenocele, adenofibrosis adenalgia
adipo- 	 adip-	fat	adipocele, adipochrome adipectomy, adipoid
adreno- 	 adren-	adrenal glands	adrenolytic, adrenomegaly adrenarche, adrenitis
aero- 	 aeri- aer-	air	aerobiosis, aerocele aeriferous, aerify aerodontia, aerosis, aerotitis
albumino- 	 albumin-	a whitish protein	albuminolysis, albuminorrhea albuminuria
algo- 	algio- alg-	pain	algolagnia, algometer, algiomotor algesthesia
alkali- 	 alkal	potash	alkaligenous alkalemia, alkaloid
allo- 	 all-	other	allocentric, allogamy allergy
allotrio- 	 allotri-	strange	allotriogeustia allotriodontia, allotriuria
alveolo- 	 alveol- alveo-	trough, channel, cavity, pit	alveolotomy alveolalgia, alveolitis alveobronchiolitis

Prefix	Other Forms	Meaning	Examples
ambi-		around, both	ambidextrous, ambilateral, ambiopia
amblyo-	ambly-	dull, blunted	amblyoscope amblyacousia, amblyopia
ameba			See amoebo-.
amino-	amin-	ammonia	aminoaciduria aminosis, aminuria
amnio-	amni-	inner fetal membrane	amniocentesis, amniorrhexis amnioma
amoebo-	amoeb- amebi- amebo- ameb-		amoebocyte amoebiasis amebicide, amebiform amebocyte amebiasis, ameboid
ampho-	amphi-	around, both	amphogenic, amphotony amphicelous
amygdalo-	amygdal- amygda-	tonsil	amygdalopathy amygdalitis, amygdaloid amygdalith
amylo-	amyl-	starch	amylorrhea amylemia, amyloid
an-	a-	negative	See a-.
ana-		again, up, intensive	analysis, anaphoresis, anatomy
ancon-		elbow	anconagra, anconitis
andro-	andr-	male, man	androgenous andriatrics
angino-	angin-	narrow, tight, constricted	anginophobia anginoid, anginose
angio-	angi-	blood vessel	angioblastm angionoma angiitis (also, angitis)
aniso-	anis-	unequal	anisocoria, anisogamy anisodont, anisopia
ankylo-	ankyl-	stiffness	ankylocolpos, ankylodactylia ankylotia, ankylosis
ante-	antero-	before	antechamber, anteflexion anterodorsal, anteroventral
anthropo-	anthrop-	man; mankind; human being	anthropology, anthropotomy anthropoid
anti-	ant-	against	antianemic, antipyogenic antacid, antophthalmic
antro-	antr-	cavity, antrum, sinus	antrobuccal, antrocele, antronasal antritis, antrodynia
anus-	ano-	anus	anusitis anogenital, anovesical
aorto-	aort-	aorta	aortoclasia, aortorraphy aortalgia, aortarctia, aortectasis
apico-	apic-	apex, tip, summit	apicolysis, apicotomy apicectomy
apo-		away	apocrine, apogee apophysis, apoplexy
aqua	aque	water	aquagenic, aquapuncture aqueduct
arachno-	arachn-	spider	arachnodactyly arachnitis, arachnoid

Prefix	Other Forms	Meaning	Examples
archeo-	arche- archi- arch-	first, beginning, original	archeocortex, archeokinetic archegonium, archesperm archiblast, archigaster archenteron
arterio-	arteri- arter-	artery	arteriomalacia, arteriopathy arteriagra, arteriectopia arteritis
arthro-	arthr-	joint	arthrocentesis, arthroplasty arthralgia, arthritis
astro-	aster-	star	astroblast, astrocyte asteroid
atelo-	atel-	incomplete	atelocardia, atelocephalous atelencephalia
atreto-	atret-	not perforated	atretocephalus, atretogastria atretopsia, atreturethria
audio-	audito-	hearing	audiometer auditognosis
auri-		ear	aurinasal, auripuncture, auriscope
auto-	aut-	self	autoblast, autodermic autopsy
auxo-		to increase	auxocardia, auxocyte, auxotroph
axio-	axi- axo- axono-	axis	axiobuccal, axiolabial, axioplasm axifugal, axilemma axodendrite, axofugal, axopetal axonometer, axonopathy
azoto-	azot-	nitrogen	azotometer, azotorrhea azotemia
balano	balan-	glans clitoridis, glans penis	balanocele, balanoplasty balanitis
baro-	bar- bary-	weight, heaviness	barognosis, barometer, barotaxis baresthesia barylalia, baryphonia
baso-	basi-	base	basocytosis, basophil basiotic
batho-	bath- bathy-	deep	bathomorphic, bathophore bathesthesia bathycardia
bi-	bin-	two	bifurcate, bigeminy, bilateral binocular, binotic
bili-		bile, gall	biligenesis, bilirachia, biliuria bilirubin
bio-	bi-	life	biogenesis, biology biome, biopsy, biosis
blasto-	blast-	bud, germ	blastocyte, blastomere blastoma
blenno-	blenn-	mucus	blennogenic, blennorrhea blennadenitis, blennemesis
blepharo-	blephar-	eyelid	blepharoplegia, blepharoptosis blepharitis, blepharoncus
brachio-	brachi-	upper arm	brachiocephalic, brachiocrural brachialgia
brachy-		short	brachychronic, brachystasis
brady-		slow	bradycardia, bradyesthesia

Prefix	Other Forms	Meaning	Examples
broncho-	bronch- bronchio-	windpipe	bronchogenic, bronchogram bronchitis, bronchadenitis bronchiocele, bronchiospasm
bucco-		cheek	buccocervical, buccolingual
bulb-	bulbi- bulbo-	bulb	bulbitis, bulboid bulbiform bulbocavernous
burso-	burs-	bag, pouch	bursolith, bursotomy bursectomy, bursitis
caco-	cac-	bad, abnormal, diseased	cacogeusia, cacomelia cacodontia, cacosmia
calcin-	calc- calci-	stone, calcium, limestone	calcinosis calcemia calciferous, calcify, calcipexy
calori-	cale- calo-	hot, heat, warmth	calorifacient, calorigenic calefacient caloradiance
campto-	campo-	bent, curved	camptocormia, camptodactylia campospasm
cancro-	cancr- cancri-; cancero-	cancer	cancrology; cancroid cancriform; cancerogenic
cantho-	canth-	corner of eye	cantholysis, canthoplasty canthectomy, canthitis
capillaro-	capillar-	hair, capillary	capillaropathy, capillaroscopy capillaritis
carcino-	carcin-	cancer	carcinogen, carcinolysis carcinemia
cardio-	cardi- card-	heart	cardiocentesis, cardiogram cardialgia, cardiectomy carditis
carpo-	carp-	wrist	carpopedal, carpoptosis carpectomy, carpitis
caryo-			See karyo.
cata-	cat- kata-	down, negative	catabasis catoptrics, cathode kataphraxis
ceco-	cec-	blind, blind gut	cecocele, cecopexy cecectomy, cecitis
celli-	celluli- cellul-	room, cell	cellicolous, celliferous cellulifugal, cellulipetal cellulitis
celo[1]	celi- cel-	belly, hollow, cavity	celophlebitis, celoschisis celiagra, celialgia celenteron, celitis
celo[2]	kel-	hernia, tumor	celosomia kelectome
centro-	centr-	center, point	centrocyte, centromere centrencephalic
cephalo-	cephal-	head	cephalocele, cephalopathy cephalalgia, cephalodynia
cerato-	kerato- kerat-	horn, cornea	ceratocele, ceratohyal keratophakia, keratoplasty keratalgia, keratitis

Prefix	Other Forms	Meaning	Examples
cerebro-	cerebri- cerebr-	brain	cerebromalacia, cerebromeningitis cerebrifugal, cerebripetal cerebritis, cerebroma
cervico-	cervic-	neck; uterus	cervicobrachial, cervicoplasty cervicitis, cervicodynia
cheilo-	cheil-	lip, edge, rim	cheiloangioscopy, cheiloplasty cheilectomy, cheilitis
chiro-	chir- cheiro- cheir-	hand	chiroplasty, chiropractic chiragra cheirognostic, cheirospasm cheiralgia
chloro-	chlor-	green	chloropenia, chloroplast chloremia, chloroma, chloruresis
cholo-	chole- chol-	gall, bile	cholochrome, chololithiasis cholecyst, cholelith cholagogue, cholemesis, cholemia
chondro-	chondr-	cartilage	chondromalacia, chondroplast chondralgia, chondrosis
chordo-	chord- cord-	cord, string	chordopexy, chordotomy chordectomy, chorditis cordectomy, corditis
chorio-	chor-	membrane	chorioblastoma, choriocele choroid
chromato-	chromo- chrom-	color	chromatoblast, chromatophore chromocyte, chromoplast chromesthesia, chromopsia
chrono-	chron-	time	chronognosis, chronotropic chronaxy
chylo-	chyl- chyli-	gastric juice	chylocele, chylocyst, chyloderma chylemia, cylosis chylifacient, chliferous, chyliform
circum-	circa-	around	circumanal, circumcision, circumoral circadian
cleido-	cleid-	collarbone, clavicle	cleidocostal, cleidocranial cleidagra, cleidarthritis
coleo-		vagina	coleoptosis, coleotomy
colon-	colo- col-	colon (lower intestine)	colonitis colocentesis, coloptosis colectomy, colitis
colpo-	colp-	hollow, vagina	colpocele, colposcope colpalgia, colpatresia

com- (before b, m, and p)	Assimilations and
	  elisions
	co- (before vowels and
	  h)
	col- (before l)
	con- (before c, d,
	  f, g, j,
	  n, s,
	  t, v)
	cor- (before r)
		with, together	combine
			commasculation, complication
			coaxial, coitus, coossify
			cohesion
			collapse, collateral
			conception, condensation
			confluent, congelation, conjugate
			connexus, consensual
			contagion, convection
			corrugator

condylo-	condyl-	rounded projection of a bone	condylotomy condylectomy, condyloid

Prefix	Other Forms	Meaning	Examples
conio-	coni-	dust, spore	coniophage, coniology, coniotomy coniosis
contra-		against	contrafissure, contraindication
copro-	copr-	dung, feces	coprohematology, coprology copremia, coproma
corneo-	corni-	horn; cornea	corneoblepharon, corneocyte cornification
cortico-	cortic-	external layer; cortex	corticopleuritis, corticotroph corticectomy, corticoid
costo-	costi- cost-	rib, side	costochondral, costoclavicular costiferous, costispinal costalgia, costectomy
coxo-	cox-	hip	coxofemoral, coxotomy coxalgia, coxitis
cranio-	crani-	skull	craniocele, craniomalacia craniectomy, craniostosis
cryo-	cry-	cold	cryobiology, cryocautery cryalgia, cryesthesia
crypto-	crypt-	hidden	cryptodidymus, cryptogam cryptectomy, cryptitis, cryptorchism
cyano-	cyan-	blue	cyanogen cynaopsia, cyanosis
cyclo-	cycl-	circle, cycle	cyclogeny, cyclophoria cyclitis, cyclosis
cysto-	cyst-	sac, bladder	cystoblast, cystolith cystitis, cystoid
cyto-	cyt-	cell	cytoblast, cytochrome cytoid, cyturia
dacryo-	dacry-	tear, as in teardrop	dacryocyst, dacryolith dacryagogic, dacryoma
dactylo-	dactyl-	finger, toe	dactylography, dactylospasm dactylalgia, dactylitis, dactylodynia
de-		away, down, from, intensive	deactivate, decomposition desaturate, descending
demo-		people	demography
dendri-	dendr-	tree	dendriform dendraxon, dendroid
denti-	dent-	tooth	dentifrice, dentilabial dentagra, dentoid
dermato-	dermat- dermo- derm-	skin	dermatocyst, dermatoarthritis dermatalgia, dermatitis dermoblast, dermophyte dermoid
desmo-	desm-	ligament, band	desmocyte, desmogenous desmalgia, desmectasis, desmitis
deutero-	deuter-	second	deuteropathy, deuteroplasm deuteranopia, deuteranomalous
dextro-	dextr-	to the right	dextrocardia, dextrogastria dextraural, dextrocular
di-		two	diarthric, dibasic, digastric dimetria, dimorphic
dia-	di-	across, through	diagnosis, diameter, diascope dieresis, diuresis

Prefix	Other Forms	Meaning	Examples
diabeto-		diabetes	diabetogenous, diabetograph diabetology
diaphragm-		wall, partition	diaphragmalgia, diaphragmodynia
dicho-		twofold	dichogeny, dichotomy
dictyo-	dicty-	net	dictyokinesis, dictyospore dictyoma
didym-		twin, testicle	didymalgia, didymitis, didymodynia
digiti-		finger, toe	digitform, digitigrade
diplo-	dipl-	two, twofold	diploblastic, diplomyelia diploid, diplopia
dipso-	dips-	thirst	dipsogen, dipsomania dipsosis
dis-	dif- (before f) di- (before g, l, r, v)	apart, away, out	dislocation, dispense diffraction, diffuscate digest, digestion dilate, dilution direct divergent, divulsion
disco-	disc- disko- disk-	disk	discoblastic, discopathy discitis, discoid diskography diskectomy, diskitis
disto-		distant, remote	distobuccal, distogingival distolabial, distopupal
dolicho-		long	dolichocephalic, dolichomorphic
dolori-		pain	dolorific, dolorifuge, dolorimeter
dormi-		sleep	dormifacient
dorso-	dorsi- dors-	back of body	dorsolateral, dorsolumbar dorsiduct, dorsispinal dorsalgia
dromo-		course, current	dromograph, dromotropic
duodeno-		duodenum	duodenocolic, duodenostomy
dynamo-		power	dynamogenesis, dynamophore
dys-		wrong, bad, abnormal	dysacousia, dysentery
e-			See ex-.
ec-			See ex-.
echino-	echin-	prickly	echinocyte, echinoderm echinoid, echinosis
echo-		echo, returned sound	echocardiogram, echomimia
eco-		home, surroundings	ecology, economy, ecosite
ecto-	ect-	outside	ectoblast, ectoglia, ectoplasm ectethmoid
ectro-		congenitally absent	ectrodactyly, ectrophalangia
ef-			See ex-.
elasto-	elast-	setting in motion	elastometer, elastoplastic elastoid, elastosis
eleo-		oil	eleometer, eleopathy
embolo-	embol- emboli-, embo-	plug, wedge (lit., to throw in)	embololalia, embolophrasia embolemia, embolectomy emboliform embolalia
embryo-	embry-	growing	embryoblast, embryocardia embryoma, embryulcia

Prefix	Other Forms	Meaning	Examples
emeto-		to vomit	emetocathartic, emetogenic
en-		in	enchondroma
	em- (before b, m, p, ph)		embolism, embryo emmenia empathy emphlysis
	er- (before r)		errhine
encephalo-	encephal-	brain	encephalocele, encephalogram encephalalgia, encephalitis
endo-	end-	within	endophlebitis, endosperm endadelphos, endangiitis
endocrino-	endocrin-	secreting internally	endocrinogram endocrinoma, endocrinosis
entero-	enter-	intestine	enterocele, enterocentesis enteradenitis, enteralgia, enteritis
ento-	ent-	inside, within	entoblast, entocele, entocornea entiris
epi-	ep-	after, at, on, over, on the outside, anterior, beside, besides, among; to, upon	epidermis, epiglottis, epistasis epaxial, epencephalon
epiplo-	epipl-	omentum	epiplocele, epiploitis epiplomphalocele, epiploscheocele
episio-		vulva	episioplasty, episiorrhaphy, episiotomy
ergo-		work	ergogenic, ergometer
eroto-		sexual desire	erotogenic, erotomania
erythro-	erythr-	red	erythroblast, erythroclast erythropia, erythrosis
eso-		inside	esophoria, esotropia
esophago-	esophag-	alimentary canal	esophagocele, esophagomycosis esophagalgia, esophagitis
esthesio-		feeling, perception	esthesiogenesis, esthesiography
ethmo-	ethm-	sieve, strainer	ethmocranial, ethmonasal ethmoid
eu-		well	eupepsia, euphoria, euthanasia
eury-		wide	euryblepharon, eurycephalic, euryopia
ex-	Elisions and assimilations e- (elided before b, c, d, g, j, l, m, r, v) ec- (before c, s, t, z) ef- (before f)	out, away from, without	excretion, expel, extension ebullition, ecaudate edentia, egesta, ejecta elation, eliminate, emission erosion, eversion, evulsion eccentric, ecstatic, ectopia, eczema effeminate, efferent, effluvium
exo-		outside, outer, outer part	exopathic, exophytic
extero-		outside	exteroceptor, exterogestate
extra-		outside, besides	extracarpal, extracellular
facio-		face	faciocervical, facioplasty, facioplegia
fascio-	fasci-	band	fascioplasty, fasciorraphy fasiectomy, fasciitis
febri-		fever	febricide, febrifugal
fecal-	feca-	bodily excrement	fecaloid, fecaloma fecalith
femoro-		thigh bone	femorocele, femoroiliac

Prefix	Other Forms	Meaning	Examples
ferro-		iron	ferrokinetics, ferroprotein
feto-	feti-	offspring, fetus	fetometry, fetoplacental feticide
fibro-	fibr-	fiber	fibrocartilage, fibrocyte fibroid, fibroma, fibrosis
filo-	fili-	thread	filopodium, filopressure filiform
fistulo-	fistul-	tubelike passage	fistuloenterostomy, fistulotomy fistulectomy
fungi-	fung-	mushroom, fungus	fungicide, fungistasis fungemia
funi-	funis-	umbilical cord	funiform funisitis
galacto-	galact- (	milk	galactocele, galactorrhea galactoma, galactagogue
gameto-	gamet- gamo-	marriage, sexual reproduction	gametocide, gametocyte gametangium, gametoid gamobium, gamogony
ganglio-	gangli-	ganglion, knot	ganglioblast, ganglioglioma gangliform, gangliectomy, gangliitis
gastro-	gastr-	stomach	gastrodermis, gastropathy gastralgia, gastritis
geno-		producing	genoblast , genotoxic, genotype
geronto-	gero- ger-	old age	gerontophilia, gerontotoxon geroderma, geromorphism geriatrics, gerodontia
gingivo-	gingiv-	gums	gingivoanxial gingivolabial gingivalgia, gingivitis, gingivosis
glio-	gli-	glue	glioblastoma, gliocyte, gliosome glioma, gliosis
glosso-	gloss- glotto- glott-	tongue	glossocele, glossoplasty glossagra, glossitis glottography, glottology glottitis
gluco-	gluc-	sugar	glucogenic, glucopenia glucagon, glucemia, glucose
glyco-	glyc-	sugar	glycohemia, glycorrhea glycemia, glycuresis
gnatho-	gnath-	jaw	gnathoplasty, gnathoschisis gnathalgia, gnathitis
gonado-	gono- gone-	seed, sperm	gonadogenesis, gonadopathy gonocele, gonocyte gonecystitis, gonepoiesis
gony-	gon-	knee	gonycampis, gonyoncus gonagra, gonarthritis, gonitis
granulo-	granul-	small grain	granulocyte, granulopenia granulitis, granuloma
gravido-	gravito- gravi-	heavy; pregnant	gravidocardiac, gravitometer gravimetric, gravistatic
gyneco-	gyne- gyno- gyn-	woman	gynecomorphous, gynecology gyneduct, gynephobia gynogenesis, gynophore gynandroid, gynatresia

Prefix	Other Forms	Meaning	Examples
gyro-	gyr-	circle, ring	gyrochrome, gyrospasm gyrectomy, gyrencephalic, gyroma
halo-	hal-	salt	halodermia, halogen haloid
haplo-	hapl-	simple, single	haplopathy, haploscope haploid, haplopia
hapto-	haph- haphe-	touching	haptoglobin haphalgesia haphephobia
hecto-		hundred (multiples of)	hectoliter, hectometer
helco-	helc-	sore, ulcer	helcology, helcoplasty helcoid, helcoma
hemato-	hemat- hemo- hem-	blood	hematoblast, hematocolpos hematoid, hematoma hemoconia, hemocyte hemagogue, hemangioma
hemi-		half	hemiglossal, hemiplegia
hepato-	hepat-	liver	hepatobiliary, hepatogenic hepatitis, hepatodynia
hepta-	hept-	seven	heptachromic, heptavalent heptatomic (second form: atom)
hernio-	herni-	protrusion, hernia	hernioplasty, herniotomy hernioid
hetero-	heter-	other, different	heteroblastic, heterosexual heterauxesis, heterodont
hexa-	hex-	six	hexabasic, hexachromic, hexadactylic hexatomic (second form: atom)
hidro-	hidr-	sweat, perspiration	hidropoiesis, hidrorrhea hidradenitis, hidrosis
histo-	histio-	web, body tissue	histoclastic, histolysis histioblast, histiocyte
holo-	hol-	whole, entire	holoblastic, holocrine holarthritis, holergastic
homo-	homeo- hom-	same, resembling	homogeneous, homosexual homeochrome, homeocyte homaxial, homergy
hormono-	hormon-	impetus, impulse	hormonogenesis hormonagogue, hormonosis
hyalo-	hyal-	glass, glassy	hyalogen, hyalomere hyalitis, hyaloid
hydro-	hydr-	water	hydrocele, hydrocephaly hydragogue, hydraulics
hymeno-	hymen-	membrane	hymenology, hymenorrhaphy hymenectomy, hymenitis
hyper-		above, beyond, extreme, excessive	hyperactive, hyperalgia hyperergy, hypertrophy
hypno-	hypn-	sleep	hypnobatia, hypnotherapy hypnoid, hypnosis
hypo-	hyp-	under	hypochondriac, hypometabolism hypaxial, hypalgia
hypso-	hypsi- hyps-	high, height	hypsokinesis hypsicephalic hypsodont

Prefix	Other Forms	Meaning	Examples
hystero- hyster-		uterus, womb	hysterocele, hyserolith hysteralgia, hysteroid
iatro-		healing, physician	iatrogenic, iatrology
ichor-		wound; fluid from a sore	ichoremia, ichorrhea
ichthyo- ichthy-		fish, fishlike	ichthyocolla ichthyoid, ichthyosis
ictero-		jaundice	icterogen, icterohepatitis
ideo-		form, appearance, idea	ideogenetic, ideokinetic
idio-		one's own	idioblast, idioglossia
ileo- ile-		ileum (lower abdomen)	ileocecal, ileocolitis ileitis
ilio-		ilium, iliac region	iliocostal, iliofemoral
in-¹	Assimilations il- (before l) im- (before b, m, p) ir- (before r)	in, into, on	incision, infriction, insertion illinition imbibition, immersion, implant irradiation, irrigation, irruption
in-²	Assimilations il- (before l) im- (before b, m, p) ir- (before r)	negative	invalid illegible, illusion imbecile, immune, imperforation irrational, irreducible, irregular
inio- ini-		occiput; back of head	iniodymus, iniopagus iniencephalus
infra-		beneath	infraclaviciar, infracostal
inguino- inguin-		groin	inguinocrural, inguinoscrotal inguinodynia
ino- in-		fiber	inoblast, inocyte initis
insulino- insulin- insul-		island, islets	insulinogenesis, insulinopenic insulinemia, insulinoma insulitis, insuloma
inter-		among, between	intercarpal, interfeminium
intra- intro-		within	intervascular, intravenous introitus, introjection
iodo- iod-		violet	iododerma, iodophilia iodemia, iodopsin
irido- irid-		iris (of eye)	iridokinesis, iridotomy iridectomy, iriditis
ischio- ischi-		hip, haunch	ischiocele, ischiopubic ischialgia, ischiodynia
ischo- isch-		suppressing	ischocholia ischemia, ischuria
iso-		equal, same	isobody, isocoria, isochronic, isotope
jejuno- jejun-		empty	jejunoplasty, jejunostomy jejunectomy, jejunitis
juxta-		adjacent to, adjoining	juxtacrine, juxtaintestinal
kali- kal-		potassium, potash	kaligenous, kalimeter kalemia
karyo- (also spelled caryo-)	kary- caryo-	nucleus of a cell	karyoblast, karyochrome, karyocyte karyapsis caryokinesis
kerato- (also spelled cerato-)	kerat- cerato-	horn	keratomycosis keratalgia, keratoma ceratohyal

Prefix	Other Forms	Meaning	Examples
keton-		keton	ketonemia, ketonuria
	keto-		ketogenesis, ketoplasia
kilo-		1,000 (in multiples)	kilocalorie, kilogram, kilometer
kine- (also spelled cine-)	kin-		kineplasty, kinescope kinanesthesia
labio-		lip; vulva	labiocervial, labiolingual
lacto-		milk	lactogenic, lactorrhea
	lacti-		lactiferous, lactigenous
lalo-		speaking	lalognosis, lalopathy
lamino-		layer	laminogram, laminoplasty
	lamin-		laminectomy, lamninitis
laparo-		loin, flank	laparocele, laparoscopic
	lapar-		laparectomy
laryngo-		larynx (windpipe)	laryngophony, laryngospasm
	laryng-		laryngalgia, laryngitis
latero-		side	lateroduction, laterotorsion
leio-		smooth	leiodermia, leiomyoma
lenti-		lens; pea-shaped	lenticonus, lentiglobus
	lent-		lentectomy, lentitis
	lenso-		lensometer, lensopathy
lepto-		small, thin, weak	leptocyte, leptodermous
	lept-		leptodontous
leuko-		white	leukoblast, leukocyte
	leuk-		leukemia, leukodontia, leukoma
	leuco-		leucocyte, leucotomy
	leuc-		leucitis
levo-		left; left-hand	levocardia, levoversion
lieno-		spleen	lienocele, lienomalacia, lienopathy
	lien-		lienitis
linguo-		tongue	linguodental, linguonasal, linguopulpal
	lingui-		linguiform
lipo-		fat	lipoblast, lipocele, lipocyte
	lip-		lipemia, lipoid, lipoma
litho-		stone	lithoclast, lithoscope
	lith-		lithagogue, lithoid, lithuria
lobo-		lobe	lobomycosis, lobotomy
	lob-		lobectomy, lobitis
lochio-		vaginal discharge	lochiocolpos, lochiorrhagia
logo-		word	logoplegia, logospasm
	log-		logamnesia
lumbo-		loin, lumbar	lumbocostal, lumbodorsal
	lumb-		lumbodynia
lympho-		water; fluid (of the body)	lymphocyte, lymphopoiesis
	lymph-		lymphadenitis, lymphangial
macro-		large, long	macroesthesia, macrognathia
	macr-		macradenous, macronychia
mal-		ill, abnormal, bad	maladjusted, malalignment, malaria
malac-		soft	malacoma, malacosis
mammo-		breast	mammogram
	mamm-		mammalgia, mammectomy, mammitis
masto-		breast	mastocytoma, mastocytosis
	mast-		mastadentitis, mastitis

Prefix	Other Forms	Meaning	Examples
maxillo-	maxill-	jawbone; upper jaw	maxillodental, maxillojugal maxillectomy, maxillitis
meato-		passage	meatometer, meatorrhaphy
meco-	mecy-	length	mecocephalic, mecometer mecystasis
medio-	medi-	middle	mediocarpal, mediolateral medicephalic, medifrontal
medullo-	medull-	marrow	medulloblast medullectomy, medullitis, medullosis
mega-	meg- megalo- megal-	great size, large	megacephalic, megalocyte megalgia megalophallic, megalopodia megalopsia
meio-			See mio-.
melano-	melan-	black, dark	melanoderma, melanoglossia malanoid, melanoma
melo-	mel-	limb	melodidymus melagra, melalgia
melono-	melo- mel-	cheek	melonoplasty meloplasty, meloschisis melitis, melotia
meningo-	mening-	membrane	meningocele, meningocyte meningitis, meninguria
meno-	men-	month (menstruation)	menolipsis, menopause menacme, menalgia
mento-	ment-	chin	mentolabial, mentoplasty mentagra
mero-	mer-	a part	meroblastic, merocrania meropia
mero-	mer-	thigh	merocele, merocoxalgia meralgia
meso-	mes-	middle	mesocardia, mesoderm mesenchyma, mesodont
meta-	met-	after, along with, among, behind, between, beyond; in anatomical terms, equivalent to *dorso* back	metabolic, metacarpal metestrus, metonymy
metro-	metr-	womb	metrocampis, metrocele metrectomy, metrodynia
micro-	micr-	small	microcephaly, microscope micracoustic, microxycyte
milli-		1,000 (in fractions)	milligram, millisecond
mio-	mei- mi-	less, decreasing	miodidymus meiosis miopus, miosis
miso-	mis-	hate	misogamy, misogyny misandria, misanthropia
mito-	mit-	thread	mitogenesis, mitoschisis mitapsis, mitosis
mono-	mon-	only, sole, single	monoplegia, monosome monacid, monorchid
morpho-	morph-	form, shape	morphogenesis, morphology morphallaxis, morphosis

Prefix	Other Forms	Meaning	Examples
muco-	mucin- muc-	mucus	mucocele, mucocolpos, mucoderm mucinoid, mucinuria mucitis, mucoid
multi-		many, much	multicuspidate, multicystic
myco-	myc- myceto- mycet-	fungus	mycoderma, mycohemia mycosis mycetocyte, mycetogenic mycethemia, mycetoma
myelo-	myel-	marrow; spinal cord	myelography, myelopathy myelalgia, myeloid
myo-	my-	muscle	myoblast, myocardia myalgia, myatrophy, myectomy
myringo-	myring-	drum membrane (the membrana tympani)	myringodermatitis, myringorupture myringectomy, myringitis
myxo-	myx-	mucus	myxofibroma, myxolipoma myxedema, myxoma
nano-	nan-	dwarf	mannocephalia, nanocormia nanoid, nanophthalmos
narco-	narc-	stupor, numbness	narcohypnia, narcoleptic narcosis
naso-	nas-	nose	nasoantral, nasolacrimal nasitis
necro-	necr-	dead body, corpse	necromania, necrotomy necrectomy, necropsy, necrosis
nemato-	nemat-	nematode worm	nematoblast, nematocyst, nematology nemathelminth, nematoid
neo-	ne-	new, strange	neocyte, neonatal nearthrosis, neencephalon
nephro-	nephr-	kidney	nephrocele, nephrotomy nepradenoma, nephrectomy
neuro-	neur-	nerve	neuroblast, neuroglia neuralgia, neuroma
neutro-		neither, neutral	neutropenia, neutrophilia, neutrotaxis
noct-		night	noctambulation, nocturia
noni-		nine, ninth	nonigravida, nonipara
normo-		normal	normoblast, normocapnia, normocyte
noso-	nos-	disease	nosology, nosotrophy nosencephalus, nosetiology
noto-	not-	back (of body)	notochord, notomelous notalgia, notencephalia
nucleo-	nucle-	nucleus	nucleofugal, nucleoplasm nucleoid, nucleosis
nycto-	nyct-	night	nyctohemeral, nyctophilia nyctalgia, nycturia
nympho-	nymph-	labia minora	nymphomania, nymphotomy nymphitis, nymphoncus
ob-	Assimilations oc- (before c) op- (before p)	against, toward, opposite	obfuscate, obliterate, obtuse occiput, occlude, occult oppilation
occipto-		back of head	occiptocervical, occipitoparietal
ochro-		sallow, paleness	ochrodermia, ochronosis
octa-	octi-	eight, eighth	octavalent octigravida

Prefix	Other Forms	Meaning	Examples
oculo-		eye	oculocardiac, oculocutaneous oculofacial, oculospinal
odonto-	odont-	tooth	odontoblast, odontoclasis odontagra, odontalgia
odoro-	odori-	smell	odorography odoriferous, odoriphore
odyno-	odyn-	pain	odynolysis, odynophagia odynacusis
olecran-		elbow	olecranarthritis, olecranarthropathy
oleo-		oil	oleocalcareous, oleocyst
oligo-	olig-	few, scant, small	oligodactylia, oligospermia oligemia, oliguria
omento-	oment-	fat skin covering	omentopexy, omentoplasty omentitis, omentectomy
omni-		all	omnipotence, omnivorous
omo-	om-	shoulder	omocephalus, omoclavicular omagra, omodynia
omphalo-	omphal-	navel, umbilicus	omphalorrhea, omphalotripsis omphalectomy, omphaloma
onco-	onc-	mass, swelling	oncocyte, oncogenesis, oncology oncoma, oncosis
oneiro-	oneir-	dream	oneirogenic, oneiroscopy oneirodynia, oneirogmus
onycho-	onych-	nail of finger or toe	onychauxis, onychoclasis onychalgia, onychitis
oo-		egg	ooblast, oocyte, ookinesis, oosperm
oophoro-	oophor-	bearing of ova	oophorohysterectomy oophoralgia, oophoritis
ophthalmo-	ophthalm-	eye	ophthalmocele, ophthalmoscope ophthalmagra, ophthalmectomy
opistho-	opisth-	behind, backward, back (of the body)	opisthocheilia, opisthognathism opisthotic, opisthorchiasis
opsono-	opsoni-	opsonin	opsonometry, opsonophilia opsonification
opto-	opti-	eye	optoblast, optometry opticiliary
orbito-		circle; eye socket	orbitonasal, orbitotomy
oro-	ora- ori-	mouth, opening	orolingual, oronasal oralogy orifice
orchio-	orchi- orchido- orchid-	testicle	orchiopexy, orchiotomy orchialgia orchidometer orchidalgia, orchidoncus
orexi-		appetite	orexigenic
organo-	organ-	organ, implement	organogenesis, organoleptic organoid, organonymy
ortho-	orth-	straight	orthograde, orthomelic, orthopedic orthodontic orthoptic
oscheo-	osche-	scrotum	oscheocele, ocheolith, oscheoplasty oscheitis, oscheoncus, oscheoma
osmo-	osm-	smell, odor	osmoceptor, osmometer osmesthesia osmidrosis

Prefix	Other Forms	Meaning	Examples
osmo-		impulse, osmosis	osmogen, osmophilic, osmotaxis
osseo-	ossi-	bone	osseofibrous, osseomucin ossifluence, ossiphore
osteo-	oste- ost-	bone	osteoarthritis, osteochondroma ostealgia, osteoncus ostalgia, ostemia
oto-	ot-	ear	otoantritis, otocleisis, otoscope otagra, otalgia
oulo-	oul- ulo- ul-	gums	oulorrhagia oulectomy, oulitis ulocarcinoma ulectomy, ulitis
ovario-	ovari- ovar- ovi- ovo- ov-	ovary, egg	ovariocyesis, ovariotomy ovarioncus ovaritis ovicide, oviduct, oviform ovotestis ovalbumin, ovoid
oxy-	oxi-	sharp, keen, pointed	oxyblepsia, oxycephalia oxigram, oximeter
ozono-	ozo-	stench	ozonometer, ozonophore ozochrotia, ozostomia
pachy-		thick	pachyderma, pachyglossia pachygnathous, pachymeningitis
palato-	palat-	roof of mouth, palate	palatoglossal, palatognathous palatitis
palin-	pali-	backward, again, repetition	palindromic, palinrrhea palikinesia, palistrophia
pan-	pano- panto-	all	panchromatic, pancreas panophobia, panoptosis pantophobia, pantoscopic
pancreato-	pancreat-	pancreas	pancreatolithiasis, pancreatolysis pancreatalgia, pancreatectomy
papillo-	papill-	nipple	papillocarcinoma, papilloretinitis papillectomy, papilledema, papillitis
papulo-	papuli- papul-	pimple, papule	papulopustular papuliferous papuloid, papulosis
para-	par-	beside, beyond, opposite, abnormal, irregular	paracentesis, paramastoid paralgia, parergasia, parorexia
parasito-	parasit-	parasite	parasitogenic, paarasitology parasitemia, parasitosis
parieto-	pariet-	wall	parietofrontal, parietomastoid parietitis
patello-	patell-	kneecap	patellofemoral patellalgia, patellectomy
patho-	path- (before vowels)	disease	pathogenesis, pathognomic pathergy, pathodontia, pathosis
pectori-	pectoro- pector-	chest	pectoriloquy pectorophony pectoralgia
pedo-	ped-	child	pedology, pedomorphism pederast, pediatrics

Prefix	Other Forms	Meaning	Examples
pedo-	pedi-	foot	pedometer, pedopathy pedialgia, pedicure
pelvio-	pelvi-	pelvis	pelvioplasty, pelviotomy pelvimeter, pelviscope
peno-	peni- pen-	penis	penoscrotal penischisis penitis
penta-	pent-	five	pentadactyl, pentavalent pentatomic
pept-	pepto-	digestion	peptoid peptogenic, peptolysis
per-		through, across, intensive	peracute, perception, pernasal
peri-		around	periarthric, pericardium, periphery
perineo-		perineum	perineocele, perineoplasty
peritoneo-	peritone- periton-	peritoneum	peritoneocentesis, peritoneopexy peritonealgia peritonitis
pero-		maimed	perobrachius, perosplanchia
petro-	petri- petr-	stone; part of temporal bone	petrosphenoid petrifaction petroleum
phaco-	phac- phak-	lens; also, a spot on the body, or freckle	phacocele, phacocyst phacitis, phacoid phakitis, phakoma
phago-		to eat, swallow	phagocyte, phagolysis
phalang-		phalanx; bones of the digits	phalangectomy, phalangitis
phallo-	phalli- phall-	penis	phallocampsis, phallorrhea phalliform phallalgia, phallitis, phallodynia
phanero-	phaner- pheno-	showing	phanerogenetic, phaneroscope phanerosis phenology, phenotype
pharyngo-	pharyng-	pharynx (throat)	pharnyngocele, pharnyngolith pharnyngitis, pharnyngodynia
pheno-			See phanero.
phlebo-	phleb-	vein	phleboclysis, phlebosclerosis phlebalgia, phlebitis
phlogo-	phlog-	burning, feverish, inflammation	phlogocyte, phlogotherapy phlogosis
phono-	phon-	sound	phonogram, phonophore phoniatrics, phonopsia
phoro-		carrying	phoroblast, phorocyte phorology, phorotone
photo-	phot-	light	photogenesis, photokinesis photalgia, photodynia, photopia
phreno-	phren-	diaphragm	phrenocolic, phrenoglottic phrenalgia, phrenectomy, phrenitis
phymato-	phymat-	tumor	phymatology phymatoid, phymatosis
physio-	phys-	physical growth	physiogenesis, physiolysis physiatrics
physo-	physali-	gas, air	physocele, physometra physaliferous, physaliform

Prefix	Other Forms	Meaning	Examples
phyto-	phyt-	a plant	phytogenesis, phytonosis phytoid, phytosis
picro-		bitter	picrogeusia, picrotoxin
piesi-	pies- piezo-	pressure	piesimeter piesesthesia piezogenic, piezometer
pilo-	pili- pil-	hair	pilocystic, pilomotor piliform, pilimiction pilosis
pimelo-	pimel-	fat	pimelorrhea pimelitis, pimelosis
pinealo-	pineal-	cone; pineal body	pinealoblastoma, pinealocyte pinealectomy, pinealoma
placento-	placent-	placenta	placentogenesis, placentology placentoid, placentoma, placentitis
plano-	plani-	a plane; sole of the foot	planocellular, planoconvex planigram, planithorax
plano-	plan-	to wander	planocyte, planomania planuria
plasma-	plasmo-	to form	plasmacyte, plasmasome plasmogen, plasmolysis
platy-		flat, broad	platycephalic, platyrrhine
pleo-	pleio-	more, excessive, multiple	pleochromatism, pleomastia pleiochromia
plessi-	pless-	stroke, paralysis	plessigaph, plessimeter plessesthesia
pleuro-	pleur-	pleura, rib, side	pleurobrachia, pleurotomy pleuralgia, pleuritis
plexo-	plexi- plex-	network	plexogenic, plexometer plexiform, pleximeter plexectomy, plexitis
pluri-		more	pluriceptor, plurilocular pluripara, pluripotent
pneo-		breath, breathing	pneogaster, pneoscope
pneumato-	pneumat-	air, gas, respiration	pneumatocele pneumatosis, pneumaturia
pneumo-	pneumono- pneumon-	lung	pneumocardial, pneumocentesis pneumorrachis, pneumorrhagia pneumonotomy pneumonitis
podo-	pod-	foot	podology podagra, podiatrist
poikilo-	poikil-	varied, mottled, irregular	poikiloblast, poikilocyte poikilosmosis
polio-	poli-	gray	polioclastic, poliomyelitis poliosis
poly-		many, much	polydactylia, polyspermia
polypo-	polyp-	polyp	polypotome, polypotrite polypectomy, polypoid
poro-	por-	passage, pore	porocele, porotomy poradenitis, porosis
post-	postero-	after, behind	postnasal, postnatal, postoral posteroclusion

Prefix	Other Forms	Meaning	Examples
posthio-	posthe- posth-	foreskin (of penis or clitoris)	posthioplasty posthetomy posthitis
pre-		before (in time or place)	precardium, prenatal, prevesical
presbyo-	presby-	old	presbyophrenia presbyacusia, presbyopia
primi-	prim-	first	primigravid, primiparous primordial
pro-		before (in time or place)	procheilon, progamous, prolapse
procto-	proct-	anus, rectum	proctocolitis, proctoptosis proctagra, proctalgia, proctectasia
prosopo-	prosop-	face	prosopoplegia, prosoposchisis prosopalgia, prosopectasia
prostato-	prostat-	prostate gland	prostatorrhea prostatalgia, prostatectomy
proto-	prot-	first	protoblast, protoplast, protospasm protanopia, protoxide
pseudo-	pseud-	false	pseudoangina, pseudocide pseudopsia, pseudosmia
psycho-	psych- (before vowels)	mind	psychogeustic, psychometry psychalgia, psychiatry, psychosis
psychro-		cold	psychroalgia, psychroesthesia
ptyalo-	ptyal- ptya-	saliva, spittle	ptyalorrhea ptyalagogue, ptyalectasis ptyalith
pubo-	pubio- pub-	becoming an adult	pubofemoral, puboprostatic pubioplasty, pubiotomy pubarche
pulmono-	pulmon- pulmo-	lung	pulmonology pulmonectomy, pulmonitis pulmolith, pulmometer
pulpo-	pulpi- pulp-	pulp (of the tooth)	pulpotomy pulpifaction pulpalgia
pupillo-	pupill-	pupil (of eye)	pupillograph, pupillotonia pupillatonia
puro-	puri-	pus	purohepatitis, puromucous puriform
pyelo-	pyel-	pelvis	pyelocutaneous, pyelonephrosis pyelectasia, pyelitis
pygo-	pyg-	rump, buttocks	pygodidymus, pygomelus pygalgia
pykno-	pykn-	thick, compact	pyknocardia, pyknocytosis pyknemia, pyknosis
pyloro-	pylor-	pylorus (lower orifice of the stomach)	pyloroplasty, pyloroptosis pyloralgia, pyloritis
pyo-	py-	pus	pyocele, pyocyst, pyogenesis pyemesis, pyoid, pyuria
pyro-	pyr- pyreto-	fever, fire	pyroclastic, pyrolysis, pyrotherapy pyrosis pyretogenesis, pyretology
quadri-	quadr-	four; fourfold	quadriceps, quadrigeminal quadrangle

Prefix	Other Forms	Meaning	Examples
quarti-		fourth	quartipara
quinque-		five	quinquecuspid
quinti-		fifth	quintipara
rachio-		spine	rachiocentesis, rachiometer
	rachi-		rachialgia, rachicentesis
	rach-		rachitis
radico-		root	radicotomy
	radiculo-		radiculopathy
	radicul-		radiculalgia, radiculectomy
radio-		ray; spread out	radioactive, radiology, radioscopy
rami-		branch	ramification
	ram-		ramitis
re-		back, again; intensive	reaction, recess, relapse, retraction refrigerant
recto-		rectum	rectocele, rectoclysis, rectoplasty
	rect-		rectalgia, rectectomy
reno-		kidney	renogastric, renoprival
	reni-		renicardiac, renipuncture
reto-		net (retina)	retothelium
	reti-		retiform
	retino-		retinoblasytoma, retinomalacia
	retin-		retinectomy, retinitis, retinosis
retro-		back, behind, backward	retroaction, retrocursive retrograde, retropulsion
rhabdo-		rod, stick	rhabdomyoma
	rhabd-		rhabdoid
rhaebo-		crooked	rhaebocrania, rhaeboscelia
	rhaeb-		rhaebosis
rheo-		flowing	rheometer, rheophore
	rhe-		rheostosis
rheumato-		flux (excessive flow)	rheumatogenic, rheumatology
	rheumat-		rheumatalgia, rheumatoid
	rheuma-		rheumapyra
	rheum-		rheumarthritis
rhino-		nose	rhinopathy, rhinoscope
	rhin-		rhinalgia, rhinesthesia, rhinitis
rhizo-		root	rhizomelic, rhizotomy
	rhiz-		rhizoid, rhizodontropy
rhodo-		red	rhodogenesis, rhodophylactic
rhytido-		wrinkle	rhytidoplasty
	rhytid-		rhytidectomy, rhytidosis
rubro-		red	ruprospinal
	rubri-		rubriblast, rubricyte
	rube-		rubefacient
saccharo-		sugar, sucrose	saccharolytic
	acchari-		sacchariferous
sacro-		sacrum	sacroiliac, sacrotomy sacrioperineal, sacrouterine
	sacr-		sacralgia, sacrarthrogenic
salpingo-		tube	salpingocele, salpingoplasty
	salping-		salpingectomy, salpingitis
sanguino-		blood	sanguinopoietic, sanguinopurulent
	sangui-		sanguicolous, sanguivorous

Prefix	Other Forms	Meaning	Examples
sapro-	sapr-	rotten	sapronosis, saprophilous sapremia, saprodontia
sarco-	sarc-	flesh	sarcoblast, sarcocyst, sarcopenia sarcoid, sarcoma, sarcosis
scapulo-	scapul-	shoulder blade	scapulohumeral, scapulopexy scapulagia, scapulectomy
scato-	scat-	dung, fetal matter	scatoscopy scatemia, scatoma
scelo-	scel- skel-	leg	scelotyrbe scelalgia skelalgia
schisto-		split, divided	schistocyte, schistomelia
schizo-	schiz-	to split, divide	schizocephalia, shizophrenia schizoid, schizosis
scirrh-		hard; hard tumor	scirrhoid, scirrhoma
sclero-	scler-	hard; the sclera	scleroderma, sclerometer scleradenitis, scleritis, scleroma
scoleco-	scolec-	worm, appendage, twisted	scolecology scolecitis, scolecoid
scopo-		to examine, to see	scopograph, scopolagnia
scoto-	scot-	darkness	scotophilia, scotoscopy scotopia
scroto-	scrot-	testicle pouch	scrotocele, scrotoplasty scrotectomy, scrotitis
sebo-	sebi-	tallow, fat, oil	sebolith, seborrhagia sebiferous, sebiparous
semen-	semini-	semen, sperm, seed	semenoma (or, seminoma) seminiferous
semi-		half	semiflexion, semiplegia
sensori-	sensi-	perception, sense	sensorimotor, sensorimuscular sensigenous, sensimeter
septa-	septi-	seven	septavalent (or, septivalent)
septico-	septi- septic-	to rot, decay	septicopyemia septimetritis, septineuritis septicemia
septo-	sept-	fence, wall	septonasal, septoplasty septectomy
sero-	ser-	whey; watery substance	seroculture, serology seralbumin, seroma
sex-	sexi- sexti-	six	sexdigitate sexivalent sextipara
sialo-	sial-	saliva	sialocele, sialocele, sialolith sialaden, sialitis, sialosis
sidero-	sider-	iron	sideroblast, siderocyte, sideropenia siderosis
sinistro-	sinistr-	left (as opposed to right)	sinistrocardia, sinistrocerebral sinistraural, sinistrocular
sino-	sinus- sinu-	hollow, fold (sinus)	sinoatrial, sinobronchitis sinusitis sinuoid
sito-	sitio-	food	sitotherapy, sitotropism sitiology

Prefix	Other Forms	Meaning	Examples
skia-		shadow	skiagram, skiametry
socio-		companion	socioacusis, sociogenic, sociotherapy
somato-	somat- som-	body	somatopathic, somatoscopy somatalgia somasthenia, somesthesia
somni-	somn-	sleep	somnifacient, somniloquence somnambulance
sono-		sound	sonogram, sonolucent
spermato-	spermo- sperm-	seed; sperm	spermatoblast, spermatocele spermoblast, spermotoxic spermacrasia
spheno-	sphen-	wedge	sphenocephaly, sphenometer sphenoid, sphenosis
sphero-	spher-	ball, globe	spherocyte, spherospermia spheresthesia, spheroid
sphinctero-	sphincter-	that which draws tight	sphincterolysis sphincteralgia, sphincteritis
sphygmo-	sphygm-	pulse	sphygmogram, sphygmometer sphygmoid
spino-	spini- spin-	spine	spinocellular, spinocortical spinifugal, spinipetal spinalgia, spinitis
spiro-[1]	spir-	breath, breathing	spirophore, spiroscope spiradenitis
spiro-[2]	spir-	turning, wrapping, coiling	spirochete spiradenoma, spiroid
splanchno-	splanchn-	entrails, viscera	splanchnocele, splanchnolith splanchnectopia, splanchnodynia
spleno-	splen-	spleen	splenocleisis, splenogenous splenauxe, splenceratosis
spondylo-	spondyl-	vertebra	spondylodesis, spondylotomy spondylizemia, spondylodynia
spongio-	spongi-	sponge	spongioblast, spongiocyte spongiform, spongiitis
sporo-	spor- spori-	seed	sporoblast, sporocyst sporangium, sporont soporiferous, sporiparous
squamo-		scale, plate	squamocellular, squamoparietal
staphylo-	staphyl-	bunch of grapes (uvula)	staphyloderma, staphyloplasty staphylagra, staphylectomy
stato-	stasi-	standing	statocyst, statolith stasimorphy
stearo-	steari- steato- steat-	fat, tallow	stearopten steariform steatocele, steatogenesis, steatolysis steatitis, steatoma
steno-	sten-	narrow	stenocardia, stenostomia stenosis
sterco-	stercor-	feces, dung	stercolith stercoremia, stercoroma
stereo-	stere- ster-	solid	stereoagnosis, stereoanesthesia stereopsis steroid

Prefix	Other Forms	Meaning	Examples
sterno-		breastbone, sternum	sternocostal, sternotomy
	stern-		sternalgia, sternoid
stetho-		chest	stethometer, stethoscope
	steth-		stethalgia, stethemia
stomacho-		stomach, opening	stomachoscopy
	stomach-		stomachalgia
stomato-		mouth, opening, orifice	stomatogastric
	stomat-		stomatitis
	stoma-		stomacace
stropho-		to twist	strophocephaly, strophosomus
	strepho-		strephopodia
strumi-		goiter	strumiform
	strum-		strumectomy, strumitis
stylo-		pillar	styloglossus, stylopodium
	styl-	the styloid	stylosteophyte
	styli-	process of the temporal	styliform
sub-	Assimilations and Elisions	below, near, almost, moderately	subacute, subconscious
	suf- (before f)		suffer, suffusion
	sup- (before p)		suppression, suppuration
	sus- (before pe)		suspension
	su- (before s)		suspiration
sucros-		sugar	sucrosemia, sucrosuria
	sucro-		sucroclastic
super-		above, beyond, extreme	superovulation
	sur- (varies)		surcingle, surexitation
	supra-		suprapubic, suprarenal
syn-	Elisions and assimilations	with, together; union, association	synapsis, syncholia, syndrome
	sy- (often before s, z)		synthesis
	syl- (before l)		systole, syzygy
	sym- (before b, m, p, ph)		syllepsis
	sys- (before s)		symbiosis, symmetry
			sympathetic, symphalangia
			syssarcosis, syssomus
syringo-		pipe, duct, tube, fistula	syringobulbia
	syring-		syringadenous
tabo-		to waste away	taboparesis
	tabi-		tabification
tachy-		swift	tachycardia, tachyphrasia
talo-		ankle	talocrural, talofibular, talotibial
	tali-		taliped
tarso-[1]		ankle	tarsomegaly
	tars-		tarsalgia, tarsectopia
tarso-[2]		edge of eyelid	tarsomalacia, tarsotomy
	tars-		tarsectomy
taxo-		arrangement, order	taxology, taxonomy
tecto-		cover, skin	tectocephaly, tectospinal
tele-[1]		end	teledendrite, telemitosis
	teleo-		teleology
	telo-		telobiosis, telocentric, telogliac
	tel-		telangion, telencephalon
tele-[2]		afar, distant	teleceptor
	tel-		telalgia, telesthesia

Prefix	Other Forms	Meaning	Examples
temporo-		time, timely	temporoauricular, temporofrontal
	tempo-	temple (of the body)	tempolabile, tempostabile
teno-		tendon	tenodesis, tenolysis
	ten-		tenalgia, tenectomy, tenodynia
	tendo-		tendolysis, tendoplasty
	tendon-		tendonitis
	teno-		tenodesis, tenofibril
	tenon-		tenonectomy, tenonitis
	tenonto-		tenontophyma
	tenont-		tenontodynia, tenontitis
terato-		monster	teratoblastoma, teratocarcinoma
	terat-	(abnormal fetus)	teratoid, teratosis
terti-		third	tertigravida, tertipara
testi-		male gonad; testicle	testicond
	testo-		testopathy
	test-		testalgia, testectomy, testitis
tetano-		spasm, tetanus	tetanometer, tetanotoxin
	tetan-		tetanoid
	tetani-		tetaniform, tetanigenous
tetra-		four	tetragenous
	tetr-		tetracid, tetraster
thalamo-		inner chamber	thalamocortical, thalamocortical
	thalam-	(thalamus)	thalamectomy, thalamencephalon
thanato-		death	thanatology
	thanat-		thanatoid, thanatopsia
theco-		case, sheath, repository	thecostegnosis
	thec-		thecitis, thecodont, thecoma
thelo-		nipple	thelorrhagia
	thele-		theleplasty
	thel-		thelalgia, theloncus, thelitis
thely-		female	thelyblast, thelygenic, thelytocia
thermo-		heat	thermolysis, thermometer
	therm-		thermalgia, thermesthesia
thigmo-		touch	thigmotaxis, thigmotropism
	thigm-		thigmesthesia
thoraco-		chest	thoracocentesis
	thorac-		thoracalgia, thoracodynia
thrombo-		clot	thromboclasis, thrombopenia
	thromb-		thromboid, thrombosis
thymo-[1]		thymus	thymocyte, thymolysis
	thym-		thymectomy, thymoma
thymo-[2]		mind	thymogenic, thymoleptic
thyro-		shield (thyroid)	thyrocele, thyrolytic
	thyr-		thyroid
tibio-		shinbone	tibiofemoral, tibiotarsal
	tibi-		tibialgia
toco-		childbirth	tocograph, tocometer
	toko-		tokodynagraph
tono-		tone, tension	tonoclonic, tonometry
	ton-		tonaphasia
tonsillo-		tonsil (orig.., almond)	tonsillolith, tonsillopathy
	tonsill-		tonsillectomy, tonsillitis
	tonsil-		tonsillith

Prefix	Other Forms	Meaning	Examples
topo-		place	topognosis, topology
	top-		topesthesia, toponym
torsi-		twisting	torsiversion
	torti-		torticollis, tortipelvis
toxico-		poison	toxicology
	tox-		toxemia, toxoid
	toxi-		toxicide, toxiferous
	toxic-		toxicoid
	toxo-		toxogen
trachelo-		neck; neck of an organ	trachelocele, trachelology
	trachel-		trachelectomy, trachelitis
tracheo-		windpipe	tracheocele, tracheoscopy
	trache-		trachealgia, tracheitis
trachy-		rough	trachyonychia, trachyphonia
trans-		through, across, beyond	transamination, transanimation
			(note differences)
			transplantation, transsexual
traumato-		wound, injury	traumatogenic, traumatology
	trauma-		traumatherapy, traumatropism
tri-		three	triangle, tricellular, triceps
tricho-		hair	trichocardia, trichoschisis
	trich-		trichalgia, trichoid
tropho-		nutrition	trophoblast, trophopathy
	troph-		trophedema, trophont
tubo-		tube	tuborrhea, tubouterine, tubvaginal
	tub-		tubectomy
tumori-		tumor	tumorigenesis
	tumor-		tumorectomy
tympano-		eardrum	tympanocentesis, tympanotomy
	tympan-		tympanitis, tympanosis
typho-		fog, stupor; typhoid	typhogenic
	typh-		typhoid
typhlo-		cecum; blind gut	typhlocele, typhlopexy
	typhl-		typhlectomy, typhlitis
ulceri-		ulcer, abscess	ulcerogenic, ulcerogranuloma
ulo-			See oulo-.
ulo-		scar, cicatrix	ulodermatitis, ulotomy
	ule-		ulectomy, ulerythema
ultra-		beyond	ultramotivity, ultrasonic
uni-		one	unicuspid, uniseptate, uniovular
urano-		roof of mouth; palate	uranoplasty, urnaoplegia
	uranisco-		uraniscochasm, uraniscolalia
urethro-		urethra	urethrocele, urethroplasty
	urethr-		urethralgia, urethrectomy
uro-		urine	urogenital, urolith
	ur-		uragogue, uremia
utero-		uterus, womb	uterogestation
	uter-		uteralgia, uteritis, uterodynia
uveo-		uvea (part of the eye)	uveoencephalitis, uveosleritis
	uve-		uveitis
uvula-		uvula	uvulaptosis
	uveo-		uveoplasty
	uvul-		uvulectomy, uvulitis

Prefix	Other Forms	Meaning	Examples
vaccino-	vaccini-	cow; vaccine	vaccinogen, vaccinostyle vacciniform
vagino-	vagin-	sheath (vagina)	vaginocele, vaginocutaneous vaginectomy, vaginitis
vago-	vag-	wandering (nerve) (vagus)	vagogram, vagomimetic vagitis
valvulo-	valvul- valvo- valvi-	membranous fold	valvuloplasty, valvulotomy valvulitis valvotomy valviform
varico-	varici- varic-	enlarged vein	varicoblepharon, varicocele variciform varicoid, varicomphalus
vaso-	vasi- vas-	vessel (usually, blood vessel)	vasostomy, vasotomy vasifaction, vasiferous vasectomy
venini-		poison	veneniferous, veneific
veno-	vene- veni- ven-	vein	venoclysis, venotomy venesuture, venesection venipuncture, venisuture venectasia, venectomy
ventro-	ventri-	abdomen, belly	ventroscopy, ventrotomy ventricumbent, ventriduct
vermi-		worm	vermicide, vermiform, vermifugal
vertebro-	vertebr-	vertebra	vertebrochondral, vertebrocostal vertebrarterial, vertebrectomy
vesico-	vesicul-	bladder, sac, blister	vesicocele, vesicoclysis vesiculectomy, vesiculitis
vestibulo-	vestibul-	cavity, entrance	vestibulopathy, vestibulitis, vestibulotomy
vibro-	vibri-	vibration, shaking	vibrocardiogram vibrosis
viro-	viri- vir-	poison	viropexis, virific viremia
viscero-	viscer-	internal organs of body	viscerogenic, visceropleural visceralgia
vulvo-	vulv-	external female genitalia (vulva)	vulvovaginal vulvectomy, vulvitis
xantho-	xanth-	yellow	xanthoderma, xanthophyll xanthosis, xanthuria
xeno-	xen-	stranger, foreign	xenogenesis, xenomenia xenophthalmia, xenorexia
xero-	xer-	dry	xerocheilia, xeroderma xeroma, xerophthalmia
xipho-	xiph-	lit., sword xiphoid process	xiphocostal, xiphopagus xiphodynia, xiphoid
zoo-	zo-	animal	zoology, zoophilism zoanthropy, zooid
zygo-	zyg-	yoke, joined	zygodactyl zygoma, zygosis
zymo-	zym-	ferment, leaven	zymogenesis, zymolysis zymoid

Appendix C
Suffixes and Common Endings

Suffixes are those word elements that come at the end of a word to modify its meaning and usually its part of speech.

Even though not all these word endings are properly suffixes, they all occur so often in medical terminology, it was felt that they should be included for easy reference. See the family to which they belong in the regular thesaurus for their etymological background and their attachment to other words.

Suffix	Other Forms	Meaning	Examples
-abdominal		pertaining to the abdomen	dorsabdominal
-acanthoma		prickly tumor	adenoacanthoma
-aceous		having the quality of	saponaceous
-acousia		pertaining to hearing	amblyacousia, echoacousia
-acrasia	-acratia	lack of self-control	copracrasia gonacratia
-ad		toward	cephalad, caudad
-adenitis		gland inflammation	blennadenitis blepharadenitis
-agnosis		lack of knowledge	acousmatagnosis, baragnosis
-agogue		leading	galactagogue, sialagogue
-agra		seizure	anconagra, cardiagra
-algia	-algesia	pain	angialgia, cardialgia cephalgia, neuralgia cryoanalgesia
-alveolar		pertaining to a cavity	dentoalveolar
-amnesia		forgetting	acousmatamnesia
-amnion		membrane	schizamnion
-anal		pertaining to the anus	ileoanal, ischioanal
-angiectasis		dilatation of a blood vessel	cholangiectasis
-angiology		study of blood vessels	cardioangiology
-angioma		tumor of a blood vessel	chondroangioma chorioangioma
-angiosis		blood vessel condition	glomangiosis
-angium		blood vessel	gametangium
-anomaly		irregular	deuteranomaly
-anterior		forward	sacroanterior
-anthropy		pertaining to man	misanthropy
-antritis		sinus inflammation	nasoantritis, otoantritis
-aortic		pertaining to the aorta	pulmoaortic
-apheresis		removal	hemapheresis, cytapheresis
-apophysis		growth, offshoot	neurapophysis pleurapophysis
-apsis		touching	karyapsis, synapsis
-apraxia		failure	neurapraxia
-aqueous		pertaining to water	chylaqueous
-arche		first, beginning	adenarche, menarche
-arctia		narrow	aortarctica, bronchiarctia
-arrhythmia		rhythm disturbance	bradyarrhythmia
-arthria	-arthric	joint condition	coxarthria monarthric, polyarthric
-arthritis	-arthritic	inflammation of joints	acroarthritis antiarthritic
-arthropathy		joint disease	coxarthropathy

Suffix	Other Forms	Meaning	Examples
-arthrosis		joint condition	clinarthrosis, dysarthrosis
-asia, -asis			See -iasis.
-asthenia		lack of strength, weakness	angiasthenia, cardiasthenia
-ataxia		disorder, irregularity	acroataxia, cardiataxia
-atelia		incomplete	cardiatelia
-atresia		imperforation	colpatresia, hysteratresia proctatresia
-atrophia		lack of nourishment	cystatrophia, hepatatrophia trichatrophia
-aulic		pertaining to a pipe	hydraulic
-aural	-auricular	pertaining to the ear	dextraural interauricular
-auxesis	auxe, -auxis	increasing	bradyauxesis, iridauxesis entereauxe, myelauxis
-axial		pertaining to the axis	equiaxial, gingivoaxial
-basia		pertaining to walking	brachybasia
-be	-bic	life	aerobe aerobic
-biliary		bile condition	atrabiliary, hepatobiliary
-biosis	-biotic	condition of life	abiosis, orthobiosis microbiotic
-blast	-blastic	germ	adenoblast, neuroblast panblastic
-blastoma		tumor of a cell	androblastoma, glioblastoma
-blennorrhea		flowing of mucus	dacryoblennorrhea
-blepharia	-blepharic	eyelid condition	atretoblepharia macroblepharia hygroblepharic
-blepsia		pertaining to vision	oxyblepsia
-bol		throwing	embolism (em- is prefix)
-brachial	-brachia	pertaining to the arm	cervicobrachial abrachia, macrobrachia
-bronchial		pertaining to the windpipe	vesiculobronchial
-bronchitis		inflammation of the windpipe	fibrobronchitis pleurobronchitis
-bry		growing, full of life	embryonic (em- is prefix)
-buccal		pertaining to cheek	antrobuccal, cervicobuccal distobuccal
-bulbar		pertaining to a bulb	circumbulbar, ischiobulbar urethrobulbar
-byon		plug	rhinobyon
-cace		bad, abnormal, diseased	archicarp, arthrocace
-calcanean	-calcaneal	pertaining to the heel bone	astragalocalcanean talocalcaneal
-campis		bent, curved	gonocampsis, osteocampsis
-capnia		carbon dioxide	normocapnia
-carcinogen		cancer-producing	hepatocarcinogen
-carcinoma		cancerous tumor	cheilocarcinoma osteocarcinoma
-cardia		a condition of the heart	brachycardia aerendocardia
-cardiac		pertaining to heart	abdominocardiac
-catharsis		a cleansing	autocatharsis

Suffix	Other Forms	Meaning	Examples
-caudal		pertaining to the tail	cephalocaudal
-cecal		pertaining to blindness	centrocecal
-cele	-coele	swelling, tumor, hernia	balanocele, craniocele aerocele, astrocoele
-cele		belly, hollow	hemocele
-celia		pertaining to the belly	schistocelia
-cenosis		emptying, evacuation	lithocenosis
-centesis		puncture	amniocentesis, arthrocentesis cordocentesis, rachicentesis
-centric		pertaining to the center	allocentric, anthropocentric
-cephalic	-cephaly	pertaining to the head	brachiocephalic bathrocephaly
-ceptor		receiving, taking	baroceptor, beneceptor receptor
-cerastic	-kerastic	mixed	cytocerastic cytokerastic
-cere		wax	adipocere
-cerebellum		brain	archeocerebellum
-cerebral		pertaining to the brain	maculocerebral
-cervical		pertaining to the neck	basiocervical, buccocervical
-chalasis	-chalasia	relaxation	arthrochalasis blepharochalasis cardiochalasia
-cheilia		condition of the lips	atelocheilia, brachycheilia microcheilia, opisthocheilia
-cheiria		condition of the hands	atelocheiria
-chiasmatic		crossing	opticochiasmatic
-cholia		bile condition	albuminocholia
-chondral		pertaining to cartilage	costochondral, osteochondral
-chondritis		cartilage inflammation	arthrochondritis inochondritis
-chondroma		cartilage tumor	fibrochondroma
-chorion	-chorial	fetal membrane	allantochorion amniochorial
-chronometer		measurement of time	algesichronometer
-chysis		pouring	pyechysis, rachiochysis
-cide	-cidal	to kill	cytocide, germicide cancericidal, cellulicidal
-ciliary		pertaining to the eyebrow	nasociliary, opticociliar
-cinesia	-kinesis	pertaining to movement	allocinesia allokinesis
-ciput		head	centriciput, occiput, sinciput
-cision		cutting	circumcision, excision
-cladic		branching	heterocladic, homocladic
-clasis	-clasia -clast -clastic	breaking	bacterioclasis alveoloclasia, aortoclasia chondroclast, cranioclast histioclastic
-cle		small	corpuscle, muscle
-cleisis	-cleidal	closing	colpocleisis, rhinocleisis sternocleidal
-clepsis		pertaining to stealing	amnioclepsis
-clonus		turmoil	blepharoclonus

Suffix	Other Forms	Meaning	Examples
-clysis		drenching	coloclysis, enteroclysis
-cnemia		pertaining to the leg	platycnemia
-coccus		berry-shaped bacterium	chondrococcus, gonococcus
-colic		pertaining to colon	cecocolic, hepatocolic
-collis		pertaining to the neck	brevicollis
-coloboma		defect	iridocoloboma
-colous		dwelling in, inhabiting	cellicolous, sanguicolous
-colpitis		inflammation of the vagina	cervicocolpitis
-colpos		vagina	aerocolpos
-colpotomy		vagina incision	celiocolpotomy
-cond		hidden	testicond
-coria		pupil condition	anisocoria, platycoria
-cormia		pertaining to the torso	camptocormia, nanocormia
-cortex	-cortical	rind, shell, covering pertaining to the cortex	archicortex cerebrocortical
-costal		pertaining to ribs, side	chondrocostal
-coxalgia		pain in the hip	sacrocoxalgia
-coxitis		inflammation of the hip	sacrocoxitis
-crania	-cranion -cranium	pertaining to the cranium	platycrania opisthocranion basicranium
-crescent		growing	excrescent
-crotic		pertaining to the pulse	bradycrotic
-crural		pertaining to the leg	astragalocrural, brachiocrural
-ctony		to kill	embryoctony
-cubital		pertaining to the forearm	brachiocubital
-cule		small	molecule
-cumbent		lying down	latericumbent
-cuspid		point	quadricuspid
-cutaneous		pertaining to skin	enterocutaneous mucocutaneous
-cyanin		the color blue	bilicyanin, cholocyanin
-cyclic		pertaining to a cycle	endocyclic, polycyclic
-cyesis		pregnancy	oocyesis, pseudocyesis
-cyllosis		a crooking, crippling	brachiocyllosis
-cyphos	-kyphosis	humped	ithycyphos scoliokyphosis
-cyrtosis		curvature	thoracocyrtosis
-cyst	-cystia -cystic	sac, bladder bladder condition	dacryocyst atretocystia fibrocystic
-cyte		cell	adipocyte, gangliocyte
-cytopenia		cell deficiency	basocytopenia
-cytosis		cell condition	koilocytosis, leukocytosis
-dactylia	-dactylous -dactyly	condition of the fingers or toes	camptodactylia anisodactylous cephalodactyly, ectrodactyly
-dental	-dentinal	pertaining to teeth	labiodental amelodentinal
-derma	-dermia -dermic	skin condition	leucoderma, pachyderma acanthokeratodermia hypodermic

Suffix	Other Forms	Meaning	Examples
-dermatitis		skin inflammation	actinodermatitis
-desis	-desma	binding	arthrodesis, syndesis cytodesma, kinetodesma
-diastasis		separation	blepharodiastasis
-diastole		dilatation	bradydiastole
-didymus		twin, testicle	cryptodidymus heterodidymus
-dinia		dizziness	scotodinia
-distal		pertaining to distance	buccodistal
-donesis		tremor	iridodonesis
-dorsal		pertaining to back	cervicodorsal
-drome	-dromic	running, course	auxodrome palindromic
-ducent	-duct -duction	leading	abducent, adducent oviduct deorsumduction
-duodenal		pertaining to the duodenum	aortoduodenal
-dynamia		power condition	ataxiadynamia
-dymus		twin	cephalodymus
-dysplasia		abnormal development	arthrodysplasia
-dysrhythmia		abnormal rhythm	bradydysrhythmia
-ectasia	-ectasis	dilatation, widening	aortectasia, cardiectasia arteriectasis, bronchiectasis
-ectomy		excision	amygalectomy appendectomy
-ectopia		out of place	adenectopia , angiectopia
-ectropion		a turning aside	cheilectropion
-edema		swelling	angioedema, cephaledema
-edonic			See hedonic-.
-elcosis (elision of -helcosis)	-helcosis	ulceration	carcinelcosis, enterelcosis keratohelcosis, masthelcosis
-elosis		to roll	blepharelosis
-embolus		obstruction	atheroembolus
-emesis	-emetic	vomiting	blennemesis, copremesis hematemesis, sialemesis
-emia (elision of -hemia)	-hemia	blood condition	anemia, hypoglycemia acardiohemia
-emphraxis		stoppage	adenemphraxis salpingemphraxis
-empyesis		suppuration	arthrempyesis
-encephalia	-encephalic	brain condition	atelencephalia centrencephalic
-enchysis		injection	cirsenchysis
-enteric		pertaining to the intestines	aortoenteric
-enteron		intestines	archenteron, celenteron
-enthesis		a placing in	allenthesis
-ereisis		a rising up	arthroereisis
-eremia		want of, absence	choroideremia, irideremia
-ergic	-ergy	pertaining to work, action	adrenergic iathergy
-erotic		pertaining to sexual desire	autoerotic
-erysis		dragging away	phacoerysis

Suffix	Other Forms	Meaning	Examples
-escent	-escence	becoming	adolescent (adolescence) alkalescent (alkalescence) convalescent
-esis		action or process	enuresis plasmapheresis
-esophagal		pertaining to the esophagus	brachyesophagus
-esthesia	-esthetic	feeling, perception	acroesthesia, anesthesia anesthetic
-eurysis		widening	colpeurysis
-exeresis	-exairesis	excision	neurexeresis phleboexairesis
-facial		pertaining to the face	basifacial, dolichofacial
-facient	-fact -faction	making	algefacient, calefacient artefact bilifaction
-fenestria		pertaining to an opening	craniofenestria
-ferous	-ferent	bearing	aeriferous, chyliferous efferent
-fibroma		fibrous tumor	adipofibroma
-fibrosis		fiber condition	angiofibrosis
-fibular		pertaining to the fibula	astragalofibular
-fic	-fication	making	soporific aerification, saccharification
-flect	-flection	bending	dorsiflect deflection, reflection
-form		shape, form	anginiform, ossiform
-fuge	-fugal	fleeing	arthrifuge, vermifuge axofugal, cellifugal
-fy		making	acidify, aerify
-gamy	-gamic -gamous	marriage	anisogamy agamic heterogamous
-gastria	-gastric	a condition of the stomach	aerogastria, arachnogastria aortogastric, nasogastric
-gen	-genesia -genesis -genic -genous	producing, originating from	allergen, cryogen algogenesia adipogenesis bronchiogenic, cryogenic aerogenous
-genia		pertaining to the jaw	opisthogenia
-gerous		producing, bearing	calcigerous, proligerous
-geustia		pertaining to taste	ageustia, allotriogeustia amblygeustia
-gingival		pertaining to the gums	buccogingival
-glia		glue	astroglia, neuroglia
-globus		ball, globe, sphere	keratoglobus
-glossia		pertaining to the tongue	ankyloglossia, baryglossia schistoglossia
-glyphic		pertaining to carving	dermatoglyphics
-gnathia	-gnathous -gnathism	pertaining to the jaw	atelognathia, brachygnathia anisognathous, eurygnathous opisthognathism
-gnomy		knowing, discerning	pathognomy, physiognomy

Suffix	Other Forms	Meaning	Examples
-gnosis		knowledge	auditognosis, diagnosis
	-gnostic		chirognostic, diagnostic
-gonium		seed, germ	archegonium
	-gone		androgone
-gram		writing, recording	cardiogram
-graft		bud, shoot, sprout	autograft
-graph		writing, recording	mammograph
	-graphy		mammography
-gravida		heavy; pregnant	multigravida, primigravida
-gryposis		a crooking, hooking	arthrogryposis
			dactylogryposis
-gynic		pertaining to female sex	hologynic
	-gynist		misogynist
-gyria		turning	schizogyria
	-gyric		cephalogyric, oculogyric
-haphia		pertaining to touch	anhaphia
	-aphia		amblyaphia
-hedonic		pertaining to pleasure	anhedonic
	-edonic (h is elided)		algedonic
-helcosis			See -elcosis.
-hemic	-hemia (see -emia)	pertaining to blood	autohemic
-hepatic		pertaining to the liver	adipohepatic, cardiohepatic
-hexia		condition	osthexia
-hexis		habit	osteocachexia
-hidrosis		pertaining to sweating	bromhidrosis, chromhidrosis
-hieric		pertaining to the sacrum	platyhieric
-hodic		pertaining to a path	panthodic
-ia		condition of	algophilia
-iac		related to	cardiac, insomniac, maniac
-iasis		condition	elephantiasis, phlebolithiasis
	-asis		psoriasis
	-asia		euthanasia
-iatria		healing	odontoiatria
	-iatric		geriatric, psychiatric
	-iatrics		andriatrics, bariatrics
-icterus		pertaining to jaundice	splenicterus
	-icteric		anicteric, antiicteric
-ilitis		inflammation of the hip	sacroiliitis
-ischemia		blood suppression	myoischemia
-ischia		suppression	galactischia
-ischiac		pertaining to the hip	rectischiac
-ism		state; condition;	alcoholism, eroticism
		fact of being;	erythrism, globulism
		process or result of an action	priapism
-itis		inflammation	arthritis, bursitis, tendonitis
-ize		treat by a particular method	alkalinize, azotize
-izemia		pertaining to depression	spondylizemia
-karyon		kernel	archikaryon
-keratoma		cornea tumor	angiokeratoma
-kerkic		pertaining to the radius	brachykerkic
-kinesis		movement	allokinesis, calciokinesis
	-kinesia		allokinesia
	-kinetic		angiokinetic, biokinetic

Suffix	Other Forms	Meaning	Examples
-kleisis		closure	arthrokleisis
-knemic		pertaining to the shin	brachyknemic
-kurtic		pertaining to a convex	platykurtic
-kyphosis	see -cyphos		
-labial		pertaining to the lips	dentilabial, buccolabial
-labile		perishable, unstable	coctolabile, hydrolabile
-lacrimal		pertaining to tears	nasolacrimal
-lacunia		hollow, gap	craniolacuna
-lagnia		lust	algolagnia, coprolagnia
-lalia		speaking, babbling	allolalia, barylalia, idiolalia
-lamellar		pertaining to a plate, layer	fibrolamellar
-lapaxy		evacuation	litholapaxy
-laryngeal		pertaining to the larynx	intralaryngeal thyrolaryngeal
-lateral		pertaining to a side	basilateral, unilateral
-lecithal		pertaining to egg yolk	centrolecithal, medialecithal
-lemma		husk, rind, sheath	basilemma
	-lemmic	pertaining to a sheath	sarcolemmic
-lental		pertaining to the lens	cerebellolental
-lepsy		seizure	epilepsy, narcolepsy
	-leptic		organoleptic, polyleptic
-leptynis		attenuation	iridoleptynsis keratoleptynsis
-leukemia		white blood cell condition	erythroleukemia pseudoleukemia
-lexia		word, speech	alexia, bradylexia, dyslexia
-limia		pertaining to hunger	bulimia
-lineal		pertaining to lines	brevilineal, longilineal
-lingual		pertaining to the tongue	alveololingual
-lipoma		fatty tumor	angiolipoma, fibrolipoma
-liposis		fatty condition	cardiomyoliposis
-lith		stone, calculus	cardiolith, cholelith
	-lithiasis	stony condition	bronchiolithiasis
-lobular		pertaining to a lobe	centrilobular
-logy		scientific study of	adenology, neurology
-loquy		speech	caverniloquy
-lordosis		bending backward	ithylordosis
-loxia		slanting	odontoloxia
-lymphitis		lymph inflammation	adenolymphitis angiolymphitis
-lysis		loosening, setting free	angiolysis, myolysis
	-lytic		auxolytic, biolytic
-malacia		soft	craniomalacia, osteomalacia
-mania		madness	dipsomania, pyromania
-mastia		breast condition	anisomastia
-mastigote		a flagellate	amastigote, choanomastigote
-maxillary		pertaining to the jawbone	inframaxillary, oromaxillary
-medullary		pertaining to marrow	cerebromedullary
-megaly		great, large, extreme	acromegaly, angiomegaly gastromegaly, nephromegaly
-meiotic		decreasing	postmeiotic, premeiotic
-melanosia		dark condition	cardiomelanosis

Suffix	Other Forms	Meaning	Examples
-melic		pertaining to a limb	camptomelic
	-melia		anisomelia, megalomelia
	-melus		cephalomelus
-menia		pertaining to menstruation	cephalomenia, ischomenia
-menorrhea		menstruation	algomenorrhea
-mere		part	adenomere
	-meric		anisomeric
	-merism		allomerism
-meter	-metry	measure	thermometer, stereometry
	-metric		calorimetric, gravimetric
-meningitis		inflammation of the membranes	arthromeningitis cerebromeningitis
-meria		pertaining to the leg	platymeria
-metra		uterus	hematometra, pyometra
-mimetic		imitation	adrenomimetic
-miosis		degeneration	osteomiosis
-mittent		sending	intermittent
	-mission		intromission
-mnesia		remembering	amnesia, hypomnesia
-molecular		pertaining to molecules	equimolecular
-morph		shape, form	mesomorph
	-morphic		bathomorphic, endomorphic
	-morphous		andromorphous
-motor		pertaining to motion	arteriomotor
	-motility		cardiomotility, neurimotility
-myalgia		muscle pain	fibromyalgia
-myces		fungal condition	myelomyces
	-mycetes		ascomycetes, schizomycetes
	-mycin		erythromycin
	-mycosis		balanoposthomycosis
-myelia		pertaining to bone marrow	hydromyelia
-myelitis		marrow inflammation	neuromyelitis, osteomyelitis
-myitis		muscle inflammation	fibromyitis
-myoma		muscle tumor	adenomyoma
-myopathy		muscle disease	cardiomyopathy
-myoplasty		formation of muscle	cardiomyoplasty
-myositis		muscle inflammation	celiomyositis
-myotomy		incision of muscle	cardiomyotomy
-narcosis		numbness	electronarcosis
	-narcotic		antinarcotic, subnarcotic
-narial		peretaining to the nostrils	internarial, postnarial
-nasal		pertaining to the nose	aurinasal, internasal
	-nasial		basinasial
	-nasion		opticonasion
-natal		pertaining to birth	antenatal, neonatal
-necrosis		pertaining to death	arterionecrosis atheronecrosis
-nector		fastening	atrionector, cardionector
	-nectin		fibronectin
-nephric		pertaining to kidney	cardionephric, paranephric
-nephritis		inflammation of kidney	lithonephritis
-nephrosis		kidney condition	hydronephrosis
-nervia		nerve condition	acardionervia

Suffix	Other Forms	Meaning	Examples
-neural	-neuric	pertaining to nerves	adenoneural, cardioneural mononeuric, polyneuric
-neuralgia		nerve pain	arthroneuralgia
-neuritis		nerve inflammation	actinoneuritis
-neurosis		nerve condition	cardioneurosis
-nomy		pertaining to law, customs	bionomy
-nyxis		pricking, puncturing	hyalonyxis, scleronyxis
-ode		road, path	cathode, diode
-odontalgia		pain in the teeth	aerodontalgia, barodontalgia
-odontia		condition of teeth	allotriodontia, orthodontia saprodontia
-odynia		pain	cardiodynia, gastrodynia
-oid	-ode -oitic	form, shape	adenoid, cystoid, lymphoid nematode chondroitic
-ol		oil	cholesterol
-olisthesis		slipping	spondylolisthesis
-oma		mass, tumor	branchioma, lymphoma
-omatoid		similar to a tumor	sarcomatoid
-omphalus	-omphalos	navel	hydromphalus cirsoomphalos
-onychia		pertaining to nails	leukonychia, schizonychia
-oncus		tumor, swelling	adenoncus, phalloncus
-ophryon		eyebrow	mesophyron
-opia	-opsia -opsy	eye or vision condition	anisopia, chloropia erythropsia, etretopsia autopsy
-ophthalmopathy		eye disease	arthroophthalmopathy
-ophthalmus	-ophthalmia	eye eye condition	cryptophthalmus adenophthalmia
-oral		pertaining to the mouth	intraoral, peroral
-orchidism		pertaining to the testicles	cryptorchidism
-ose		sugar, starch	galactose, glucose
-osis	-ose	condition	acidosis, fibrosis, psychosis adenose
-osmia		pertaining to smells	autosmia
-osseous		pertaining to bone	fibro-osseous
-osteitis		bone inflammation	arthrosteitis, endosteitis
-osteoid		similar to bone	dentinosteoid
-osteoma		bone tumor	endosteoma, fibro-osteoma
-osteosis		bone condition	angiosteosis, parosteosis
-otic	-otia	pertaining to the ear	basiotic, opisthotic ankylotia, pachyotia
-otitis		ear infection	barotitis
-ous		full of	squamous
-pachynsis		thickening	blepharopachynsis
-pagus		fixed, firmly set	craniopagus, ischiopagus
-palatine		pertaining to roof of mouth	nasopalatine
-paludism		malaria	cardiopaludism
-papular		pertaining to pimples	maculopapular
-paresis		weakness, relaxation partial paralysis	angioparesis, enteroparesis myoparesis, taboparesis

Suffix	Other Forms	Meaning	Examples
-parous		producing, bearing	albuminiparous, oviparous
-path		disease	psychopath
	-pathy		andropathy, osteopathy
-pedal		pertaining to the foot	capitopedal, carpopedal
-pellent		driving, pushing	repellent
-pelvic		pertaining to the pelvis	intrapelvic
	-pellic		brachypellic, leptopellic
-penia		lack of, need	calcipenia, leucopenia
			sarcopenia
-pepsia		pertaining to digestion	bradypepsia
	-peptic		dyspeptic
-petal		seeking	cellulipetal, corticipetal
-pexis		fixation	adipopexis, calcipexis
	-pexia		adipopexia, collopexia
	-pexy		funiculopexy, hepatopexy
-phagy		pertaining to eating	allotriophagy
	-phagia		bacteriophagia, bradyphagia
	-phagic		lipophagic
	-phagous		biophagous
-phakia		lens condition	keratophakia
-phany		showing, appearing	androphany
	-phania		menophania
-pharyngeal		pertaining to the pharynx (throat)	glossopharyngeal
			nasopharyngeal
-pharyngitis		inflammation of throat	adenopharyngitis
			nasopharyngitis
-phasia		pertaining to speech	cataphasia, heterophasia
-phil		affinity for something	aerophil
	-philia		algophilia, opsonophilia
	-philic		hemophilic
-phimosis		a muzzling	blepharophimosis
-phlebitis		inflammation of a vein	celophlebitis
-phlysis		eruption	galactophlysis
-phobia		fear of	agoraphobia
	-phobe		homophobe
-phone		sound;	audiophone, cardiophone
	-phonic	pertaining to sound	stereophonic
	-phonia		baryphonia, lamprophonia
-phore		being borne, carried	aerophore, antrophore
	-phoresis		adiaphoresis, diaphoresis
	-phoria		anisophoria, exophoria
	-phoric		cryophoric
	-phorous		adenophorous, cystophorous
-phose		light	antrophose, centraphose
-phragm		enclosure, wall	diaphragm
	-phragma		inophragma
-phrax		enclosure, stoppage	emphraxis
-phrenia		condition of the mind	bradyphrenia, oligophrenia
	-phrenic		schizophrenic
-phthisis		wasting away	limophthisis
-phthoria		corruption	blastophthoria
-phygous		arresting	galactophygous

Suffix	Other Forms	Meaning	Examples
-phylactic	-phylaxis	protection, guarding	cryophylactic, prophylactic dermatophylaxis, prophylaxis
-phyll	-phyllum	leaf	chlorophyll, xanthophyll blastophyllum
-phyly		tribe	blastophyly, histophyly
-phyma		swelling, tumor	arthrophyma, tenontophyma
-phyte	-physis -phytic	plant (pathological growth)	arthrophyte, osteophyte hypophysis holophytic
-phythisis		wasting away	ophthalmophythisis
-piesis		pressure	anisopiesis, otopiesis
-plakia		pertaining to plates	erythroplakia, leukoplakia
-planesis	-plania -plany	wandering	phacoplanesis arterioplania, galactoplania angioplany
-plasia	-plasm -plast -plasty	form; surgical formation of	leukoplasia, fibroplasia alloplasm, protoplasm protoplast angioplasty, cranioplasty
-plectrum		anything to strike with	auscultoplectrum
-plegia	-plegic	stroke, paralysis	blepharoplegia, cardioplegia cephaloplegia, prosopoplegia quadriplegic
-pleura	-pleural	side (of body)	aeropleura hepatopleural
-plication		process of folding	cecoplication
-pnea		breath, breathing	bromopnea, orthopnea
-pneumatic		pertaining to air, respiration	cardiopneumatic
-pneumonic		pertaining to the lungs	hepatopneumonic
-podia		pertaining to the feet	atelopodia, megalopodia
-poiesis	-poietic	making, producing	angiopoiesis, hematopoiesis hidropoietic, nephropoietic
-pontine		pertaining to a bridge	bulbopontine
-pore		passage, pore	blastopore, myelopore
-poreia		pertaining to walking	opisthoporeia
-porosis		pore condition	chondroporosis, osteoporosis
-portal		entrance, gateway	hepatoportal
-posthitis		inflammation of the prepuce	balanoposthitis
-posy		drinking; intake of fluids	oligoposy
-praxis	-pragia	performance	echopraxis bradypragia
-preputial		pertaining to the prepuce	balanopreputial
-privia	-privic -prival	deprived of	calciprivia chloroprivic adrenoprival
-proctia	-proctic	pertaining to the anus	ankyloproctia, enteroproctia periproctic
-prosopia	-prosopic	condition of the face	ateloprosopia brachyprosopic
-psychic	-psychalia	pertaining to mind	cenopsychic algopsychalia
-pten		volatile	eleopten, stearopten

Suffix	Other Forms	Meaning	Examples
-ptosis	-ptosia	falling	archoptosis, mastoptosis aortoptosis, cardioptosia
-ptyis		to spit, expectorate	albuminoptysis
-pubic		becoming an adult	infrapubic, ischiopubic
-pulmonary		pertaining to the lungs	aorticopulmonary cardiopulmonary
-pupillary		pertaining to the pupil	iridopupillary oculopupillary
-purulent		pertaining to pus	fibropurulent sanguinopurulent
-pyelitis		inflammation of the pelvis	calcipyelitis
-pyosis		pus condition	arthropyosis, celiopyosis
-pyra		fire, fever	lochiopyra
-rachidia	-rhachidian	spine condition	atelorachidia encephalorhachidian
-renal		pertaining to the kidneys	arteriorenal, cardiorenal
-rhacia		spine condition	bilirhachia
-rhage	-rrhagia	bursting forth	hemorrhage balanorrhagia, blennorrhagia
-rhaphy		suture, seam	angiorrhaphy, cheilorraphy
-rhea		flowing, discharging	diarrhea, menorrhea
-rhexis		breaking; rupture	amniorrhexis, metrorrhexis
-rhine	-rhinal -rhinia	pertaining to the nose	leptorrhine basirhinal atretorrhinia, brachyrhinia
-sacral		pertaining to the sacrum	craniosacral
-salpingitis		inflammation of a tube	adenosalpingitis oophorosalpingitis
-sarcoma		flesh tumor	angiosarcoma, fibrosarcoma myosarcoma, osteosarcoma
-scapular		pertaining to the shoulder blade	cervicoscapular costoscapular
-schesis		retention	hidroschesis, lochioschesis
-schisis	-schism	splitting, fissure	cranioschisis, penischisis odontoschism
-scirrhus		hard	mastoscirrhus
-sclerosis		hardening	arteriosclerosis craniosclerosis
-scoliosis		twisting, bending	cnemoscoliosis
-scope	-scopic -scopy	view, examine	microscope skiascopic cardioscopy
-scrotal		pertaining to the testicle pouch	abdominoscrotal penoscrotal
-sepsis	-sepia -septic	putrid, rottenness	chroniosepsis colyseptic
-septal		pertaining to the septum	nasoseptal
-serous		pertaining to serum	fibrtoserous
-sialia		pertaining to saliva	asialia
-site		food	autosite
-skelic		pertaining to the leg	brachyskelic
-solvent	-solution	loosening	dissolvent dissolution

Suffix	Other Forms	Meaning	Examples
-some		body	chromosome
	-somatic		leptosomatic, psychosomatic
	-somia		celosomia
-somnia		pertaining to sleep	dyssomnia, insomnia
-sparaxis		a tearing	dermatosparaxis
-spasm		involuntary contraction	bronchiospasm, campospasm
	-spastic		angiospastic
	-spastia		coleospastia
-spermal		pertaining to seed (sperm)	angiospermal
	-spermia		oligospermia
-sphenoid		wedge-shaped	basisphenoid
-sphere		ball, globe	centrosphere, chromosphere
-sphygmia		pertaining to pulse	bradysphygmia
	-sphyxia		asphyxia, acroasphyxia
-spinal		pertaining to the spine	cerebellospinal
-spiral		pertaining to a spire	bulbospiral
-splanchnia		pertaining to the viscera	perosplanchnia
-spondylia		pertaining to the vertebrae	platyspondylia
-spore		seed	macrospore, zygospore
-stabile		stable, resisting	coctostabile, hydrostabile
-staphyline		pertaining to the uvula	brachystaphyline
-stasis		stoppage	coprostasis, iridostasis
	-stasia		menostasia
-static		standing, halting	cariostatic, hydrostatic
-staxis		dripping	bronchostaxis, menostaxis
-stenosis		narrow condition	aortostenosis
			bronchiostenosis
			rhinostenosis
-steresis		loss of	glossosteresis, halisteresis
			iridosteresis, ovariosteresis
-sternia		chest condition	koilosternia
-sthenia		strength abnormality	asthenia
	-sthenic		anisosthenic
-stomy		mouth, opening	angiostomy, hepatostomy
	-stomia		atelostomia
-strepsis		twisting	arteriostrepsis
-strophe		pertaining to twisting	angiostrophe
-synechia		binding together	blepharosynechia
-tabes		wasting away	craniotabes
-tachometer		measurement of speed	cardiotachometer
-taraxis		confusion	chronotaraxis
-taxis		arrangement	angiotaxis, centrotaxis
	-taxia		acroataxia
-thel		nipple	coelothel
-thenar		palm of hand	opisthenar
-therapy		treatment	crymotherapy, hydrotherapy
-therm	-thermy	heat	isotherm, diathermy
-thesis		a placing	prosthesis, synthesis
	-thesia		allesthesia
-thlipsis		pressure	neurothlipsis, oncothlipsis
-thoraic		pertaining to the thorax	cervicothoraic
-thrix		hair	monilethrix, sclerothrix

Suffix	Other Forms	Meaning	Examples
-thrombus		clot	cardiothrombus
-thymia		condition of the mind	cyclothymia, schizothymia
-tibial		pertaining to the shin	astragalotibial
-tocia		pertaining to childbirth	bradytocia
-tomy		incision	amniotomy, phlebotomy
	-tome	a cutting instrument	adenotome
-tonia		relating to tone, tension	acromyotonia
	-tonic		auxotonic, cardiotonic
-topy		relating to place	idiotopy
	-topia		heterotopia
-torsion		twisting	ectorsion, levotorsion
-torus		protuberance	keratotorus
-toxic		poisonous	bacteriotoxic, psychotoxic
	-toxin		adrenotoxin
-tresis		perforation	lithotresis
	-tresia		sphenotresia
-tribe		crushing	angiotribe, cephalotribe
	-tripsis		apotripsis, entripsis
	-tripsy		lithotripsy
-trichous		pertaining to hair	holotrichous
	-trichia	hair condition	oligotrichia
-trope		turn, turning	neurotrope
	-tropia		cyclotropia
	-tropic		arthrotropic, hepatotropic
	-tropism		barotropism, sitotropism
-trophy		nutrition, growth	anomalotrophy, hypotrophy
	-trophic		angiotrophic, brephotrophic
	-trophia		atrophia, bradytrophia
-trypesis		boring (a hole)	cephalotrypesis
			craniotrypesis
-tympanic		pertaining to the eardrum	craniotympanic
	-tympanal		aerotympanal
-ulcia		to draw, to pull	embryulcia
-uresis		voiding of urine	alginuresis, diuresis
-urethria		urethra condition	atreturethria
	-urethral		bulbourethral
-uria		urine condition	bradyuria, oliguria, polyuria
-uterine		pertaining to the uterus	cervicouterine, vesicouterine
-vaginal		pertaining to the vagina	subvaginal
-valent		worth	heptavalent
-vascular		pertaining to blood vessels	cardiovascular, fibrovascular
-venous		pertaining to veins	arteriovenous
-vergence		turning	deorsumvergence
-version		turning	cardioversion
-vesical		pertaining to the bladder	cervicovesical, vaginovesical
-vesicular		pertaining to the bladder	maculovesicular
-vorous		pertaining to eating	lactivorous, sanguivorous
-vesical		pertaining to bladder	cervicovesical
-xanthoma		yellowish tumor	fibroxanthoma
-xesis		scraping	arthroxesis
-zemia		pertaining to loss	androgalactozemia
-zyme		fementation	angiozyme

List of Works Consulted

Becker, E. Lovell, Sidney I. Landau, Alexandre Manuila, *International Dictionary of Medicine and Biology*, 1986.

Chabner, Davi-Ellen, *The Language of Medicine*, Third Edition. Philadelphia: W. B. Saunders Company, 1985.

Chabner, Davi-Ellen, *Medical Terminology: A Short Course*, Third Edition. Philadelphia, W. B. Saunders Company, 2003.

Churchill' Illustrated Medical Dictionary. New York: Churchill Livingstone, 1989.

Dorland's Illustrated Medical Dictionary, 31ˢᵗ Edition. Philadelphia: W. B. Saunders Company, 2007.

Dox, Ida, Biagio John Melloni, Gilbert M. Eisner, *Melloni's Illustrated Medical Dictionary*. Baltimore: Williams & Wilkins, 1985.

Erlich, Ann, and Carol L. Schroeder, *Medical Terminology for Health Professions*, 4ᵗʰ Edition. Albany, NY, Delmar, 2001.

Glanze, Walter D., Kenneth N. Anderson, Lois Anderson, eds., *The Mosby Medical and Nursing Encyclopedia*. New York: New American Library, 1985.

Hamilton, Betty, and Barbara Guidos, *The Medical Word Finder, A Reverse Medical Dictionary*. New York: Neal-Schuman, 1987.

Miller, Benjamin F., and Claire Brackman Keane, *Encyclopedia and Dictionary of Medicine, Nursing, and Allied Health*. Philadelphia: W. B. Saunders. 1987

Sloane, Richard, *The Sloane-Dorland Annotated Medical-Legal Dictionary*. St. Paul: West Publishing Company, 1987.

Stedman's Medical Dictionary, 28th Edition. Baltimore: Lippincott Williams & Wilkins, 2006.

Taber's Cyclopedic Medical Dictionary, Edition 14, Illustrated. Philadelphia: F. A. Davis Company, 1993.

Thomson, William A. R., *Black's Medical Dictionary*. New York: Barnes & Noble, 1972.

Urdang's Dictionary of Current Medical Terms for Health Science Professionals. New York: Wiley, 1981.

Various Internet Resources.

Walton, John, et al., editors, *The Oxford Companion to Medicine*. New York: Oxford Publishing Company, 1986.

Webster's Medical Desk Dictionary. Springfield, Mass.: Merriam-Webster, 1986.

A Thesaurus of Medical Word Roots